Oxford Textbook of

Public Health Palliative Care

Oxford Textbook of
Public Health Palliative Care

EDITED BY

Julian Abel
Director, Compassionate Communities, UK

Allan Kellehear
Clinical Professor, College of Nursing and Health Sciences, University of Vermont, USA

OXFORD
UNIVERSITY PRESS

OXFORD
UNIVERSITY PRESS

Great Clarendon Street, Oxford, OX2 6DP,
United Kingdom

Oxford University Press is a department of the University of Oxford. It furthers the University's objective of excellence in research, scholarship, and education by publishing worldwide. Oxford is a registered trade mark of Oxford University Press in the UK and in certain other countries

First Edition published in 2022

Impression: 2

Published in the United States of America by Oxford University Press
198 Madison Avenue, New York, NY 10016, United States of America

British Library Cataloguing in Publication Data
Data available

Library of Congress Control Number: 2021950723

ISBN 978–0–19–886299–4

DOI: 10.1093/med/9780198862994.001.0001

Printed and bound by
CPI Group (UK) Ltd, Croydon, CR0 4YY

Contents

SECTION 3
Basic practice methods

SECTION 4
Population-based approaches

SECTION 5
Evidence base

SECTION 6
Education and training

SECTION 7
Conclusion

Editors

Julian Abel, MB, ChB, is Director of Compassionate Communities UK and a retired palliative care physician. Julian developed an interest in the public health approach to palliative and end of life care during his clinical years, running projects at local, regional, and national levels. He was Vice President of Public Health Palliative Care International. He is co-author of the book *The Compassion Project* (2020), based on the Frome model of compassionate communities and an enhanced model of primary care. He is co-author of a number of papers about different aspects of public health palliative care. His papers have appeared in *BMJ Supportive & Palliative Care*, *British Journal of General Practice*, *Annals of Palliative Medicine*, and others.

Allan Kellehear, PhD, FAcSS, is a Clinical Professor in the College of Nursing and Health Sciences at the University of Vermont, USA. He is also an honorary professor at McMaster University in Canada, and at the University of Bradford and Durham University in the UK. Allan established the world's first university-based, public health palliative care unit in Australia in the 1990s (La Trobe University) and is widely known for two early foundation texts in the field, *Health Promoting Palliative Care* (1999) and *Compassionate Cities: Public Health and End of Life Care* (2005). He has since co-edited two further volumes to advance practice understanding of this field: *International Perspectives on Public Health and Palliative Care* (2012), with Libby Sallnow and Suresh Kumar, and *Compassionate Communities: Case Studies from Britain and Europe* (2016), with Klaus Wegleitner and Katarina Heimerl.

Contributors

Julian Abel, MB, ChB, Director, Compassionate Communities UK, St Martin, Cornwall, UK

Samar Aoun, MPH, PhD, Perron Institute Research Chair in Palliative Care, University of Western Australia and Perron Institute for Neurological and Translational Science, Perth, Australia; Adjunct Professor, La Trobe University, Melbourne, Australia

Nikki Archer, RGN, MSc Nursing, Supportive Care Director, St Giles Hospice, West Midlands, UK

Luc Deliens, PhD, Professor of Palliative Care Research, Director of the End-of-Life Care Research Group, Vrije Universiteit Brussel, Brussels; Ghent University, Ghent, Belgium

Pati Dzotsenidze, MD, PhD, Assistant Professor, Faculty of Medicine, Georgian National University, Tbilisi, Georgia

Polly Edmonds, MBBS, FRCP, Consultant in Palliative Medicine, Palliative Care Team, King's College Hospital NHS Foundation Trust, London, UK

Andrea Grindrod, PhD, BEdSt, RN, Projects Manager and Senior Research Fellow, Public Health Palliative Care Unit, La Trobe University, Melbourne, Australia

Mark A. Hazelwood, MSc, Chief Executive, Scottish Partnership for Palliative Care, Edinburgh, UK

Emilio Herrera Molina, MD, MPH, MBA, President of New Health Foundation, Seville, Spain; Global Chief Health Officer of Keralty (gCHO) and President of Keralty Foundation, Miami, FL, USA

Emma Hodges, DBA, Chief Executive Officer, St Giles Hospice, West Midlands, UK; Honorary Lecturer at Keele University and Business Support Director for Compassionate Communities, UK

Mary Hodgson, MA, MRes, PhD, FRSA, Community Action Lead, St Christopher's Hospice, London, UK

Debbie Horsfall, PhD, Professor of Sociology, School of Social Sciences, Western Sydney University, Sydney, Australia

Aliki Karapliagkou, PhD, Lecturer in Sociology, University of Bradford, Bradford, UK

Allan Kellehear, PhD, FAcSS, Clinical Professor, Department of Nursing, College of Nursing and Health Sciences, University of Vermont, Burlington, VT, USA; Emeritus Professor, University of Bradford, UK

Helen Kingston, MBBS, MRCGP, General Practitioner, Frome Medical Practice, Somerset, UK

Kathy Kortes-Miller, PhD, MSW, Associate Professor and the Director of CERAH, School of Social Work, Director, Centre for Education and Research in Aging and Health (CERAH), Lakehead University, Thunder Bay, ON, Canada

Suresh Kumar, MBBS, Dip PallMed, MA, Director, WHO Collaborating Centre for Community Participation in Palliative Care and Long Term Care, Institute of Palliative Medicine, Kerala, India

Philip J. Larkin, PhD, RN, Kristian Gerhard Jebsen Chair of Palliative Care Nursing, Palliative and Supportive Care Service, Lausanne University Hospital and University of Lausanne, Lausanne, Switzerland

Rosemary Leonard, PhD, Professor of Social Capital and Sustainability, School of Social Sciences, Western Sydney University, Sydney, Australia

Silvia Librada Flores, MSc, Compassionate Community Program Director and Innovation and Research Manager in Palliative Care and Compassionate Communities, New Health Foundation, Seville, Spain

Dan Malleck, PhD, Professor, Department of Health Sciences, Brock University, St. Catharines, ON, Canada

Denise Marshall, MD, CCFP, FCFP, Professor, Palliative Medicine, Division of Palliative Care, Department of Family Medicine, McMaster University, Hamilton, ON, Canada

Catherine Millington-Sanders, MBBS, FRCGP, Kingston CCG EOLC Clinical Lead, South West London Sustainability Transformation Plan EOLC Clinical Lead; Difficult Conversations Co-Founder and National Clinical Lead, RCGP/ Marie Curie National Clinical End of Life Care Champion, RCGP/Marie Curie Daffodil Standards, UK

Jason Mills, RN, BN (Hons), MCHMed, PhD, FACN, FHEA, Senior Lecturer, Curriculum Leader, Faculty of Health & Education, Torrens University, Brisbane, Australia

Shyla Mills, RN, BN, MPallCare, MPH, Chief Executive Officer, Palliative Care Queensland, Brisbane, Australia

Kerrie Noonan, BA(Psych), MPsych(Clinical), PhD, GCBA, MAPS, Director, Death Literacy Institute; Adjunct Research Fellow, School of Social Sciences, Western Sydney University, Sydney, Australia

Charles Normand, DPhil, Professor of the Economics of Palliative Care and Rehabilitation, Cicely Saunders Institute, King's College London, UK; Professor Emeritus, Trinity College Dublin, Dublin, Republic of Ireland

Manjula Patel, PhD, Chief Executive, Murray Hall Community Trust, Sandwell, UK

Rebecca M. Patterson, MA, Director of Good Life, Good Death, Good Grief., Scottish Partnership for Palliative Care, Edinburgh, UK

Sally Paul, MSW, PhD, Senior Lecturer, School of Social Work and Social Policy, University of Strathclyde, Scotland, UK

Katherine Pettus, PhD, Senior Advocacy and Partnerships Director, IAHPC, Houston, TX, USA

Holly Prince, HBSW, MSW, PhD (Cand.) Project Manager, Centre for Education and Research on Aging & Health, Lakehead University, Thunder Bay, ON, Canada

Jairam Kamala Ramakrishnan, MRCPsych, MPH, Honorary Consultant in Public Health & Liaison Psychiatry, Institute of Palliative Medicine, India; Honorary Senior Lecturer in Psychological Medicine, University of Auckland, Auckland, New Zealand

Heather Richardson, RGN, RMN, MA, PhD, is the CEO of St Christopher's Hospice, London; Honorary Professor in Palliative Care, Lancaster University, Lancaster, UK

John P. Rosenberg, RN, BN, MPallC, PhD, Senior Lecturer, School of Nursing, Midwifery and Paramedicine, University of the Sunshine Coast, Caboolture, Australia

Bruce Rumbold, PhD, Associate Professor, Public Health Palliative Care Unit, La Trobe University, Melbourne, Australia

Libby Sallnow, PhD, Honorary Senior Clinical Lecturer and Palliative Medicine Consultant, St Christopher's Hospice and Marie Curie Palliative Care Research Department, University College London, London, UK

Joseph Sawyer, MBBS, MSc, Alzheimer's Society funded Academic Clinical Fellow in Palliative Medicine, Marie Curie Palliative Care Research Department, University College London, London, UK

Mark Spreckley, DrPH, MRes, MBA, MSc, Senior Lecturer, Institute of Health & Social Care, London South Bank University, London, UK

Kelli I. Stajduhar, RN, PhD, FCAHS, Professor, School of Nursing, Research Fellow, Institute of Aging and Lifelong Health, University of Victoria, Victoria, BC, Canada

Bonnie Tompkins, BPH (Public Health), Council Member, Public Health Palliative Care International, ON, Canada

Steven Vanderstichelen, PhD, Senior Researcher, Coordinator of the Compassionate Communities Centre of Expertise, Vrije Universiteit Brussel, Brussels, Belgium

Julia Verne, MBBS, MSc, PhD, FFPH, Head of Health and Social Care Epidemiology, Clinical Lead for Palliative and End of Life Care, Office for Health Improvement and Disparity, DHSC, UK

Gail Wilson, MSc, Deputy Clinical Director, St Luke's Hospice, Plymouth, UK

Abbreviations

ACE	adverse childhood experience
ABCD	Asset-Based Community Development
CiP	capability in practice
CAEOL	Caring at End of Life
CDAS	Centre for Death and Society
CCC	Compassionate City Charter
COVID-19	coronavirus disease 2019
DLI	Death Literacy Index
eHealth	electronic health
EHR	electronic health record
EMR	electronic medical record
ePRO	electronic patient-reported outcome
EOL	end of life
EAPC	European Association for Palliative Care
GMC	General Medical Council
HPPC	Health-Promoting Palliative Care
HPPCS	health-promoting palliative care school
HPS	health-promoting school
HELP	Healthy End of Life Project
HIV	human immunodeficiency virus
HRBA	human rights-based approach
ICT	information and communication technology
IAHPC	International Association for Hospice and Palliative Care
IoT	internet of things
JRCPTB	Joint Royal College Physicians Training Board
LGBTQTS+	lesbian, gay, bisexual, transgender, queer, and Two-Spirited
LEND	Listen, Empathy, Notice, and Do
LMICs	low- and middle-income countries
MOOC	massive open online course
MND	motor neurone disease
NHS	National Health Service
NGO	non-governmental organization
PGD	prolonged grief disorder
PHPC	Public Health Palliative Care
PHPCI	Public Health Palliative Care International
SAC	Specialty Advisory Committee
UN	United Nations
VR	virtual reality
WSU	Western Sydney University
WHO	World Health Organization
WHPCA	Worldwide Hospice Palliative Care Alliance

Introduction

Julian Abel and Allan Kellehear

Why this book and why now?

This is a book about the public health approach within palliative care. Often when we think about 'public health' it is more usual to think about palliative care as part of the public health system—similar to the hospitals, nursing homes, and community clinics but also the broader supports for population health such as sewerage and water purification systems or workplace health and safety. In universities, we often think of public health in terms of the surveillance sciences—epidemiology, health services research, computer modelling, or the bench sciences devoted to understanding disease. But in this volume of contributors, we are specifically addressing a newer and less recognized aspect of public health—public health practice methods such as education, health policy, community development, and social ecology. We are also specifically examining the role of the 'new' public health, sometimes also known as health promotion. Health promotion is a major departure from the emphases on surveillance, disease, and health services by placing its gaze and efforts on practice solutions, health and well-being, and community and civic involvement in healthcare—in this case, palliative care. This *Oxford Textbook of Public Health Palliative Care* is an introduction to this dimension of practice.

The health promotion side of palliative care is necessarily new. Modern palliative care emerged in the 1960s, partly as a response to the isolation of the dying and the bereaved, but partly also as an urgent effort to move clinical practices at the end of life from cure to comfort care. Symptom management, new forms of health services specific to care of the dying and their families, and reimagining new ways to involve family and community were needed. Much has been achieved for these aims in these early years.

However, the matter of how to involve the community has often been eclipsed by the need to establish the credibility of the clinical practice. 'Community' often became places from which to recruit volunteers, raise funds and awareness of the new service, and locations to deliver new forms of day care or home care. The direct service emphasis had gradually distorted our understanding of 'community' by often making this appear singular rather than plural, by making it appear as target and receiver rather than partner and participant, by locating it on the periphery of care instead of understanding its necessary and central position.

In the last 20 years, health-promoting palliative care—the 'new' public health in palliative care—has grown strongly throughout the world, with many leading policy and practice innovations now making their way into the academic and professional literatures. There is now an international association, an international journal, an international conference series, numerous books and doctoral dissertations, and the inevitable wave of critique and reply that signals the arrival of a new perspective that has become part of our established offer, policies, and debates. The time is ripe for an international textbook reference work. It is our intention, alongside the contributors in this book, to provide that introductory reference.

Reimagining palliative care

The predominant medical model of palliative care has left out too many people and has been limited in its scope. Palliative care, in contrast to much of healthcare, has largely been viewed as primarily a profession-led concern. It is professions who are central to the care of dying, the bereaved, and their families. The focus on late dying and early bereavement has led to a dominance of medical, nursing, and psychological professions and services with small recognition and far fewer resources invested in the longer, more crucial journey of care provided by communities—neighbourhoods, schools, workplaces, faith groups, local governments, social media, friendship networks. The people in these places are more than bystanders at the end of life. They are also far more, and must be far more, than volunteers managed by a health service. The longer part of dying, and the far longer part of grieving, occurs across a swathe of civic and local community settings, and it is in that longer experience and those multiple settings that we must recognize and promote the future of palliative care.

The professional and direct service emphases have also meant that our understanding and practices of care have largely created a 'one-way' model—professionals and their volunteers provide everything there is—or nothing. This is partly a legacy of believing or acting as if the important part of palliative care is the medical and nursing care. In fact, most of the important part of dying and its care is psychological, social, and spiritual—and in those matters the people most able and best positioned are the natural social networks inherent for most people living and leaving a life in society. Everyone has a potential role to play in the provision of palliative care, as long as we remember that most of that provision is non-medical, for the vast majority of time.

This is a lesson and principle well understood in the broader public health domain and the reason why all schools, workplaces, local governments, churches, temples, and mosques, as well as neighbourhoods and industries play important roles in healthcare. It is why safety belts are built into motor vehicles, why we try to use condoms or bicycle helmets, why there are health and safety guidelines in supermarkets and in offices around the world, why people volunteer to guide at children's road crossings, or become 'safety houses', join Neighbourhood Watch programmes, or give up smoking and take up regular exercise. Health is everyone's responsibility. We all play a small part because we must (by law) or we want to (ethically for the social good). Public health palliative care reconnects us with this broader public health vision of civic participation and provision.

A whole population, whole life approach

The public health principles of palliative care always promote a whole population approach. Not only does a public health gaze examine the patterns of disease, illness, disability, or injury across a population, but it also plans a whole population approach to their prevention, harm reduction, and necessary treatment and care. That approach means more than the supply of professionals and services because historically we have seen whole populations as not only patients but also providers of care for each other. This is the central reason why direct provision of health services has never been sufficient to the first aims of prevention and harm reduction. The core public health strategies, and values, of health promotion, health equity, public health ethics, and health policies have meant that poverty alleviation, social justice, and the problem of social difference, access, and inequality, remain first causes to champion in public health history and advocacy. Public health palliative care brings those concerns to the provision of care at the end of life and so this volume describes these concerns too.

For unless clinical forms of palliative care are able to connect with public health concerns that take them beyond a narrow focus on health services and symptom science, the problem of care of the dying, the bereaved, and caregivers will continue to resemble models of late care and crisis management. Only by understanding and acting with and alongside community and civic partners will palliative care be able to begin to address its early vision of 'whole person care' and achieve meaningful aspirations for quality and continuity of care at the end of life. Many of the keys to accomplishing this vision and these desires lie outside of face-to-face patient care—in the partnerships found in community allies, social sector care professions, policy development, and health services redesign.

Moreover, the challenges of accessing the palliative care services we offer are great and ever widening—to ethnic and religious minorities, to lower- and middle-income nations, to the marginalized in prisons, those living on the streets and alleys of countless cities, and to those whose identities are hidden from us though they face us directly. Any hopes we have to develop our care models in more compassionate ways to serve that human diversity lie in a more critical and decentred set of sympathies and sensibilities so long associated with an affluent and professional gaze. The values and practices, and not merely the academic sciences of public health, can help us achieve, and move more closely to this vision of care for a whole population, whole life approach to palliative care.

Themes in the book

In the service of arguing and advocating for this whole population, whole life, practice approach for palliative care, we open the book with a series of chapters examining some of the compelling reasons why this approach is essential. The chapters here look closely at the demographic and epidemiological drivers that make a public health practice approach essential to newer ways of doing palliative care. We also look at the international policy context and examine some of the key developments and tensions for a new public health palliative care. Other chapters examine the economic evidence and arguments, the sociological reasons, and the practice rationale for a public health palliative care.

The next section discusses basic concepts—what exactly is the so-called new public health? Where and how did it emerge from the recent history of palliative care ideas and practices? What is the meaning of 'health' and 'well-being'? When public health voices in palliative care speak of 'prevention', 'harm reduction', 'early intervention', or 'participatory relations', what is meant by these different terms and phrases, and how are they to be understood and applied in the practice of palliative care?

Section 3 of the book addresses the basic practice methods. Major methods are introduced, clarified, and described. There are chapters on community development, a public health strategy so often operating under the more popular label of 'compassionate communities'. This is followed by a chapter on social ecology, a public health approach in palliative care so often going under the more popular name of 'compassionate cities'. Thereafter, other chapters address methods of public education (health and death literacy), health policy, health promotion, health-promoting clinical practice methods, and digital applications for public health palliative care.

Section 4 of the book examines population-based approaches, including health service redesign, the end of life experiences of grief and loss, and of equity-orientated care. The final chapter in this section concerns palliative care provision in resource-poor nations.

Section 5 examines the evidence basis of public health palliative care. Chapters here summarize the existing evidence for the effectiveness of public health palliative care across a multiple range of practice domains. Contributors to this section also identify and explore the evidence of 'naturally occurring social networks' and the corresponding evidence for their effectiveness. This section concludes with a review of the complexities and challenges in the collection of evidence for public health palliative care effectiveness, especially for large-scale civic interventions in general.

Section 6 addresses the challenges of education and training in this field. The section starts reflectively with a chapter on pedagogy—what is the learning philosophy that should guide professional education for public health palliative care? The role of public health palliative care in education is given a special exploration for how this might work with children in the context of schools. The idea of the health-promoting palliative care school is introduced in this section. Next, the recent review and revision of the palliative medical curriculum is described and explored for how the new curriculum has integrated the new public health palliative care for the training of the next generation of UK palliative care physicians. Finally, the range and the strengths and limitations of the numerous 'toolkits' offered internationally are described and examined.

We finish this book in Section 7 with a final reflection on the challenges for palliative care as it attempts to embrace a public health vision of practice. We reflect on the necessary shift from a service and clinical model of care for the dying and their caregivers, to a more inclusive model. This is a future model not merely defined by cause of death, age, or diagnosis, but one that works for all people including those near and far, young and old, disadvantaged or disenfranchised, and in local or international settings. This is because the human impulse behind all care at the end of life is best realized through the social practice of compassion—a care for the other that is shared with others.

SECTION 1

The case for public health palliative care

1

Demographic and epidemiological challenges

Julia Verne

Introduction

The past three decades have seen unprecedented demographic change in the world with populations in both industrialized and middle- to low-income countries ageing rapidly. As populations age, the cause of death changes and chronic diseases of affluence, such as diabetes, heart disease, and cancer, and diseases of old age, such as dementia, become the major causes of death (Worldwide Hospice Palliative Care Alliance, 2020). These kinds of deaths are preceded by longer periods of physical and mental deterioration and accompanying dependency on others. At the same time, there has been a reduction in birth rates and unprecedented migration both within countries and across countries, much driven by economic considerations as well as war. This means that family sizes are shrinking and there are fewer young people to care for the ageing population. Specialist palliative care has tended to focus on the support of cancer patients and their families although recent years have seen a change in this with increasing interest in support for people dying from other chronic conditions such as respiratory conditions (Public Health England, 2019; Worldwide Hospice Palliative Care Alliance, 2020).

Although the populations of industrialized countries have seen significant ageing of their populations, similar changes have been experienced in developing and middle-income countries, albeit more slowly. With this worldwide demographic change, the causes of death and serious illness prior to death have changed (World Health Organization, 2011). As life expectancy increases, the elderly population tend to suffer increased numbers of comorbidities, including frailty and dementia.

The *Global Atlas of Palliative Care* has estimated that over 56.8 million people may need palliative care. While more patients worldwide are now receiving palliative care than at the time of the first edition of this volume in 2014, increasing from 16,000 services caring for 3 million patients to over 25,000 services caring for over 7 million patients, this still means that only about 12% of the need is being met (Worldwide Hospice Palliative Care Alliance, 2020). Prior to the coronavirus disease 2019 (COVID-19) pandemic, 68.9% (36.5 million people) of palliative care need in adults worldwide was associated with a non-communicable disease (Worldwide Hospice Palliative Care Alliance, 2020). Communicable diseases such as HIV/AIDS, haemorrhagic fever, and tuberculosis accounted for 24.4% while injuries—an important cause of death worldwide—accounted for only 6.2% (Centeno and Arias-Casais, 2019). Although the largest single disease group accounting for adult palliative care was cancer, conditions such as HIV, cerebrovascular diseases, and dementia were the most common diseases associated with under-provision or no provision of palliative care (Centeno and Arias-Casais, 2019).

In high-income countries, it is the elderly (aged 75 years and older) who comprise the majority of people who die (Worldwide Hospice Palliative Care Alliance, 2020). In England, for example, 68.2% of those who die are aged 75 years or older at death (Public Health England, 2018, 2020e). Indeed, 39.8%, die aged 85 years or older at death. The size of this group is rapidly growing because of demographic change, both due to increased life expectancy and the ageing of the 'baby boom' population who were born after the Second World War. Over the next two decades, the number of people aged 85 years and older in England will double and those aged 100 years and older will quadruple. The UK is now defined as an 'ageing society' and by 2035 it will become a 'super-aged society' based on the proportion of the population aged 65 years and older (Eurostat, 2021).

While the proportion of people who die in England aged 75 or older has changed little over recent years, rapid increases in life expectancy have meant that mortality and overall numbers of deaths temporarily reduced over the past two decades. However, both mortality and overall numbers of death have been rising rapidly and it is the elderly and very elderly who are contributing to a large projected rise in numbers of deaths (Etkind et al., 2017). In England and Wales combined, annual deaths are projected to rise by 25.4% (from 501,424 in 2014 to 628,659 by 2040). Fig. 1.1 shows how the age distribution at death is predicted to change with increasing numbers of deaths occurring at older ages.

In England, it was estimated that, prior to the COVID-19 pandemic, between 69% and 82% of people who die could benefit from some form of palliative care to support their end of life care needs,

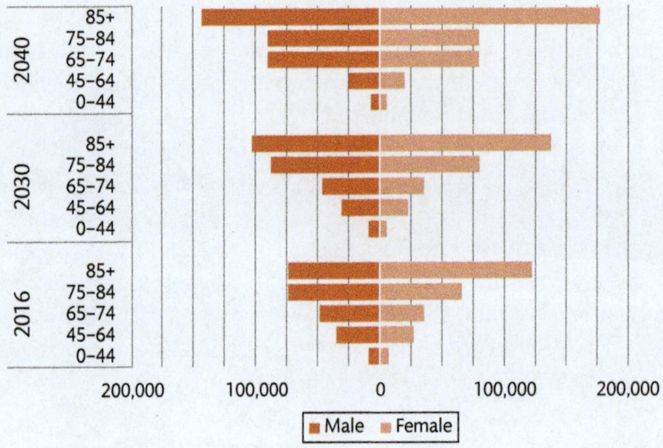

Fig. 1.1 The age distribution of deaths projected for future years.

although not necessarily specialist palliative care (Murtagh et al., 2014). This type of care would include symptom relief for pain, breathlessness, and terminal agitation. It also includes support in the three other domains of psychological, social, and spiritual/existential needs at the end of life. It was similar to the estimate of 75% by Gomez-Batiste and colleagues (2014), based on chronic disease prevalence, that argued that almost everyone who does not have an 'unexpected' death, may need at least some element of palliative care.

Etkind and colleagues (2017) have projected that if age- and sex-specific proportions of people with palliative care needs were to remain the same as in 2014, in England and Wales the number of people requiring palliative care would be expected to grow by 25.0% (from 375,398 to 469,305 people/year) by 2040. However, as described previously, if this upward trend in the number of deaths in recent years continues, the increase will be by 42.4% (161,842 more people/year, total 537,240). Importantly, Etkind and colleagues (2017) have shown, using disease-specific projections, that dementia and cancer will be the main causes of death for which palliative care will be needed in the future. Dementia-related deaths are predicted to increase from 59,199 to 219,409 deaths per year by 2040 and cancer deaths to increase from 143,638 to 208,636 deaths by 2040 in England and Wales. The increase in deaths from dementia has important implications for involvement by the individual in decisions about their care and therefore exertion of their autonomy if they lose mental capacity (Nuffield Council on Bioethics, 2009). Healthcare systems must now start to adapt to the age-related growth in deaths from chronic illness, by focusing on integration and boosting of palliative care across healthcare and social care disciplines. Much of the professional palliative and end of life care will be provided by non-specialists in primary care and in social care. However, the vast majority of that future care, in terms of hours and tasks, will be provided by families and their communities. Countries with similar demographic and disease changes will likely experience comparable rises in professional and community needs (Eurostat, 2021).

It is a sobering fact that the projected 160,000 increase in people in England and Wales who may need palliative care by 2040 is slightly more than the increase of over 125,000 deaths due to COVID-19 over the first year of the pandemic for the UK as a whole; also taking into account other causes of mortality, the number of deaths rose to 695,000 during 2020 (Etkind et al., 2017; Statista.com, 2021). This made 2020 the deadliest year (number of deaths) since 1918, at the height of the Spanish influenza pandemic; however, as can be seen, demographic change alone would have made 2040, just 20 years away, the deadliest year since 1918 if not for the COVID-19 pandemic (Etkind et al., 2017).

The specific care needs of people towards the end of their life are influenced by their underlying illnesses. There have been reductions in the number of people dying from stroke and heart disease, especially between 75 and 84 years of age, and the number of people dying with dementia recorded as an underlying or contributory cause of death has increased considerably. In some regions of England, one in four people die with dementia (Public Health England, 2018, 2020e). The future will see this trend continue, with even more people at the end of their life suffering from dementia due to the expected increase in the number of people dying in their late eighties or later.

The change in underlying and contributory causes of death associated with ageing impacts the pattern of decline prior to death. Unlike cancer patients for whom the terminal phase is frequently predictable, older adults, especially with non-cancer morbidity including dementia, are more likely to experience a period of increasing limitations to daily living punctuated by serious episodes of acute illness which lead to stepwise decline or what has been termed 'prolonged dwindling' (Lynn and Adamson, 2003). A study by Ennis and colleagues (2015) found that half (50.3%) of the residents in a study of 38 care homes in Southern England died of what was described as 'dwindling', 26.2% from a terminal condition, 19.2% from an acute condition, and 4.2% had a sudden death.

Age affects place of death because of the increasing prevalence of comorbidities with age and need for care by others. Older adults account for the majority of people who die in hospital: 67.8% of deaths in hospital occur in people aged 75 years and older at death, while 37.2% are aged 85 years and older at death. The age profile of deaths in hospital reflects the age profile of deaths in the population (Public Health England, 2020d). Although many elderly people would prefer to die in their own home, or a hospice, very few achieve this. They account for the highest proportion of deaths in care homes as this is where many live (Public Health England, 2020e). Yet a care home is reported to be the least preferred place of death (Calanzani et al., 2014). Currently about one in four people die in care homes (Public Health England, 2020e). If the numbers of people dying, especially at older ages and with dementia, increase, then the number of care home beds required will increase based on current usage (Bone et al., 2018). Although on average one in four people die in care homes, in England there is wide unwarranted variation by local healthcare administration areas (Public Health England, 2018). Prior to the COVID-19 pandemic, the proportion of all people who died aged 75 years and older in a care home varied between 10% and 43% (Public Health England, 2018, 2020e). This, in part, was related to variations in care home provision across the country, once adjusted for the population over the age of 75 years. However, variation in availability of beds only accounts for around 30% of the variation seen in the proportion of people who die in care homes. This indicates that other factors are important including length of time spent in the care home prior to death and the ratio of nursing to residential homes in each area.

Another example of unwarranted variation in the way people are cared for in the healthcare system prior to death is in the number of hospital admissions prior to death even if the person dies in the community. Two-thirds of people who die in England have a hospital admission in the final 90 days of their life and on average, one in 14 (6.9%) had three or more emergency hospital admissions during the last 90 days of life (Public Health England, 2020c). However, the risk of multiple admissions varies geographically. Many of the patients with multiple admissions are elderly and this primarily reflects inadequate arrangements to care for them in the community and absence of clear indications from patients, in advance care plans, as to whether they want these transfers (Public Health England, 2020d). There is good evidence that multiple transfers between home/care home and hospital at the end of life is very distressing to patients and their families (Hanratty et al., 2014).

Interestingly, the difference in the age at death between males and females is projected to reduce, with females making up 55% of people dying aged 85 or older in 2040 compared to 62% in 2016. This narrowing of the age at death between males and females means that the number of elderly people living alone may reduce and care may need to focus more on frail couples than frail individuals. This will introduce a new dynamic as it may be the shared priorities for autonomy of a couple, along the lines of 'til death do us part', rather than individual priorities of elderly people that healthcare and social care will have to consider more frequently in the future (Turner et al., 2016).

Social implications of the changing demography and epidemiology

Recent sociodemographic trends have not only seen an increase in the number of people dying, and an increased age at death, but also subsequent changes in cause of death and increased dependency on others for care for prolonged periods before death. In addition, the number of younger people of working age who could help care for the elderly at the end of life is, in many countries, reducing. The relationship between the numbers of elderly who may need caring for, and the numbers of people of working age who could potentially care for them is described by the 'dependency ratio' (Eurostat, 2020). Dependency ratio calculation is complex as it depends on the age profile of the population, birth rate, life expectancy, and inward and outward migration.

Across Europe, the last few years have been a time of unprecedented migration especially from the East of Europe to the West. For example, about 3 million young people left Romania to work in Western Europe, leaving few behind to care for their elderly, but other countries such as England have benefited from inward migration from Eastern Europe, especially Poland and Romania, to staff care homes (Business Review, 2019). Interestingly, the COVID-19 pandemic has triggered considerable reversal of this migration. Dependency ratios (ratio of people aged $\geq$65 years to people of working age) are, in general, increasing across high-income countries, Currently, the European Union average is 29.9%. However, the countries with the highest rates, such as Italy at 34.8%, have significant challenges in the workforce to care for the elderly (Eurostat, 2021). Across Europe the shortage of people to care for the elderly presents significant challenges to the protection and preservation of their autonomy as they approach the end of life.

Sociodemographic trends have led to other challenges for those approaching the end of life in many countries, these include loneliness, loss of autonomy, and anomie in the face of death. Loneliness and the absence of close family or friends to call on is another pandemic of our time. The *Atlas of Variation for Palliative and End of Life Care in England* (Public Health England, 2018) demonstrated the proportions of elderly people aged 65 years and older who live alone in their own homes varies from 25% to 45% by local authority (local government area). The number of people living alone increases with age and by the time people reach the age of 85 years, almost 60% of those in their own homes live alone (Public Health England, 2018). Many of those living alone may also do so in poverty (Verne et al., 2018). A study in 2018 found that local authorities reported a 70% increase in the preceding 3 years in what are commonly known as paupers' funerals, also known as public health funerals, paid for by the local authority—when a person, usually elderly, dies alone with no resources to pay for their funeral and no traceable family (ITV.com, 2018).

Elderly people living alone may have no family, the family may have moved away for work or family reasons and may or may not support their elderly relative. A recent study in which the chapter author was a co-author, asked members of the general population aged 45 years and over whether they had anyone to count on for regular help if the need arose. It found that 12% reported that they felt they had no relative, friend, or neighbour that they could count on and 19% claimed there was just one person. In contrast, 37% claimed there were two to four people they thought they could count on and 33% thought there were five or more people. This highlights that around a third of the older adult population may find themselves without family or community support if they were to require support for end of life care. The rates were higher in London and for those who did not belong to religious or community groups (Tapp et al., 2019).

Living alone at home and social isolation may exacerbate suffering for the elderly person in the psychological, social, and spiritual domains and presents additional challenges for the delivery of comprehensive palliative care especially in people's own homes. The loss of autonomy is greater when there is no one to call on for help and the individual becomes dependent on state provision of healthcare and social care. Depression is common and may even lead to a wish to hasten death (Rurup et al., 2011; van Wijngaarden et al., 2015). These demographic changes and social isolation of older adults, compounded by their deteriorating health and increased dependency, underpins the increasing numbers of elderly cared for and dying in care homes.

Many of the recent demographic changes have witnessed a parallel decrease in religiosity and other social traditions, practices, and knowledge about dying, death, and bereavement. These changes have compounded the widespread prevalence and experience of anomie. Many people may now simply not know how they could exert their autonomy around dying and death. In our survey of over 3500 people, we found that 37% of 45–65-year-olds and 30% of 70–79-year-olds said that they had not thought seriously about end of life care planning. This dropped to 18% in those aged 80 years or over, however, still leaving one in five at this advanced age not seriously thinking about end of life care (Tapp et al., 2019). There is accumulating evidence that not knowing what to think or do about death or avoiding thinking and talking about it are major challenges for all concerned (Borgstrom and Walter, 2015). It for this reason that charity-led events such as 'What Matters Most' (What Matters Conversations, 2020) or the 'National Day of Reflection' (Marie Curie, 2021) (1 year from the first COVID-19 lockdown) are important in prompting thought and discussion and hopefully planning. As discussed later in this chapter, the media coverage of the COVID-19 pandemic may have done more to combat anomie than any state- or charity-funded public health palliative care health promotion campaigns.

Impacts on autonomy and dignity

One principle of both public health practice and palliative and end of life care is the promotion of individual autonomy and participation in decision-making. Under Article 12 of the International Covenant on Economic, Social and Cultural Rights and Article 7 of the International Covenant on Civil and Political Rights, 'all member countries of the United Nations are obliged to safeguard patients at the end of life against pain and suffering, allowing them to die with dignity'. Interpretations of the role of dignity of the dying patient as a human rights issue have been limited to a focus on ensuring patients die without suffering pain and other terminal symptoms. Dignity may also relate to self-determination. Elderly patients are extremely vulnerable to losing their autonomy as they approach the end of life because of physical and mental frailty.

While the United Nations has recognized that elderly people need special attention to protect their human rights (Mahler, 2017), there is no published literature to date on the specific human rights of elderly people at the end of life. Physical frailty alone reduces the individual's ability to take autonomous actions even in the most basic daily tasks and forces reliance on others, for example, professional and family carers (Agich, 2003). However, it is the high prevalence of loss of mental capacity in elderly patients due to dementia-like conditions which really impacts their autonomy and leaves them especially vulnerable to potentially paternalistic decision-making by others (Sales, 2014). Autonomy is not simply about arranging practical issues related to care (Van Brussel, 2014). Autonomy is important to people approaching the end of life for an optimal sense of psychological well-being, retaining identity and sentience as long as possible, as well as retaining at least some control over physical, social, and spiritual matters where these are considered important to them. Dignity and duty, especially not to be a burden, emerge as strong reasons for exerting autonomy in elderly people (Van Brussel, 2014).

There should not be a blanket assumption of lack of mental capacity in a patient with a degenerative brain condition but for each decision, large or very small, the patient's capacity to make it should be reviewed and every effort made to make it possible for them to participate using simple language, non-verbal cues, or returning to the decision on another occasion (General Medical Council, 2010).

Impact of the COVID-19 pandemic on a public health approach to palliative and end of life care

Monitoring demographic change and its impact on the epidemiology of disease over time is useful. However, wars and pandemics have an immediate effect on causes of death and patterns of delivery of palliative and end of life care. The COVID-19 pandemic has been extraordinary in its impact not only in the huge excess death toll from COVID-19 but also the impact of the pandemic on excess deaths from other conditions. By the third week of March 2021 there had been 2,684,093 COVID-19-related deaths reported to the World Health Organization COVID-19 dashboard (World Health Organization, n.d.).

In England and Wales, the excess deaths were markedly increased in hospitals and care homes during both the first and the second wave of the pandemic but have been continuously greater in people's private homes since the start of the pandemic. Deaths in care homes increased by 220%, while home and hospital deaths increased by 77% and 90%, respectively. Hospice deaths fell by 20%. Additional deaths were among older people (86% aged ≥75 years), and most occurred in care homes (56%) and at home (43%) (Office for National Statistics, 2021). The deaths in care homes have highlighted previous inadequacies in palliative and end of life care support for the staff and residents of care homes. Greater support for care homes through closer collaboration with primary care, specialist palliative care services, and community geriatricians is needed for now and for future pandemics (Gordon et al., 2020).

However, not only have there been greater numbers of people dying to care for, under radically different circumstances than normal, and more bereaved relatives suffering difficult and traumatic bereavements (Kentish-Barnes et al., 2015) with the typical grief associated with death and dying, but it has been suggested that there will also be novel grief processes, linked to social isolation or self-blame around causing infection or not being able to attend funerals (Wallace et al., 2020). Importantly, there has been huge media attention on the plight of those dying in care homes where, in England, normally about a fifth to a quarter of the population die. Similarly, the issue of inequalities has been raised and the risks and special need for care for marginalized groups and especially those with vulnerabilities at the end of life, for example, those with learning disabilities (Public Health England, 2020a, 2020b).

The COVID-19 pandemic has, par excellence, demonstrated that palliative and support care can act in synergy with active treatment attempting to save lives. The lived experience of clinicians hoping for (and doing) the best while planning for the worst has been broadcast out to the nation day after day.

While the death and toll from long COVID-19 has been catastrophic and there is likely to be a vast number of people suffering psychological problems post COVID-19 (Kentish-Barnes et al., 2015; Wallace et al., 2020), the media coverage of dying, death, and bereavement may result in a seismic change in public knowledge, attitudes, and preparedness for death which national campaigns such as 'Dying Matters' (Hospice UK, 2021) could only dream of.

The COVID-19 pandemic has thrust scenes of dying in every setting from intensive care units to care homes, death, loss, and bereavement into everyone's living room through endless media coverage at every hour of the day or night during the past year, leading to an unexpected and even relentless process of socializing aspects of palliative and supportive care. It has highlighted the fragility of life, the need to face and discuss death, and plan for its, perhaps unpredictable, eventuality. Things normally taken for granted have been suspended, such as unlimited visiting to enable a loved one who is terminally ill to say 'good-bye' and 'I love you', to hold hands and say 'I am sorry', or to attend funerals, or meet with family and friends and community to observe rites and derive support. This means that each of us perhaps reflects more on the need to talk about our own or loved one's death to prepare 'just in case' and tell each other what is important to us (What Matters Conversations, 2021). Breaking bad news to relatives, and especially when this had to be done by phone or video link, has been vividly exposed by reporters, capturing the words said and the emotional turmoil on both sides of the conversation. What normally happens hundreds of thousands of times in a year in private and more often face to face has been shown to the public.

Similarly, the impact, albeit many times magnified, of loss and grief on members of the public and indeed of caring for dying patients on frontline health and social care personnel has been explicitly shown. The pandemic, inadvertently, has communicated more to the general public about death and dying, the need to plan for potential death and tell your loved ones that you love them in case at the critical moment it will not be possible, and about the importance of social support.

Moreover, the role of each individual in the care of the dying and after death has been exposed from the doctors and nurses in hospital or at home, or carers in care homes who care for the dying, break bad news, and comfort the bereaved, through the hospital porters and mortuary technicians to funeral directors. The charities, too, despite huge financial losses due to the inability to fund raise, have played their roles in providing support and information to the public, especially those which support the bereaved, and campaigned at a governmental level to acknowledge the impact of the pandemic on the population. The National Day of Reflection (Marie Curie, 2021), organized on the first anniversary of national lockdown, was one such example to engage the nation to show solidarity with those who had lost their loved ones not only to COVID-19 but other causes during the year.

The COVID-19 pandemic has highlighted the very small specialist palliative care workforce but also the ability of other medical specialists, nurses, and social care workers to provide the majority of end of life care including breaking bad news conversations with family and friends. The plight of care home residents approaching the end of life, in particular, has been highlighted during the pandemic, particularly their frailty and dependence on others prior to death.

The increasing need for a public health palliative care

Until the COVID-19 pandemic, the population of the world had been continuing to age, with many industrialized nations moving into the 'super aged' demographic description. In some countries, like England, the total number of people dying had been increasing, pre COVID-19, as the baby-boomers, born after the Second World War, age and their age at death had been steadily increasing. This had radically changed the profile of the conditions from which and with which people die, impacting the trajectory of decline before death, the ability to accurately predict the end of life, and the specific medical, psychological, social, and spiritual needs of the dying population. Moreover, increasing numbers of elderly people are dying with diminishing family and/or community support and significant numbers with extreme loneliness and no one to call upon for help except professionals. A slow 'dwindling' course towards death had become common, marked by episodes of acute illness and deterioration. The majority of people who die experience months or years of loss of physical and mental capacity prior to death and increasing dependence on others with a subsequent diminishing scope for making autonomous decisions. While death in hospital has reduced over the past decade, institutions, hospitals, and care homes are still, in England, the commonest place of death (Public Health England, 2020e). The high prevalence of loss of mental capacity to be involved in decision-making associated with dementia makes the issue of advance care planning even more critical.

While these epidemiological and demographic changes have deepened the public health understanding of the new needs for palliative and end of life care, especially with respect to the importance of the non-specialist medical and social care contributions to the care of the dying—particularly in the care home sector and at home, as the majority of people die in older age and of non-cancer conditions—they have also led to a distancing of the public from death and dying and led to anomie with respect to death, dying, and bereavement.

The COVID-19 pandemic has opened a public discussion about what is important to the dying and their families with a recognition of the importance of human interaction and the psychosocial context of dying ('what matters to me'). Indeed, while medical and social care staff have been active bystanders in providing care, it is the personal nature of death as the last chapter of an individual's life and the importance of family and community that has so moved people around the world and emphasized why a wider scope for the understanding of death and dying and care at a population level is so important.

The COVID-19 pandemic has strengthened the rationale and importance for a public health approach to end of life care and support before and after death. In particular, historical and recent changes to our demography and epidemiology have highlighted the value of three important features of public health palliative care as a palliative care practice.

Firstly, public health palliative care considers a dying individual not solely as a medical patient seen only through the lens of their disease and failing organs but as a valued, integrated member of social networks within a community, both real and/or virtual, until their death. Caregivers and the bereaved have social networks that are crucial to mobilize for the purposes of health and well-being and in tackling their circumstance-related morbidities and risk of mortality. The sheer pressure of global numbers—in those who are ageing and in the comorbidities of their ageing—suggest severe limits to the professional capacity of direct service provision. Only through partnerships with the civic sectors of the wider society (from schools, workplaces, or local governments), and with local community supports (from neighbourhoods, family networks, or social media), will palliative care cope with the rising demands for access, equity, quality, and continuity of care at the end of life. Clinical services by teams of professionals can only be part of this solution, and in the context of the above-mentioned tide of demographic numbers, a small part.

Secondly, we now observe important changes to our usual public health approach that move our priorities from one heavily invested in surveillance assessments of population need and focusing on discreet and narrow interventions to an equal sociological emphasis on new and existing population practices for support. Community development practices—partnerships with healthcare and social care services with local communities using their own assets of people power—long viewed as the only solution for low-income national health approaches, are now finding new homes inside the affluent economies of resource-rich nations. The limits to professional services are being increasingly recognized, now underlined by the COVID-19 crisis, as being further impetus for reinvigorating the methods used in other areas of public health outside palliative care—health and end of life literacy, place-based approaches such as compassionate communities, civic health and social policy development, primary care redesign, and partnership working across civic and health and social care sectors.

Finally, public health palliative care mobilizes not just health or social services, whether state or insurance funded, but social capital to care for the dying and their loved ones up to and after death. The definition and the practice of continuity of care is now being revised to include a deeper understanding of community—not simply as sites for services—but as partners. The idea of 'social capital' as the generation and support for community resilience, support, and trust is being explored by public health approaches for its value in attaining the original vision of 'whole person' care at the end of life because there can be no adequate addressing of the 'whole person' without a detailed understanding of 'person-in-community'. Social, psychological, and spiritual care is now shifting away from mere occupational understandings and responses to patients, to a position where communities and neighbourhoods can play clear and sustainable roles for each other at the end of life and beyond. Public health palliative care is evolving from merely surveillance and intervention work for healthcare in general to embracing cooperative practices and partnerships for end of life care.

Conclusion

As Dr Tedros Adhanom Ghebreyesus, Director General, World Health Organization, wrote in his foreword to the second edition of the *Global Atlas of Palliative Care*, 'The COVID-19 pandemic has highlighted the importance of palliative care in all health care systems. The need for relief from severe suffering, the difficult decision making, and complicated grief brought on by the pandemic are exactly the types of problems that palliative care was designed to help address' (Worldwide Hospice Palliative Care Alliance, p. 10).

In a sense, this very public exposé of dying, death, and bereavement may result, once the pandemic recedes, in the reclaiming of death, dying, and bereavement by everyone. Palliative care may finally become a civic responsibility and not just solely a professional one. The future may be ripe for new partnerships and cooperation between local communities and the professional services that live and work among them. In this historical context and consequence, the future looks bright.

REFERENCES

Agich, G. 2003. *Dependence and Autonomy in Old Age: An Ethical Framework for Long Term Care.* Cambridge: Cambridge University Press.

Bone, A., Gomes, B., Etkind, S. N., Verne, J., Murtagh, F., Evans, C. J., et al. 2018. What is the impact of population ageing on the future provision of end-of-life care? Population-based projections of place of death. *Palliative Medicine,* **32**, 329–336.

Borgstrom, E. and Walter, T. 2015. Choice and compassion at the end of life: a critical analysis of recent English policy discourse. *Social Science & Medicine,* **136–137**, 99–105.

Business Review. 2019. Romania's emigrant population is the fifth largest in the world and growing, OECD report finds. [Online] Available at: https://business-review.eu/news/romanias-emigrant-population-is-the-fifth-largest-in-the-world-and-growing-oecd-report-finds-203223

Calanzani, N., Moens, K., Cohen, J., Higginson, I. J., Harding, R., Deliens, L., et al. 2014. Choosing care homes as the least preferred place to die: a cross-national survey of public preferences in seven European countries. *BMC Palliative Care,* **13**, 48.

Centeno, C. and Arias-Casais, N. 2019. Global palliative care: from need to action. *Lancet Global Health,* **7**, e815–e816.

Ennis, L., Kinley, J., Hockley, J., and McCrone, P. 2015. The cost of providing end of life care for nursing care home residents: a retrospective cohort study *Health Services Management Research,* **28**, 16–23.

Etkind, S., Bone, A. E., Gomes, B., Lovell, N., Evans, C. J., Higginson, I. J., et al. 2017. How many people will need palliative care in 2040? Past trends, future projections and implications for services. *BMC Medicine,* **15**, 102.

Eurostat. 2020. Old age dependency ratio increasing in the EU. [Online] Available at: https://ec.europa.eu/eurostat/web/products-eurostat-news/-/DDN-20200713-1

Eurostat. 2021. Population (demography, migration and projections). [Online] Available at: https://ec.europa.eu/eurostat/web/population-demography-migration-projections/data/database

General Medical Council. 2010. Treatment and care towards the end of life: good practice in decision making. [Online] Available at: https://www.gmc-uk.org/ethical-guidance/ethical-guidance-for-doctors/treatment-and-care-towards-the-end-of-life

Gomez-Batiste, X., Martínez-Muñoz, M., Blay, C., Amblàs, J., Vila, L., Costa, X., et al. 2014. Prevalence and characteristics of patients with advanced chronic conditions in need of palliative care in the general population: a cross-sectional study. *Palliative Medicine,* **28**, 302–311.

Gordon, A., Goodman, C., Achterberg, W., Barker, R. O., Burns, E., Hanratty, B., et al. 2020. Commentary: COVID in care homes—challenges and dilemmas in healthcare delivery. *Age and Ageing,* **49**, 701–705.

Hanratty, B., Holmes, L., Lowson, E., Grande, G., Addington-Hall, J., Payne, S., et al. 2012. Older adults' experiences of transitions between care settings at the end of life in England: a qualitative interview study. *Journal of Pain and Symptom Management,* **44**, 74–83.

Hospice UK. 2021. Dying matters. [Online] Available at: https://www.dyingmatters.org/

ITV.com. 2018. ITV news investigation finds 70% rise in 'paupers' funerals'—with some councils preventing relatives attending. [Online] Available at: https://www.itv.com/news/2018-06-15/itv-news-investigation-finds-70-rise-in-paupers-funerals

Kentish-Barnes, N., Chaize, M., Seegers, V., Legriel, S., Cariou, A., Jaber, S., et al. 2015. Complicated grief after death of a relative in the intensive care unit. *European Respiratory Journal,* **45**, 1341–1352.

Lynn, J. and Adamson, D. 2003. *Living Well at the End of Life: Adapting Health Care to Serious Chronic Illness in Old Age.* Santa Monica, CA: Rand Corporation.

Mahler, C. 2017. What is the situation with human rights of the elderly? UN Open-ended Working Group on Ageing—review and prospects. *Zeitschrift fur Gerontologie und Geriatrie,* **50**, 281–286.

Marie Curie. 2021. National day of reflection. [Online] Available at: https://www.mariecurie.org.uk/get-involved/day-of-reflection

Murtagh, F., Bausewein, C., Verne, J., Groeneveld, E. I., Kaloki, Y. E., and Higginson, I. 2014. How many people need palliative care? A study developing and comparing methods for population-based estimates. *Palliative Medicine,* **14**, 49–58.

Nuffield Council on Bioethics. 2009. *Dementia: Ethical Issues.* London: Nuffield Council on Bioethics. Available at: https://www.nuffieldbioethics.org/wp-content/uploads/2014/07/Dementia-report-Oct-09.pdf

Office for National Statistics. 2021. Deaths registered weekly in England & Wales, provisional: week ending 19 March 2021. [Online] Available at: https://www.ons.gov.uk/peoplepopulationandcommunity/birthsdeathsandmarriages/deaths/bulletins/deathsregisteredweeklyinenglandandwalesprovisional/weekending19march2021

Porta i Sales, J. 2014. [Palliative care and human rights.] *Medicina Paliativa,* **21**, 45–47.

Public Health England. 2018. Atlas of variation for palliative and end of life care in England. [Online] Available at: https://fingertips.phe.org.uk/profile/atlas-of-variation

Public Health England. 2019. The 2nd atlas of variation in risk factors and healthcare for respiratory disease in England. [Online] Available at: https://fingertips.phe.org.uk/profile/atlas-of-variation

Public Health England. 2020a. COVID-19: deaths of people with learning disabilities. [Online] Available at: https://www.gov.uk/government/publications/covid-19-deaths-of-people-with-learning-disabilities

Public Health England. 2020b. Disparities in the risk and outcomes of COVID-19. [Online] Available at: https://assets.publishing.service.gov.uk/government/uploads/system/uploads/attachment_data/file/908434/Disparities_in_the_risk_and_outcomes_of_COVID_August_2020_update.pdf

Public Health England. 2020c. Emergency admissions in the 3 months before death. [Online] Available at: https://www.gov.uk/government/publications/emergency-admissions-i n-the-3-months-before-death

Public Health England. 2020d. Older people's hospital admissions in the last year of life. [Online] Available at: https://www.gov.uk/government/publications/older-peoples-hospital-admissions-in-the-last-year-of-life

Public Health England. 2020e. Palliative and end of life care profiles. [Online] Available at: https://fingertips.phe.org.uk/profile/end-of-life

Rurup, M., Deeg, D. J., Poppelaars, J. L., Kerkhof, A. J., and Onwuteaka-Philipsen, B. D. 2011. Wishes to die in older people: a quantitative study of prevalence and associated factors. *Crisis,* **34**, 194–203.

Statista.com. 2021. Weekly number of excess deaths in England and Wales from week ending January 5, 2018 to week ending March 19, 2021. Available at: https://www.statista.com/statistics/1131428/excess-deaths-in-england-and-wales/

Tapp, A., Nancarrow, C., Morey, Y., Warren, S., Bowtell, N., and Verne, J. 2019. Public responses to volunteer community care: propositions for old age and end of life. *PLoS One,* **14**, e0218597.

Turner, M., King, C., Milligan, C., Thomas, C., Brearley, S. G., Seamark, D., et al. 2016. Caring for a dying spouse at the end of life: 'It's one of the things you volunteer for when you get married': a qualitative study of the oldest carers' experiences. *Age Ageing,* **45**, 421–426.

Van Brussel, L. 2014. Autonomy and dignity: a discussion on contingency and dominance. *Health Care Analysis,* **22**, 174–191.

van Wijngaarden, E., Leget, C., and Goossensen, A. 2015. Ready to give up on life: the lived experience of elderly people who feel life is completed and no longer worth living. *Social Science & Medicine,* **138**, 257–264.

Verne, J., Pring, A., and Bowtell, N. 2018. Living alone, in poverty and loneliness–challenges for pensioners wishing to be cared for and die at home in England. *Palliative Medicine,* **32**, 3–330.

Wallace, C., Wladkowski, S. P., Gibson, A., and White, P. 2020. Grief during the COVID-19 pandemic: considerations for palliative care providers. *Journal of Pain & Symptom Management,* **60**, E70–E76.

What Matters Conversations. 2020. What matters most charter. 2020. [Online] Available at: https://www.whatmattersconversations.org/2020-charter

World Health Organization. n.d. WHO coronavirus (COVID-19) dashboard. [Online] Available at: https://covid19.who.int/

World Health Organization. 2011. Global health and aging. [Online] Available at: https://www.who.int/ageing/publications/global_health.pdf

Worldwide Hospice Palliative Care Alliance. 2020. *Global Atlas of Palliative Care,* 2nd ed. London: Worldwide Hospice Palliative Care Alliance. Available at: http://www.thewhpca.org/resources/global-atlas-on-end-of-life-care

2

International palliative care policy: public health in relation to the 'new' palliative care

Philip J. Larkin

Introduction

This chapter has two broad aims. Firstly, it explores why a public health approach is globally relevant for the future of palliative and end of life care and considers the risk to the discipline if this approach is undervalued. Secondly, it poses the question 'Does international palliative care policy exist and why is it important?' Certainly, policy informing the facets of palliative care development does exist and the case for its need is well made. Global distribution and availability of palliative care has been assessed using a number of indicators (Arias et al., 2019; Clark et al., 2020). Building on revised work from an initial assessment in 2006 (T. Lynch et al., 2013), Clark and colleagues (2020) demonstrate that despite endorsement by key players in world health such as the World Health Organization (WHO), 87% of the global population are still unable to access palliative care when they need it. Service need does not seem to match policy demand and Clark and colleagues question the effectiveness of current global strategies. If this assertion is true, what does this mean for our response as a palliative care community?

The chapter also introduces the notion of a 'new' palliative care. The contemporary discourse on 'serious health-related suffering' (Knaul et al., 2018; Sleeman et al., 2019) has brought the arguments for a public health palliative care approach to the fore. This has challenged palliative care to move beyond a useful and important localized clinical service for those dying from cancer to a more socially conscious and politicized approach to addressing the needs of vulnerable populations. As will be discussed, agencies such as the International Association for Hospice and Palliative Care (IAHPC), the Worldwide Hospice Palliative Care Alliance (WHPCA), and the European Association for Palliative Care (EAPC) have taken up this challenge, focusing their initiatives on the public health agenda and offering different perspectives based on their varied target audience. A challenge to this is to ask whether the differing foci of these agencies contribute to or inhibit the evolution of the public health message and if a more cohesive approach is needed.

The term 'palliative and end of life care' (sometimes called PEoLC) is used deliberately throughout this chapter. Despite the benefit of early intervention offered in tandem with active treatments, for most people, the exposure to palliative and end of life care is synonymous with end of life care and death. For many people in low- and middle-income countries (LMICs), early intervention and treatment options are limited or unattainable. To offer a counter balance between the political ideal and the patient reality, the phrase is used here to capture that essential and necessary part of the palliative and end of life care spectrum. Both remain an essential part of the public health palliative care approach.

Beginning with a presentation on the evolution of the public health message and the unique contribution of the palliative care agencies, the chapter argues that public health palliative care risks losing gains already made if interagency collaboration to seek common goals and objectives is not strengthened. Further, suggesting that a human rights argument in itself is insufficient to ensure political changes, a case will be made that a social justice framework has the potential to achieve greater accountability from those charged with the delivery of a public health palliative care approach. Finally, examples of initiatives and projects which have situated the public health message in the language of social justice—equity, compassion, and care—will be presented.

The evolution of a public health palliative care: a global challenge

The IAHPC provides an excellent resource in terms of the many conventions, treaties, position statements, and civil society initiatives which have been developed over many years to address the need to relieve pain and suffering in the global population (https://hospicecare.com). These include, for example, multilateral treaties on the management of narcotic drugs which have informed the call for essential medicines to alleviate pain and the safe use and distribution of opioids to the same effect. Undoubtedly, there has been a concerted and laudable effort on the part of global palliative care agencies to address the inequities which currently exist and to secure a place for palliative care as a part of health provision for all citizens. Overall, efforts have resulted in some success, appropriately targeted to unmet need, and with a particular focus on LMICs.

Recent publications such as the second edition of the *Global Atlas of Palliative Care* by the WHPCA in partnership with the WHO attest to the significant need for palliative care where despite improvements since the first edition in 2014, only between 12% and 14% of the global population in need receive the service (exponentially higher in LMICs) (WHPCA, 2020). However, it may be insufficient to assume that the challenges faced in LMICs is only due to poverty, deprivation, or poor management and governance of resources. A critical view of the development of palliative care over the last 50 years since St Christopher's hospice first opened might suggest that we still lack a clear vision and definition of what palliative care is, for whom, and when. A range of directives and policies have attempted to address this but a final and concrete outcome seems somewhat elusive and has led to a divergence of opinion along two broad lines: (1) clinicians who wish to assure that palliative care as a medical/clinical discipline is legitimized and seen as an essential component of healthcare provision, and (2) a wider community response (which also includes clinicians) who promote advocacy and lobbying as a model for global equitable access, incorporating national and international social and political movement to achieve this.

There is evident overlap between these two lines of thought but, on balance, it would seem that the current discourse favours the latter socio-political approach to enhance palliative care for all, with a focus towards where palliative care is underdeveloped or even non-existent. However, it would be fair to say that disparate views remain and a space for dialogue is needed to enable a clear vision for the future. Perhaps, also, there is a divide between (1) and (2) in terms of geography; the arguments for palliative care as a recognized specialist practice being more evident in those countries where palliative care integration is more established, in contrast to countries where palliative care development is limited. This is not to say that efforts have focused only on the ill-termed 'third world'.

Some of the 53 countries within the WHO European Region in need of palliative care development have benefitted from the work of agencies such as the EAPC (https://www.eapcnet.eu/) the IAHPC, and the WHPCA (https://www.thewhpca.org/). Open Society Foundations (https://www.opensocietyfoundations.org/) have been particularly influential in establishing leadership programmes to support local and national programmes and change has been effective. However, some aspects of palliative care are under threat, even in countries where palliative care is well established. Recent concerns suggest the UK hospice model seems under threat, partly through challenges of integration within the healthcare systems and separate funding structures, but more recently closure of services due to lack of staff and resources ('End-of-life care is under serious threat', 2019). A need for revision of the hospice models seems necessary for its survival. It is notable that some European developments such as the highly effective WHO palliative care development project in Catalonia, Spain (Ela et al., 2014), argued strongly for an integrated care model with statutory services in contrast to the charitable funding structure associated with the British model and this has been favoured in many European countries with varying degrees of success, depending on the structure of the health system and political will.

Of course, charitable donation features at some point in many international palliative care developments but the experience of the UK model and the challenges it faces are a warning to the wider community. In developing locally responsive services, there is an equal need to provide clear and distinct messages of the added value of palliative care for the healthcare system and avoid risk of further fragmentation. Independence comes at a cost and for the future of palliative care, sustainability and integration are key determinants of success. Embracing a public health approach to palliative care is an important step on this road.

Although projects such as that in Catalonia, previously mentioned (Ela et al., 2014), have consistently argued for public health palliative care and indeed, demonstrated its care and cost benefits, in recent years, this has become more visible, notably with work which has championed the ideal of a global palliative care approach to address 'serious health-related suffering' (Knaul et al., 2018; Sleeman et al., 2019). Of course, this ideal is based on earlier seminal work which challenged the somewhat paternalistic vision of end of life to a health promotion-orientated approach to palliative care, addressing equity of access, delivered in a timely fashion and at the place of choice of the person in need, and challenging the professionalization (or medicalization) of dying (Sallnow et al., 2016).

However, the report in *The Lancet* by Felicia Knaul and colleagues entitled 'The Lancet Commission on Palliative Care and Pain Relief— findings, recommendations, and future directions' (Knaul et al., 2018) appears to have been a catalyst from which much of the current debate on universal health coverage and the need for coherent care packages to address serious health-related suffering stems. An important element of this work is that it blends the need for clinical and, in some cases, disease-specific approaches to care (e.g. through the work of global cancer agencies) with the wider systemic solution-based approach for implementation. Collaboration is clearly key to addressing global unmet need.

Have we achieved a public health approach to palliative care?

Public health palliative care has been described as 'a term that can be used to encompass a variety of approaches that involve working with communities to improve people's experience of death, dying and bereavement' (Archibald et al., 2016, p. 1). The seminal work by Kellehear (1999) into health-promoting palliative care and later, compassionate communities (Kellehear, 2013) championed the idea that a social model of care speaks better to the range of social, cultural, and economic factors which influence the experience of living and dying than predominant disease-orientated models. Certainly, current discourse around palliative and end of life care would fit well with this revised vision of public health.

Dzingina and Higginson (2015) describe the evolution of public health from its older hierarchical, professionally dominated, and 'top-down' model to one which sought to embrace more effective community engagement and social responsibility. This resonates with the shift in palliative care towards the larger health challenges in society including chronic illness, the specific needs of an ageing population, and dementia care, all of which reflect global epidemiological and societal needs. The role of public and patient involvement, which seems critical to this more inclusive and egalitarian approach, is also evidenced in the relation to palliative care, if more notable in research than practice (Johnson et al., 2021). However, although public and patient involvement has developed well in the UK, the concept is new in many other countries and so the idea of service users' voices in the co-creation and evaluation of service provision and engagement has some way to go.

There is a growing body of literature about the need to embrace a public health approach to palliative and end of life care and the specific benefit of universal health coverage as a way to target services to those most in need, in a cost-effective and affordable way, and so alleviate unnecessary suffering. One example by Da Lima and Pastrana (2016) provides a constructive account of the added value of a public health approach to address the reality of death, dying, and inequity. It raises a number of interesting points noted across the literature, not least the evidence of unmet need, need for clear policy and direction, and monitoring systems. What is notable here, as in other policy documents related to public health palliative care, is the need to explain (or re-explain) what palliative care is and does.

Despite the fact that the modern hospice/palliative care movement proposed by Cicely Saunders (1918–2005) and internationally emulated by others is now well established, there seems to a consistent need in the literature to redescribe and reframe what palliative care is. Of course, the fact is that the reach of palliative care globally is inequitable and there is a significant imbalance between those in need and those who benefit from access and care (Knaul et al., 2018), and it remains a concern that clear messaging about the benefit at population level seems elusive. Each reframing of the description risks a distortion in the message or at least a loss of the 'sound-bites' which policy makers need in order to grasp the essentials quickly. This may not just be about messaging but more about how health systems perceive that message when planning and allocating resources, identifying priorities, and the fundamental value they place on palliative and end of life care in the context of their overall health strategy. The more complex the message, the less likely it will be understood and it may be important for the palliative care community to take stock of why this message is so hard to deliver and what methods are needed to frame future dialogue about the discipline. The public health palliative care approach touches on a number of dimensions which need to be incorporated in the messaging and the following brief oversight give a sense of the complexity in understanding the role and function of palliative and end of life care today.

Palliative care as a human right: is it enough?

The idea of palliative care as a human right has been proposed by a number of clinicians in palliative care (Brennan, 2007; Gwyther et al., 2009). Ezer and colleagues (2018) identify how agencies such as Human Rights Watch (http://www.hrw.org) and Open Society Foundations have championed the human rights agenda in palliative and end of life care and how in particular Human Rights Watch reported both the challenges and achievements, though few, to implementation of palliative care and pain relief in different countries. The EAPC 'Lisbon Challenge' (later, the Prague Charter) also called on governments to acknowledge the right to palliative care through policy and action, notably access to essential medication and education and training for clinicians (Radbruch et al., 2013). A more recently published 2018 supplement to the *Journal of Pain and Symptom Management* provided a series of papers edited by Callaway and Foley (2018), including that of Eser and colleagues (2018) offering a concise discussion on the evolution of the public health model and why it was important then and relevant now. The series of papers presented a range of perspectives and concrete international examples of how a public health approach has benefited the development of palliative care. The approach, which also frames the work of the EAPC described previously and the WHO roadmap for palliative care (Callaway et al., 2018; Eser et al., 2018), was based on three distinct principles:

- Palliative care should be considered a public health issue.
- Palliative care is a basic human right.
- Lack of access to pain relief and essential medicines is a form of cruel, inhuman, and degrading treatment.

Despite the fact that various bodies and organizations including the United Nations, through their Sustainable Development Goals programme, and the WHO have regularly called on governments and states to address care for those with palliative and end of life care needs including equitable access to essential medicines (Martin-Moreno et al., 2008; Callaway and Foley, 2018; Callaway et al., 2018; Eser et al., 2018; Maetens et al., 2019), the 2014 World Health Assembly resolution 67.19 is considered a turning point in the call for the integration of palliative care through global health and partnership strategies (World Health Assembly, 2014). The resolution charged the WHO with ensuring the 'strengthening of palliative care as a component of comprehensive health care throughout the life course' (World Health Assembly, 2014, p. 3). Member states were urged to take responsibility for the inclusion of palliative and end of life care in their systems and the Director General was requested to ensure integration and to develop and strengthen evidence-based guidelines. The resolution gave the WHO a right to raise compelling arguments why countries should adopt the strategy and focus efforts towards palliative and end of life care for their population. Citizens had the (human) right to optimal care to ease suffering. Although there is evidence that the resolution was seen as largely positive by stakeholders based on WHPCA global data already cited, the overall impact of the World Health Assembly resolution 67.19 has been minimal to date and there remain a number of gaps and problems still to be addressed (Knaul et al., 2018; Carrasco et al., 2021).

The first problem is that human rights are notoriously difficult to 'police' and as was seen in the response to the World Health Assembly resolution cited by Carrasco and colleagues (2021), a lack of rigorous indicators or processes to monitor implementation meant that some countries did not respond effectively and that opportunities were lost. Clark and co-workers (2019) present an interesting ecology of global palliative care implementation and determine that palliative care is 'lower in countries with high levels of political corruption, infant mortality, deaths by infectious diseases, and weak democracy' (p. 793). One of the risks of imposing palliative care in situations of instability is that it may be seen as a cheaper alternative to expensive and ill-distributed disease-modifying treatments than an integrated package of care (Selwyn, 2008).

Therefore, decisions on whether palliative care is an important component of care are not just not based on a laudable belief in a human right but in the reality of political and economic governance. A question posed, therefore, is whether human rights are enough? An alternative approach which may have greater strength in political terms is to consider palliative and end of life care in terms of social justice. Academics in this field of social science, such as Kathleen Lynch (Lynch et al., 2009), have argued that equality (of access) is based on three components; love, care, and solidarity. In effect, relationships and community have a strong impact on how care is given and received. This also reflects issues of gender and power which equally impact the political sphere of palliative and end of life care, such as the expected role of women as caregivers and the neoliberal, bureaucratic (or indeed corrupt) nature of healthcare delivery, highlighted by Clark and colleagues (2019). Lynch argues that a social justice framework is a more tangible model on which care and political response to inequity can be judged. This does not mean that human rights are not important. The work of Human Rights Watch would indicate its essential value to equity but may imply that in a new and divergent field such as palliative and end of life care, a more structured approach which can be measured and monitored is needed to support the human rights discourse to make any long-lasting significant change and impact.

Palliative care: evolving definitions and lost opportunities

Perhaps a further challenge that has been an evident thorn in the side of palliative care development is a lack of consensus on definition. The original definition proposed by the WHO in 1990 clearly focused on a specialist medical practice relative to trajectory of disease, pain and symptom control, and a focus towards end of life care at a time when active or curative care was no longer possible but including death, dying, and bereavement (WHO, 1990). Although this was the *sine qua non* for palliative care practitioners for many years, criticism of its overt cancer-orientated focus and limited relevance to changing demographics of ageing and chronic disease led to a shift in definition in 2002, emphasizing that palliative care was an approach to care which could be delivered across a range of settings in which people experience palliative and end of life care, including the possibility of early intervention. The suggestion that it was as an approach to, rather than specialist care was not well received by some countries where efforts had focused on recognizing palliative medicine as a specialist practice including university-based education at undergraduate and postgraduate level. The early days of the revised definition led to disquiet and a perceived risk of dilution of the message of palliative care for patients and families and its added value to care.

In 2021, the debate on definition remains unresolved. Reflecting the social justice approach to equity noted earlier and the fact that previous definitions did not seem to account for the social determinants of health including social networks, gender, and culture, there has been a more recent call for a further revision of definition which moves away from reductionist disease-centred frameworks to an advocacy model which encourages normalization of palliative care within healthcare systems to address health-related suffering. The IAHPC has focused particular attention towards the need for political engagement and effective communication if true integration of palliative care is to be achieved. The call for this definition to replace the current WHO definition has gained traction, not least because it addresses some 'real-world' truths about caring for people at the end of life. One example is the acknowledgement that patients and families are partners in care, rather than just recipients of care. A second is that most people in need of palliative care, particularly in LMICs, are unlikely to receive specialist palliative care but can benefit from generalist support. Further, palliative and end of life care can be given with minimal training. However, most important is the reference to wider social determinants that impact the experience of dying, including access to essential medications, the need for legislation and policy to ensure the right to access, and financial recognition by insurance systems.

It would seem that this third definition has greatest resonance with the aims and objectives of the public health approach to palliative care. It offers a thoughtful and reflective position which takes the important elements of previous definitions and tries to situate them within a more globally responsive and realistic focus for best practice. Yet, the 2002 definition remains in force despite compelling arguments to the contrary. Perhaps one reason for this is the predominance of the biomedical model of health which places less value on the social determinants of health. Further, the current positioning and somewhat diverse vision and scope of the three key global organizations (EAPC, IAHPC, and WHPCA) may have inadvertently obscured the opportunity to harness the momentum of the World Health Assembly resolution 67.19 together. There are clear reasons why each developed their specific mandate but for the future, it may be that a common voice and vision may service palliative and end of life better.

Whereas the WHPCA and IAHPC focus on global palliative and end of life issues and its concomitant challenges, the EAPC, as an non-governmental organization of the Council of Europe, has a mandate to the European region, working through member organizations and providing a platform for those working in the field. With a strong clinician base, their work has been instrumental in improving palliative and end of life care through practice education and research across the EU which is itself complex in its definition and scope. In contrast, the WHPCA proposes a global commitment based on the principle of universal health coverage, empowering national associations to strengthen their mission, and advocates at a global level for policy change. The IAHPC has its origins in the US and the International Hospice Institute and the American Academy for Hospice and Palliative Medicine. Advocacy and leadership are key elements of its approach, highlighting specifically the issue of serious health-related suffering in its vision.

Evidently, each organization needs to focus on its own mandate to ensure it meets the expectations of its members and subscribers. There is some evidence of collaboration across certain aspects (e.g. IAHPC grants to attend EAPC congresses, a link between the EAPC and the WHPCA through the work of the EAPC director across both groups, and a past president of the EAPC is currently president of the IAHPC). There has been change and it is notable that the contemporary language expressed across all three key players reflects political and advocacy strategies to ensure that palliative and end of life care is placed on the strategic health agenda of governments and agencies. Sadly, however, the lack of consensus on definition is troubling and there is an urgent need for greater and more formal engagement between the organizations to address this and other critical issues to strengthen the cohesive message for change.

The public health palliative care agenda: key messages for the global community

Other groups beyond the individual organizations noted here have strongly influenced the political global landscape of palliative and end of life care and/or contributed to their vision in supporting international initiatives. One example, the Pain & Policies Studies Group, has reported its influence on access and regulation of opioids, key to the delivery of optimal pain management, over a 20-year period (Cleary and Maurer, 2018). Through national and international collaborations, this group makes particular reference to a public health approach through balancing access and availability of pain relief medication, notably opioids, with measures to avoid exploitation and abuse. An international pain policy fellowship has been developed across a number of LMICs where local healthcare professionals with leadership potential to act as change agents at national level were identified to promote the use of and legislation for opiate use. Evaluation of this initiative demonstrates a positive outcome in terms of opioid consumption; increased evidence of national strategies, education, and training; and distribution and monitoring. Early fellows have become mentors to others as the programme has expanded. As such, the work of the Pain & Policies Studies Group provides a strong example of success in establishing a public health approach to address serious health-related suffering. However, it also demonstrates the complexity of initiatives needed to assure a cohesive and successful outcome. This needs infrastructure and resources and, moreover, partnerships. The Pain & Policies Studies Group, demonstrate how academic, clinical, and social agencies can come together to effect change.

Given the fact that palliative care applies across the age spectrum and is not only associated with an elderly frail population, the needs of children warrant mention here. An important part of the policy development that has taken place to date regards the situation of children with palliative care needs. Although the number of children requiring palliative care is clearly less than adults, approximately 7% of the global population or up to 21 million children worldwide (Knaul et al., 2018; Marston et al., 2018), the range of chronic, life-limiting, and rare disease encompassed in children's palliative care brings its own complexity in terms of identification of need and establishment of appropriate service provision. The International Children's Palliative Care Network (ICPCN), founded in 2005, has championed the unique needs of children with life-limiting illness as distinct from the adult population (https://www.icpcn.org/). Through a range of policy statements and position papers as well as partnerships with the other agencies, the ICPCN works at a global level to bring paediatric palliative care practitioners, service providers, and organizations together under an umbrella of advocacy, strengthened evidence base to inform best practice, and networking. In effect, it situates itself as a global leader to bring the diverse groups involved in children's palliative care together and do so through the adoption of the public health approaches advocated by other agencies: communication, advocacy, research, education, and strategic development at local and national levels (presented through the acronym CARES). The fact that global agencies have included children's palliative care in establishing data regarding demographic estimation of need (Knaul et al., 2018) is important and inclusion of children's palliative care as an optional track in EAPC congresses demonstrates a commitment to advancing care for children and families through research and education.

These initiatives are important to ensure that the wider benefit of palliative and end of life care for children and families is secured and dialogue between the key agencies is essential to assure responsive messages to policy makers so that the discussion is about all citizens, not just adults or children. The ICPCN strategic plan 2019–2023 make a number of points which are of equal importance to all. The first is that advocacy does not just evolve. It needs training and so initiatives to promote training opportunities for practitioners to incorporate advocacy as a core element of practice are important. There is a case that advocacy is so important in the public health agenda that it warrants specific personnel with this skill set. This is the case for the IAHPC who has an appointed advocacy officer. Certainly, having such expertise has enabled the voice of palliative and end of life care to be heard at the appropriate political tables and by those who influence our global healthcare agenda. However, there has also been a long-term global message that palliative and end of life care is everyone's business and if so, advocacy is one tool which has the potential to effectively strengthen that message. At the very least, the inclusion of advocacy as a part of undergraduate and postgraduate palliative and end of life care curricula development may help establish how change can be fostered from a 'bottom-up' rather than 'top-down' approach.

Therefore, a second element is education. The WHO public health model (Stjernswärd et al., 2007) indicates the value of education as part of its tripartite strategy for public health and this has figured largely in palliative and end of life care initiatives to develop better understanding of its benefits to the wider healthcare community. Evidence demonstrates how education in palliative and end of life care is supported by partnerships between clinical and academic providers. This attests to the need to provide curricula or at least call for the inclusion of palliative and end of life care in existing curricula as part of the dissemination of knowledge to equip practitioners to provide effective clinical care. To some extent, the education agenda has flagged the 'specialist–generalist' debate. The proposed revision of definition promoted by the IAHPC (Radbruch et al., 2020) notes that palliative care can be delivered with 'basic palliative care training'. Many excellent education initiatives such as those provided by the African Palliative Care Association (https://www.africanpalliativecare.org) demonstrate how the principles of palliative and end of life care can be embedded into clinical care, even with scarce resources and limited funding. Further, the 'professionalization of dying' (Kellehear, 1999) is challenged when communities can demonstrate how they can come together to provide the best care possible even in adverse and challenging circumstances. Of course, at different levels of integration, needs change and so there are equal calls to enhance the scope of education to include professorial appointments which can offer leadership and direction to embed the palliative and end of life care message in undergraduate and postgraduate curricula (Paal et al., 2019). Actually, both general and specialist education are essential for sustainability and future workforce planning.

The third element, but perhaps the most important is communication. Given the diversity which exists in terms of the definition of palliative and end of life care, it would seem that there is an urgent need to condense and coalesce the message for the wider community. The use of technology and digital platforms to extend the reach of messaging is critical and indeed, the coronavirus pandemic has demonstrated how effective this can be. The potential to develop online methods for communication strategies needs further structure and investment. Again, in as much as advocacy warrants expertise not usually found with the clinical service provider cohort, communication needs experts to guide and shape the language of palliative and end of life care to ensure succinct delivery and avoid confusion in word and deed. The debate around assisted suicide and euthanasia offers one example where language used to describe key elements of the palliative care approach, such as dignity, have been appropriated to describe different approaches to life's end. This is a separate debate beyond the scope of this chapter but the need to be able to provide clear descriptions of what palliative care is and what purpose it serves (as well as whom it serves) is vital for the future of the discipline.

Public health palliative care: when it works well

An exhaustive discussion on the many positive achievements that the public health palliative care approach has engendered is not possible. However, some 'seminal' projects speak to the elements which make up this approach and address many of the points raised so far: community engagement, equity and rights, and sustainability. Among many examples are those reported by Callaway and Foley (2018) with reports from central and eastern Europe as well as more global studies such as those in Rwanda, South Africa, Vietnam, and Mongolia. All clearly espouse the public health palliative care message with varying levels of success. Special mention of the work of *Casa Sperantei* in Romania led by Professor Daniela Mosiou is warranted, having developed a national network of palliative care clinical and educational opportunities supported by Open Society Foundations and the World Bank (Mosoiu et al., 2018). Their work has demonstrated the transformative potential of palliative care to a resource-limited health service to improve standards of care and do so with a model of cost efficiency. Two further examples proposed here from India and Colombia demonstrate the potential that a public health palliative care approach can bring to the widest dimension of the population and make the case how public health palliative care must be underpinned by the desire to strengthen social justice measures to empower communities who may be considered vulnerable.

The Kerala project: 20 years of experience in Malappuram

The development of palliative care services in Kerala, India, is one of the most visible examples of how palliative and end of life care can address the needs of a community even in a situation of poor resources. The vision of Dr Suresh Kumar and the Pain and Palliative Care Society that existing medical structures could not meet the needs of the population who would warrant palliative and end of life care, led to the establishment of the Neighbourhood Network of Palliative Care, a clinician and volunteer-based service reaching up to 2500 people a week and making palliative care accessible and affordable. The strong focus on local community volunteerism to support the limited statutory structures shifted the delivery of palliative and end of life care from a medical to a social model which values community and sees them as a resource and support network reflecting the reality of limited access to services and treatment for the majority of the population. Perhaps its success has been due to a cascade approach, whereby the district was divided into smaller units serving a limited number of 50–60 patients. The role of the volunteer, gathered across the social spectrum, was critical in terms of empowering families to develop skills for self-sufficiency and economic sustainability, while acting as a conduit with the medical and nursing services trained to provide good pain and symptom management.

Equally notable to its success was the ability to engage with local politicians and the media to spread the message and establish a change process in terms of healthcare planning, thinking, and action. Early description of the model has demonstrated its benefit and value and its potential translation across other health systems, latterly in Thailand and Sri Lanka through its social entrepreneurial focus (https://www.ashoka.org). A review published in 2018 (Philip et al., 2018) provides evidence of the benefit of this community home-based approach to palliative and end of life care, noting how the demographics of the population served had changed over the 20 years since inception and now included far fewer cancer patients and far greater numbers of patients with chronic life-limiting illness for which diversity in skills and competences would be needed to match the changing dynamics of the epidemiology of death and dying.

However, the success in Kerala has not been transplanted well to other parts of India and a number of suggestions why this should be so have included the strong social and public education models, coupled with higher than average rates of literacy in the population when compared to India as a whole. Nevertheless, the potential reach of this model, supported by its strong community engagement and public health message, offers one example of how palliative care can be transformed to better meet the needs of the population it serves.

New Health Foundation and *Todos Contigo* ('All with you'): Colombia, South America

Originally developed in Seville, Spain, under the direction of Dr Emilio Herrera-Molina, the New Health Foundation placed community at the centre of their initiative to mobilize local resources and optimize health and social care services to provide compassionate palliative and end of life care. A number of centres developed in Spain. The model comprises three elements: the need to address the cost of end of life care, to bring key players such as policy makers and clinicians to the same table as the public for the co-creation of appropriate initiatives, and to tap into the wider resources in society who would wish to contribute to societal improvements including care at the end of life. The goal of the Foundation is to develop flexible, responsive, and synergistic interventions which can adapt to the changing dynamic of needs in healthcare (https://www.newhealthfoundation.org/).

Todos Contigo (Spanish for 'All with you') is one example of a community-orientated project to enhance end of life care. Utilizing the compassionate communities experience, a range of tools and resources are made available to local communities to establish priorities, develop plans, structures, and networks for sustainability, as well as develop quality mechanisms for evaluation. Relocating to Colombia, South America, in 2015, the project has been able to develop a national palliative care programme and, through engagement with Colombian healthcare insurers, understand the healthcare of the community better (in terms of the profile of illnesses which are most likely to lead to the need for end of life care) and so provide cost-effective and sustainable models of care. *Todos Contigo* also harnesses the benefit of the volunteer approach noted earlier in the Kerala model, bringing a range of national community structures (schools, businesses, universities, etc.) to develop their vision of a *compassionate country* through a network of compassionate cities, linked through consensus recorded in their Declaration of Medellin (https://www.newhealthfoundation.org).

The approach of *Todos Contigo*, in tandem with most other community initiatives, would argue that palliative and end of life care can only be supported if the current paternalistic and overburdened system is challenged and that the focus shifts from curing to healing—a message espoused by Cicely Saunders and other in the early days of palliative care. This is a critical message for the future of public health palliative care. Perhaps, rather than starting a revolution, we are building on the foundations already laid and as suggested by T. S. Eliot in 'Little Giddings':

> And the end of all our exploring
> Will be to arrive where we started
> And know the place for the first time.
>
> (Eliot, 1942)

Conclusion

Palliative and end of life care are now part of the landscape of global healthcare, albeit with varying dimensions and opportunities. Progress has been made but sustainability lies in the hands of the leaders and champions who believe strongly in its aims and vision for a just and equitable society where people can live and die, free from pain and suffering. The next steps are both ambitious and challenging but as is proposed in this chapter, the failure to seek common ground and a shared language will inhibit the potential to transform. Steps have been taken and the palliative care community needs to support its leaders in progressing these tentative steps for the good of all citizens. At its inception, hospice and palliative care was a radical step change and its pioneers took risks to establish something in which they wholeheartedly believed. Today's visionaries should adopt that spirit to ensure we do not lose sight of our mission and vision—palliative care for all.

REFERENCES

Archibald, D., Patterson, R., Haraldsdottir, E., Hazelwood, M., Fife, S., and Murray, S. A. 2016. Mapping the progress and impacts of public health approaches to palliative care: a scoping review protocol. *BMJ Open*, **6**, e012058.

Arias, N., Garralda, E., De Lima, L., Rhee, J. Y., and Centeno, C. 2019. Global palliative care and cross-national comparison: how is palliative care development assessed? *Journal of Palliative Medicine*, **22**, 580–590.

Brennan, F. 2007. Palliative care as an international human right. *Journal of Pain and Symptom Management*, **33**, 494–499.

Callaway, M. V., Connor, S. R., and Foley, K. M. 2018. World Health Organization public health model: a roadmap for palliative care development. *Journal of Pain and Symptom Management*, **55**, S6–S13.

Callaway, M. V. and Foley, K. M. 2018. The International Palliative Care Initiative. *Journal of Pain and Symptom Management*, **55**, S1–S5.

Carrasco, J. M., Inbadas, H., Whitelaw, A., and Clark, D. 2021. Early Impact of the 2014 World Health Assembly Resolution on Palliative Care: a qualitative study using semistructured interviews with key experts. *Journal of Palliative Medicine*, **24**, 103–106.

Clark, D., Baur, N., Clelland, D., Garralda, E., López-Fidalgo, J., Connor, S., et al. 2020. Mapping levels of palliative care development in 198 countries: the situation in 2017. *Journal of Pain and Symptom Management*, **59**, 794–807.

Clark, J., Barnes, A., Campbell, M., and Gardiner, C. 2019. A life or 'good death' situation? A worldwide ecological study of the national contexts of countries that have and have not implemented palliative care. *Journal of Pain and Symptom Management*, **57**, 793–801.

Cleary, J. F. and Maurer, M. A. 2018. Pain and Policy Studies Group: two decades of working to address regulatory barriers to improve opioid availability and accessibility around the world. *Journal of Pain and Symptom Management*, **55**, S121–S134.

De Lima, L. and Pastrana, T. 2016. Opportunities for palliative care in public health. *Annual Review of Public Health*, **37**, 357–374.

Dzingina, M. D. and Higginson, I. J. 2015. Public health and palliative care in 2015. *Clinics in Geriatric Medicine*, **31**, 253–263.

Ela, S., Espinosa, J., Martinez-Munoz, M., Lasmarias, C., Beas, E., Mateo-Ortega, D., et al. 2014. The WHO Collaborating Centre for Public Health palliative care programs: an innovative approach of palliative care development. *Journal of Palliative Medicine*, **17**, 385–392.

Eliot, T. S. 1942. *Little Gidding*. London: Faber and Faber.

End-of-life care is under serious threat. [Letters] *The Guardian*, 16 September 2019. Available at: https://www.theguardian.com/society/2019/sep/16/end-of-life-care-is-under-serious-threat

Ezer, T., Lohman, D., and de Luca, G. B. 2018. Palliative care and human rights: a decade of evolution in standards. *Journal of Pain and Symptom Management*, **55**, S163–S169.

Gwyther, L., Brennan, F., and Harding, R. 2009. Advancing palliative care as a human right. *Journal of Pain and Symptom Management*, **38**, 767–774.

Johnson, H., Ogden, M., Brighton, L. J., Etkind, S. N., Oluyase, A. O., Chukwusa, E., et al. 2021. Patient and public involvement in palliative care research: what works, and why? A qualitative evaluation. *Palliative Medicine*, **35**, 151–160.

Kellehear, A. 1999. *Health Promoting Palliative Care*. Melbourne: Oxford University Press.

Kellehear, A. 2013. Compassionate communities: end-of-life care as everyone's responsibility. *Quarterly Journal of Medicine*, **106**, 1071–1075.

Knaul, F. M., Farmer, P. E., Krakauer, E. L., De Lima, L., Bhadelia, A., Jiang Kwete, X., et al. 2018 Alleviating the access abyss in palliative care and pain relief—an imperative of universal health coverage: the Lancet Commission report. *Lancet*, **391**, 1391–1454.

Lynch, K., Baker, J., Lyons, M., Feeley, M., Hanlon, N., O'Brien, M., et al. 2009. *Affective Equality: Love, Care and Injustice*. London: Palgrave.

Lynch, T., Connor, S., and Clark, D. 2013. Mapping levels of palliative care development: a global update. *Journal of Pain and Symptom Management*, **45**, 1094–1106.

Maetens, A., Cohen, J., and Harding, R. A. 2019. Public health approach to integrate palliative care into a country's health-care system: guidance as provided by the WHO. In: MacLeod, R. and Van den Block, L. (eds.) *Textbook of Palliative Care*, pp. 1–20. Cham: Springer.

Marston, J., Boucher, S., and Downing, J. 2018. International Children's Palliative Care Network: a global action network for children with life-limiting conditions. *Journal of Pain and Symptom Management*, **55**, S104–S111.

Martin-Moreno, J. M., Harris, M., Gorgojo, L., Clark, D., Normand, C., and Centeno, C. 2008. *Palliative Care in the European Union* (Report number IP/A/ENVI/IC/2007-123). Brussels: European Parliament, Economic and Scientific Policy Department.

Mosoiu, D., Mitrea, N., and Dumitrescu, M. 2018. Palliative care in Romania. *Journal of Pain and Symptom Management*, **55**, S67–S76.

Paal, P., Brandstötter, C., Lorenzl, S., Larkin, P., and Elsner, F. 2019. Postgraduate palliative care education for all healthcare providers in Europe: results from an EAPC survey. *Palliative & Supportive Care*, **17**, 495–506.

Philip, R. R., Philip, S., Tripathy, J. P., Manima, A., and Venables, E. 2018. Twenty years of home-based palliative care in Malappuram, Kerala, India: a descriptive study of patients and their care-givers. *BMC Palliative Care*, **17**, 26.

Radbruch, L., De Lima, L., Knaul, F., Wenk, R., Ali, Z., Bhatnaghar, S., et al. 2020. Redefining palliative care—a new consensus-based definition. *Journal of Pain and Symptom Management*, **60**, 754–764.

Radbruch, L., Payne, S., de Lima, L., and Lohmann, D. 2013. The Lisbon Challenge: acknowledging palliative care as a human right. *Journal of Palliative Medicine*, **16**, 301–304.

Sallnow, L., Richardson, H., Murray, S. A., and Kellehear, A. 2016. The impact of a new public health approach to end of life care: a systematic review. *Palliative Medicine*, **30**, 200–211.

Selwyn, P. A. 2008. Palliative care and social justice. *Journal of Pain and Symptom Management*, **36**, 513–515.

Sleeman, K. E., de Brito, M., Etkind, S., Nkhoma, K., Guo, P., Higginson, I. J., et al. 2019. The escalating global burden of serious health-related suffering: projections to 2060 by world regions, age groups, and health conditions. *Lancet Global Health*, **7**, e883–e892.

Stjernswärd, J., Foley, K. M., and Ferris, F. D. 2007. Integrating palliative care into national policies. *Journal of Pain and Symptom Management*, **33**, 514–520.

WHO Expert Committee on Cancer Pain Relief and Active Supportive Care and World Health Organization. 1990 . Cancer pain relief and palliative care: report of a WHO expert committee [meeting held in Geneva from 3 to 10 July 1989]. World Health Organization. [Online] Available at: https://apps.who.int/iris/handle/10665/39524

World Health Assembly. 2014. Strengthening of palliative care as a component of integrated treatment within the continuum of care. Paper presented at World Health Assembly 134th session. [Online] Available at: https://apps.who.int/iris/handle/10665/173012

Worldwide Hospice Palliative Care Alliance. 2020. *Global Atlas of Palliative Care*, 2nd ed. London: Worldwide Hospice Palliative Care Alliance. Available at: http://www.thewhpca.org/resources/global-atlas-on-end-of-life-care

3

The social nature of dying and the social model of health

Allan Kellehear

Introduction

People outside of healthcare circles often think of dying as the slow or sudden destruction of a physical life. Someone dies in a car accident or is found overdosed at home and is unable to be revived. Alternatively, someone we know has lived with cancer for a few months or years but succumbs when all treatments have failed and they 'finally' die from a 'bleed' or their heart stops. Inside healthcare circles the problem of dying is a failed resuscitation attempt or a death in the night at a care home or hospital. In palliative care we think of dying as a potentially longer matter, and healthcare staff there support a longer experience of dying with home care services, outpatient admissions, and inpatient care.

In all these examples we see 'dying' as a physical trouble with a patient's destiny in full sight even if we don't know when this might occur. In the modern world, 'dying' must have a 'medical label' to even be viewed as 'dying'. The mere process of advanced ageing is not usually seen as 'dying'. The expressed desire to kill oneself is not viewed as 'dying'. Being chronically ill with a life-threatening disease is not viewed as 'dying'. The designation of 'dying' and the mobilization of health services for its care only happens when we have a medical understanding of imminent threat. In this way, both popular and healthcare understandings of dying are inexorably tied to physical ideas of entropy and collapse.

Although the physicality of ideas about death is not new, the idea of the time before death as a mainly physical journey towards it is new and recent. The institutional and symptom science priorities privileged by palliative care have reinforced this view of dying as a physical journey notwithstanding philosophies that have attempted to balance this model of care with psychological, spiritual, and psychosocial approaches. In the end, what we place at the core of our work shapes that work. It is important to understand that this common view about the primacy of physicality at the end of life is not true.

Moving away from dominant notions about physical mortality, my aim will be to show that dying is fundamentally a social experience for those who live through it. I will argue that the social facts about dying necessitate a social model for its care. If one accepts that dying is a social experience with a physical dimension and not a physical experience with a social dimension then a reorientation of practice, research, and curriculum priorities should follow. In the service of this argument, I will first describe how dying in the human sciences has been and continues to be a diverse and contested set of ideas. I will then summarize elements of social experience that characterize most of the competing views and then introduce the 95% rule. This rule demonstrates that most of a dying person's time is a social time with clinical encounters merely occupying the ever-diminishing 5%. The next sections will describe the social model of health. I will show how this approach directly complements the care of dying by targeting the 95% rule while addressing both social determinants of health and common healthcare goals. Finally, I will focus on the public health movement in palliative care taking care to introduce the core elements that qualify it as the quintessential social model of health that places 'well-being' at the heart of what it does.

Shifting and contested understandings about dying

The study of dying conduct and experiences is very much a post-1945 endeavour although exceptions may be found in the work of earlier anthropologists such as Sir James Frazer, Bronislaw Malinowski, Arnold van Gennep, and others. Since that time, the modest field concerning itself with the time before death, the imminent confrontation with mortality, has been largely dominated by social, behavioural, and medical sciences. Unsurprisingly, when different fields study the same topic they tend to see different things, This result is what is commonly called 'epistemology'—each field draws different conclusions because their own assumptions and criteria for what counts as real or important knowledge are different. Notwithstanding this underlying cause for the different perspectives, a review of the major ones helps us understand why each of us holds the view we do and the limitations of that view in relation to alternative ones. Contextualizing our understanding in this way also helps us understand how arriving at our own view is not derived by us as a mere 'natural' or self-evident set of observations. Our views are themselves a social construction heavily shaped by the prevailing academic and professional views of the day.

Most of the different views about dying can be summarized into seven broad perspectives. (There are copious volumes of studies in each area but I cite only three or so early landmark references as illustration for these perspectives.) These theories promote and emphasize a view of dying principally as an expression of (1) agency, (2) linearity, (3) fluctuation, (4) disengagement, (5) disintegration, (6) indeterminacy, or (7) transcendence (see Kellehear, 2009).

Dying as agency

The idea that people die in control as best as they are able was first described in historical and sociological studies of suicide (Durkheim, 1952; Alvarez, 1970). People choose the time and the place of their death after determining their reasons to withdraw from life. The idea that these reasons are mostly determined by depressive mood is an ahistorical and ethnocentric one as many people choose suicide for nationalist, religious, or culture-specific reasons, most of which display altruism and clarity of thought and purpose. This idea of agency—of self-control—is also an abiding theme within both historical and anthropological observations upon the 'good death' (see McManners, 1985; Jalland, 1996; Houlbrooke, 1998). The good death was an idea about an ideal style of dying that entailed having some warning before death came so that one is able to prepare—to bid farewells, redistribute personal goods and assets, and to make preparations for the afterlife. A product of agrarian societies, it is also largely an artefact of the middle classes who were among the first to gain a longer life expectancy, wealth, and increasing sentimentality in their intimate relationships. This understanding of dying is very economically determined.

Dying as linearity

A favoured view from sociologists and anthropologists is one that portrays dying as a journey (see Van Gennep, 1969; Glaser and Strauss, 1971). Dying begins at point A and ends at point B. Dying may begin at the point of diagnosis (or prognosis) and end with the event of death itself. Dying is what happens between the end of 'normal' life (marked by a diagnosis/prognosis) and the actual death. This is often described as a period of liminality by anthropologists. This view has given rise to a number of stage theories not solely about grief but also about dying. In stage theories, it is assumed that people display particular types of emotion or behaviour initially, in the middle, and then towards the end of the period of transition. The limitation of this view of dying is that it mainly applies to slow forms of dying. Furthermore, staging creates an artificial appearance of what is normal, inadvertently creating ideas of 'deviance' and 'abnormality' in its wake. This can result in stereotypes and expectations about the 'right' way to die.

Dying as fluctuation

Dying as an uncertain and fluctuating experience is often described by gerontologists. This view of dying often draws from studies of the elderly, especially the elderly in care homes (Giacalone, 2001; Lunney et al., 2003; Sidell and Komaromy, 2003). Dying in these settings is characterized by times of health and then illness, followed by more times of health followed by other times of ill health. As each episode of illness is experienced, the return to the next phase of health is not quite as strong as the previous plateau of health. There is a steady decline but this decline has an oscillating pattern right up to the last weeks of life. The limitation of this view is that it is confined to some forms of illness and ageing and ignores the common event of sudden death, direct forms of decline, and forms of dying that have no illness associated with them. It also glosses over the problem of how such cycles of wellness and illness create and reinforce a person's perception of chronic illness and not dying in the population who experience this style of 'dying'. In other words, this description of dying strongly favours the caregiver view and not the view of the person at the centre of the experience being described.

Dying as disengagement

Favoured by sociologists, psychologists, and gerontologists, some observers believe that all dying is an experience of withdrawal (see Cumming and Henry, 1961; Kalish, 1968; Fulton, 1977). Either in suicide, ageing, or in cancer, at some point even if it is only in the last hours, dying is characterized by a withdrawal from others. This view has prompted a debate about whether this characteristic is one 'feature' or a 'whole style' of dying. It has also prompted debate about whether we are observing a withdrawal based on physical decline, a personal choice, or in fact merely a personal reaction to social withdrawal by others (Scoggins, 1971; Hochschild, 1975). The limitation of this view is that it does not address the experiences of sudden or rapid dying in accidents, disasters, wars, or catastrophic illnesses. It is also a view of dying heavily drawn and evidenced in the period close to death and not to the longer period of living with dying.

Dying as disintegration

This is the most popular theory of dying and one favoured by biologists and medical researchers. Here, dying is viewed as the slow or quick collapse of the body. The body is likened to a machine (Nuland, 1993; Lawton, 2000; Armstrong-Costa, 2004). A part or several parts of the machine break down from any number of causes. If the sequence of breakdown is unable to be arrested (through therapeutic interventions), this process of decline will inevitably lead to a catastrophic sequence of mechanical events that will eventually lead to the final collapse and extinction of conscious life. The major limitation with this view is that it mainly reflects an observer's view and not an insider's view of the experience of dying. Dying is viewed here as separate from the matter of identity. You are 'dying' when we say you are dying, not when you say you are dying. In so-called qualitative studies of this style of dying, a lack of longitudinal data and a concentration on late dying experiences and clinical sites have exaggerated physical dimensions of personal experience. The identity and experience of dying may or may not be accompanied by disintegration. For example, people may disintegrate (from a medically observed view) but not perceive themselves to be dying at all (e.g. chronic illness, survivorship identities, deniers) or they may perceive themselves to be dying but be in perfect health (e.g. death row or death camp inmates, passengers on a doomed plane or ship, premeditated suicides). This is a view of dying that privileges the onlooker or professional experience. It is an idea about dying that severs the link with personal experience or assumes it must be identical—what you see must be what they feel.

Dying as indeterminacy

These theories of dying tend to be advocated by political science and social theory observers. These theories point out a style of dying that has no obvious destination or certainty to its character (see Agamben, 1998; Noys, 2005; Kellehear, 2007). The most common examples are life in nursing homes and death camps. Nursing homes are not considered hospices despite their high death rates and despite the fact that any assessment of life expectancy must be short. Although death is imminent, that is not the reason for admission—self-admission or involuntary admission. Life becomes contingent but is this 'dying'? How much of modern dying is like this—unrecognized? The limitation of this view of dying is an over-identification of the experience of dying with circumstance and not to life stage. Furthermore, although circumstance may predict public conduct, that conduct does not define the limitation of awareness. An identity of dying may be like many other roles and experiences in life—episodic, context dependent, and hidden. Dying in these kinds of circumstances may be indeterminate but that does not mean it does not exist—its existence/awareness may merely be episodic.

Dying as transcendence

The tendency of most other theories of dying to favour both a problem-based and onlooker view of this experience has also meant that the idea of dying has rarely progressed to include positive experiences. From small groups of medical and psychological studies from intensive care, palliative care, and resuscitation medicine come observations of dying as positive transformation (see Moody, 1975; Sabom, 1982; Holden et al., 2009). This behaviour can be observed from the moment a prognosis is made and may also include post-resuscitative and deathbed visions. Patients in these circumstances may commonly report greater intimacy and love in their immediate relationships, reminiscence and meaning making, courage against fear, and positive mystical experiences not well explained by hallucination theories. The limitation of these theories is their minimizing of the experiences of suffering and loss and the lack of prevalence information that would tell us how typical these experiences are. Many of the studies of deathbed visions and near-death experiences, for example, are also observations drawn from late parts of the dying experience and not the earlier parts. Many of the mystical elements are also stereotypically associated with 'dying' but their prevalence and distribution in non-dying examples of human behaviour—shamanism, bereavement, disasters, or meditation experiences—are unexplained. This point raises a broader question about the different theories about dying: how many of these features or types of dying are really specific to dying and may these instead be characteristics of any experience which features personal rupture and social reorientation?

Common elements in theories about dying

What are the central messages within these theories of dying? First, all the major theories of dying emphasize its social nature—the control people exercise at the end of life; how the time between realization of impending death, and death itself, is a time of change; how that time may be characterized by suffering and decline but that this may not be a simple steady descent into death but an irregular back-and-forth process; how dying can be a process of personal withdrawal from other people because of the severity of illness, the need to be alone, or as a reaction to stigma or rejection; how dying can often produce physical incapacity and suffering but not always and indeed frequently not; and finally how, despite all the suffering and all the diverse personal reactions and circumstances people can exhibit, dying is often transformative and positive at different stages of the trajectory of dying and this includes right up to the last minutes of life itself. Finally, perhaps most crucially, the physical element of dying cannot always convince its bearer of its journey any more than health can guarantee self-protection against the will to die. In the end, even when the identity has accepted imminent death through a series of physical prompts and reminders the overriding experience of dying is characteristically and overwhelmingly social in its nature.

We see common elements between and behind all these seven elements—the inexorable link between personal reaction and the social world of the dying; the power struggle between (1) those who observe and care for dying and (2) the personal experience of dying as experienced by the dying themselves. We see how traditional human science views of dying consistently privilege social action, social behaviour, and social experience over descriptions of physical collapse and suffering. Indeed, some theories, such as those from political sciences and social theory, lament the emphasis on physicality in descriptions of dying at all because these obscure other forms of dying and therefore other insights into the confrontation with mortality.

Eclipsed from medical view and insight are the conscious dying experiences of those who are not ill and not commonly found in clinical sites—the suicides and murders, the inmates of death row and death camps, those with short life expectancies in the minutes or hours on doomed flights, ships, or buildings, and those who go to war and don't return, and those who experience sudden death on the streets or in surgery but do return to speak of their experiences. Though we may not meet most of these in palliative care, the insights we learn from these other experiences of dying must be included in our learning if we are to truly understand the full range and determinants of the human confrontation with death.

Furthermore, although few dismiss the physical nature of dying—from any source—most agree that it is the personal and social reactions towards the prospect of death that are the major determinants of the experience. This is the key underlying reason why some people are terminally incapacitated but don't view themselves as 'dying' and other people are in good health but know they are about to die. The shift in identity and experience is the core element in our study and care of the dying. The physical experience of dying is a necessary but not sufficient condition to create 'the experience of dying'. However, the social experience of dying is both a necessary and sufficient condition to create the physical experience of dying. This principle underlines the social nature of dying.

When we cross-compare all these different perspectives about the human confrontation with death we are able to draw three key insights. First, that positive experiences occur just as commonly alongside negative ones. To make that assessment we must take the long view of living with dying that frequently is the larger part of dying outside of healthcare institutions. In this context, I am not merely referring to non-illness forms of dying but also illness forms of dying outside of episodes of direct professional care—those hours, days, weeks, or years when no healthcare professional is around in the daily life of the dying person.

Secondly, the physical constraints of suffering do not mainly determine the behavioural or emotional outcomes. It is the reactions to catastrophic news or suffering that are key to the sequence of behaviour and emotion we see associated with 'dying conduct'—whether this is news derived from a poor prognosis or engine failure on a transatlantic flight. And personal identity and reaction in its turn is shaped and determined largely by the social supports one has at the time and then subsequently in the journey towards expected death (Kellehear, 2014).

Finally, although the total experience of dying enjoys a certain overlapping 'reality' from those who experience it first hand and those who experience it vicariously as carers and onlookers, those experiences are not identical in crucial ways. The dying experience is not best summed up by onlooker accounts whether these accounts are derived from medical, family, or other witness accounts. This observation has repeatedly emerged not merely in review of different academic perspectives about personal reactions to the approach of death but also by comparing first-person accounts with those of observers' accounts of dying and death.

Where people really die: understanding the 95% rule

Although most of us who work in palliative care acknowledge that the social world of the dying person is a crucial part in the support of that person, that recognition is not supported by the institutional culture of modern healthcare. For example, Wright and McSherry (2013) report that nurses spend approximately 1 hour and 20 minutes in an 8-hour shift on face-to-face interactions with patients—about 5% of their time. This finding confirmed an identical earlier finding about nurses (Hendrich et al., 2008). The figures for doctors are worse. In the UK and the US, the amount of time an average doctor in primary care spends face-to-face with an individual patient is between 13 and 15 minutes (Gottschalk and Flocke, 2005; Brodwin and Radovanovich, 2016). In hospitals, the interactional element of patient care runs to similar form at 13% or 14%—residents spend more time on their computer than with patients (Wenger et al., 2017; Chaiyachati et al., 2019). These figures for doctors translate inversely to less than 1% of patient time from their point of view.

Professional contact with patients and family is not that much better in formal palliative care contexts. The average home visit by a doctor is estimated to be around 40–60 minutes (National Institute for Health and Care Excellence, 2018). If we take the more generous estimate, this means that on the occasion when a doctor does visit at home, this will represent 4.17% or less than 5% of a patient's entire day again. This more extended time for home visits parallels those by nurse practitioners even in dementia care contexts where the range is between 30 and 50 minutes, depending on the 'procedure'—again less than 5% of a patient's day, on the day of the visit with, obviously, the weekly average falling and reducing that percentage (Doyle et al., 2017).

In economic assessments of palliative home care, Wenk (2006) estimated optimal visits at twice a week and nursing also twice a week with four counselling or psychology visits a month. This was (a rather ideal and optimal) averaging out of visitations depending on the intensity of the assistance and depended on many factors—the type and stage of disease progression and the geographical access issues, and so on (Wenk, 2006). If we use Wenk's overall assessment of visits by an assortment of healthcare professionals during any average week of palliative care under optimal circumstances (for the health service), and we assume all the professional visits last the full hour, visits for 5 hours per week are possible but that still constitutes an average of less than 5% of a patient's time in any single day, per month. What then does palliative care offer in the other 95%?

Overall, as a generalizable principle, we can say—and say conservatively—that dying people spend less than 5% of any one day in front of a doctor or nurse. Even this estimate is only true on the days that a doctor or nurse visits outside of an inpatient facility. For dying patients, their caregivers, and the bereaved, this will always mean that over 95% of their time is spent alone, with friends and other family, with neighbours or work colleagues, with animal companions, or with the internet or the television. I describe this situation as the 95% rule.

And yet there is almost no attention in the main palliative care journals about 'interventions' or contributions that palliative care services might make into these social groups and networks. Much of the social in our psychosocial aspirations revolve around direct service provision by chaplains, counsellors, or volunteers and seldom the civic and neighbourhood networks that make up 95% of the patient's and caregiver's worlds at the end of life. The time that volunteers or chaplains spend with dying people—day to day and over the course of dying—is little better than other more clinical colleagues. 'Visits' are just that—episodic and brief. Central to any discussion about why this emphasis has occurred, and continues to occur, has to do primarily with the health service model underlying contemporary palliative care.

Most of the debate about models of healthcare revolve around the proportionate professional understanding and policy and funding emphasis on biomedical models of health versus a social model of health. In palliative care, for example, how much research is dedicated to symptom science over social research given that much of a patient's and family's felt experience is actually of social origin? How much of the health services research emphasis in palliative care in our journals is about assessing inter-professional working (including with volunteers), trials of different intervention pathways to advance care plans or access to pharmacy, assessing types of available care, and endless assessments of patient–doctor communication? There remains a dearth of studies about meaning-making, sources of effective support in the 95% spaces where people live and die, trials of new approaches and practices for the enhancement of well-being, or civic experiments that link primary care or palliative care to partnership working with business or schools, for examples. Biomedical models place most of their emphasis on crisis and symptom management and not on prevention and harm reduction of the negative social determinants of health and well-being. Correspondingly, biomedical models commonly neglect the promotion of the positive social determinants for health and well-being if these cannot be supplied by specific professionals and delivered episodically in the clinical services manner. This pattern of emphases is a reflection of the broader healthcare system, values, and priorities.

The policies of our broader healthcare systems exacerbate and strengthen these priorities. Although direct healthcare services are believed to be responsible for less than half of all health outcomes—between 15% and 43%—it is this system that receives the lion's share of funding growth. Spending on the social determinants of health—poverty, housing, crime prevention, public education, income support—continue to be cut relative to healthcare expenditure. This paradox is also reflected in the worldwide prevention budget which runs at around 5% of all healthcare budgets (Centre for Progressive Policy, 2019).

Features of a social model of health

The only model of care which directly addresses most healthcare needs including those of dying people and their families is a social model of health. A social model of health addresses the social nature of dying. Yuill and colleagues (2010) argue that there are five features of a social model of care:

1. A social model of health is not an alternative to a medical model but it is a serious reorientation of those priorities that places the social character of the dying, death, bereavement, and caregiving issues at the centre of any care actions and policies. A social model of health recognizes the importance and value of biomedicine and direct health service provision but it is not overwhelmingly *the* most important provision. It is one important thing but not the over-riding important thing in healthcare. Physical palliation needs are crucial but they do not, indeed cannot, occupy the core work of care of the dying if one accepts that the characterizing feature of dying is social.
2. A social model of health recognizes that all health is enabled or inhibited by the social context. Social context has a major impact on individual experience, conduct, and choice; the effectiveness of any medical care provided; and the creation, maintenance, and sustainability of continuity of care. The most common ways that we think about context is to remember the impacts of culture, ethnicity, gender, or social class but other influences are just as crucial and often less visible. Some of these less visible influences are social support networks, housing and transport access, health and end of life literacy, employment status and conditions, circumstances of stigma, isolation, and social exclusion.

   Although we sometimes think of many of these influences as affecting 'minorities', this is a pop sociology myth. It is true that some so-called minority groups do experience great hardship because of their cultural status (e.g. gypsies and other travellers, prisoners, or people of colour), but many other people who are not so obvious in population health terms also struggle and are disadvantaged by their own social circumstances and these can erode quality of life, access to services, continuity of care, or even life expectancy as much as these other groups. The elderly, the socially isolated, remote rural residents, the lonely and friendless, and those without access to public education and therefore any literacy about dying, bereavement, or caregiving are key among these common examples.
3. A social model of health also recognizes that culture not only determines how health and disease—and ageing, death, dying, grief, and caregiving—are seen and managed but also experienced. And by 'culture' we are referring to *all* national or religious traditions not just those from ethnic or migrant groups. In this context, the reference to 'culture' includes all our—and our own—assumptions and values about life and death, illness and health, dignity and shame, pride, honour, and dependency and autonomy, and a host of other small and large things we often do not reflect upon in our often busy and highly distracted, daily lives. 'Culture' is not all about 'the other'.
4. A social model of health also recognizes that health is a political matter. Political choices, processes, and policies determine health in crucial ways that have major impacts on the distribution of health and illness (epidemiology) and the national, regional, and local pattern of services (access and quality). In other words, political processes have a major impact on the social determinants of health. And when we speak about the 'social determinants of health' we are not merely referring to the clinical epidemiology of dying but equally importantly its social epidemiology—the pattern and distribution of loneliness, depression, anxiety, unemployment, social isolation, stigma, social rejection and aversion, sexual dysfunction, drug and alcohol abuse, lost school or work days, suicides, and sudden deaths. Quality health services are a necessary but not sufficient condition to ameliorate the social morbidities of living with dying unless the health services approach is embedded in a social model of healthcare.
5. Finally, a social model of health recognizes that other voices matter. Health is *not* a wholly determined matter for medicine but other health and social care interests must determine what is important in health and well-being as well as illness and accident prevention, and logically, in ageing, dying, death, grief and bereavement, and in caregiving in the community. This observation about the political economy of healthcare is not a call for the overturning of medical dominance. Rather, the political economy identified in a social model of health recognizes the importance of partnerships with civic and social care colleagues in tackling the challenges of health, illness, and mortality in our communities throughout history and into our future. Quality and access to healthcare at the end of life—as in other areas of life—is not achievable without partnerships with civic institutions (local government, workplaces, schools) and communities (neighbourhoods, personal and social media) that govern and underpin the 95% of the daily life of the dying person, their carergivers, and the bereaved.

The social model of health has often travelled under a number of different names—social medicine, community medicine, social health, preventive medicine, and of course public health (Germov, 2016). The term 'public health' has a tendency to be misunderstood as indeed do all the other synonyms such as social medicine or community medicine. Public health is often identified with *all* health and social care efforts within a society to tackle health, disease, disability, and accidents. This meaning of public health ranges from legislation to protect people from food poisoning and faulty building construction or car design, to the training and distribution of healthcare professions, the building of hospitals, and the adequacy of national water purification and sewerage processes.

However, the phrase public health is also used more specifically in academic and clinical circles to refer to a range of surveillance sciences—epidemiology, health services research, demography, population biology, health social sciences, bioethics, computer and mathematical modelling, and a variety of bench sciences. These disciplines are most commonly found in university departments. However, in local governments, local and international non-governmental organizations, and in academic departments with a special interest in social models of health (e.g. social work, nursing, and health promotion) the phrase 'public health' refers principally to a set of methods of practice.

These practices include health promotion, community development, social ecology, public education (health literacy), social and health policy development, environmental action and political advocacy, legal studies, participatory action, community partnerships, and social marketing. This collection of methods also often goes under the name of the 'new' public health principally for two reasons:

1. It prioritizes health and well-being over disease and illness, and
2. It prioritizes practice and solution identification over surveillance and problem identification. 'Public health palliative care', the 'public health approach to palliative care', 'health-promoting palliative care', or the 'compassionate community/cities' movement are all synonyms for the new public health approach in palliative care. This is the social model of health as it is specifically applied to palliative care.

Public health palliative care: a social model of health

Public health palliative care is a social model of health because it reflects the main themes within that model. These are (1) an emphasis on the social determinants of health while living with ageing, dying, caregiving, and grief and bereavement; (2) an emphasis on practice methods in public health as equal priority alongside clinical practice methods; (3) an emphasis on cultural awareness that minimizes anguish about social differences by employing a participatory style of working rather than assuming the traditional 'expert' stance of authority and paternalism; (4) an emphasis and awareness of the politics of health that means working equally for prevention and health-promotion sciences and priorities alongside those from clinical management; and (5) recognizing and working with other voices in the health, social care, civic, and community contexts of practice.

Social determinants of health

The quality of a person's or family's life while dying or caregiving is determined by the strength of their social support networks. Although chaplaincy, social work, or counselling services can help—especially for those with few supports and for those in acute crisis—most of the time spent by any one dying person or single family will be in community. It is therefore important to recognize and to work to promote community development in any area/region where a primary care or palliative care service operates.

Strengthening community ties is about promoting and advocating the need for greater neighbourhood supports and greater civic engagement and responsibility by workplaces, schools, faith groups, or local government to identify and support those ageing, living with life-limiting illness, caregiving, and bereavement. Sometimes this will mean lending support and encouragement to volunteer groups but the actions of volunteers do not define nor exhaust the limits of 'community' action. Civic organizations should all have policies and prescribed actions that define how they will contribute to their students, teachers, managers, employees, parishioners, or members how they will look after one another in end of life circumstances. Also, Neighbourhood Watch groups should not limit themselves to crime prevention. All communities need to remember that end of life care—like health—is everyone's responsibility and primary and palliative care services can provide a leadership role in the promotion of a vision that tackles loneliness, social isolation, depression, lost school days, or even suicide. The social epidemiology at the end of life cannot be merely defined as a health services problem or its management success will always be elusive.

Emphasis on practice methods

Whether we are referring to primary care or palliative care in the field of practice, or whether we are referring to university departments of palliative care or public health, the development, testing, and dissemination of practice methods are crucial in addressing the social determinants of health at the end of life. Problem assessments by health services or epidemiological research are meaningless beyond a handful of academic pundits unless these are accompanied by equal effort and energy into solutions-based programmes of work. The arts of community development—of working with people in neighbourhoods or the local government or the faith groups—to create the necessary supports for ageing, dying, caregiving, and grieving will be essential. The arts of social ecology—being mindful about how physical and social environments can shape health-promoting behaviour will also be important. Public education—promoting health and end of life literacy—is crucial in reducing fear and enhancing resiliency in the community, among families, and among those dying and grieving. The development of health-promotion ideas and strategies are also crucial—the promotion of experiences of health and well-being are the best methods for the prevention and harm reduction of the social morbidities associated with ageing, dying, caregiving, and loss and grief. But at all times, a clinical harm reduction strategy towards our patients and families must not exhaust our palliative care actions because the greater challenge will be the development of practices for health and well-being.

Emphasis on cultural awareness

Because each of us is limited by our twin experiences of education and upbringing, we need to learn about the values and early experiences that shape other people's roads to happiness or despair, or vulnerability and resilience. This is not easily learned by simply asking. Important things in a person's life are usually only shared when trust is earned first. This is just as true of our patients as it is for our colleagues in health, social, or civic care. For the purposes of developing a plan of social action, this trust and knowledge about another requires a participatory working style. Community development therefore is not merely 'community work' or 'community-based' services. It is working with communities and not on communities. This will often mean arriving together at a joint understanding of a set of problems and a joint agreement about how to go about addressing these. Some public health palliative care clinicians engage directly in this process of participation. Other clinicians and services are unable to do this for a range of reasons so instead employ a community development worker. If community development workers are employed than most of these colleagues will know they are not creating a service but creating areas of sustainable, self-interested support networks for their community—whether these may be neighbourhoods or workplace/school place policies.

Emphasis on the politics and policies of social health

If the limits of palliative care—and the limits of healthcare—are to be defined by the location of a service provider, palliative care will never penetrate beyond most urban areas or certainly only provide elementary services when they do. Many rural areas are grateful they are able to be visited by a community nurse with some palliative care training or experience. How one compares this kind of 'access' with 'access' in a large city is questionable. Once again, the question of whether we view palliative care as something which addresses the physical challenges of dying or whether this is a social model of care is highlighted in this example. Clearly, a public health palliative care approach does not set its limits to acute care provision as its minimum standard but rather on ideas about prevention, harm reduction, early intervention, and the promotion of health and well-being. Since most of these are social matters, a public health palliative care approach must go against the limited understandings of the broader healthcare system of formulating its ideas about 'access' in terms of 'services' alone. In this way, the need to work with cultural awareness—whether this be in terms of the local Vietnamese community or an isolated part of rural Scotland—has less to do with how to get a doctor or a nurse into those spaces and much more to do with how to encourage and mobilize the use of local community and civic assets to meet the goals of good palliative care as a social model of health.

Emphasis on other voices

The realization of the importance of cooperation with sectors and communities that are outside the 'palliative care team' is a reminder of the importance of partnership working and the value of social networks. Just as it is important for primary or palliative care teams to have partnerships with social work or chaplaincy colleagues or to have links with bereavement or cancer support groups, so too it is equally important to have these with actual neighbourhoods, local governments, and businesses or schools in the same way. Partnerships with these kinds of networks have been shown to reduce health service use (Age UK, 2014; Cronin, 2016; Abel et al., 2018), helping to manage the demand pressures on general practitioner services or accident and emergency services. They have also been shown to reduce morbidities and raise health standards in a range of disease-specific groups (O'Mara-Eves et al., 2013; Sallnow et al., 2016). In this way, the public health palliative care goals of reducing social morbidities and promoting health and well-being are only served not simply by employing practice methods but also in applying these with important civic others or in encouraging them to employ these for the greater health and social care good. In this way, cooperation means partnerships means social models of working.

Conclusion: a well-being approach to end of life care

The short modern history of palliative care has continually emphasized 'whole person' care—care of the physical, psychological, social, and spiritual aspects of living with dying, caregiving, and bereavement. However, the leadership profile, the professional composition, and the funding priorities of contemporary palliative care have placed most of the emphasis on the clinical side of managing and supporting those human experiences. Palliative care services are overwhelmingly led by clinicians—of any stripe. It is rare for palliative care services to be led by businesses, local governments, housing associations, schools, or even volunteers. It is not unheard of, but it remains rare and exceptional. The core elements of our vision in palliative care have been clinical with a heavy emphasis on clinician-to-patient or clinician-to-family interactions. The social world of dying, caregiving, and grief is both wider and deeper than these narrow corridors of insight and experience.

Despite the emphasis on health or whole person care in lofty national and international policy documents, most palliative care funding goes to health services and not to trade unions, employer groups, or school groups, to develop their own palliative care approaches for the workers, students, or teachers in their charge. As we have seen in this chapter already, there is great irony in this set of priorities. In these ways, the funding priorities of palliative care somnolently follow the lead of global clinical priorities and not those of public health and certainly not those with social health priorities. Yet it is also true that a social model of health is gathering pace among global health priorities every day. This is because our broader theories and policies about the very nature of health have not really changed since 1948 when the World Health Organization first described its own understanding of this idea.

The World Health Organization definition of health is tautological. Health is asserted to be a positive state of complete physical, mental, and social well-being (Medical News Today, 2020). And well-being in its turn is commonly defined in terms of its dimensions in health—physical, mental, spiritual, and social health. Despite the fact that 'health' or 'well-being' are employed as synonyms for each other, both definitions begin with identifying its determinants—beginning first with personal assets such as a person's social background—and then going on to emphasize personality and social networks. Of course, all these 'assets' themselves determine each other and in that way are 'dynamic'—each feeds the other in a back-and-forth manner. When in equilibrium and balance, they can generate happiness and life satisfaction. When one dimension comes under increasing challenge, all other dimensions become threatened until resolution. Without resolution all other dimensions remain under 'stress' (Dodge et al., 2012).

The task of a health-promoting palliative care therefore is to recognize that these four dimensions are not merely sites for services—but equally importantly as sites where social cultivation and growth must take place for the sake of patient health and well-being. Visitation by volunteers or by social care professionals will always be insufficient for the task because it is the social milieu of the patient and family that requires the actual change, support, and development. Wherever the patient and their caregivers find themselves—whether this be at clubs, workplaces, schools, in local government areas or local neighbourhoods, on social media, or in front of the television set—the promotion of well-being through social supports and helpful information *must take place at these sites*. This is the precise technical meaning of 'community development'. For our professional services in palliative care then, community development means partnership working with neighbourhoods and civic sectors of the local area. It also implies one further implication and this can seem conceptually and practically counterintuitive.

Palliative care is not primarily a symptom science. Palliative care does not merely palliate. Palliation is merely one function of our science. The broader aim of palliative care is the promotion of health and well-being at the end of life. The challenging task before us when delivering on our promise for whole person care is to recognize the following fact: 'whole person care' for any individual patient or caregiver must logically mean 'whole community care'. This is because the life-giving sources of health and well-being are best found not in professional services alone, but more abundantly and more steadfastly among our friends and families, in our places of spirit and stillness, and our sites of work, play, and prayer. Palliative care is a well-being science.

REFERENCES

Abel, J., Kingston, H., Scally, A., Hartnoll, J., Hannam, G., Thomas-Moore, A., et al. 2018. Reducing emergency hospital admissions: a population health complex intervention of an enhanced model of primary care and compassionate communities. *British Journal of General Practice* **68**, e803–e810.

Agamben, G. 1998. *Homo Sacer: Sovereign Power and Bare Life*. Palo Alto, CA: Stanford University Press.

Age UK. 2014. *People, Place, Purpose: Shaping Services Around People and Communities Through the Newquay Pathfinder*. Age UK Cornwall and Isle of Scilly.

Alvarez, A. 1970. *The Savage God: A Study of Suicide*. New York: Bantam.

Armstrong-Costa, A. 2004. *Living and Dying with Cancer*. Cambridge: Cambridge University Press.

Brodwin, E. and Radovanovic, D. 2016. Here's how many minutes the average doctor actually spends with each patient. *Business Insider UK*, 6 April.

Centre for Progressive Policy. 2019. *Beyond the NHS: Addressing the Root Causes of Poor Health*. London: Centre for Progressive Policy.

Chaiyachati, K. H., Shea, J. A., Asch D. A., Liu, M., Bellini, L. M., Dine, C. J., et al. 2019. Assessment of inpatient time allocation among first year internal medicine residents using time-motion observations. *JAMA Internal Medicine*, **179**, 760–767.

Cronin, P. 2016. Compassionate communities in Shropshire, West Midlands, England. In: Wegleitner, K., Heimerl, K., and Kellehear, A. (eds.) *Compassionate Communities: Case Studies from Britain and Europe*, pp. 30–45. Abingdon: Routledge.

Cumming, E. and Henry, W. E. 1961. *Growing Old: The Process of Disengagement*. New York: Basic Books.

Dodge, R., Daly, A. P., Huyton, J., and Sanders, L. D. 2012. The challenge of defining wellbeing. *International Journal of Wellbeing*, **2**, 222–235.

Doyle, C., Setoya, N., Goeman, D., and Kayama, M. 2017. The role of home nursing visits in supporting people living with dementia in Japan and Australia: cross national learnings and future system reform. *Health Systems & Reform*, **3**, 203–213.

Durkheim, E. 1952. *Suicide*. London: Routledge & Kegan Paul.

Fulton, R. 1977. The sociology of death. *Death Education*, **1**, 15–25.

Germov, J. 2016. *Second Opinion: An Introduction to Health Sociology*, 6th ed. Melbourne: Oxford University Press.

Giacalone, J. A. 2001. *The US Nursing Home Industry*. Armonk, NY: ME Sharpe.

Glaser, B. and Strauss, A. L. 1971. *Status Passage*. London: Routledge & Kegan Paul.

Gottschalk, A. and Flocke, S. A. 2005. Time spent in face-to-face patient care and work outside the examination room. *Annals of Family Medicine*, **3**, 488–493.

Hendrich, A., Chow, M. P., Skierczynski, B. A., and Zhenquiang, L. 2008. A 36-hospital time and motion study: how do medical-surgical nurses spend their time? *The Permenente Journal*, **12**, 25–34.

Hochschild, A. R. 1975. Disengagement theory: a critique and proposal. *American Sociological Review*, **40**, 553–569.

Holden, J., Greyson, B., and James, D. (eds.) 2009. *The Handbook of Near-Death Experiences: Thirty Years of Investigation*. Santa Barbara, CA: ABC-CLIO.

Houlbrooke, R. 1998. *Death, Religion and the Family in England, 1480–1750*. Oxford: Clarendon Press.

Jalland, P. 1996. *Death in the Victorian Family*. Oxford: Oxford University Press.

Kalish, R. 1968. Life and death: dividing the indivisible. *Social Science & Medicine*, **2**, 249–259.

Kellehear, A. 2007. *A Social History of Dying*. Cambridge: Cambridge University Press.

Kellehear, A. (ed.) 2009. *The Study of Dying: From Autonomy to Transformation*. Cambridge: Cambridge University Press.

Kellehear, A. 2014. *The Inner Life of the Dying Person*. New York: Columbia University Press.

Lawton, J. 2000. *The Dying Process: Patients' Experiences of Palliative Care*. London: Routledge.

Lunney, J. R., Lynn, J., Foley, D. J., Lipson, S., and Guralnik, J. M. 2003. Patterns of functional decline at the end of life. *Journal of the American Medical Association*, **289**, 2387–2392.

McManners, J. 1985. *Death and the Enlightenment*. Oxford: Oxford University Press.

Medical News Today. 2020. What is good health? [Online] Available at: https://www.medicalnewstoday.com/articles/150999

Moody, R. A. 1975. *Life After Life*. Covington, GA: Mockingbird.

National Institute for Health and Care Excellence. 2018. Chapter 6. GP-led home visits. Emergency and acute medical care in over 16s: service delivery and organization. NICE guidelines 94. [Online] Available at: https://www.nice.org.uk/guidance/ng94/evidence/06.gpled-home-visits-pdf-4788818467

Noys, B. 2005. *The Culture of Death*. Oxford: Berg.

Nuland, S. B. 1993. *How We Die*. London: Chatto & Windus.

O'Mara-Eves, A., Brunton, G., McDaid, D., Oliver, S., Kavanagh, J., Jamal, F., et al. 2013. Community engagement to reduce inequalities in health: a systematic review, meta-analysis and economic analysis. *Public Health Research*, **1**, 4.

Sabom, M. B. 1982. *Recollections of Death: A Medical Investigation*. New York: Harper & Row.

Sallnow, L., Richardson, H., Murray, S. A., and Kellehear, A. 2016. The impact of a new public health approach to end-of-life care: a systematic review. *Palliative Medicine*, **30**, 200–211.

Scoggins, W. F. 1971. Growing old: death by instalment plan. *Life Threatening Behavior*, **1**, 143–147.

Sidell, M. and Komaromy, C. 2003. Who dies in care homes for older people? In: Katz, J. S. and Peace, S. (eds.) *End of Life in Care Homes: A Palliative Approach*, pp. 43–57. Oxford: Oxford University Press.

Van Gennep, A. 1969. *The Rites of Passage*. Chicago, IL: University of Chicago Press.

Wenger, N., Mean, M., Castioni, J., Marques-Vidal, P., Waeber, G., and Garnier, A. 2017. Allocation of internal medicine resident time in a Swiss hospital: a time and motion study of day and evening shifts. *Annals of Internal Medicine*, **166**, 579–586.

Wenk, R. 2006. Palliative home care. In: Bruera, E., Higginson, I., Ripamonti, C., and von Gunten, C. (eds.) *Textbook of Palliative Medicine*, pp. 277–284. Boca Raton, FL: Hodder Arnold.

Wright, S. and McSherry, W. 2013. How much time do nurses spend on patient care? *Nursing Times*, **109**, online issue.

Yuill, C., Crinsin, I., and Duncan, E. 2010. *Key Concepts in Health Studies*. London: Sage.

4

Palliative care

The new essentials

Julian Abel, Allan Kellehear, and Aliki Karapliagkou

Introduction

In a previous paper (Abel and Kellehear, 2016) we examined the potential for reshaping palliative care services by applying the principles of the public health approach to end of life care. The public health model of palliative care has shown promising evidence of effectiveness (Kumar, 2007; O'Mara-Eves et al., 2013; Cronin, 2015; South, 2015; Sallnow et al., 2016). The social justice basis for this approach responds to the crucial need for equity of care irrespective of age, background, diagnosis, or cause of death. This chapter describes a practical model that redesigns and reshapes palliative care services, by inviting and organizing the coordination and interaction between specialist palliative care, generalist palliative care, compassionate communities, and the civic approach to end of life care. The first part of this chapter describes the four components of the proposed model in order to define the core terms of reference for this discussion. We will then describe how the four components can work together, in order to promote issues of importance to health and well-being at the end of life—not solely for the dying patient, but also for caregivers, and the bereaved. The final part of the chapter makes recommendations for changes in professional service organization and social practices, starting from changes within the organization and operations of the core components.

Palliative care components

Health services around the world are organized differently. The key components of care entailed in the model may be found to a greater or lesser extent in all. The challenge for respective palliative and end of life care services is to fulfil the functions of the model we describe according to the needs of their local organizational and community structures.

Specialist palliative care

There is no single or clear definition of specialist palliative care (Pastrana et al., 2008). The World Health Organization (2020) defines palliative care as 'an approach that improves the quality of life of patients and their families facing the problem associated with life-threatening illness, through the prevention and relief of suffering by means of early identification and impeccable assessment and treatment of pain and other problems, physical, psychosocial and spiritual. This definition comes as a subheading under 'Cancer' and does not make a specific reference to non-cancer terminal diagnoses and conditions. It also does not differentiate between specialist and generalist palliative care and does not include bereavement as a routine aspect of palliative and end of life care.

Many countries recognize palliative care as a medical speciality with training programmes equivalent to other accredited specialities, or at least subspecialities. Similarly, there are recognized training programmes for specialist palliative care nurses. The domains of care involved are broad and inclusive of physical, social, psychological, and spiritual needs. The boundaries between specialist and generalist are not clear and are dependent on local practice and custom. Specialist knowledge is particularly called into use in those people who have particularly complex end of life needs.

Inpatient specialist palliative care is commonly but not exclusively provided in hospices. Outpatient care is supported through the use of specialists from multiple fields, including doctors, nurses, physiotherapists, spiritual and psychological counsellors, occupational therapists, social workers, and others.

Specialist palliative care support teams are present within many hospitals in the UK, acting as an advisory service. The proportion of hospital inpatients who need specialist palliative care is difficult to estimate and determine. What we do know is that non-cancer patients are under-represented in specialist palliative care, although they have comparable needs to cancer patients (Luddington et al., 2001).

Ethnic minority community members, older people, and marginal groups (e.g. homeless populations) have also been documented to escape timely referral to specialist palliative care services (Ahmed et al., 2004). By and large, in those countries that have palliative care recognized as a specialty, the care provided is mainly for patients with a cancer diagnosis who have complex needs with symptom control problems.

Generalist palliative care

Generalist palliative care can be defined by exclusion—it is not a medical specialty, and involves care at the end of life that is not provided by specialist palliative care teams. It includes care provided by all health and social care professionals who look after people who are dying and those who are bereaved. The issue of who provides generalist palliative care depends upon each individual country's healthcare system, its organization, and its regulations. In the UK, most hospital specialities look after terminally ill patients, and may be supported to a greater or lesser extent by in-hospital specialist palliative care teams. Outside the hospital setting, care is coordinated by primary care teams, consisting of general practitioners, trained nursing staff, social workers, and nursing staff who give physical hands-on care.

Compassionate communities

Compassionate communities are the networks of support in neighbourhoods and communities surrounding those experiencing death, dying, caregiving, and loss. Conceptually and practically, these networks have been defined by 'inner' and 'outer' circles of care and community resources (Horsfall et al., 2012; Abel et al., 2013). The 'inner' circles of care typically consist of between three and ten people who are closely related to the person with the illness. They usually provide personal (physical) care, as well as companionship and psychological and emotional support. The 'outer' circles of care consist of between five and 50 people or more, with an average number of 16 (Horsfall et al., 2015). The 'outer' circle is not focused exclusively on the patient but often helps with the 'stuff' of life—the shopping, the cooking, the cleaning, lifts to and from hospital appointments, gardening, dog-walking, as well as providing valuable love, laughter, and friendship. In a study of family caregiving for cancer patients, the average number of hours per week spent on these tasks was 62 (Rowland et al., 2017)—a sizeable proportion of which could be shared with community members, neighbours, and friends within the network.

Support from communities, involving people not included in the inner and outer circles, is included within the context of compassionate communities. This type of support might be directly related to the challenges of death, dying, loss, and care giving and might include volunteer groups and third-sector organizations. It also includes making use of the vast array of activities and resources that are often commonly found in communities. Community development, which aims at building community resources, is part of the process of strengthening compassionate communities, commonly using ground up participatory methodologies. People become more connected—or reconnected—to their communities by linking their personal lives with new social activities and networks that were previously unknown to, or little used by, them—book clubs, walking clubs, coffee mornings, gym classes, befriending groups, and more. Patients, families, and friends may all benefit from using these rich resources.

Civic end of life care

Professional services, such as specialist or generalist palliative care, give and receive support from communities to enhance their respective tasks of support for people with life-limiting illness and their caregivers. In the same way, communities or neighbourhoods require support from civic sectors to effectively undertake their responsibilities towards people with end of life care needs. Professional support is incomplete without community support, especially in matters to do with quality and continuity of care. In the same way, community support cannot offer continuity or quality of care without civic participation and cooperation from public sectors and institutions—schools, workplaces, or places of worship. This is quite simply because these are the key social institutions inhabited by the very neighbours, family members, or friends offering support to the dying or the bereaved. It is, therefore, crucial to recognize that neighbourhood caregivers are not faceless social entities but rather actual employees, students, worshipers, shoppers, and club members. The civic component of end of life care recognizes this foundational inter-dependency as the very support basis of community care, and mobilizes actions that support end of life care in public institutions.

Although there are potentially numerous ways to involve business or schools in end of life care, the Compassionate City Charter (Kellehear, 2016) provides a succinct and ready-made tool for embedding this approach. The Charter includes action recommendations for schools, workplaces, churches and temples, trade unions, cultural centres, hospices, and care homes, among others. Reorientation of healthcare towards civic partnerships, as described in the Ottawa Charter of Health Promotion (World Health Organization, 1986) is a consistent part of the public health approach to end of life care. A variety of incentive schemes to promote participation from the different social and cultural sectors, and an annual memorial parade, are all part of the actionable aspects of engaging people at the broadest community level in end of life care. The Charter does not define how it should be put into practice. This is something that is different in local contexts and depends upon who owns the initiative of becoming a Compassionate City, as well as how the Charter is adapted for different national circumstances. However, the principles apply across the globe. In the context of communities, the word 'city' is etymologically associated with its core social element—the citizen—and is taken from the Latin root word *civitas*, which describes shared civic responsibilities that transcend traditional tribal barriers (such as those of gender, 'race', or social class), a common purpose, and a sense of community.

Palliative care: interdependency

The interdependency model proposes a way of integrating the processes and operations of the four basic components—specialist palliative care, generalist palliative care, compassionate communities, and civic end of life care—that make up palliative and end of life care. Their effective coordination aims at improved well-being at the end of life for every citizen affected by a life-limiting condition.

In Fig. 4.1, each component is represented by a cog which is united by a chain joining them all. Together, they work to drive up the benefits of the hierarchy of well-being at the end of life, which we describe in Fig. 4.2. The absence of any one of the cogs means that the promotion and reproduction of well-being is disrupted, and the clinical and public health effectiveness in addressing the comorbidities associated with dying, caregiving, or loss will be undermined.

Having understood that it is the seamless union of all four components that sustains end of life care, we will make suggestions on how professional services can reshape and reorganize within the framework of a complete end of life care system with public health priorities. The linkage between the cogs and the mutual participation in joint initiatives is needed in order to be able to realistically provide end of life care and bereavement support for all, irrespective of age, background, and diagnosis.

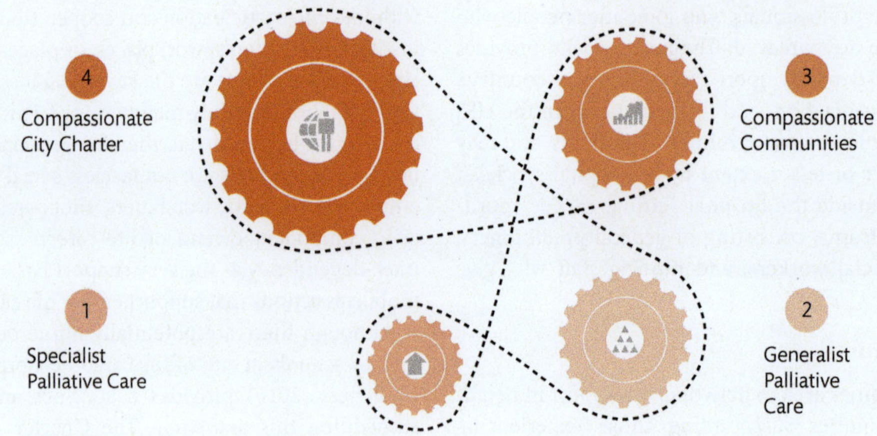

Fig. 4.1 Palliative care, the interconnected web.
Reproduced with permission from Abel, J., Kellehear, A. & Karapliagou, A. 2018. Palliative care—the new essentials. *Annals of palliative medicine*, 7, S3–S14.

Fig. 4.2 portrays 'The hierarchy of well-being' representing both the negative consequences of poor care (generated by individual but disjointed palliative and end of life care components), and the ideal positive outcomes (generated by individual but cooperating palliative and end of life care components). The left-hand side column describes the social and clinical epidemiological consequences and poor health service and social care and support. The right-hand side column describes the equivalent positive outcomes. Many of the poor outcomes we commonly associate with the dying or bereavement journey—such as depression, loneliness, or 'compassion fatigue'—overlap or are better explained as system failures in professional service or social support systems. However, without an optimal level of public health practice in end of life care—the interconnected web as we describe them here—it is not easy to distinguish between the pure social and psychological consequences of facing mortality and loss, on one hand, and the polluting social and psychological consequences of poor care, on the other.

The challenge in building collaborative partnerships between the four key components of palliative and end of life care, and coordinating their respective processes, is that the practice represents an innovation with multiple readjustments. Regular, face-to-face contact between organizations and practitioners that are often siloed into their separate departments is needed. Compassionate communities, for example, can struggle to access the domain of professional practice, gain acceptance, and establish effective communication that will allow them to take a more active role in care. Civic engagement in end of life care is not yet fully understood in societies where healthcare is perceived as a professional responsibility.

This means that significant domains of care and support are left untapped. Professional services alone cannot fill these gaps. The roles and practices of professional, community, and civic care are naturally complementary and not mutually exclusive. Care in general, and palliative and end of life care in particular, is achieved through the mutual efforts of specialist and generalist palliative care, community care, and civic end of life care. The interconnected web proposes actions for the expansion of their collaboration, aiming to improve inclusion of specific needs, as well as citizens who find themselves marginalized in care. The rest of this chapter considers

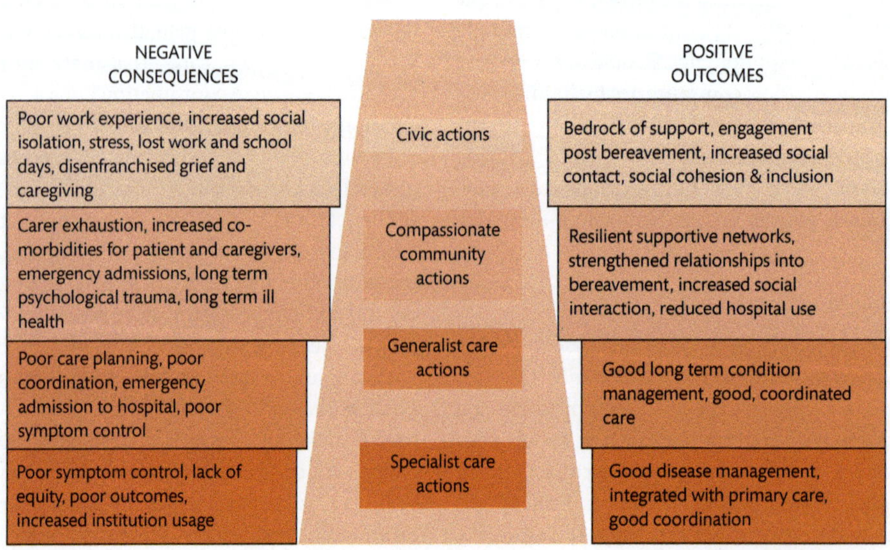

Fig. 4.2 The hierarchy of well-being.
Reproduced with permission from Abel, J., Kellehear, A. & Karapliagou, A. 2018. Palliative care—the new essentials. *Annals of palliative medicine*, 7, S3–S14.

the reassessment of roles and properties of each of the components, and offers recommendations for their adaptation, aiming to bridge their practices and promote greater inclusion in care.

Specialist palliative care recommendations

Current specialist palliative care services fulfil a variety of functions ranging from inpatient specialist palliative care beds in hospices and hospitals, outpatient services, community visiting, advice and support for primary care and the community, and in-hospital teams for symptom control and advice. Carers' feedback from the VOICES 2015 survey (Office for National Statistics, 2015) clearly demonstrates the impact and benefits of high-quality palliative care. In particular, for those patients who receive hospice care, the feedback about the quality of care is almost always excellent.

This can be in stark contrast to the experience of end of life care in other settings—hospitals or communities—where specialist services may be limited (Mitchell, 2002; Smith et al., 2003; To et al., 2011). This is particularly, but not exclusively, the case in non-cancer terminal illnesses (To et al., 2011; Seow et al., 2014), people of lower socioeconomic background, and diverse communities who tend to benefit less from specialist palliative care services in hospital settings (Currow et al., 2008). Opportunities for advance planning and building of supportive networks are often missed, resulting in crises which precipitate unplanned admissions to hospital—as in the case of heart failure patients who fail to receive advance planning and specialist palliative care services early in their illness (Small et al., 2009). The marked difference in home and hospital death rates between those with a diagnosis of cancer and those with non-cancer terminal illnesses—cancer patients are more likely to die at home (National End of Life Care Intelligence Network, 2021)—is a consequence of lack of identification of the final phase of terminal illness, and lack of specialist palliative care in the community among the latter.

The reorganization of specialist palliative care services relies upon the basic principle that supportive communities can do much of what is currently being done by professional specialist teams. Outpatient care and community specialist care can form partnerships with informal caring networks to enable terminally ill patients to spend time or die at home. A strong and resilient supportive community is better able to cope with the stresses and strains of caring for someone who is dying. Examples of how this is done come from Australia, where a networking approach to palliative care in the community has been adopted (Horsfall et al., 2015; Horsfall and Higgs, 2017; Horsfall et al., 2017). Building strong networks means that patients can be looked after at home with members of the 'inner' circle of care being trained in caring skills, such as manual handling and medication administration. Strong 'outer' circles within the caring networks support those closer to the person who is dying in a variety of ways. They may take care of simple everyday tasks and provide respite and emotional support. Specialist palliative care teams therefore need to develop the skills of how to map networks of support, identify strengths and weaknesses, and be able to work with families and friends to further strengthen what is already present.

Similarly, the adoption of the civic approach to end of life care and the implementation of the Compassionate City Charter creates awareness about end of life care needs and provisions of support in the spaces and environments where citizens socialize, work, study, and engage in various activities. Citizens who engage with the end of life and its care, and are encouraged to do so by the very social sectors and public institutions they interact with on a daily basis, are more likely to form partnerships with professional healthcare services and assist in the delivery of care in the community. The attitude of compassion and practical support that they encounter in school, work, society, club, or centre of worship will be transferred to private sectors where palliative and end of life care can be burdensome and isolating. It is incumbent upon specialist palliative care to be an active participant, if not a leader, in implementation of the Compassionate City Charter. They play an important role in education around death literacy, helping communities in all settings to develop the necessary skills.

Once strong social networks are in place, it is possible to consider changing the roles and functions of specialist palliative care services to enable the formation of partnerships with community and civic sectors and supports (Box 4.1).

In the UK, all residents have access to primary care services. This means that general practitioner services are notified of all deaths, including the place where death occurred. This creates the possibility of ensuring universal coverage of palliative care through review of each death. However, not all health services have primary care teams, and not everyone has access to healthcare. The key challenge in these circumstances is to build reliable health systems that provide equity of care to all who need it. Solutions to these problems are place dependent. Generic solutions often do not fit individual circumstances. Aiming for the key function of universal coverage should be an aspiration for all palliative care teams.

Box 4.1 Recommendations for changes to specialist palliative care

- Reduced specialist palliative care in-patient beds as the need for them decreases with increasing care at home.
- Routine use of network mapping and network enhancement for all clinical staff.
- Training in understanding of network mapping and network enhancement for all involved in end of life care, including non-clinical staff, volunteers, hospice shops, and fundraising teams.
- Training in care at end of life, such as manual handling and administration of injections at the end of life for supportive community networks.
- Participation in multidisciplinary meetings with primary care teams.
- Participation in starting and supporting compassionate community initiatives, including the Compassionate City Charter.
- Changing job plans so that specialist palliative care advice and support available in the community on a 24-hour basis through the use of video technology.
- Availability of a same-day or next-day visiting service of specialist palliative care nurses or doctors, if needed.
- Use of community development workers as a routine part of clinical teams.
- Participation in the after-death audit for every patient who dies to establish whether the final phase of illness was identified early. This can be assessed by the extent to which care planning was completed, whether network enhancement and linkage to community resource took place, and end of life medication was available at the time of death. In addition, referral of relatives to community support bereavement networks should be offered as a matter of routine. If these steps have not taken place, then opportunities for how this could have happened need to be sought for continuous service improvement.

Generalist palliative care recommendations

Generalist palliative care takes place in different settings, in hospitals, in primary care, and in the community. The complexity of generalist palliative care makes it difficult to predict and organize into concrete processes and therapeutic practices. The final phases of life may go unrecognized, undermining people's chances to receive advance care planning for better symptom control. Characteristically, there is little concurrence among medical and nursing staff over which individual patients have palliative care needs. Concurrence is only increased with proximity to death (Gott et al., 2001). In cases where death is sudden, such as with heart disease, any opportunities to carry out advance planning are often missed, and death may result after a hospital admission, to the distress of patients and caregivers (Small et al., 2009).

Emergency admissions to hospital without recognition of end of life care needs equally undermines the opportunity to build resilient networks and prepare for care at home. Aggressive treatments in a situation of crisis and lack of communication with healthcare professionals can lead to distressing experiences for relatives and friends, which have long-term consequences, and impact bereavement (Wright et al., 2008). Finally, the coordination of care can be problematic—general practitioners express discomfort about their ability to perform palliative care adequately (Mitchell, 2002). When supported by specialist palliative care teams their effectiveness increases, and patients are able to benefit from palliative care support, including social care prior to an acute crisis. Inadequate care of the terminally ill negatively impacts their bereaved caregivers. Adverse circumstances at the time of death complicate bereavement experiences and lead to longer-term poor health outcomes (Stroebe et al., 2007).

Generalist palliative care, even more so than specialist palliative care, is often called to deal with acute crisis situations, particularly in the absence of advance planning. Being reliant on professional care alone means that when this care is not available, it can be quite challenging to help and support in an effective way (Box 4.2). A collaborative approach between health and social care has been recommended as a way to deal with limited resources (Larkin et al., 2012). Adopting a community and civic approach to end of life care adds to the suggested partnership.

A compassionate community approach looks for support within the patients' own networks. If community resource building has taken place, there may also be support groups that could provide some kind of help in the short term while supportive networks are being built, and while health and social care mobilize their own resources. The coordination of care requires a specific initiative facilitated by a community development worker embedded within the clinical care team. Longer-term resilient network building is best started early in the patient's journey. Equipping networks with skills in caregiving and pain control should be routine for everyone identified as being at the end of life. The training needed does not have to be given by professionals, but can be community led, by groups who have already had training and experience in caring for someone who has died.

Box 4.2 Recommendations for changes to generalist palliative care

- Routine use of network mapping and network enhancement for those at the end of life.
- Early identification of people at the end of life, irrespective of diagnosis.
- Linkage to community resource through schemes such as social prescribing.
- Use of service directories of local resources seen in social prescribing schemes.
- Review of every death in an after-death audit, looking for opportunities to learn how earlier recognition of the final phase of illness could have improved outcomes.
- Setting up bereavement peer support groups and linkages to community groups of support and common interest.
- Participation in the Compassionate City Charter implementation.
- Develop pathways to easy access to advice from specialist services through a timely specialist review, irrespective of diagnosis.
- Community development workers are to be part of the clinical team.

Clinical compassionate community skills

For both specialists and generalists alike, knowledge of the interdependency of the different components of palliative care has to be supported by how to make use of this in clinical practice, down to the level of one-to-one patient contact. Assessments of people's supportive networks should be a routine part of assessment. This assessment forms the basis of any compassionate community intervention, helping to identify which sphere of action is most needed in an individual's journey.

Post assessment, interventions can be conceptualized into three categories. The first is for those people who are well enough and self-motivated enough to be connected to community resources. This requires local knowledge of community activity, such as those contained on resource directories such as that of Health Connections Mendip (https://healthconnectionsmendip.org/). This includes resources not directly limited to palliative and end of life care, such as the usual activities and interests to be found in any community. The second level of intervention is network enhancement, a clinical skill that takes practice and expertise. When people's networks show signs of lack of resilience, drawing together resources from the inner, outer, and community circles helps to build resilience and combat loneliness. Overcoming obstacles such as a sense of being a burden, maintaining privacy and dignity, and thinking that support is limited to hands-on care are common issues which will need solutions. The third level of intervention relates to skilling up networks to be able to manage the demands of caring. The medical management of end of life, particularly the last few days, is often straightforward if it is well coordinated. Caring networks benefit a lot from learning the tasks of physical care, which can easily be taught. Generalist and specialist palliative care services should set their services up so that these skills are taught to families and carers as a matter of routine. Not only do services have to set up education opportunities, clinicians will need to make this subject a routine part of their discussions, particularly because the levels of support will change as illness severity worsens. It is therefore an ongoing conversation which responds to caring networks' needs.

Compassionate communities recommendations

Reorganization of palliative care services is dependent upon the development of collaborative relationships with compassionate communities. Compassionate communities rely upon the principle of civic responsibility to care for those undergoing the experiences of death, dying, loss, and care giving. Their formation can be initiated by healthcare services or community and charitable organizations alike. Supportive networks formed within the framework of compassionate communities may contain anywhere between ten and 100 people. This is an enormous community resource that makes a difference between a successful, resilient network that can look after someone throughout the course of their illness, and that of a weak network that results in a hospital admission during a crisis.

A community development programme initiated by healthcare services can add value and enhance available resources and support. This is particularly important for people who have limited naturally occurring networks. Development of supportive networks and community resources for end of life care requires the employment of a community development worker. If this resource is to be available to both primary care teams and hospitals, the community development worker needs to be integrated into the clinical teams. Building relationships and common working practices requires collaboration on joint initiatives. Community development by its very nature cross-cuts multiple organizations and services. A compassionate community initiative functions as an interdisciplinary and participatory activity, helping healthcare services transcend boundaries that reinforce exclusion and limit care.

The last phase of life presents increased care needs and can lead to unplanned admissions to a care institution in a situation of crisis. Nursing homes may take on much of the burden of end of life care. Building strong resilient networks can provide a community solution to this particular problem (Box 4.3).

People who develop strong supportive networks at the end of life establish relationships that last for years (Horsfall et al., 2015). A sense of 'togetherness' that comes from participation in social networks and recognition as a person who is caring for someone with a life-limiting condition, and, therefore, grieving, also helps to alleviate the fundamental problems of social isolation and loss experienced during bereavement (Sjolander and Ahlstrom, 2012). These are issues that adversely impact health in the long term, causing psychological morbidities and increased mortality (Stroebe et al., 2007; Sjolander and Ahlstrom, 2012; Holt-Lunstad et al., 2015).

Bereavement is associated with worse health outcomes indicated by the presence of physical symptoms and increased use of medical services (Stroebe et al., 2007). It has been estimated that bereavement impacts hospital inpatient days, and adds to the cost of healthcare services by between £16.2 million and £23.3 million per year. The same study found that in the long term (2 years post loss), bereaved people were still distressed, and more likely than non-bereaved individuals to be out of work. If we also take into consideration the economic, social, and psychological consequences of bereavement, the overall impact is likely to be considerable (Bonanno and Kaltman, 2001; Valdimarsdóttir et al., 2005). It is not a coincidence then that during the early days and months of death, there is an increased mortality risk among the bereaved—depending upon experiences of caring and circumstances of death (Christakis and Iwashyna, 2003; Stroebe et al., 2007).

Box 4.3 Recommendations for building compassionate communities

- Employment of community development workers in primary care to assist people with end of life care needs in building supportive networks. Their work includes mapping of existing support and setting up new groups where there are gaps and unattended needs. Community development workers can run a friendship cafe, giving people with similar needs the opportunity to network and ask questions. They may also set up a peer support bereavement drop-in session. Healthcare professionals should be trained in supporting these natural caring networks and their formation.
- Community development workers are to be made part of the clinical team caring for people at the end of life.
- Training programmes in network mapping and network enhancement. These should be for professionals and community members alike.
- Community training programmes, such as Last Aid, in skills needed to look after people at the end of life. These should include manual handling and pain relief medication administration, including subcutaneous medication.
- Look for opportunities to support the use of community-led 'what matters' and advance planning conversations within the networks built to sustain community end of life care.
- Develop a directory of resources that support end of life care in the community, and are available to all citizens—the public and professionals alike. This directory needs to be regularly updated.
- Develop programmes that train community members to support the end of life and its care. Schemes such as Compassionate Neighbours (https://compassionateneighbours.org/) serve such purposes efficiently. Community members trained in the use of public resources for the benefit of patients with end of life care needs play similar roles. Their presence helps people to be signposted to the supports they need most. Community programmes also encourage social cohesion and the formation of communities bound by compassion—their members look out and support one another.

Civic end of life care recommendations

> Compassionate Cities are communities that publicly recognize these populations, and these needs and troubles, and seek to enlist all the major sectors of a community to help support them and reduce the negative social, psychological and medical impact of serious illness, caregiving, and bereavement. A Compassionate City is a community that recognizes that care for one another at times of health crisis and personal loss is not simply a task solely for health and social services but is everyone's responsibility. (Kellehear, 2016, p. 80)

The domains of caring for someone at the end of their life are not limited to homes, local neighbourhoods, or healthcare institutions. The experiences of caring are also not limited to solely the main carer but extend through whole caring networks and communities. These experiences are carried through into our wider social domains and activities—our workplaces, schools, places of worship, and countless other social institutions. These social worlds underline and cradle our spiritual experience—our experiences of meaning-making in the face of everyday life and personal crises—and we carry them with us wherever we are. Furthermore, in population health terms, each of us will experience loss and bereavement multiple times in our lifetime. This naturally means we need to find ways of helping and supporting those undergoing these experiences at an everyday level. We need to ensure that when death, dying,

Box 4.4 Recommendations for building civic actions

- Identification of key civic leaders to form a steering committee for a Compassionate City.
- Look for philanthropic, government, and private sources of support, as well as administrative support for the committee.
- Link the steering committee with the compassionate communities programme leaders.
- Create a steering committee in collaboration with schools, workplaces, places of worship, and other public sectors.
- Regularly engage social media and cultural centres to stimulate death, caregiving, and grief and bereavement projects.
- Link the steering committee with key health services representatives (specialist and generalist palliative care) and work within a common framework of community networking using thorough databases and directories of community supports.
- The steering committee will develop a set of action plans based on the Compassionate Cities Charter.

caregiving, and loss visit us that—wherever we are, and whoever we are—satisfactory support will be found in all the relevant life worlds that we inhabit.

The Compassionate City Charter (Kellehear, 2016) is a succinct way of organizing a purposeful programme of civic action oriented towards the end of life. The Charter is drawn from the principles of the Ottawa Charter for Health Promotion (Kellehear, 1999). The key point in the implementation of the Charter is that most of the individual action points need to be part of an ongoing programme. This does not have to be done all at once but plans do need to be put in place to make sure all the necessary actions are commenced at some point. Some actions may be less relevant for some communities—for example, some communities may not have prisons or refugees. In these cases, adopting communities may need to examine what vulnerable or marginalized groups need instead to be considered in their local area. Art galleries or museums may not be crucial in a particular city or town but other cultural sites and activities may be more relevant. Each community will need to carefully consider how the Charter may need to be modified to create the most effective and impactful civic actions that support their local communities in their participation for end of life care.

There is no single right way of instigating and implementing civic action, including use of the Compassionate City Charter. The key component is enthusiasm of a core group of individuals or institutions who want to take an initiative forward. Ideally, as broad a coalition as possible should be involved. This can prove to be difficult with slow-moving bureaucracies or engaging elected representatives when these change on a regular basis. It is sometimes necessary to begin a project on a small scale and gradually expand it to become more inclusive. In addition, what works in one place will not necessarily work in another, which means that each area will need to find its own solutions of how to run a civic programme (Box 4.4).

Conclusion

Academic and clinical textbooks on palliative medicine commonly promote a model of care that is professional led and health services oriented. There is little emphasis on the importance of the role of community and social relationships in healthcare at the end of life (Holt-Lunstad et al., 2015). Given that social relationships are a major determinant of health, finding ways of integrating this into routine healthcare is important for medicine as a whole and palliative care in particular. Community and civic models of action and how these may be partnered and synergized with professional action have been far less common. When the 'social' aspects of care are advocated, recommendations and discussions often focus upon support groups or 'psychosocial' actions that reduce or confine community involvement to volunteer services or small-scale neighbourhood supports.

We have argued that a health-promoting palliative care service—one designed and fit for purpose as a population health model—must embrace a cooperative model of practice and service design that seamlessly fuses the different levels of clinical and community expertise. This means that it is essential for palliative care to realize a cooperation between specialist and generalist palliative care services, working in partnership with local communities, and the broader civic sectors of society that support and sustain those communities. Each individual sector acting in isolation will not work for palliative and end of life care. Rather, the recognition of their inter-dependence, and effective cooperation will enhance each individual part—specialist and generalist palliative care, compassionate communities, and compassionate cities. Death, dying, loss, and caregiving will be a repeated experience for all of us. We want the best for ourselves and the people we know and love. Together, we can do this across whole populations.

REFERENCES

Abel, J. and Kellehear, A. 2016. Palliative care reimagined: a needed shift. *BMJ Supportive & Palliative Care*, **6**, 21–26.

Abel, J., Kellehear, A., and Karapliagou, A. 2018. Palliative care—the new essentials. *Annals of Palliative Medicine*, **7**, S3–S14.

Abel, J., Walter, T., Carey, L. B., Rosenberg, J., Noonan, K., Horsfall, D., Leonard, R., Rumbold, B., and Morris, D. 2013. Circles of care: should community development redefine the practice of palliative care? *BMJ Supportive & Palliative Care*, **3**, 383–388.

Ahmed, N., Bestall, J., Ahmedzai, S. H., Payne, S., Clark, D., and Noble, B. 2004. Systematic review of the problems and issues of accessing specialist palliative care by patients, carers and health and social care professionals. *Palliative Medicine*, **18**, 525–542.

Bonanno, G. A. and Kaltman, S. 2001. The varieties of grief experience. *Clinical Psychology Review*, **21**, 705–734.

Christakis, N. A. and Iwashyna, T. J. 2003. The health impact of health care on families: a matched cohort study of hospice use by decedents and mortality outcomes in surviving, widowed spouses. *Social Science & Medicine*, **57**, 465–475.

Cronin, P. 2015. Compassionate communities in Shropshire, West Midlands, England. In: Wegleitner, K., Heimerl, K., and Kellehear, A. (eds.) *Compassionate Communities: Case Studies from Britain and Europe*, pp. 30–45. Abingdon: Routledge.

Currow, D. C., Agar, M., Sanderson, C., and Abernethy, A. P. 2008. Populations who die without specialist palliative care: does lower uptake equate with unmet need? *Palliative Medicine*, **22**, 43–50.

Gott, C. M., Ahmedzai, S. H., and Wood, C. 2001. How many inpatients at an acute hospital have palliative care needs? Comparing the perspectives of medical and nursing staff. *Palliative Medicine*, **15**, 451–460.

Holt-Lunstad, J., Smith, T. B., Baker, M., Harris, T., and Stephenson, D. 2015. Loneliness and social isolation as risk factors for mortality: a meta-analytic review. *Perspectives on Psychological Science,* **10**, 227–237.

Horsfall, D. and Higgs, J. 2017. Palliative care. In: Tasker, D., Higgs, J., and Loftus, S. (eds.) *Community-Based Healthcare: The Search for Mindful Dialogues*, pp. 123–132. Rotterdam: Sense.

Horsfall, D., Leonard, R., Rosenberg, J. P., and Noonan, K. 2017. Home as a place of caring and wellbeing? A qualitative study of informal carers and caring networks lived experiences of providing in-home end-of-life care. *Health & Place,* **46**, 58–64.

Horsfall, D., Noonan, K., and Leonard, R. 2012. *Bringing Our Dying Home: Creating Community at End of Life.* Research Report. University of Western Sydney.

Horsfall, D., Yardley, A., Leonard, R., Noonan, K., and Rosenberg, J. P. 2015. *End of Life at Home: Co-Creating an Ecology of Care.* Research Report. Sydney: Western Sydney University.

Kellehear, A. 1999. Health-promoting palliative care: developing a social model for practice. *Mortality,* **4**, 75–82.

Kellehear, A. 2016. The Compassionate City Charter: inviting the cultural and social sectors into end of life care. In: Wegleitner, K., Heimerl, K., and Kellehear, A. (eds.) *Compassionate Communities: Case Studies from Britain and Europe*, pp. 76–87. Abingdon: Routledge.

Kumar, S. K. 2007. Kerala, India: a regional community-based palliative care model. *Journal of Pain and Symptom Management,* **33**, 623–627.

Larkin, M., Richardson, E. L., and Tabreman, J. 2012. New partnerships in health and social care for an era of public spending cuts. *Health & Social Care in the Community,* **20**, 199–207.

Luddington, L., Cox, S., Higginson, I., and Livesley, B. 2001. The need for palliative care for patients with non-cancer diseases: a review of the evidence. *International Journal of Palliative Nursing,* **7**, 221–226.

Mitchell, G. K. 2002. How well do general practitioners deliver palliative care? A systematic review. *Palliative Medicine,* **16**, 457–464.

National End of Life Care Intelligence Network. 2021. Palliative and end of life care profiles. [Online] Available at: http://www.endoflifecare-intelligence.org.uk/profiles/CCGs/Place_and_Cause_of_Death/atlas.html

Office for National Statistics. 2015. *National Survey of Bereaved People (VOICES): England, 2015.* London: Office for National Statistics.

O'Mara-Eves, A., Brunton, G., McDaid, G., Oliver, S., Kavanagh, J., Jamal, F., Matosevic, T., Harden, A., and Thomas, J. 2013. Community engagement to reduce inequalities in health: a systematic review, meta-analysis and economic analysis. *Public Health Research,* **1**, 4.

Pastrana, T., Jünger, S., Ostgathe, C., Elsner, F., and Radbruch, L. 2008. A matter of definition—key elements identified in a discourse analysis of definitions of palliative care. *Palliative Medicine,* **22**, 222–232.

Rowland, C., Hanratty, B., Pilling, M., Van Den Berg, B., and Grande, G. 2017. The contributions of family care-givers at end of life: a national post-bereavement census survey of cancer carers' hours of care and expenditures. *Palliative Medicine,* **31**, 346–355.

Sallnow, L., Richardson, H., Murray, S. A., and Kellehear, A. 2016. The impact of a new public health approach to end-of-life care: a systematic review. *Palliative Medicine,* **30**, 200–211.

Seow, H., Brazil, K., Sussman, J., Pereira, J., Marshall, D., Austin, P. C., Husain, A., Rangrej, J., and Barbera, L. 2014. Impact of community based, specialist palliative care teams on hospitalisations and emergency department visits late in life and hospital deaths: a pooled analysis. *BMJ,* **348**, g3496.

Sjolander, C. and Ahlstrom, G. 2012. The meaning and validation of social support networks for close family of persons with advanced cancer. *BMC Nursing,* **11**, 17.

Small, N., Barnes, S., Gott, M., Payne, S., Parker, C., Seamark, D., and Gariballa, S. 2009. Dying, death and bereavement: a qualitative study of the views of carers of people with heart failure in the UK. *BMC Palliative Care,* **8**, 6.

Smith, T. J., Coyne, P., Cassel, B., Penberthy, L., Hopson, A., and Hager, M. A. 2003. A high-volume specialist palliative care unit and team may reduce in-hospital end-of-life care costs. *Journal of Palliative Medicine,* **6**, 699–705.

South, J. 2015. *A Guide to Community-Centred Approaches for Health and Wellbeing.* London: Public Health England.

Stroebe, M., Schut, H., and Stroebe, W. 2007. Health outcomes of bereavement. *Lancet,* **370**, 1960–1973.

To, T., Greene, A., Agar, M., and Currow, D. 2011. A point prevalence survey of hospital inpatients to define the proportion with palliation as the primary goal of care and the need for specialist palliative care. *Internal Medicine Journal,* **41**, 430–433.

Valdimarsdóttir, U., Helgason, Á. R., Fürst, C. J., Adolfsson, J., and Steineck, G. 2005. Need for and access to bereavement support after loss of a husband to urologic cancers: a nationwide follow-up of Swedish widows. *Scandinavian Journal of Urology and Nephrology,* **39**, 271–276.

World Health Organization. 1986. *The Ottawa Charter for Health Promotion: First International Conference on Health Promotion, Ottawa, 21 November 1986.* Geneva: World Health Organization.

World Health Organization. 2020. Palliative care – key facts. [Online]. Available at: https://www.who.int/news-room/fact-sheets/detail/palliative-care

Wright, A. A., Zhang, B., Ray, A., Mack, J. W., Trice, E., Balboni, T., Mitchell, S. L., Jackson, V. A., Block, S. D., and Maciejewski, P. K. 2008. Associations between end-of-life discussions, patient mental health, medical care near death, and caregiver bereavement adjustment. *JAMA,* **300**, 1665–1673.

SECTION 2
Basic concepts and theory

5

A history of public health palliative care

Bruce Rumbold

Introduction

This chapter outlines some of the dynamic networks of people and projects affiliated with the field we now call public health palliative care (PHPC). Rather more than an academic or practice discipline, PHPC can be better appreciated in historical terms as a social movement within the wider palliative care field itself. PHPC is interested in reforming not only specific systems of end of life care but also the societies that support them. Social movements have ambitious aims, and people participate in them because the ideas and approaches being promoted make sense of their experience, or give shape and substance to their discontents and aspirations, and offer options for practical action (Blumer, 1994). Social movements invite people's allegiance as well as interest. Any story about a social movement concerns the actors as well as the ideas they bring, the responsiveness or resistance of the hearers, and the activities that result (Krinsky and Crossley, 2014). In what follows I will indicate how collaborative relationships as well as common interests have shaped the PHPC story so far.

As will soon become evident, the overall story of PHPC contains various accounts that ideally should be told by different narrators. The story here follows the beginnings in Australia of what has become, through its international spread, the PHPC movement. I track its growth through the collaborations reported at the international conferences that began in 2009, and reflect upon its coordination through the PHPCI Council. There is already extensive documentation of many of these collaborations. I make no attempt to review all of this literature, but will rather point to sources where it may be found.

The core texts of the PHPC movement—*Health Promoting Palliative Care* (HPPC) (Kellehear, 1999a) and *Compassionate Cities* (Kellehear, 2005)—come from work undertaken at La Trobe University, Melbourne, Australia, at the turn of the current century. As this volume shows, these foundational models have been supplemented and enriched as other strands of knowledge and experience have been woven in over the past decade in particular. This richness and diversity will be needed in the decade to come as global societies undergo fundamental change not only through the aftermath of the coronavirus disease 2019 (COVID-19) pandemic but also the continuing impact of climate change, of which the pandemic is but one instance. At the moment, however, it is the pandemic that has brought to public consciousness the importance of an ethic of the common good in order to live with social change. This ethic is integral to PHPC practice. I believe that the approaches to care foreshadowed in PHPC strategies such as compassionate cities and compassionate communities will be fundamental to building societies of the future, not just in order to provide end of life care but to maintain a viable social fabric in the face of radical disruption.

Beginnings: health-promoting palliative care

The hospice movement engaged with one version of public health in the 1980s as hospice programmes around the world, in search of reliable continuing funding, and hoping to expand the reach of their programmes, began to negotiate a place within their national healthcare systems. The details of these negotiations depended on the nature of those health systems, but common features were the requirement that hospices justify their processes and measure their outcomes in the terms set by each healthcare system, adjust their staffing profiles to resemble those of other healthcare disciplines, and see their local communities less as collaborators and more as consumers.

Palliative care emerged from this 'mainstreaming' of hospice care (Rumbold, 1998) and began to embed end of life care within healthcare systems, securing funding and extending access. But it also marginalized aspects that had been central to the hospice approach, particularly the contribution of local communities, and gave priority to clinical care over social and civic dimensions of care. It failed to capture what had been key aspects of the earlier hospice movement—its accountability to and reliance upon practical support from local communities. Comparing the healthcare discipline of palliative care with the hospice movement from which it emerged, Allan Kellehear (1999a) identified, as underdeveloped areas in palliative care, social science and public health perspectives, social and spiritual aspects of care, early-stage care, and care for those with life-threatening (not just terminal) illness. He argued that a more comprehensive way of bringing hospice into the healthcare system would be to use a new public health, not solely a health services, framework. In *Health Promoting Palliative Care* (Kellehear, 1999a), he shows how this might be carried out, and how a public health framework could restore aspects of care marginalized through mainstreaming. He used the foundational health promotion framework, the Ottawa Charter (World Health Organization (WHO), 1986), which in dialogue with the hospice tradition and its goal of health at the end of life manifested in a good death, and hence created the core strategies of HPPC:

1. *Facilitate education* and information for health, dying, death, and loss.
2. *Facilitate social supports* both personal and community.
3. *Develop personal skills* that add value to people's ability to cope and develop alongside their experiences of dying, death, and loss.
4. *Encourage palliative care services* to re-orientate towards health promotion rather than simply confine themselves to clinical service offerings.
5. *Combat death-denying health policies* and attitudes in the general community, media, and community health colleagues and services.

It's important to note that this model was developed during a key transition for palliative care in Victoria, Australia. The state government had agreed to fund palliative care as an integral part of the healthcare system. It had decided to tender services for all eight health regions in order to standardize the various community-based programmes that had developed over the previous decade or so and redefine service boundaries to ensure state-wide coverage. Inevitably this process disrupted the existing programmes. Some found themselves in competition over territory, while all needed to revise their service models to meet the conditions of the tender. Consequences included competition between services that had previously collaborated, and reorientation of accountability from local communities towards central government.

This was the context in which Allan Kellehear devised the HPPC model and approached the Victorian Department of Health to fund a Palliative Care Unit at La Trobe University that would implement the initial vision of HPPC. His advocacy resulted in 3 years of project funding on the directive of the minister, who overrode advisors who saw this public health approach as incommensurate with the new palliative care system they had just devised. The Unit was commissioned to undertake service, teaching, and research (Kellehear, 1999b), and the selection of the staff and design of the programme was targeted towards the underdeveloped areas of the health services approach to palliative care. Allan was appointed as professor of palliative care. I was half-time lecturer alongside my continuing position in practical theology with the Melbourne College of Divinity. A health promotion position was shared between two cancer survivors with recent lived experience of serious illness. The Unit offered a health promotion and education programme, 'Life Support', for people living with life-threatening illness, subjects in social approaches to dying, death, and grief at both undergraduate and postgraduate level, and a range of bespoke training opportunities for palliative care staff and community groups. Allan engaged with the palliative care system at a range of levels in advocacy, training, and policy development. Our research interests at first focused on further conceptual development of a public health approach, and findings were communicated through academic publications, media appearances, and more accessible publications such as newspaper columns and edited narrative collections.

Reception of the model and programme by palliative care practitioners was mixed. Some saw HPPC as diverting attention from the clinical services believed to be the core business of palliative care, with a few arguing that 'we're already doing this'. Others saw value in the emphasis on community engagement but found no capacity within their service to adopt the model. A few pointed to a lack of evidence supporting HPPC initiatives: there was at that stage very little attention paid to consumer perspectives on the care received. Others again, however, found that the HPPC model articulated concerns about the transition they were experiencing as palliative care practitioners, and some of these began to develop local strategies to engage their communities. And, in some instances, the enthusiasm they brought to these innovations provoked the scepticism of colleagues: social movements can evoke resistance as much as they attract.

At the end of the 3-year project period, the La Trobe University Unit received recurrent funding support from government, enabling expansion of both the teaching and service programmes. Our health promotion work shifted so that we were less providers, more facilitators, supporting practitioners to develop HPPC as part of their own programmes. In 2003, the Victorian Department of Health funded a 4-year programme, 'Strengthening Palliative Care in Victoria through Health Promotion', which allowed the Unit to support and mentor part-time health promotion workers in three regional palliative care services to develop HPPC programmes appropriate to each region. One project struggled to establish itself, due in part to several unanticipated changes in the health promotion role: although in introducing some key workers to HPPC the project shaped their ongoing contribution to palliative care in Victoria and beyond. Another project based in a community health centre managed to embed HPPC criteria in quality assurance tools. A third, in the Hume Region, became a demonstration project as a result of the diversity and reach of the community collaborations it was able to elicit (Kellehear and Young, 2007; Salau et al., 2007). Strategies and resources developed by the team in the Hume Region have permeated widely both nationally and internationally. The project ultimately was not sustainable in its own region due to the illness of key players and because—ironically—a new state government palliative care funding model made it impossible to maintain the service's health promoting structure. Nevertheless, demonstration projects were important in helping stimulate practical expressions of HPPC ideas in a number of locations elsewhere in Australia and overseas.

The story of the first 10 years of work in Australia is outlined in more detail in the proceedings of the first international conference (Rumbold, 2012b). I have gone into some detail about the Strengthening Palliative Care project because the paradigmatic nature of the Hume Region response provided some fascinating examples of community partnerships, developed strategies and tools that are now widely used around the globe, and clarified many issues involved in implementing the HPPC approach. But the Strengthening Palliative Care project experience overall also points to the vulnerability of project-based implementation, both in terms of effectiveness and sustainability. Since then, the Unit has facilitated other multisite projects, with similar outcomes: some sites experience unanticipated disruption due to external organizational factors or events in key workers' lives; others produce new possibilities and insights. In the latter case, a key factor is nearly always the involvement of one or more champions, people with a clear vision and vocational commitment to the work. Published accounts are inevitably biased towards what has worked rather than what hasn't. Now that there is a decade or more of publications and conference reports on HPPC projects, it is evident that some have flourished, while others have failed to thrive. How many more—as with aspects of the Strengthening Palliative Care project—have not made it to publication at all?

The mixed reception of HPPC among palliative care practitioners has already been mentioned, but it was soon evident that palliative care services receptive to HPPC and wishing to implement it found a similarly varied response within their local communities. There were always people interested in and willing to be engaged with end of life issues, but often they needed more support than services were able to provide. Sometimes community groups that might have been able to provide that support did not see end of life issues as their business. From a public health perspective, therefore, the question arises as to what sort of community will see end of life care as everyone's concern? What sort of community will partner with palliative care and other end of life services, rather than simply expect professional services to meet all needs when they arise (and find that expectation impossible)? This of course points to the classic public health strategy of healthy settings, and Allan used this in a second book, *Compassionate Cities* (Kellehear, 2005), which applies the healthy settings/healthy cities model put forward by the WHO in 1980 to end of life issues. As with HPPC, he stresses that health must address dying and grieving. He also assumed that compassion, the fundamental social emotion as Nussbaum (1996) calls it, will connect citizens in mutual concern. Clearly, compassion is strongly linked with social inclusion, a fundamental determinant of health. As is typically the case with the asset-based approach of PHPC, compassion reframes the problem-based literature on social exclusion in terms of social inclusion.

UK engagement

For much of the first decade of this century HPPC literature came mainly from Australia. Even that was sparse, as proponents here were focused more on implementing ideas than writing about them. Nevertheless, some UK colleagues, sociologists, and palliative care practitioners for the most part, were aware of this HPPC literature, and its relevance was heightened as the National Health Service (NHS) developed a framework for high-quality care of all adults approaching the end of life. The strategy, launched in 2008 (Department of Health, 2008a), drew upon the experience of voluntary hospices that had operated since the late 1960s; the NHS End of Life Care Programme (2004–2007) that had developed tools such as the Gold Standard Framework for primary care and the Liverpool Care Pathway for the last days of life; the Marie Curie Delivering Choice programme which took a whole system approach to end of life care; and a series of innovative practice projects that offered their insights to the consultation. The strategy was developed under the leadership of the clinical leads of the End of Life Care Pathway groups of all 12 English strategic health regions.

The NHS strategy made no reference to public health approaches, but it did point consistently to the role of community in supporting quality end of life care. This in turn led to the formation of Dying Matters (http://www.dyingmatters.org), a wide-ranging coalition of public, private, and voluntary organizations, led by the National Council for Palliative Care, with a brief to 'support changing attitudes and behaviours in society towards dying, death and bereavement'. This information and resource-sharing site continues to have a major role in supporting community-based practice.

The practical introduction of public health approaches to frame community practice in the UK clearly required a catalyst and Allan Kellehear filled that role. When he left La Trobe University for the University of Bath to take up a chair and the position of director of the Centre for Death and Society (CDAS) in late 2006, he was renewing links with the well-established sociology of death and dying network in the UK more than the palliative care sector. The emphasis on caring communities in the national End of Life Strategy, however, prompted various palliative care leaders to invite him to speak at conferences, consultations, and symposia. It became clear at these events that many people had read the HPPC texts, and were interested in the ideas, but needed something more to facilitate action. For potential activists, Allan's public oratory provided that something more, while the act of gathering together to hear Allan speak enabled participants to identify fellow travellers and explore possibilities for collaboration. Some of these encounters helped catalyse or consolidate significant projects in England and Scotland including later policy developments in those countries in both palliative care and public health (National Palliative and End of Life Care Partnership, 2015; Scottish Public Health Network, 2015; NHS Shetland, 2019).

One of these was the Good Death project, led by Professor Edwin Pugh, one of the early clinical leads involved in the End of Life Care Strategy, in partnership with North East Public Health and Teesside University Compassionate Communities Unit (Conway, 2012). Citizens' consultations over a 3-month period were the basis for developing a Good Death Charter that outlined proposals for the kind of care and support that people who are dying, their families, and their carers should expect to receive. The Charter was intended to guide health, social care, voluntary groups, and others who plan and provide end of life care or support (https://www.dyingmatters.org/news/nhs-north-east-publishes-good-death-time-think). The Teesside University Unit oversaw and evaluated implementation.

Another sort of initiative in the UK emerged as the Murray Hall Community Trust recognized in the HPPC model synchronicity with their work with chronically and terminally people across the life course in marginalized communities in the midlands. The Trust adopted a compassionate communities framework, identified common ground in a range of other projects across the UK (Barry and Patel, 2013), and has continued to provide a lead in developing the movement through the national charity Compassionate Communities UK (https://www.compassionate-communitiesuk.co.uk).

The shifting terminology in these last two paragraphs points to another factor contributing to the interest in PHPC, naming compassion as the ethical imperative underlying a public health approach. While the Hume Region team in Australia had begun to use the term 'compassionate communities' to describe their community development work, it was not until a few years later that this became a common descriptor for HPPC practice, particularly in England. A possible explanation for adopting the term is that interest in compassionate care linked PHPC with other contemporary discussions of compassion (Rumbold, 2012a). One of these was the NHS enquiry that identified compassion as absent from care in mid-Staffordshire, and the subsequent naming of compassion as a core value in the NHS Next Stage Final Review (Department of Health, 2008b) and then the NHS Constitution. The other, more global conversation arose from Karen Armstrong's 2008 Charter for Compassion (https://charterforcompassion.org/charter) that was promoted both to neighbourhood groups and national governments around this time.

Scotland pursued a path parallel to developments in England, but the Scottish Government's *Living and Dying Well: A National Action Plan for Palliative and End of Life Care in Scotland* (NHS Scotland, 2008) reflected the overall intention of NHS Scotland that healthcare incorporate community consultation and co-design. The authors of *Living and Dying Well* were explicit about 'the exploration of ideas and issues for addressing palliative and end of life care from a public health and health promotion perspective' and set up a working group to do this under the leadership of Scott Murray, a Professor of General Practice at the University of Edinburgh. Scott had encountered HPPC in a visit to Melbourne, and invited Allan to present at a working group conference in Edinburgh in 2009 which generated enthusiasm and support to adopt HPPC as a response to the public health goal of *Living and Dying Well* (Haraldsdottir et al., 2010). Scotland has thus developed an effective integration of health and community care, with Scott Murray continuing to provide leadership in Scotland and at a global level on the integration of palliative care and community experience in primary care.

Allan's keynote presentation at a 'Help the Hospices' (now Hospice UK) conference led to an encounter that has had an enduring impact on the PHPC movement. Suresh Kumar—a palliative care doctor from India—introduced himself after the presentation and invited Allan to India to see the Neighbourhood Network programme in Calicut (Kozhikode) that he'd designed and led since 2004. Suresh had not previously encountered PHPC literature, but his programme already implemented the core ideas and values of a compassionate communities approach (Kumar, 2012). Allan's visit in 2008 led Allan, Suresh, and Libby Sallnow, who had undertaken an earlier palliative medicine residency with Suresh, to the idea of holding an international conference in Calicut, both to make the Neighbourhood Network programme more widely known and to focus the interest in public health approaches that was now coming from many parts of the globe.

In the UK, the 3 years leading up to the first international conference had been particularly productive for public health approaches to end of life care. Policy frameworks provided by NHS England and NHS Scotland facilitated collaborations as practitioners saw the potential for developing compassionate communities approaches or recognized that they were already engaged in some respects in public health approaches. These policies also saw palliative medicine more involved than it had been in Australia, and ensured early adoption of public health strategies and development of resources by peak bodies. Research networks were set up across a range of government and third-sector services and universities. Not all the early UK initiatives outlined by Conway (2012) have survived, but many more have subsequently emerged and become sustainable through affiliation with Compassionate Communities UK and Public Health Palliative Care International (PHPCI).

The way public health approaches to palliative care have been transmitted and implemented shows that the PHPC story is a story about a social movement: the networks that formed in Australia, and even more so in the UK, can be seen as a collective arising from unrest or dissatisfaction with the status quo of palliative care and a desire for a new way of being, leading to collective action designed to bring about societal change (Brown et al., 2004). Allan Kellehear has been a node in most of these networks, but as a leader who catalyses the multiple initiatives, not one who attempts either to create or manage them. The strength of compassionate communities as a social movement is its capacity to mobilize innovative action in end of life care, as did the hospice movement before it. And herein lies one of the current challenges to PHPC: how to bring about societal change without being constrained by processes like those that saw hospice mainstreamed and captured within healthcare systems.

As the first international conference was held, the emerging field of PHPC was taking shape around several themes:

- PHPC is a practice, a body of knowledge, an aspiration or intention that draws upon many strands of prior knowledge and practice, and provides a conceptual frame that validates and permits new approaches to end of life care.
- It provides a radical critique of palliative care. It sees its origins in the hospice movement that catalysed diverse community developments in end of life care at the edges of health systems of the day. It seeks to reclaim aspects lost as those community projects were drawn into mainstream health.
- It also provides a radical critique of traditional public health ideas by insisting that the organized effort of care must include the experiences of death, dying, and grief and loss.
- It provides a radical critique of traditional public health ideas by insisting that the organized effort of care must include community and not just professional, government-endorsed health services, and not merely for those in good health or transitory ill health. A distinctive characteristic of PHPC is that it includes care in all its civic dimensions (Karapliagou et al., 2018, p. 1).

International conferences and development of public health palliative care

Over the past decade, the international conferences have provided a way to track the development of PHPC in terms of both geographical and conceptual reach. Noonan and colleagues (2020) have mapped the conference themes and on this basis projected the next decade's conceptual and practice developments. Here, I want rather to focus on the participants, particularly on the way successive conferences have linked new people with different backgrounds of practice and enquiry into the PHPC movement. It would also be possible to identify occasional or declining connection with the movement, but the focus here is on engagement that has been sustained.

Calicut, Kerala, India, 2009

The first international conference, set up largely by invitation from the organizers Allan, Libby, and Suresh, highlighted the Neighbourhood Networks model, and provided an overview of practice in various parts of the world (Sallnow et al., 2012). The majority of participants came from projects or programmes already mentioned in the story, but a few delegates from Africa and South America also attended. In essence, the conference showcased possibility, through the various initiatives outlined in the overview, but most powerfully through its setting. The Neighbourhood Network demonstrated an end of life programme embedded in the community, with collaboration between community groups and healthcare providers intrinsic to its operation. For us first-world participants, the contrast with our healthcare-centric Western palliative care models was both confronting and exciting. It was inspiring to see fundraising driven by schoolchildren, neighbourhoods cooperating to employ a nurse, and opioids collected from the local corner store.

Another important initiative that was beginning to take shape at this time in New South Wales, Australia, was a partnership between the Home Hospice programme (presented in Kerala by Manion et al., 2012) and Western Sydney University (WSU). A grant from Cancer Council NSW in 2008 not only evaluated Home Hospice performance but proceeded more generally to look at informal care networks supporting people to die in place. A salient feature was that participants were recruited through the community, not through health services: the project studied natural networks where health services contributed to, but did not manage, overall care. This project produced the *Bringing Our Dying Home* report (Horsfall et al., 2011), and the work was further expanded through an Australian Research Council Grant awarded in May 2011. John Rosenberg, currently President of PHPCI, joined the research team for the Australian Research Council project, which produced the *End of Life at Home: Co-Creating an Ecology of Care* report (Horsfall et al., 2015) as well as a number of peer-reviewed articles. The social network enhancement studies of the WSU 'Caring at the end of life' group have influenced and informed many subsequent community development programmes.

A further Australian initiative emerging in 2010 was the GroundSwell Project (https://www.thegroundswellproject.com/) set up to facilitate community-based creative arts explorations of end of life themes. Three months after their chance meeting on a Melbourne street, Kerrie Noonan, a participant in Kerala and a member of the WSU team, and Peta Murray, an arts and health academic and playwright, launched the not-for-profit organization that continues to provide education, project support, and advocacy in partnership with a range of civic, educational, and business groups.

Dhaka, Bangladesh, 2011

The second conference in Dhaka in 2011 was designed by the local conference committee as an intervention to support establishing palliative care in Bangladesh, with a significant proportion of the programme presenting clinical practice issues relevant to the emerging national system. Among the small international contingent was a group from Limerick, Ireland, who lobbied successfully to host the third conference in 2013. Staff at Milford Hospice, Limerick, had found in HPPC an approach consistent with their existing practice and their aspirations, exploring it further with Allan and also with me in a 2010 visit when their project design was well advanced. Their compassionate communities project had started in 2011 (McLoughlin and Ratigan, 2016) and their widely used animated promotion video 'Bill United' premiered at the Dhaka conference. Dhaka also saw the first public presentation of the Western Sydney University social networks project outlined previously.

Meanwhile, back in the UK, another project exploring a local solution to community care at the end of life was being developed by Julian Abel, a palliative care physician with Weston Hospice and the Weston Area Health Trust, in collaboration with colleagues in CDAS Bath (Abel et al., 2011). Julian had been in contact with Allan prior to the latter's departure to Dalhousie University, Nova Scotia, Canada, in 2011 and had become aware of the social networks project at WSU. He and a colleague made a trip to Australia late in 2012 to explore network enhancement with WSU and visit the La Trobe University Unit, leading to the circles of care model (Abel et al., 2013) being presented in an article involving Weston, CDAS, WSU, and La Trobe staff. Julian's affiliation with the PHPC movement brought not only further links into palliative medicine networks, but his strong background as an activist and advocate for social renewal. His subsequent partnership with Allan has had not only national, but global influence in advancing the PHPC movement.

Limerick, Ireland, 2013

The Limerick conference, organized and led by Kathy McLoughlin, Jim Ratigan, and others at the Milford Care Centre in Limerick, proved to be a watershed event in the expansion of the PHPC movement (https://phpci.org/phpc13). It was in Limerick that a number of the people who have in recent years become key researchers and advocates first linked with the movement. Further, it was at the Limerick conference that an international working group was set up to develop a constitution that would enable a council to be appointed at the next conference in 2015.

Luc Deliens, with a medical sociology background like Kellehear, was an invited keynote speaker at Limerick, and presented there some of the work of the End of Life Research Group (https://endoflifecare.be/) based at the Free University of Brussels and Ghent University, Belgium. As the founder and director of this group, Luc had already assembled a strong team of social scientists researching end of life care services not only in Belgium but across Europe and beyond. The public health/population health approach of the group (Cohen and Deliens, 2012) complements the conceptual and practice-oriented programmes already gathered under the PHPC umbrella, and the focus on evidence contributed by Luc, Joachim Cohen, and others continues to benefit a number of international PHPC collaborations.

Emilio Herrera, a Spanish palliative care physician with a background in population health, came to the Limerick conference months after founding the New Health Foundation (http://www.newhealthfoundation.org/), recognizing the synchronicity between the neighbourhood support model he was planning to build and compassionate communities ideas. The New Health Foundation has subsequently implemented a major project based around the Compassionate City Charter in Seville, where already several thousand citizens have been trained to provide or facilitate the end of life care of hundreds of palliative patients and their families. The Foundation's approach can be described as integrated palliative care (Herrera Molina et al., 2017), but it is a whole system integration that incorporates practical community care and support, not merely a health service integration. As with the circles of care model, the person at the end of life is at the centre, surrounded by family, friends, personal caregivers, and volunteers. The next circle includes public and private health services. The Foundation has also extended its work to other cities and regions in Spain, and supports projects in Colombia, Brazil, Argentina, and Mexico.

Carol Tishelman and Olav Lindqvist, also present at the Limerick conference, had encountered HPPC through Annette Street, visiting from La Trobe University, and explored the ideas further through their continuing collaboration when she and Olav, then a postdoctoral fellow, were visiting researchers in the La Trobe University School of Nursing. A visit to the team in Hume Region, Victoria, Australia, prior to the Limerick conference was particularly influential for them both. In the weeks before she departed Australia, Carol developed a proposal for a major competitive Swedish government research grant, entitled 'Integrating palliative care, health promotion and public health: the DöBra program'. She, and Olav as a co-investigator, were successful in their application, and the programme commenced in 2015 at the Karolinska Institutet, Sweden, where Carol is Professor of Innovative Care. DöBra (Lindqvist and Tishelman, 2016) used action research methods and pioneered end of life applications of design thinking (EBCD or experience-based co-design) to work with a wide range of partners in the general community including arts organizations, specific client groups such as elder care, and health services. Networks were built across the whole of Sweden, including among Indigenous groups and practitioners in the far north. Olav's sudden death in 2018 was a major personal loss not only to his family and colleagues in the DöBra project team, but also to the extended PHPC community. Carol has also provided the impetus for an informal international research collaboration that conducts workshops associated with EAPC and PHPC conferences (Sallnow et al., 2016).

Also present at Limerick was Klaus Wegleitner from Alpen-Adria University in Austria. As with the other European delegates identified here, Klaus came to Limerick on the basis of common ground between PHPC approaches and the work being undertaken with colleagues in developing caring communities in Austria, Germany, and Switzerland. This work was grounded in a German-language literature on organizational cultures of dying, health promotion, and systems approaches. In searching the English literature, they identified the synchronicity of their approach with compassionate communities and social network enhancement.

Klaus and his colleagues combined these insights to inform a demonstration project that began in 2013 in Landeck, Austria, a town of 8000 residents (Wegleitner et al., 2016b, 2020). The three-phase structure encompassed the whole system of care in Landeck: first, mapping the existing culture of care, including both formal and informal networks; second, collaborating in designing initiatives to strengthen those networks and enhance resources; and third, implementing initiatives and planning for sustainability. The focus was not on palliative care as such, but rather on the systems of care that support people throughout their lives, exploring how these systems can continue to be effective at the end of life. Social networks were shown to create a 'third social space' between private households and institutional care, but maintaining this space involved resisting the privatization of care that splits care between commercial and private provision.

The German-speaking researchers bring further theoretical and conceptual depth to PHPC conversations, particularly around the philosophy, organizational structure and politics of caring societies, analysis of the 'third social space', and framing conversations about care and decision-making as practising ethics (Wegleitner et al., 2016a; Schuchter and Heller, 2018).

Denise Marshall, a family medicine and palliative care physician from Canada, was given a copy of *Compassionate Cities* by a mentor Mary Lou Kelley, who suggested the approach would meet the needs articulated by Indigenous communities in a large Canadian palliative care enquiry in which both were involved. Mary Lou thought it gave an international language, terminology, and framework for what they were doing and wanted Denise's input. Denise says 'It was truly epiphanal for me to read that book. ... it gave substance to something deep within me that I could now name as the essence of what I felt I was missing from my work. In my own personal life I was and am a passionate social activist—and yet, until I read [*Compassionate Cities*] I hadn't connected that part of my soul to my actual work in palliative care' (personal communication, 2021).

Early in 2013, Denise travelled from her base at McMaster University in Ontario to meet Allan in Nova Scotia. There she heard about the Limerick conference and attended as part of her study leave. Since then she has applied her social activism to the Canadian palliative care community, recruiting colleagues and catalysing initiatives that have featured in subsequent conferences, particularly in Ottawa in 2017.

From the 250 delegates I have singled out for attention six people. Clearly many more stories could be told. But these six bring between them networks spanning more than 20 nations and a rich background of research and practice experience. They illustrate how the Limerick conference strengthened PHPC as a practice-based social movement and also reinforced its research dimensions.

Bristol, UK, 2015

The fourth international conference (https://phpci.org/phpc15) consolidated the new connections made in Limerick and showcased a number of research and practice developments around the world. Projects that were beginning or simply being proposed in 2013 now reported on progress, while further projects were introduced. The number and range of delegates demonstrated the increasing reach and variety of the PHPC movement. Among them were 20 Canadians, who successfully lobbied for the next conference to be held in Canada.

Two important organizational initiatives emerged in Bristol. One was the appointment of the inaugural council of the PHPCI, incorporating representatives of key regions across the globe, with Allan Kellehear as chair. The other was the launch of the Compassionate Cities Charter (http://phpci.org/tools), which engaged a number of civic organizations with the conference.

The Charter demonstrates and facilitates an important shift within PHPC, from basing initiatives in palliative care to undertaking projects that begin outside the health system. The Compassionate City Charter outlines the sort of social structural transformation needed for compassionate communities to emerge within that city. It highlights the way public policy needs to be permissive, providing space for civic action, while resourcing the institutions that will support such action. Ways in which the Charter can facilitate the interaction of civic institutions with specialist and general palliative care have been outlined by Abel and colleagues (2018) and Kellehear (2016).

Another milestone project commenced soon after the Bristol conference. The Compassion Project (Abel et al., 2018) in Frome, Somerset, UK, built upon the 2010 findings of Cronin and colleagues

(2016) who assisted local communities by training free-standing volunteer networks to support the most frail and vulnerable in their midst. The focus of Cronin's team was on improving social connection, but they found consistently that after-hours call-outs to general practitioner services or trips to emergency departments declined significantly in the areas where these trained volunteers operated.

The Compassion Project centred on the sole general practitioner practice in Frome that cares for a population of around 28,000 people. That is, unlike many PHPC predecessors, the Frome project is based in primary care, not palliative care. The story has been told in detail in *The Compassion Project* (Abel and Clarke, 2020) in a narrative infused with public health concepts but using virtually none of its terminology! Another of the published accounts also avoids public health language, choosing rather the language of primary care (Abel et al., 2018). The intervention involved rigorous identification of all those in need, not limited by age or diagnosis, followed by care planning and referral to a community development service for goal setting and social network enhancement. This service, Health Connections Mendip, was established as part of the project. Participants were selected by 'clinical impression': that is, palliative patients were part of the mix, not treated as a separate cohort. The Frome project combines capacity building with social network enhancement. The general practitioner clinic works in partnership with Health Connections Mendip, which is operated by community development workers. Health Connections Mendip generates and maintains a comprehensive Mendip Directory, offers one-on-one care planning, and trains and supports volunteer community connectors. Thus, the health connectors (community development workers) are the bridge between clinic and community, while community connectors are conversation partners/promoters of the programme. The research team was able to demonstrate over a 3-year period a 14% reduction of unplanned admissions to emergency departments, compared with a 28.5% increase in the remainder of Somerset.

Like the Landeck and WSU projects, the Frome project illustrates how community development differs from volunteering, and how network enhancement develops existing assets rather than trying to substitute them. These projects also work with a continuing care system, not simply one that has been set up around end of life issues. A distinctive contribution of Frome, however, has been attention to the impact of community development on health system operations and costs, an issue deserving more attention from PHPC practitioners (Collins et al., 2021). And the contrasting published accounts show how stories about the same project can be crafted quite differently for different audiences.

Another important affiliation that commenced after the Bristol conference arose from a meeting between Allan Kellehear and Xavier Gomez-Batiste, professor of palliative care in the University of Vic, Barcelona, Spain, and director of the WHO Collaborating Centre for Public Health Palliative Care Programmes (http://ico.gencat.cat/ca/inici). Xavier is internationally known for his work in developing a population-based palliative care system in Catalonia. He invited Allan to Barcelona for a week, then set up a collaboration to implement and evaluate the Compassionate City Charter in Vic (Gomez-Batiste et al., 2018). He and his group bring not only a substantial record of practice and research in end of life care, but also long-established links with the WHO.

Ottawa, Canada, 2017

The Ottawa conference (https://phpci.org/phpc17) showcased the rapid growth of PHPC awareness and practice in Canada (Marshall and Kortes-Miller, 2018), that has wherever possible pursued integration by 'overlaying' PHPC theory of practice onto existing initiatives with funding and momentum rather than competing to establish new PHPC-specific projects. This approach can introduce end of life care as an integral part of public health work with marginalized or underserved populations. The effectiveness of such approaches that co-design services with their community stands in contrast to those that attempt outreach by extending existing clinical services.

The Frome project was of course highlighted at the Ottawa conference, while a significant further development in global responses to the Compassionate City Charter was demonstrated as a delegation from Taiwan attended the conference prior to the signing of the 2017 Taipei Declaration for Health Promoting Palliative Care (Huang et al., 2018). Palliative care services across Taiwan wish to commit to greater partnerships with their community around matters of social support, public education about death and dying (death literacy), and health promotion for end of life care. The declaration was launched at Taiwan's International Symposium on Palliative Care in December 2017. A month earlier, Allan Kellehear had been an invited guest at a series of meetings with government ministers, members of the Ministry of Health and Welfare, and superintendents of the public hospital system in Taipei. The centre piece for that week-long event was a 1-day seminar and workshop on compassionate communities/cities.

Blue Mountains, Australia, 2019

The 2019 conference (https://phpci.org/phpc119) reflected its Australian location with a strong focus on practical community engagement in the workshops and concurrent sessions. Australian PHPC has been largely pragmatic, and many recent projects are based in local communities in partnerships with a variety of care providers, not limited to healthcare or palliative care services. An arts-based enquiry was incorporated both within and alongside the programme, and plenary sessions included Indigenous keynote presenters from both Australia and Aotearoa New Zealand. Public health perspectives on bereavement had a higher profile (Aoun et al., 2015), and another keynote address reminded us that settings include the built environment—that creating well-being through urban planning and urban design can provide public health end of life care opportunities (Donovan, 2017).

Another theme coming into clearer focus at Ottawa and the Blue Mountains was the way in which a public health perspective can critique end of life projects that have been shaped by palliative care services alone. Understanding the social determinants of health and the way health inequalities arise from social inequalities helps explain the limited reach of palliative care programmes. For more than 20 years, mainstream palliative care has identified the need to engage with unreached populations but has in practice struggled even to include illnesses other than cancer, let alone groups alienated by professional services. A PHPC approach can provide a way forward by beginning in an exploration of the needs of marginalized or excluded groups rather than promoting previously developed services they might be able to access.

Looking out from the conference centre we could see the forested slopes of the Blue Mountains rolling out to the horizon. Less than 4 months later, this view comprised scorched tree trunks, burnt soil, and ash, a sign of environmental, social, and existential challenges to come, including the pandemic that would lead to the postponement of the 2021 conference.

So where are we now?

In this chapter, the growth of PHPC has been described as the emergence of a social movement. As the movement has grown in size, extended its reach, and increased its diversity, it has become embedded in people and places, expressed in cities and communities, and promoted in a range of media both old and new. The initial goal of the movement of reforming end of life care through engaging a community's informal caring networks continues to progress. But the work done to develop community engagement has identified a series of strategies and skills that can be applied well beyond the domain of end of life care. PHPC strategies can create healthy settings using a community's assets and on that community's terms. As these communities change, flexible integration models that link the community's informal networks of care with formal services can adapt to the changing circumstances. The coming years offer opportunity for consolidation of the gains already made by the PHPC movement, but they will also test the movement's capacity to adapt to change as, together with most aspects of our global infrastructure, we encounter the disruption of the climate emergency that is already upon us.

Organizing the movement

In the past decade, some organizational structure has been introduced into the PHPC movement, first through the international conferences and now the PHPCI Council and associated national chapters and related non-governmental organizations. In a little over 20 years, PHPC has grown from being a small group in Melbourne with short-term funding into an international network with members in dozens of countries. While this international network, PHPCI, began by recruiting individual members, it is currently exploring ways in which those memberships can be organized through national networks. For some members of PHPCI, PHPC is the primary focus of their work, while for others, PHPC ideas enhance their work in complementary domains. PHPCI provides a flexible structure that enhances national and international collaborations, supports emerging practitioners and researchers, and both assembles and validates PHPC knowledge and information.

The first two international conferences were held in cities in the so-called global south, but all subsequent conferences have been located in the global north. This global north or first-world dominance was not intended at the beginning: rather, at the first conference the idea of alternating between first- and two-thirds world venues was discussed. To move towards a global perspective and greater inclusion, PHPC as a movement needs to continue to move beyond its current first-world, English-speaking dominance. The international conferences provide a place to begin this process, and various conference committees have already made efforts, through scholarships and invitations to speakers, to include global south participants. There are resourcing problems with organizing international conferences in global south venues, currently mitigated to some extent by virtual conference formats, but these problems could be addressed—appropriately for PHPC—by partnerships between a global south venue and a global north supporter. Hopefully such north–south partnerships would lead to further collaborations and mutual learning around practice and research. As the movement is now creating formal networks at international and national levels to link the increasing number of informal networks associating themselves with the movement, it may be time to consider how strategies for network enhancement apply to the movement itself.

This international network is not only diversifying but changing. A number of the original leaders are nearing or entering retirement, and new, younger leaders are completing their professional or academic qualifications and developing practice and research innovations. With changing membership and further degrees of organization, the movement overall now faces questions about how to balance this organizational structure with the individual and collaborative agency that has generated the PHPC movement in the first place.

Integrated public health end of life care

Social movements typically distinguish themselves from their surroundings in order to transform them. Hence, Cicely Saunders, reflecting on hospice care as a social movement, could say that 'we moved out of the NHS … so that attitudes and knowledge could move back in' (Saunders, 1981, p. 4). In retrospect, the cost of moving programmes back in was considerable—the losses incurred in returning hospice to the mainstream is what catalysed the PHPC movement. But as PHPC has, during its development, operated on the edges or outside the immediate orbit of palliative care, possibilities for convergence, rather than moving back in, have become apparent.

The place where old and new movements meet is consumer experience. For the hospice movement, then HPPC, a key starting point for reform was people's actual experience of end of life care. In both instances, healthcare systems marginalized or ignored aspects of that experience important to dying people, their families, and their friends. One of the ways that PHPC insights have diffused into the mainstream, I would suggest, is that over the past decade in particular, palliative care service guidelines have increasingly sought to take consumer experience into account. They have, however, done so, for the most part, by collecting data from consumers on their experience, or involving a representative consumer on a reference group, then proceeded to design health service responses to those consumer needs that are of central interest to palliative care practitioners, despite the evidence showing that a comprehensive model of care must take very seriously both health service provision and social network support. Although integrated palliative care guidelines acknowledge the need to involve communities and unpaid caregivers, in practice most service models continue to be designed within the boundaries of the health system (van Beek et al., 2016; Mondejar-Pont and Ramon-Aribau, 2019). Sometimes this health service approach is even called a public health contribution to end of life care. For example, a 2016 review of 'opportunities for palliative care in public health' (de Lima and Pastrana, 2016) makes no reference to the approaches represented in this textbook, instead focusing solely on health system responses. In many jurisdictions, this tension between health services and PHPC perspectives continues (Gallagher and Marshall, 2020). Public health approaches in a PHPC perspective focus less upon identifying patient and family perspectives to which services should develop a response, more upon building systems of care that allow active participation of people and their social networks in the care provided at end of life. That is, public health approaches to palliative care pay attention not only to integrating care within health services but also to connecting informal care—a dying person's existing social networks and local community assets—with the care provided by the formal services. By doing this, a public health approach extends issues such as management, accreditation, and governance beyond the health sector alone. End of life care systems, to be effective, must not only recognize this 'patient and social network' but ensure that professional care, service delivery, and policy enhance the care provided by the person's social network. The unfortunate reality of most health service programmes is that they can actively disrupt rather than support this network (Horsfall et al., 2013). To use the circles of care image again, a comprehensive model needs to encourage activists within each of the circles, and partnerships across them need to be similarly inclusive, in order to avoid situations where one part of the system is working on, rather than with, another.

It is important to emphasize that, while PHPC critiques end of life care models that limit themselves to health service delivery, it is not trying to set up an alternative system. The goal of PHPC is not to create another discipline to complement or rival palliative care but to promote a framework that can, through cross-sectoral partnerships, create a comprehensive, integrated model for end of life care for all. This involves reforming existing models of care so that they permit and encourage active collaboration of formal and informal caregivers. In general, the failure to integrate formal and informal approaches to care arises not from an unwillingness to consider this approach (Siouta et al., 2016), but from a lack of recognized strategies to achieve it. Developing such strategies is PHPC's focus, and at present most development takes place within a compassionate communities paradigm. Scaling up compassionate communities projects into system-wide programmes, however, presents its own challenge. Many of these projects have recruited a community, working with groups that are not necessarily representative of the whole population. At its worst, a compassionate community can be owned by privileged people using the strategy to enhance their own care. All such projects should aspire to a population health perspective that takes into consideration the common good—how can insights and assets generated here be made more widely available? And a population approach should avoid hegemony—how can our programme be made available to all?—choosing the harder route of co-design. The hegemonic approach is reflected in a number of current palliative care conversations about expanding services to other population groups without exploring why palliative care may not be an answer to these groups' end of life needs, or understanding why palliative care itself has become so circumscribed. So compassionate communities has shown itself to be a persuasive paradigm for some activists and communities, but still needs to incorporate social inclusion concepts and strategies lest it be another casualty of the inverse care law which states that interventions designed to reduce inequality may in fact increase it as resources are captured by those with the highest health literacy.

To be sustainable and effective, compassionate communities interventions need to take place within societies that aspire to equitable participation of all citizens and whose governance values collaboration and enhances social inclusion. The Compassionate City Charter articulates a civic framework within which inclusive compassionate communities can be sustained, and end of life care finds a place as part of the broader systems of care in everyday life. This shift in the focus of care can be seen in some of the key studies mentioned previously—Frome (Abel and Clarke, 2020), Landeck (Wegleitner et al., 2020), and Viv (Gomez-Baptiste et al., 2018)—which demonstrate how care at end of life is provided by the same networks that have provided care throughout life.

Envisioning the future

If there is one lesson to be learned from this history it is that, to achieve its goals, PHPC must resist the path taken by the hospice movement when it made a principal alliance with healthcare. As the Compassionate City Charter exemplifies, comprehensive reform of end of life care requires wide-ranging partnerships, as indeed does public health in general. Fran Baum asserts that 'Public health [should join with] the voices that are arguing for a return to public policies that seek to promote civil society, encourage an investment in the social fabric of communities, and protect the environment' (Baum, 2002, p. 526). Like public health itself, PHPC has implicit within it a particular view of civil society and of politics, and the partnerships that are needed. It also shares the fundamental dilemma described by Ilona Kickbusch: 'Major health issues and major health determinants [are deliberated] in fora to which the public health community has little or no access, and is not prepared for—such as foreign policy, security policy, economic policy, and trade policy' (2006, p. 6).

I would suggest that, to achieve its reformist goals and to contribute further to a civil society that faces unprecedented challenges in coming years, the PHPCI network needs to open itself even more to the political scientists, philosophers, ethicists, economists, and urban planners (among others) who participate in some of these key social change movements. Ideally this means developing partnerships with other reformist movements that have values in common: movements with policies that put care at the centre (Tronto, 2013), nurture human agency (Nussbaum, 2013), and take seriously the fundamental importance of human mortality, vulnerability, and uncertainty in the shaping of society and culture (Monbiot, 2017).

Preparing for the future

The social and environmental conditions, and hence the healthcare systems that PHPC will seek to address in the future, will differ from those described in this story to date. The COVID-19 pandemic is already changing patterns of work and social behaviour, and has given a new prominence to public health voices and their message that health is everyone's responsibility. It has also, through the stories of bad deaths, consolidated ideas about what a good death might be. Through the social disruption that has occurred, space has been created for people to think about what matters in life—what is a good life—and what sort of society we wish to be, and world we wish to inhabit. The pandemic has, for many, given greater prominence to moral, ethical, and political perspectives that have too often been left implicit in health promotion and community development, and neglected in political discourse in general.

The COVID-19 pandemic has reinforced the importance of public health readiness and the way this is reliant on healthy settings. The interdependent community that is needed in pandemic times must be developed prior to the pandemic. To deal with the future already upon us, ethical action for the common good needs to be embedded in social life. This is the context of the assertion I made at the beginning of this chapter. The PHPC movement, with its ethic of compassion and commitment to the common good, points not only towards strategies to reform end of life care. It also demonstrates, with other partners, values and methods fundamental to building societies able to deal with the disruption that is to come as we emerge from this pandemic and face further, even more pressing, demands of climate change.

REFERENCES

Abel, J., Bowra, J., Walter, T., and Howarth, G. 2011. Compassionate community networks: supporting home dying. *BMJ Supportive & Palliative Care*, **1**, 129–133.

Abel, J. and Clarke, L. 2020. *The Compassion Project*. London: Aster.

Abel, J. and Kellehear, A. 2016. Palliative care reimagined: a needed shift. *BMJ Supportive & Palliative Care*, **6**, 21–26.

Abel, J., Kellehear, A., and Karapliagou, A. 2018. Palliative care—the new essentials. *Annals of Palliative Medicine*, **7**, S3–S14.

Abel, J., Kingston, H., Scally, J., Hartnoll, J., Hannam, G., Thomson-Moore, A., et al. 2018. Reducing emergency hospital admissions: a population health complex intervention of an enhanced model of primary care and compassionate communities. *British Journal of General Practice*, **68**, e803–e810.

Abel, J., Walter, T., Carey, L., Rosenberg, J., Noonan, K., Horsfall, D., et al. 2013. Circles of care: should community development redefine the practice of palliative care? *BMJ Supportive & Palliative Care*, **3**, 383–388.

Aoun, S., Breen, L., Howting, D., Rumbold, B., McNamara, B., and Hegney, D. 2015. Who needs bereavement support? A population-based survey of bereavement risk and support need. *PLoS One*, **10**, e0121101.

Barry, V. and Patel, M. 2013. *An Overview of Compassionate Communities in England*. London: Murray Hall Community Trust and National Council for Palliative Care.

Baum, F. 2002. *The New Public Health: An Australian Perspective*. Melbourne: Oxford University Press.

Blumer, H. 1994. Social movements. In: Lyman, S. (ed.) *Social Movements: Critiques, Concepts, Case-Studies*, pp. 60–83. New York: New York University Press.

Brown, P., Zavestoski, S., McCormick, S., Mayer, B., Morello-Frosch, R., and Gasior Altman, R. 2004. Embodied health movements: new approaches to social movements in health. *Sociology of Health and Illness*, **26**, 50–80.

Cohen, J. and Deliens, L. (eds.) 2012. *A Public Health Perspective on End of Life Care*. Oxford: Oxford University Press.

Collins, A., Brown, J., Mills, J., and Philip, J. 2020. The impact of public health palliative care interventions on health system outcomes: a systematic review. *Palliative Medicine*, **35**, 473–485.

Conway, S. 2012. Public health developments in palliative care in the UK. In: Sallnow, L., Kumar, S., and Kellehear, A. (eds.) *International Perspectives on Public Health and Palliative Care*, pp. 85–97. London: Routledge.

Cronin, P. 2015. Compassionate communities in Shropshire, West Midlands, England. In: Wegleitner, K., Heimerl, K., and Kellehear, A. (eds.) *Compassionate Communities: Case Studies from Britain and Europe*, pp. 78–104. London: Routledge.

De Lima, L. and Pastrana, T. 2016. Opportunities for palliative care in public health. *Annual Reviews in Public Health*, **37**, 357–374.

Department of Health. 2008a. *End of Life Care Strategy: Promoting High Quality Care for all Adults at the End of Life*. London: Department of Health.

Department of Health. 2008b. *High Quality Care for All: NHS Next Stage Final Review*. London: Department of Health.

Donovan, J. 2017. *Designing the Compassionate City: Creating Spaces Where People Thrive*. London: Routledge.

Gallagher, E. and Marshall, D. 2020. Framework on palliative care in Canada. *Canadian Family Physician*, **66**, 642–643.

Gómez-Batiste, X., Mateu, S., Serra-Jofre, S., Molas, M., Mir-Roca, S., Amblàs, J., et al. 2018. Compassionate communities: design and preliminary results of the experience of Vic (Barcelona, Spain) caring city. *Annals of Palliative Medicine*, **7**, S32–S41.

Haraldsdottir, E., Clark, P., and Murray, S. 2010. Health-promoting palliative care arrives in Scotland. *European Journal of Palliative Care*, **17**, 130–132.

Hererra-Molina, E., Librada, S., Angel, M., Jadad-Garcia, T., Rodriguez, Z., and Jadad, A. 2017. The New Health Foundation: transforming palliative care. *European Journal of Palliative Care*, **24**, 122–124.

Horsfall, D., Leonard, R., Noonan, K., and Rosenberg, J. 2013. Working together-apart: exploring the relationships between formal and informal care networks for people dying at home. *Progress in Palliative Care*, **21**, 331–336.

Horsfall, D., Noonan, K., and Leonard, R. 2011. *Bringing Our Dying Home: Creating Community at End of Life*. Research Report. Sydney: University of Western Sydney.

Horsfall, D., Yardley, A., Leonard, R., Noonan, K., and Rosenberg, J. 2015. *End of Life at Home: Co-Creating an Ecology of Care*. Research Report. Sydney: University of Western Sydney.

Huang, S. J., Yu-Chiao, H., Woung, L. C., Lee, O. K., Chu, D. C., Huang, T. C., et al. 2018. The 2017 Taipei Declaration for Health-Promoting Palliative Care. *Journal of Palliative Medicine*, **21**, 581–582.

Karapliagou, A., Kellehear, A., and Wegleitner, K. 2018. The public health end-of-life care movement: history, principles and style of practice. In: Lloyd-Williams, M. (ed.) *Psychosocial Issues in Palliative Care: A Community Based Approach for Life Limiting Illness*, 3rd ed., pp. 1–22. Oxford: Oxford University Press.

Kellehear, A. 1999a. *Health Promoting Palliative Care*. Melbourne: Oxford University Press.

Kellehear, A. 1999b. Health-promoting palliative care: developing a social model for practice. *Mortality*, **4**, 75–82.

Kellehear, A. 2005. *Compassionate Cities: Public Health and End of Life Care*. London: Routledge.

Kellehear, A. 2016. The Compassionate City Charter: inviting the social and cultural sectors into end of life care. In: Wegleitner, K. Heimerl, K., and Kellehear, A. (eds.) *Compassionate Communities: Case Studies from Britain and Europe*, pp. 162–184. London: Routledge.

Kellehear, A. and Young, B. 2007. Resilient communities. In: Monroe, B. and Oliviere, D. (eds.) *Resilience in Palliative Care: Achievement in Adversity*, pp. 223–238. Oxford: Oxford University Press.

Kickbusch, I. 2006. Mapping the future of public health: action on global health. *Canadian Journal of Public Health,* **97**, 6–8.

Krinsky, J. and Crossley, N. 2014. Social movements and social networks: introduction. *Social Movement Studies,* **13**, 1–21.

Kumar, S. 2012. Public health approaches to palliative care: the Neighbourhood Network in Kerala. In: Sallnow, L., Kumar, S., and Kellehear, A. (eds.) *International perspectives on public health and palliative care*, pp. 98–109. London: Routledge.

Lindqvist, O. and Tishelman, C. 2016. Going public: reflections in developing the DöBra research program for health-promoting palliative care in Sweden. *Progress in Palliative Care,* **24**, 19–24.

Manion, H., Manion, G., and Dansie, K. 2012. Discovering options: an Australian initiative in the care of the dying. In: Sallnow, L., Kumar, S., and Kellehear, A. (eds.) *International Perspectives on Public Health and Palliative Care*, pp. 156–171. London: Routledge.

Marshall, D. and Kortes-Miller, K. 2018. Was the 5th International Public Health Palliative Care Conference 2017 Canada's tipping point? *Annals of Palliative Medicine,* **7**, S130–S134.

McLoughlin, K. and Ratigan, J. 2016. 'Join Bill United': compassionate communities in Limerick, Ireland. In: Wegleitner, K. Heimerl, K., and Kellehear, A. (eds.) *Compassionate Communities: Case Studies from Britain and Europe*, pp. 185–215. London: Routledge.

Monbiot, G. 2017. *Out of the Wreckage: A New Politics for an Age of Crisis.* London: Verso.

Mondejar-Pont, M. and Ramon-Aribau, A. 2019. Integrated palliative care definition and constitutive elements: a scoping review. *Journal of Integrated Care,* **27**, 285–304.

National Palliative and End of Life Care Partnership. 2015. *Ambitions for Palliative and End of Life Care: A National Framework for Local Action 2015–2020.* London: National Palliative and End of Life Care Partnership.

NHS Scotland. 2008. *Living and Dying Well: A National Action Plan for Palliative and End of Life Care in Scotland.* Edinburgh: The Scottish Government.

NHS Shetland. 2019. *Palliative and End of Life Care Strategy 2019–2022.* Glasgow: Voluntary Action Scotland.

Noonan, K., Sallnow, L., and Richardson, H. 2020. Ten years of public health palliative care conferences: a critical reflection for the next decade. *Progress in Palliative Care,* **28**, 78–82.

Nussbaum, M. 1996. Compassion: the basic social emotion. *Social Philosophy and Policy,* **13**, 27–58.

Nussbaum, M. 2013. *Creating Capabilities: The Human Development Approach.* Cambridge, MA: The Belknap Press.

Rumbold, B. 1998. Implications of mainstreaming hospice into palliative care services. In: Parker, J. and Aranda, S. (eds.) *Palliative Care: Explorations and Challenges*, pp. 24–34. Sydney: MacLennan & Petty.

Rumbold, B. 2012a. Compassionate care: engaging the spirit in care. *Progress in Palliative Care,* **20**, 106–113.

Rumbold, B. 2012b. Public health approaches to palliative care in Australia. In: Sallnow, L., Kumar, S., and Kellehear, A. (eds.) *International Perspectives on Public Health and Palliative Care*, pp. 52–68. London: Routledge.

Salau, S., Rumbold, B., and Young, B. 2007. From concept to care: enabling community care through a health promoting palliative care approach. *Contemporary Nurse,* **27**, 132–140.

Sallnow, L., Kumar, S., and Kellehear, A. (eds.) 2012. *International Perspectives on Public Health and Palliative Care.* London: Routledge.

Sallnow, L., Tishelman, C., Lindqvist, O., Richardson, H., and Cohen, J. 2016. Research in public health and end-of-life care: building on the past and developing the new. *Progress in Palliative Care,* **24**, 25–30.

Saunders, C. 1981. The founding philosophy. In: Saunders, C., Summers, D., and Teller, N. (eds.) *Hospice: The Living Idea*, p. 4. London: Edward Arnold.

Schuchter, P. and Heller, A. 2018. The care dialog: the 'ethics of care' approach and its importance for clinical ethics consultation. *Medicine, Health Care and Philosophy,* **21**, 51–62.

Scottish Public Health Network. 2015. *Palliative and End of Life Care in Scotland: The Rationale for a Public Health Approach.* Edinburgh: ScotPHN Report.

Siouta, N., van Beek, K., van der Eerden, M., Preston, N., Hasselaar, J. G., Hughes, S., et al. 2016. Integrated palliative care in Europe: a qualitative systematic literature review of empirically-tested models in cancer and chronic disease. *BMC Palliative Care,* **15**, 56.

Tronto, J. 2013. *Caring Democracy: Markets, Equality and Justice.* New York: New York University Press.

Van Beek, K., Siouta, N., Preston, N., Hasselaar, J., Hughes, S., Payne, S., et al. 2016. To what degree is palliative care integrated in guidelines and pathways for adult cancer patients in Europe: a systematic review. *BMC Palliative Care,* **15**, 26.

Wegleitner, K., Heimerl, K., and Kellehear, A. (eds.) 2016a. *Compassionate Communities: Case Studies from Britain and Europe.* London: Routledge.

Wegleitner, K. and Schuchter, P. 2018. Caring communities as collective learning process: findings and lessons learned from a participatory research project in Austria. *Annals of Palliative Medicine,* **7**, S84–S98.

Wegleitner, K., Schuchter, P., and Prieth, S. 2016b. Caring community in living and dying in Landeck, Tyrol, Austria. In: Wegleitner, K., Heimerl, K., and Kellehear, A. (eds.) *Compassionate Communities: Case Studies from Britain and Europe*, pp. 216–246. London: Routledge.

Wegleitner, K., Schuchter, P., and Prieth, S. 2020. Ingredients of a supportive web of caring relationships at the end of life: findings from a community research project in Austria. *Sociology of Health and Illness,* **42**, 987–1000.

World Health Organization. 1986. *Ottawa Charter for Health Promotion.* Geneva: World Health Organization.

6

The 'new' public health

Theoretical origins of public health palliative care

Mark Spreckley and Allan Kellehear

Introduction

What are the academic roots of public health palliative care? Does it matter? A public health approach to palliative care can, at least in one sense, be said to always have existed in palliative care. Palliative care has always exhibited a concern with epidemiological and health services research and a focus on health services designs and interventions. However, the phrase 'public health palliative care' is commonly employed to describe a wider set of priorities from this narrow and older meaning of public health.

This is the 'new' public health—a set of priorities derived from mainstream public health that has privileged social practice methods such as community development, public education, and civic actions. The new public health has also been characterized by an abiding concern with health and well-being as a priority—but not excluding a concern with disease or unnecessary death. There has also been a greater commitment to ethical concerns such as participatory relationships or challenges of access, equity, and social justice. Although these different priorities now commonly exist side by side in the wider health system, they have been late insights in the field of palliative care and historically slow in their professional and policy uptake.

Our aim in this chapter is to introduce the main concepts of the new public health. This is an essential task for two reasons. First, it is important to show how current ideas about community development or social ecology are linked to long-established and evidence-based ideas from the wider field of public health itself—that these concepts are not 'invented', 'novel', or 'recent' untested ideas. Second, it is important to demonstrate that the practice methods advocated for palliative care are themselves widely used and effectively deployed in many other areas of public health endeavour—from health ageing or healthy schools programmes, to mental health and disability fields, for example. We argue that the application of new public health ideas to the field of palliative care is a recent corrective to a long-standing but unbalanced focus on symptom science, health services research, and professional dominance in end of life care.

What is the 'new' public health?

The new public health has been characterized by several recurring emphases within its different work from disability, or drug and alcohol studies, or infant health and dementia care. These are 'emphases' because the new public health is a concern with community and civic actions that work separately, alongside, and within health service systems concerned with disease cure and health service interventions. They are not 'pure' alternatives but different priority sets in the general effort to support health in society.

An emphasis on 'health' and the social determinants of health

Traditionally, the definition of health has been limited to that of a state which is the opposite of death or disease, with health indicators focused on mortality and morbidity. In more recent years, health has been characterized as a positive, polar continuum of complete physical, mental, and social well-being and indicated by measures of quality of life. New public health encompasses this broader concept of health and considers the social factors that determine health.

A diverse range of social, economic, and environmental factors impact people's health and well-being. These wider, social determinants of health include gender, race/ethnicity, education, work, living and working conditions, employment status, housing conditions, proximity to hazards such as air pollution or floods, and access to social and health services. Socially and economically deprived populations experience disproportionately high levels of long-term health problems and death with the prevalence of long-term conditions increasing along with rates of multimorbidity (Blickem et al., 2018).

These challenges cannot be addressed by the healthcare system alone and instead a broader focus on creating and developing healthy and sustainable communities is required (Buck et al., 2018). Addressing these wider determinants of health has a key role to play in reducing health inequalities.

An emphasis on prevention, harm reduction, and early intervention

New public health incorporates a wide range of interventions which seek to reduce the risks to health, encompassing prevention, harm reduction, and early intervention strategies. Primary prevention aims to prevent exposure to hazards that may cause disease or injury, by changing unhealthy or unsafe behaviours and environments and increasing resistance to disease or injury should exposure occur. Some examples of these modifications include the introduction of legislation and enforcement to control the use of hazardous materials, mandating safe practices such as condom use, immunization against infectious disease, and education about healthy lifestyles.

Secondary prevention, also known as harm reduction, aims to reduce the impact of disease or injury that has already occurred, providing early detection and diagnosis at the presymptomatic stage of disease, through measures such as regular medical screening or examination, the wearing of seat belts, or the use of bicycle helmets. These measures enable effective treatments to be employed to stop progress, prevent complications, and shorten the duration or lessen the impact of the disease.

Tertiary prevention aims to reduce the impact of an ongoing illness or injury, to improve the ability to function, enhance quality of life, and increase life expectancy. It is characterized by being patient centred, adopting integrated care pathways to improve disease management. Such interventions such as cardiopulmonary rehabilitation programmes seek to stabilize the disease process and prevent sequelae of long-term impairments or disabilities.

An emphasis on a social model of health (civic participation)

Traditionally, healthcare programmes have adopted a *deficit model* approach to identifying the problems and needs of populations such as defining levels of deprivation, illness, and health-damaging behaviours. These *deficits* are addressed by the design and implementation of curative, welfare-driven services which are resource intensive, generating long-term, high-level dependence. While deficit models are important for identifying and prioritizing levels of need, they may undermine the role that individuals and communities play as active participants to create, acquire, and maintain health their own health.

An *asset-based* approach to health aims to identify those health-promoting or protective factors operating at different levels within individuals, communities, organizations, and systems that are most likely to lead to higher degrees of overall health, well-being achievement, and sustainability. Assets within a community might include existing information sources, social supports, community trust and networks, levels of volunteering, high levels of neighbourhood co-operation and organization, or strong proactive civic leadership. These assets are also sometimes known as social capital—a bank of resources that can be drawn upon not merely in times of crisis but also for the purposes of building prevention and resilience in a community (Baum and Ziersch, 2003). A key principle of an asset-based approach is to tilt the focus towards *creating* health rather than *fixing* it (Van Bortel et al., 2019).

New public health focuses on the health and well-being of the individual and their wider community, advocating multisectoral interventions that create healthy environments, reduce inequalities, and develop community assets that empower individuals and their communities to adopt healthier lifestyles and behaviours across the life course.

An emphasis on 'management' of incurable conditions

A chronic disease or illness is a condition that is slow in progression, long in duration, and void of spontaneous resolution. This type of condition often limits the function, productivity, and quality of life of someone who lives with it. It is estimated that globally one in three of all adults experience older age, undesirable lifestyle factors, and low socioeconomic status and these lifestyles have been consistently associated with the development of multiple chronic conditions (Hajat and Stein, 2018). Chronic illnesses can be characterized by stages of clinical severity, patterns of symptoms, and anticipated courses of progression.

The social and economic impact of such prevalence is greatly increased with each additional chronic condition and is often associated with increased likelihood of emergency hospital admission, in-patient stays, and the need for long-term support.

The consequence to patients includes a deterioration in quality of life, medication adherence, inability to work including financial loss, decrease in long-term symptom control, and increased dependency on carers. For the future, with a growing, ageing population, this high burden from multiple chronic conditions is projected to further increase (Hajat and Stein, 2018).

New public health strategies aim to prevent or deter the onset of disease, reduce the incidence of complications, and diminish the severity of illness. Inequalities in population health outcomes become targets to identify and address. Such measures include surveillance techniques which seek to prevent the occurrence, alter the course of a new disease, and identify those at risk. Equally, the development of comprehensive, population-based strategic plans that focus on the management of chronic illnesses is prioritized. Prominently, these plans include community-based programmes which educate and address the health and social needs of individuals living with chronic illnesses, such as we commonly see for atherosclerosis, or chronic obstructive pulmonary disease.

An emphasis on practice methods

New public health incorporates a systems-based, programmatic approach to health, introducing multiple, parallel interventions that aim to protect and promote the health status of the individual and the wider population. Practice methods focus on disease prevention, reducing inequalities and striving for social equity, while building health system capacity, stakeholder capability and participation, and ensuring efficient use of resources. New public health promotes the utilization and integration of multiple interventions. Multisectoral stakeholder involvement and community participation and cooperation is an integral feature of these practice methods. These include community development, health literacy, ecological analysis, and policymaking.

Community development enables people to work together across traditional organizational and community boundaries by organizing supporting forums, networks, and events that promote community participation and decision-making and address the divisions of social exclusion and discrimination. This collective working enables local health and social care agencies to understand, engage, and partner with the communities, contributing to political awareness about health issues that affect these communities and to act to bring positive and sustainable changes within them (Community Development Foundation, 2007).

Health literacy considers how people find, understand, evaluate, use, and communicate health information. The development of these literacy capabilities and communication skills enables the individual to appraise health information and take appropriate action towards collective health and well-being. Health literacy development may be promoted across multiple settings, including the home, school, and workplace, seeking to address the barriers to access and improve health and wellness for individuals, families, and the wider community (Vamos, 2020).

Ecological orientation stems from the recognition that most public health challenges, such as preventing heart disease by encouraging people to exercise regularly or improve their diet, are too complex to be addressed adequately from a solely personal perspective. Instead, personal understanding and actions need to be supported by more comprehensive approaches that integrate the personal skills with organizational, cultural, and community planning, support, and policy regulation (Stokols, 1996).

The active engagement and participation of communities and citizens in the policymaking process are important for effective policymaking and implementation. Such participation may take place within the context of a school, workplace, or local government (United Nations, 2007). Such practices are key to ensuring that policies are context specific, inclusive, and address the needs of the community or wider population. This form of integrated, adaptable systems approach to public health management is critical to addressing the growing complexity of individual and community needs of increasingly ageing populations with multiple, long-term conditions.

What's 'new' about all this?

New public health builds upon the historical foundations of sanitary and infectious disease control and primary healthcare approaches, by introducing and developing health promotion into health services by way of community partnerships. Public health evolved through a process of trial and error and with developing scientific and medical knowledge, events such as natural disasters have become catalysts for further development. Large-scale events such as war and natural disasters have highlighted the limits to medicine and health services and accented the need for wider community action and responsibility.

The history of public health provides a critical understanding of the field, its paradigms, and its practices. The lessons from public health history enable society to respond better in the future and avoid the mistakes of the past, particularly the reliance on solely professional responses to health, illness, disability, and injury (Beaglehole, 2004). The evolution of public health has created a legacy which is incorporated into contemporary, new public health (Awofeso, 2004). New public health is an integrative approach to protecting and promoting the multifaceted health status of both the individual and wider population, and health services and community resources, to address societal and global inequalities as a partnership for health and well-being. To accomplish that aim effectively, the new public health has drawn its knowledge and application from multiple disciplines, including the biomedical, clinical, and social sciences as well as management systems and advancing technological innovations.

Why is a 'new' public health so important?

There are five important reasons why the new public health is so important to the effective management of health and illness in a modern world. These reasons are that the new public health approach is a better fit with recent epidemiology; is a better upstream methodology for more efficient use of health services; that health as a target for public health services is logically the best form of prevention and harm reduction; that social strategies are best suited for social epidemiological troubles; and new public health ideas present the most effective approach to tackling health and well-being in a holist, systemic way—the approaches overcomes the limitations of pursuing partial solutions.

A better fit with modern epidemiology

In the past, public health was seen as a scientific discipline which studied and implemented measures to control communicable diseases. The dominant paradigm was that by addressing unsanitary environmental conditions this may prevent diseases such as cholera and typhoid. Measures of control included public health legislation relating to minimum standards for drainage sewage and refuse disposal. Likewise, the interruption of disease transmission through improved water filtration processes and vaccination became standardized disease outbreak control measures (Awofeso, 2004).

Today, the scope of public health has dramatically changed. New forms of health challenges are rising, particularly the ever-increasing, ageing population. Individuals are living longer and with complex conditions and comorbidities such as cardiovascular disease, diabetes, addictions, and the challenges of mental health. Other contemporary challenges include the rise in sedentary lifestyles, lack of physical activity, poor diet, substance abuse, and violence. New public health offers a better fit with modern epidemiology, with greater emphasis on preventing or managing disease, injuries, disabilities, and death while identifying the wider social determinants of health and promoting a healthy environment for individuals and communities.

A better upstream strategy for health services

New public health employs upstream strategies such as preventative measures for ensuring that health services are able to meet the demands of a growing population and are not overrun. Primary preventative strategies aim to promote population health and well-being and prevent disease and harm before it occurs. This is defined as an upstream approach to public health.

Evidence shows that investing in upstream population-based prevention is more effective and efficient at addressing negative health outcomes and reducing health inequalities than traditional, more downstream prevention measures (Orton et al., 2011). For example, according to the World Health Organization (WHO), on average, individual-level approaches were found to cost five times more than interventions at the population level (WHO, 2011). Other studies have demonstrated that public health interventions are significantly more cost-effective than clinical interventions (Owen, 2011).

A comprehensive public health strategy needs to include a combination of population and targeted individual preventive approaches. The most effective approach to modern public health challenges will involve looking beyond standardized or evidence-based behavioural and environmental change intervention models that target the root cause of the problem—the social determinants of health.

Health is the best form of 'prevention' and harm reduction

Prevention is about addressing the upstream causes of ill health, based on health creation, rather than the traditional downstream focus on health condition management. Promotion of healthy lifestyles and the prevention of ill health is a fundamental principle of new public health. The increasing focus on health outcomes reconfirms the priority placed on investment in the determinants of health through health promotion. New public health is based on a comprehensive understanding of the way in which lifestyles and living conditions determine health status and a recognition of the need to mobilize resources and make sound investments in policies, programmes, and health services which create, maintain, and protect health by supporting healthy lifestyles and creating supportive environments for health.

For example, consider the use of bicycle helmets to minimize the risk of serious head injury in the event of a road traffic accident. Such a preventative and harm reduction strategy can prevent death and/or reduce the need for emergency hospital admission, surgical intervention, and long-term rehabilitation. The associated costs to the individual in terms of reducing harms to physical and mental well-being, quality of life, and social and health consequences to the individual's social network, as well as the demand and economic costs to the health system can be avoided. Promoting health in this context translates to absolute harm avoidance at best and harm reduction at minimum.

From an occupational health perspective, healthcare staff such as nurses and therapists regularly apply risk assessment procedures and use equipment such as hoists to assist with the moving and handling of patients. The introduction of such health and safety practices may prevent or reduce the risk of musculoskeletal injury to staff with a consequential need for sickness absence and therapeutic intervention.

The introduction of specific health promotion policy and legislation such as the UK Manual Handling Regulations 1992 can enforce such safe systems of work (Health and Safety Executive, 2016).

Social strategies best for addressing the social epidemiology

New public health promotes the integration of community-oriented public health measures working with and for individuals and frequently in partnership with specific healthcare services. Such a collaborative approach to public health is critical for addressing contemporary health needs and the wider social determinants of health. Centralized public health agency interventions have the potential to miss the complexity of local social determinants and may even risk damaging local networks in their efforts to impose public health projects on local communities (Hardy, 2013).

In the absence of locally rooted knowledge, assessment and participation and further reinforcement of inequities among high-risk groups within the community is likely.

In contrast, community-engaged assessment and community development increases the likelihood that health-focused partnerships will address the causes of health disparities while also bolstering support for local networks and existing programmes and projects. By using existing and trusted local community networks, health concerns and policy changes that complement local knowledge and ideas may be effectively targeted (Hardy, 2013). For example, alcohol and other drug interventions have historically targeted individual-level risk factors associated with high rates of consumption and harm, such as personal age, gender, ethnicity, and socio-economic status. More recent interest has focused on identifying community characteristics that facilitate *risky* alcohol consumption and subsequent harm, for which community-level interventions are appropriate (Shakeshaft et al., 2012).

Community recovery is more than the personal recovery of community members; it is also a voluntary process through which a community uses the resolution of alcohol and other drug-related problems as a vehicle for collective healing, community renewal, and enhanced intergenerational resilience. These community strategies engage and impact individual outcomes. There are multiple pathways and styles of community recovery and renewal in which successful strategies must achieve a community and cultural fit. The process involves 'strengthening the connective tissue between those with and without such problems while restoring and sustaining the quality of community life' (Evans et al., 2013).

While community recovery can come from many different sectors such as neighbourhood organizations, health and social service agencies, educational institutions, the criminal justice system, or religious institutions, long-term recovery and community renewal is only possible when multiple sectors are involved (Evans et al., 2013).

Achieves public health 'holism'—physical, psychological, spiritual, and social

Holism is based on the premise that natural, physical, biological, or social systems and their constituent properties should not be viewed as a collection of parts, but instead, as an integrated whole (Smuts, 1926). A health system is considered to be an ensemble of all public and private organizations, institutions, and resources mandated to improve or restore health (WHO, 2007). Traditionally, such health systems have operated in organizational silos and primarily focused on the treatment of patients when they become unwell.

Traditional medical care focuses on an individual's health, viewed as a collection of signs and symptoms that are presented for diagnosis and treatment. Since much of the personal problem is frequently derived from the wider context in which a person lives and works, such an interpretation may be seen as only a partial solution and does not address causation. Such an approach does not tackle the principal causes and wider determinants of health such as socio-economic position, lack of education, or lack of employment, for example. Therefore, by only addressing one of the systems, the medical care approach is considered a partial solution.

In contrast, new public health acknowledges the importance of the relationship and synergies between the individual and his or her environment—the interpersonal, organizational, community, and policy levels of the wider social system. Such a perspective advocates a holistic and community-centred approach, where the individual who needs care is viewed and respected as a person-in-system with multidimensional needs (WHO, 2007). The biopsychosocial approach to healthcare recognizes the complex, multifaceted physical and social factors that determine individual and community health and well-being. Public health holism must address all the systems simultaneously to be effective.

Key ideas of the new public health

There have been seven major shifts to the way public health in the modern world is viewed by the professionals and academic researchers who work in this field in the last 100 years. These shifts have been prompted by recent changes in modern epidemiology and demography and in their turn these changes have prompted parallel changes to our approaches to these 'new' problems.

From disease focus to health focus

Disease occurs in an individual when the agent, host, and environment interact to create adverse conditions of health. Historically, public health was seen as a disease-focused discipline which identified and implemented measures for controlling communicable diseases, such as addressing environmental conditions and poor sanitation. The traditional definition of health, 'a state of complete physical, mental and social well-being and not merely the absence of disease or infirmity' as introduced by the WHO (1948), has in more recent years been challenged due to the unrealistic nature of the definition and the changing patterns of morbidity (Huber et al., 2011). Few people are disease free, because they may live with a viral burden, experience a slow degenerative problem such as atherosclerosis or arthritis, or may be born with a disability, but that does not mean they cannot or should not strive for health. Furthermore, as modern populations age, chronic health conditions become a 'new' normal for millions worldwide. These populations also are able to strive for health and should not be disqualified for public health attention simply because they live with disease, illness, injury, or disability with no hope of cure. In these contexts, health management and illness management are the new targets of public health.

This new definition of public health has evolved, including, 'The ability to adapt and to self-manage, in the face of social, physical and emotional challenges' (Huber et al., 2016). This definition focuses on the individual's capacity to adapt and self-manage, with active participation in health promotion and the adaptation to a healthy lifestyle. This new concept of health also supports the creation of a vision of a health-promoting society, one in which self-management and adaptation behaviours and skills are usual and normal. New public health focuses on the health of the individual and the wider population, and as such, encompasses all community and individual activities directed towards improving the environment for health, reducing factors that contribute to the burden of disease, and fostering those factors that relate directly to improved health.

The health impact pyramid (Frieden, 2010) provides a conceptual framework for observing the role and impact of health-related interventions. In this five-tier pyramid, efforts to address socioeconomic determinants are at the base.

Life expectancy is a key measure of a population's health status and is closely related to people's socioeconomic circumstances. At this level, public health measures focus on poverty reduction and improving education.

The second tier of the pyramid represents interventions that change the environmental context to make healthy options the default choice.

Examples of contextual changes that create healthier default positions include the provision of clean water, elimination of asbestos exposure, and the introduction of smoke-free legislation and taxation on tobacco, alcohol, and sugar-rich foods. Strategies which address risk factors and create healthier environmental contexts include designing community spaces which promote increased physical activity.

The third level of the pyramid represents protective interventions that do not require ongoing clinical care. Such an intervention has less impact on the population and requires reaching individuals and seeking active engagement, for example, immunization and engagement in smoking cessation programmes.

The fourth level of the pyramid represents ongoing clinical interventions such as the long-term management of chronic disease. This intervention may reduce disability and prolong life; however, the impact of these interventions across the population is limited by barriers such as lack of access, adherence and defined outcome measures.

The fifth tier represents health education, either provided during a clinical encounter with a healthcare professional or in other community-based settings. This measure is seen as the least effective type of intervention, as it is dependent on behavioural change, rather than establishing a context in which healthy choices are the default action. An example of this form of intervention is obesity management (Frieden, 2010).

In summary, interventions focusing on lower levels of the pyramid tend to be more effective because they reach broader segments of society and require less individual effort. Implementing interventions at each of the levels can achieve the maximum possible sustained public health benefit. To address the health of a population, all comprehensive public health programmes should aim to implement measures at each level of intervention, maximizing synergy, and the likelihood of long-term success (Frieden, 2015).

From medicalization to civic participation

The term *medicalization* defines a problem in medical terms, usually as an illness or disorder, and subsequently using a medical intervention to treat it. For example, the administration of a vaccination or participation in health screening is seen as the application of medical treatments or surveillance technologies on a population-wide level. Historically, medicalization was conceived as a balance between the patient and the doctor, as the two principal players. It employed a top-down model, where clinicians would treat disempowered populations (Gray et al., 2015).

In recent years, factors such as the diversifying role of stakeholders, the application of advancing technology and media, as well as the higher expectations of better-informed and more involved patients have demonstrated that actively informed and engaged patients have better outcomes (Parsons et al., 2010). Civic participation encompasses a wide range of formal and informal activities, which may directly benefit the individual and the wider population, for example, by participating in group activities such as being a member of a local sports team (exercise) or church (providing and receiving support).

In addition to the direct benefit that civic participation provides to the community, by valuing interdependence and fostering a sense of belonging, it also produces secondary health and well-being benefits for participants. Civic participation improves health by building social capital, 'features of social organization such as networks, norms, and social trust that facilitate coordination and cooperation for mutual benefit' (Putnam, 1995, p. 67).

By belonging to civic groups, participants' social networks expand, thereby making them aware of opportunities to be physically active in their community. Simply belonging to a group can improve health, with formal or informal group membership shown to increase social capital and decrease social isolation among members (Office of Disease Prevention and Health Promotion, 2020).

As a result, these groups may indirectly improve the physical and mental health of their members. Engaging in meaningful civic activities can also help individuals develop a sense of purpose, which may promote further civic participation (Baum and Ziersch, 2003). Measures of community well-being such as improved community health, educational achievement, or local economic strength depend on the level of social capital that exists within a community. A community where each citizen has the experience of being connected to those around them and knows that their safety and success are dependent on the success of all others, needs to be created.

Social capital in healthcare systems is an important factor for the delivery of high-quality, integrated, coordinated, and *effective* care. There are at least four roles for community engagement in healthcare: to determine local needs and aspirations, to promote health and reduce health inequalities, to improve service design and the quality of care, and to strengthen local accountability (Coulter, 2010).

Civic participation is not just about joining social groups, it is also about how involving formal civic institutions and organization such as workplaces, schools, local government, social media, cultural organizations such as museums and galleries, and holding festivals (fun runs, memorial services, music festivals, etc.) contributes, by policy and action, to the health and well-being of communities.

Communities as building blocks for health

Communities may be defined by where they are geographically placed and/or where people share a common identity or affinity. Community life, social connections, and having a voice in local decisions are all factors that underpin good health and quality of life. It is recognized that inequalities exist and that many people experience the effects of social exclusion or lack social support (Public Health England, 2015).

Participatory approaches to community development seek to address the social determinants of health and the marginalization and powerlessness caused by health inequalities. Such interventions are about mobilizing assets within communities, promoting equity, and increasing people's control over their health and lives.

For many people, their contribution to community life is through their work, studies, or religious membership, volunteering, representation, community leadership, and activism. There are important roles for key stakeholders such as in local government, workplaces, schools, social media, healthcare providers, and their partners in fostering community resilience and enabling individuals and communities to take more control over their health and well-being.

This may be achieved by measures such as enhancing individual capability to provide health and well-being advice, information, and support in their community. Equally, by collaboration and partnership with local services and communities, working together to identify health needs and plan and implement community projects as well as ensuring access to community resources by connecting people to practical help, group activities, and volunteering opportunities to meet health needs and increase social participation.

The role of the community plays a central role in health promotion and is a core principle of new public health. The assets within communities, such as personal skills and knowledge, social networks, and community organizations such as workplaces or schools, are building blocks for good health. Community-centred approaches are about mobilizing these social assets—these civic players—within communities so that they may promote equity and increase people's control over their own health outcomes.

From patient focus to a settings focus

According to the Ottawa Charter (WHO, 1986), 'Health is created and lived by people within the settings of their everyday life; where they learn, work, play and love.' The emphasis is on the actual physical and social environments in which people find themselves. This settings-based approach to health promotion involves a holistic and multidisciplinary method which integrates action across all risk factors. The goal is to maximize disease prevention utilizing an environmental approach. However, unlike old public health ideas that link health to the physical environment alone, the new public health envisions this environment in more social terms to include the organizational and support elements of where we work, play, and pray. The key principles of healthy settings include community participation, partnership, empowerment, and access and equity. Action to promote health through different settings can take many forms. Actions often involve some level of organizational development, including changes to the physical environment or to the organizational structure, administration, and management through policy.

Settings can be used to promote health as they are vehicles to reach individuals, to gain access to services and other supports, and to synergistically bring together the interactions throughout the wider community. 'Healthy settings' approaches have been implemented in different ways in multiple areas. Settings-based health promotion has become a central feature of efforts to promote health that recognize the significance of context. Emerging in part from a perception of an over-reliance on individualistic methods, this theoretical shift in emphasis from the individual-focused, health problems and topics based on 'risk factors' to the nature of the system and the organization, is a core part of the new public health approach (Whitelaw et al., 2001).

In practical terms, a number of key features are considered central to such activity, for example, as well as acting to develop personal competencies, there is a desire to act in various ways on policies, reshape environments, build partnerships, bring about sustainable change through participation, and develop empowerment and ownership of change throughout the setting (Whitelaw et al., 2001). Likewise, there is also a need for health promoters to develop new skills, adopt new roles, and work with new partners. For example, to identify a shift in potential health promotion roles from the traditional medical 'expert' to the 'change facilitator' or 'project manager'. Such measures seek to change public expectations of health services and encourage members of the public to take greater responsibility for their own health and well-being. This ongoing process involves organizational development, building intersectoral cooperation, negotiating and creating infrastructures requiring social skills, group leadership, organizational competencies, and project management (Lueddeke, 2016).

From one-size-fits-all to context dependency

The development, implementation, and measure of effectiveness for public health policies, programmes, and other types of intervention are strongly influenced by context. Context is taken to refer to any feature of the circumstances in which an intervention is conceived, developed, implemented, and evaluated. Understanding how interventions relate to context is critical to understanding how they work, why they sometimes fail, and whether they can be successfully adapted, scaled up, or translated from one context to another (Craig et al., 2018). Context provides us with an understanding about why an intervention impact may vary or how far effects observed in one context can be generalized to another. Those engaged in public health projects should systematically incorporate considerations of context at all stages of the project life cycle.

Within the health system, context is frequently described as a set of factors or attributes that can affect quality improvement projects, for example, through the influence of an organization's leadership, trust, or culture. The dynamic nature of context may be observed either in terms of the relationship between intervention and implementation, or between the various environmental factors that might influence it, such as political, cultural, and organizational structures (De Silva, 2014). An example of this contextual, public health management is demonstrated in the prevention of diseases such as human immunodeficiency virus (HIV) and hepatitis B within a marginalized and vulnerable population.

Drugs such as heroin and other opioids, cocaine, and methamphetamine are commonly used by injection and this route of administration has been a major source of infectious disease transmission. This behaviour is associated with crime, social breakdown, and imprisonment. More specifically, these illicit practices and criminal contexts are associated with non-sterile needle use. Methadone substitution is widely used to reduce drug dependency and needle exchange programmes provide reliable and sterile sources of needles. Because of this alternative drug and context for drug use administration, this approach has been successful in reducing the spread of such blood-borne diseases among intravenous drug users. Such detoxification in a healthier context, with follow-up programmes, are effective in reducing HIV transmission and overall rates of community drug use (Surgeon General Report, 2016).

From clinical epidemiology to social epidemiology

Epidemiology describes the pattern, distribution, and size of disease problems in human populations. Its purpose is to help understand disease processes, outcomes, and determine factors in causation. Epidemiology has evolved since the early days of the sanitation era, where the work of Chadwick identified a link between poor living standards and the spread and growth of disease. These early observations formed the foundation of modern epidemiology and surveillance (Awofeso, 2004).

Clinical epidemiology is the science of making predictions about individual patients, applying strong scientific methods to clinical reasoning and decision-making. Epidemiology is a critical requirement for the prioritized planning, implementation, and evaluation of services that seek to prevent, control, and treat disease. Epidemiology is addressing new challenges of social equity in health; this has become an important part of modern epidemiology with the growing understanding that social conditions and cultural background are key factors not only in disease incidence and prevalence, but in access to preventive and curative healthcare.

Social epidemiology is a branch of epidemiology that focuses specifically on the effects of social-structural factors on states of health. The major premise of social epidemiology is that each society forms its own distribution of health and disease. Social epidemiology proposes to identify the specific characteristics that affect the pattern of disease and health distribution in a society and to understand its mechanisms. The central theme for social epidemiology is in determining what the effects are of social factors such as social structure, culture, and environment on both individual and population health. Social epidemiology may contribute to public health by providing the indicators for social, environmental, and political intervention. New public health advocates a social epidemiological approach to promote and address population health.

Social epidemiology also identifies the adverse social outcomes of clinical patterns of disease, for example, depression, job loss, suicide, mental illness, social isolation, and loneliness. These are adverse social patterns of health that are observed by epidemiologists as the consequences and causes of other physical problems. Social inequality indicators, such as education or income, have an impact on access to healthcare as well as on utilization and quality of healthcare in different countries and across variable healthcare systems. The integration of social networks and provision of social support play a key role in influencing adherence to medical treatment, help-seeking behaviours, and utilization of health services and outcomes.

From cure strategies to management strategies

Traditionally, health systems have primarily focused on the treatment of patients when they become unwell. At the primary care level, community-based, first-contact services are delivered by a healthcare professional such as a general practitioner, dentist, or pharmacist. Secondary healthcare diagnostic and treatment services are delivered via a community hospital and tertiary care, via a specialist medical centre. Three important and inter-related challenges for contemporary public health have been identified, including the ageing nature of population demographics, the development of chronic diseases at younger ages, and socioeconomic inequalities in the distribution of multiple chronic health conditions and its effects (United Nations, 2017).

The curative model of medical care is defined as an approach to clinical medicine that narrowly focuses on the goal of 'cure'. An effective cure is contingent on an accurate diagnosis, based on knowledge and understanding of pathophysiology and clinical signs, derived from empirical research on clinical processes. This cure-oriented approach is highly invested in a scientific, biomedical approach to clinical practice (Fox, 1997). In contrast, it is recognized that other important goals exist, including that of promoting health, preventing illness and injury, restoring functional capacity, and long-term caring for those who cannot be cured.

In the UK, long-term health conditions such as heart disease, diabetes, asthma, and osteoarthritis account for the majority of general practitioner, out-patient, and accident and emergency appointments and over three-quarters of all in-patient bed days. Traditionally, this has been addressed by reactive, single, unconnected episodes of care (Department for Health and Social Care, 2018).

In contrast, the proactive management of long-term health conditions seeks to build a partnership with patients over the longer term and focus on supporting patients to self-manage. Implementation requires a whole systems approach which intervenes at community level, including the individual patient, health and social care providers, and wider organizations and agencies working with the patient (e.g. their workplace or family home) (Taylor et al., 2014). This person-centred approach to management means that the individual is positioned at the centre of their care, with their needs, preferences, health priorities, and lifestyle taken into account. Self-management support is a complex intervention and core components include the provision of education about the long-term condition, psychological strategies to support adjustment, methods to support adherence to treatment, practical support for clinical tasks and activities of daily living, and social support. These principles are an essential component to the management of multimorbidities, medicine optimization, and long-term conditions (Boxford, 2018).

Some common examples

The long-term management of an ageing population living with HIV

Over 103,000 people in the UK are currently living with HIV and more than 40% of those people accessing HIV care are aged 50 or over. With the advancement in antiretroviral drug therapy, people living with HIV may achieve a normal life expectancy (Public Health England, 2019; National AIDS Trust, 2022). However, due to the nature of the virus, and adverse side effects of medication combined with the usual process of ageing, people living with HIV may develop chronic, physical, and mental health conditions.

People with HIV are living with a complex range of physical, mental, and social health-related challenges (O'Brien et al., 2014) which may be attributed to the premature development of many complications normally associated with ageing, drug-specific toxicity, lifestyle factors, persistent inflammation, and residual immunodeficiency (Deeks and Philips, 2009). Due to the episodic nature of HIV disease, and the complex side effects of antiretroviral therapy, people living with HIV may require a range of rehabilitation approaches aimed at promoting health and wellness across the lifespan (Gahagan et al., 2012).

The British HIV Association (2013) advocates the use of a self-management approach, which like many other long-term health conditions can help people with HIV to gain confidence, skills, and knowledge to manage their own health, with resulting improvements in quality of life and independence. The design and delivery of rehabilitation services needs to take account of the dynamic and wide-ranging environmental factors and influences that may affect people living with HIV.

Based on a comprehensive knowledge synthesis, O'Brien and colleagues (2010, 2011) developed evidence-informed recommendations for rehabilitation with adults living with HIV, with a focus on older adults. These recommendations included rehabilitation professionals considering the role of extrinsic, contextual factors such as stigma and ageism, HIV disclosure, and emotional and practical social support. The role of intrinsic factors such as self-management and spirituality should also be addressed.

New public mental health management

The term *mental health* is used to describe a spectrum, from mental health problems, conditions, illnesses, and disorders through to mental well-being or positive mental health (Faculty of Public Health, 2021). In England, one in six people report experiencing a common mental health problem such as anxiety and depression over the past week and young women have emerged as a high-risk group (McManus et al., 2016). Mental illness is responsible for more occupational sickness absence than any other condition and is more common in people living alone, in poor physical health, and not employed (McManus et al., 2009).

The impact of mental health problems in childhood and adolescence may reduce educational achievement and employability as well as increase the risk of impaired relationships, drug and alcohol misuse, violence, and crime (Faculty of Public Health, 2021).

The social, physical, and economic environments in which people are born, grow, live, work, and age have important implications for mental health (Marmot, 2010). Poor mental health can lead to a 'cycle of disadvantage' that can impact negatively on the individual and wider community by causing higher levels of physical morbidity and mortality, lower levels of educational and work performance, offending behaviour, and poor community cohesion (Friedli and Parsonage, 2007). New public mental health focuses on these wider determinants of health and well-being, over the life course, and the means by which inequalities may be identified and addressed. This new public health approach views people as active citizens and co-producers with something to offer, rather than passive clients or service users. The emphasis is on 'doing with' rather than 'doing to'—empowering and enabling people to take control of their lives and supporting them to do more for themselves (Faculty of Public Health and Mental Health Foundation, 2016).

A community may be defined as a place or a socially constructed shared identity which is used to describe the relationships, values, identities, and interests that connect people, or a shared investment in a place, movement, or culture (Yerbury, 2012). Connected communities, supported through interventions designed to promote social inclusion and strengthen social networks, have the potential to make an important contribution to mental well-being within the community (Goldie et al., 2016). Such measures, intended to achieve positive mental well-being for all, need to be embedded at multiple levels across communities, including family homes; neighbourhoods, in settings such as workplaces and schools; and from within health and social care practice. Protecting and promoting positive mental health and well-being needs to become a shared and central aspiration thereby ensuring that communities reach their full potential (Goldie et al., 2016).

Ear and hearing health

Hearing loss affects over 1.3 billion people worldwide of whom it is estimated that 466 million people are currently living with disabling hearing loss and 80% of those affected are living in low- and middle-income countries (Wilson et al., 2017). By 2050 it is predicted that nearly 2.5 billion people, or one in four people, will be living with some degree of hearing loss (WHO, 2021). Hearing loss has both immediate and long-term consequences for the individual and the wider community, which includes challenges with communication and social interaction, impaired activities of daily living, education, and employment, poorer socioeconomic status, reduced mental health and well-being, and an adverse effect on quality of life (Arlinger, 2003).

The development and implementation of a national ear and hearing care strategy aims to reduce the prevalence, incidence, and impact of hearing loss through public health approaches that are integrated within the health system and wider community. The strategy addresses the key domains of hearing loss prevention, screening, and management (WHO, 2013).

Many of the causes of hearing loss may be avoided through public health strategies and clinical interventions implemented across the life span. In children, nearly 60% of hearing loss is due to avoidable causes that can be prevented through implementation of public health measures such as immunization, effective maternal and childcare practices, and the identification and management of common ear conditions. In adulthood, occupational and recreational exposure to loud noise or oxotoxic medicines are preventable causes of hearing loss (WHO, 2021).

Early identification of hearing loss and ear diseases is also key to effective management. The screening for the detection of hearing loss and related ear conditions is conducted for those individuals and communities most at risk, for example, new-born babies and infants, workers exposed to occupational noise, and older adults. Follow-up hearing assessment and ear examination may be conducted in a community or clinical setting and once hearing loss is identified, it is important that it is addressed as early as possible, and in an appropriate manner, to mitigate any adverse impact (WHO, 2021). This holistic, systems-based approach employed in the prevention and harm reduction strategies for hearing loss and impairment is characteristic of new public health approaches.

Persistence and change in public health palliative care

The aim of all public health has been identifying the patterns of health and disease, identifying their determinants both physical and social, and developing interventions to address these troubles. For most of public health history this has been performed through the application of the twin strategies of (1) employing surveillance sciences and (2) deploying professional/health service interventions. For much of the twentieth century these two dominant approaches have led to concerns about an overemphasis on disease and illness and the growth of professional dominance, especially medical dominance. The new public health has been a recent corrective to these criticisms by turning our research attention to the social determinants of health and the civic and community assets that can be marshalled to promote health and prevent health troubles.

However, two problems emerged in the early part of health promotion's history, and both of these can be traced to their origins within the longer public health history. First, the public health image of death and dying displayed no underlying nuanced understanding. Death was the enemy. Dying was medical and public health failure. Second, although gradually the health promotion movement within modern healthcare was embraced, there persisted a continual tendency to interpret 'community' in terms of local neighbourhoods alone, or to reduce interventions to behaviours, rather than to focus on structural changes related to power and politics—legislative and policy changes, or incorporation of death, dying, and bereavement into duties of care by businesses, schools, faith groups, and popular media.

These old and new legacies inside the changing nature of public health created a deep division over understandings about death and dying which contributed to the development of the 1960s hospice and palliative care movement. In hospice and palliative care, death and dying would no longer be viewed as failure but an opportunity for a new branch of healthcare to promote health and well-being at the end of life. Dying would no longer disqualify the patient from quality and continuity of care. However, the new specialism of palliative care would continue to take two older views of public health into its new life: (1) professional services would be key to health and well-being for the dying and their families, and (2) communities would be viewed as local neighbourhoods volunteering their time, usually under their professional training and supervision. Social capital became an extension of professional capital, and community assets such as volunteers, the direction of financial donations, or local community energy and activism, became appropriated as health service assets.

Health-promoting palliative care drew on recognition of the social determinants of health as well as the social epidemiology of living with life-limiting illness, advanced ageing, long-term caregiving, and grief and bereavement. The identification of the social morbidity of these experiences was front and centre. Palliative care had long recognized the central importance of health and well-being at the end of life but its achievement of this was limited to the last days and weeks and to the limited capacity of professional services to reach people in these circumstances. The new health-promoting palliative care would reorient palliative care to the importance of building and partnering with community and not just servicing or drawing further care-labour from it. Health-promoting palliative care would expand the idea of community to embrace the civic sectors of work, education, industry, local government, and media, and restore their roles as leader, partner, planner, and participant. These new roles, and for traditional palliative care, these new settings/environments, meant the balancing of clinical methods with new public health ones suited to settings—community development, public education, social ecology, policy development, social marketing, and services redesign.

Practice methods that are deployed in most fields of public health are now applied in hospice and palliative care. The concern with clinical epidemiology is balanced with a concern for social epidemiology at the end of life. The concern for a patient and the family who supports that individual is now extended to an equal concern for the community that must support both. The concern with symptom science and clinical interventions is balanced with an equal concern with for community and policy studies and their interventions. The political issue of professional capital—the education, training, recruitment, and retention needs of palliative care professionals—is balanced with an equal concern for social capital—the public education, recruitment, and retention of a cross-section of civic leaders and institutions that must support the episodic care of formal health services.

Finally, the concern with access and equity must go beyond a sole focus on outreach to one characterized by engagement, partnership, co-creation, and representation. Because a health service—palliative care or any other—is always limited by its own geographical, staffing, and financial resources, partnership is essential. Services designed without their local communities, civic leaders, and institutions identify problems and solutions for those communities at their own peril. One size does not fit all. Overcoming barriers to access, treatment adherence, or optimal outcomes lies in the ability of individual professionals and their services to understand and work with local contexts of caste, class, locality, and social and cultural difference. The extent to which these lessons and insights are learned from the new public health movement will be the measure of the effectiveness and continuing success of the new public health palliative care.

Conclusion

Societal achievements of increased life expectancy and reduced mortality from infectious and non-infectious diseases may be attributed to the evolution and legacy of public health measures that date back more than 150 years (Awofeso, 2004).

New public health eras usually arise when the dominant public health frameworks become obsolete as a result of changing health patterns and advances in health knowledge and practice (Beaglehole, 2004). For example, during the early days of the sanitation era of public health, the association between environmental conditions and their adverse effect on health outcomes was identified, leading to environmental standards for clean water and sewage disposal, and a legal framework for implementing public health interventions. These preliminary events became the foundations of modern epidemiology and surveillance.

Today, we acknowledge that all countries are at different stages of economic, epidemiological, and sociopolitical development and face varied, complex threats and challenges from the environment. A key objective for each government and ministry of health is achieving adequate health and well-being for their populations, within available and limited resources (Tulchinsky and Varavikova, 2009).

There is recognition that the traditional medical approach to managing these global challenges is limited and only offers a partial, unsustainable solution. The new public health has been and continues to be so important to the effective management of health and illness in a modern world characterized by chronic disease management including those living with life-limiting conditions.

The new public health approach is a better fit with recent epidemiology, acknowledging an ever-increasing, ageing population, a context where individuals are living—and dying—with long-term health conditions. The new public health presents the most effective approach to tackling health and well-being in a holist, systemic way working with all stakeholders for the benefit of all. New public health approaches recognize the importance of social relationships and synergies between individuals and their physical and civic environment. The recognition of these synergies and potential partnerships supports an effective healthcare system that goes beyond mere health services to make healthcare, including end of life care, everyone's responsibility. The justification for this more sociological effort is that health is and should be an end in itself, a human right, and a prerequisite for optimal human development (Frieden, 2010).

REFERENCES

Arlinger, S. 2003. Negative consequences of uncorrected hearing loss—a review. *International Journal of Audiology*, **42**, S17–S20.

Awofeso, N. 2004. What's new about the 'new public health'? *American Journal of Public Health*, **94**, 704–709.

Baum, F. and Ziersch, A. 2003. Social capital. *Journal of Epidemiology Community Health*, **57**, 320–323.

Beaglehole, R., Bonita, R., Horton, R., Adams, O., and McKee, M. 2004. Public health in the new era: improving health through collective action. *Lancet*, **363**, 2084–2086.

Blickem, C., Dawson, S., Kirk, S., Vassilev, I., Mathieson, A., Harrison, R., et al. 2018. What is asset-based community development and how might it improve the health of people with long-term conditions? A realist synthesis. *SAGE Open*, **8**, 1–13.

British HIV Association. 2014. *Standards of Care for People Living with HIV*. London: British HIV Association.

Boxford, S. 2018. What works in managing long-term conditions through enhanced primary care services? [Integrated Health and Social Care Literature Reviews.] Cordis Bright. [Online] Available at: https://www.necsu.nhs.uk/wp-content/uploads/2019/02/2018-06-ManagingLTCthoughEnhancedPrimaryCareServices-CordisBright.pdf

Buck, D., Baylis, D., and Robertson, R. 2018. *A Vision for Population Health*. London: Kings Fund.

Community Development Foundation. 2007. *The Community Development Challenge*. London: Community Development Foundation.

Coulter, A. 2010. *Engaging Communities for Health Improvement—A Scoping Study for the Health Foundation*. London: The Health Foundation.

Craig, P., Di Ruggiero, E., Frohlich, K. L., Mykhalovskiy, E., White, M., Campbell, R., et al. 2018. Taking account of context. In: *Population Health Intervention Research: Guidance for Producers, Users and Funders of Research*, pp. 9–24. Southampton: NIHR Evaluation, Trials and Studies Coordinating Centre.

Deeks, S. G. and Phillips, A. N. 2009. HIV infection, antiretroviral treatment, ageing, and non-AIDS related morbidity. *BMJ*, **338**, a3172.

Department for Health and Social Care. 2018. *Prevention is Better Than Cure—Our Vision to Help You Live Well for Longer*. London: Department for Health and Social Care.

De Silva, D. 2014. *Helping Measure Person-Centred Care—A Review of Evidence About Commonly Used Approaches and Tools Used to Help Measure Person-Centred Care*. London: The Health Foundation.

Evans, A. C., Lamb, R., and White, W. L. 2013. The community as patient: recovery-focused community mobilization in Philadelphia, 2005–2012. *Alcoholism Treatment Quarterly*, **31**, 450–465.

Faculty of Public Health. 2021. Why public mental health matters. [Online] Available at: https://www.fph.org.uk/policy-campaigns/special-interest-groups/special-interest-groups-list/public-mental-health-special-interest-group/better-mental-health-for-all/why-public-mental-health-matters/

Faculty of Public Health and Mental Health Foundation. 2016. *Better Mental Health for All: A Public Health Approach to Mental Health Improvement*. London: Faculty of Public Health and Mental Health Foundation.

Fox, E. 1997. Predominance of the curative model of medical care: a residual problem. *American Medical Association,* **278**, 761–763.

Friedli, L. and Parsonage, M. 2007. *Mental Health Promotion: Building an Economic Case.* Belfast: Northern Ireland Association for Mental Health.

Frieden, T. R. 2010. A framework for public health action: the health impact pyramid. *American Journal of Public Health,* **100**, 590–595.

Frieden, T. R. 2015. The future of public health. *New England Journal of Medicine,* **373**, 1748–1754.

Gahagan, A., Ross, E., Mann, A., and Lewellen, D. 2012. *A Scan of Policies Related to Access to Rehabilitation in Canada and the United Kingdom.* Halifax, Canada: Department of Health Promotion, Dalhousie University.

Goldie, I., Elliott, I., Regan, M., Bernal, L., and Makurah, L. 2016. *Mental Health and Prevention: Taking Local Action.* London: Mental Health Foundation.

Gray, D., Russell, G., and White, E. 2015. Medicalisation in the UK: changing dynamics, but still ongoing. *Journal of the Royal Society of Medicine,* **109**, 7–11.

Hajat, C. and Stein, E. 2018. The global burden of multiple chronic conditions: a narrative review. *Preventive Medicine Reports,* **12**, 284–293.

Hardy, L., Bohan, K., and Trotter, R. 2013. Synthesizing evidence-based strategies and community-engaged research: a model to address social determinants of health. *Public Health Reports,* **128**, 68–76.

Health and Safety Executive. 2016. *Manual Handling: Manual Handling Regulations 1992. Guidance on Regulations,* 4th ed. London: HSE Books.

Huber, M., Knottnerus, J. A., Green, L., van der Horst, H., Jadad, A. R., Kromhout, D., et al. 2011 How should we define health? *BMJ,* **343**, 4163.

Huber, M., van Vliet, M., Giezenberg, M., Winkens, B., Heerkens, Y., Dagnelie, P. C., et al. 2016. Towards a patient-centred operationalisation of the new dynamic concept of health: a mixed methods study. *BMJ Open,* **5**, 010091.

Lueddeke, G. 2016. *Global Population Health and Wellbeing in the 21st Century: Toward New Paradigms, Policy, and Practice.* New York: Springer.

Marmot, M. 2010. *Fair Society, Healthy Lives: The Marmot Review: Strategic Review of Health Inequalities in England Post-2010.* The Marmot Review. Available at: https://www.parliament.uk/globalassets/documents/fair-society-healthy-lives-full-report.pdf

McManus, S., Bebbington, P., Jenkins, R., and Brugha, T. 2016. *Mental Health and Wellbeing in England: Adult Psychiatric Morbidity Survey 2014. Executive Summary.* London: Health and Social Care Information Centre.

McManus, S., Meltzer, H., Brugha, T., Bebbington, P. E., and Jenkins, R. 2009. *Adult Psychiatric Morbidity Survey 2007: Results of a Household Survey.* Leeds: National Centre for Social Research and the Department of Health Sciences, University of Leicester, UK.

National AIDS Trust. 2022. https://www.nat.org.uk/about-hiv/hiv-statistics

O'Brien, K., Solomon, P., Trentham, B., MacLachlan, D., MacDermid, J., Tynan, A., et al. 2014. Evidence-informed recommendations for rehabilitation with older adults living with HIV: a knowledge synthesis. *BMJ Open,* **4**, 004692.

O'Brien, K., Wilkins A., Zack, E., and Solomon, P. 2010. Scoping the field: identifying key research priorities in HIV and rehabilitation. *AIDS and Behavior,* **14**, 448–458.

O'Brien, K., Wilkins, A., Zack, E., and Solomon, P. 2011. Developing clinical practice guidelines in HIV rehabilitation: process recommendations and guiding principles. *AIDS Education and Prevention,* **23**, 457–468.

Office of Disease Prevention and Health Promotion. 2020. Social cohesion. US Department of Health and Human Services. [Online] Available at: https://www.healthypeople.gov/2020/topics-objectives/topic/social-determinants-health/interventions-resources/social-cohesion

Office of the Surgeon General. 2016. *Facing Addiction in America: The Surgeon General's Report on Alcohol, Drugs, and Health.* Washington, DC: US Department of Health and Human Services.

Orton, L. C., Lloyd-Williams, F., Taylor-Robinson, D. C., Moonan, M., O'Flaherty, M., and Capewell, S. 2011. Prioritising public health: a qualitative study of decision making to reduce health inequalities. *BMC Public Health,* **11**, 821.

Owen, L. 2011. The cost-effectiveness of public health interventions. *Journal of Public Health,* **34**, 37–45.

Parsons, S., Winderbottom, A., Cross, P., and Redding, D. 2010. *The Quality of Patient Engagement and Involvement in Primary Care: An Inquiry into the Quality of General Practice in England.* London: The Kings Fund.

Public Health England. 2015. *A Guide to Community-Centred Approaches for Health and Wellbeing.* London: Public Health England.

Public Health England 2019. *HIV in the United Kingdom: Towards Zero HIV Transmissions by 2030.*

Public Health England and UCL Institute of Health Equity. 2015. *Local Action on Health Inequalities, Reducing Social Isolation Across the Life Course.* Practice Resource. London: Public Health England.

Putnam, R. D. 1995. Bowling alone: America's declining social capital. *Journal of Democracy,* **6**, 65–78.

Shakeshaft, A., Petrie, D., Doran, C., Breen, C., and Sanson-Fisher, R. 2012. An empirical approach to selecting community-based alcohol interventions: combining research evidence, rural community views and professional opinion. *BMC Public Health,* **12**, 25.

Smuts, J. C. 1926. *Holism and Evolution.* New York: Macmillan Company.

Stokols, D. 1996. Translating social ecological theory into guidelines for community health promotion. *American Journal of Health Promotion,* **10**, 4.

Taylor, S., Pinnock, H., Epiphaniou, E., Pearce, G., Parke, H., Schwappach, A., et al. 2014. A rapid synthesis of the evidence on interventions supporting self-management for people with long-term conditions: PRISMS—Practical Systematic Review of Self-Management Support for long-term conditions. *Health Service Delivery Research,* **2**, 53.

Tulchinsky, T. and Varavikova, E. 2009. *The New Public Health: An Introduction for the 21st Century,* 2nd ed. San Diego, CA: Academic Press.

United Nations. 2007. *Civic Engagement in Public Policies: A ToolKit.* New York: United Nations.

United Nations. 2017. *World Population Ageing—Highlights.* ST/ESA/SER.A-397. New York: Department of Economic and Social Affairs, Population Division, United Nations.

Vamos, S., Okan, O., Sentell, T., and Rootman, I. 2020. Making a case for education for health literacy: an international perspective. *International Journal of Environmental Research and Public Health,* **17**, 1436.

Van Bortel, T., Wickramasinghe, N. D., Morgan, A., and Martin, S. 2019. Health assets in a global context: a systematic review of the literature research. *BMJ Open,* **9**, e023810.

Whitelaw, S., Baxendale, A., Bryce, C., MacHardy, L., Young, I., and Witney, E. 2001. 'Settings' based health promotion: a review. *Health Promotion International*, **16**, 339–353.

Wilson, B. S., Tucci, D. L., Merson, M. H., and O'Donoghue, G. M. 2017. Global hearing health care: new findings and perspectives. *Lancet*, **390**, 2503–2515.

World Health Organization. 1948. Definition of health. [Online] Available at: https://www.who.int/about/who-we-are/constitution

World Health Organization. 1986. *Charter Adopted at the International Conference on Health Promotion, November 17–21 1986, Ottawa, Ontario, Canada*. Geneva: World Health Organization.

World Health Organization. 2007. *Everybody's Business: Strengthening Health Systems to Improve Health Outcomes: WHO's Framework for Action*. Geneva: World Health Organization.

World Health Organization. 2008. *The Tallinn Charter: Health Systems for Health and Wealth, 27 June 2008*. Copenhagen: WHO Regional Office for Europe.

World Health Organization. 2011. *Review of Public Health Capacities and Services in the European Region*. Copenhagen: WHO Regional Office for Europe.

World Health Organization. 2016a. *Childhood Hearing Loss: Strategies for Prevention and Care*. Geneva: World Health Organization.

World Health Organization. 2016b. Deafness and hearing loss (factsheet). [Online] Available at: http://www.who.int/mediacentre/factsheets/fs300/en/

Yerbury, H. 2012. Vocabularies of community. *Community Development Journal*, **47**, 184–198.

7 Health and well-being

Julian Abel

[There was] a strong correlation between men's flourishing lives and their relationships with family, friends, and community ... Those who kept warm relationships got to live longer and happier.

—Mineo, 2017 (on Robert Waldinger, 2015)

The key to healthy aging is relationships, relationships, relationships.

—George Vaillant, cited in Mineo, 2017

Introduction

Western healthcare is founded upon a deficit model. The aspiration for health services is that, through the good management of disease, people will live long, healthy, and happy lives. This is an attractive idea. It throws the responsibility of happiness and well-being onto the person with the illness. The professionals can identify illness through correct diagnosis, whether this is physical, social, psychological, or spiritual, and treat appropriately through the use of professional expertise and services. Diseases that cannot be cured can be managed to minimize their harm. However, managing health and well-being by focusing on harm reduction does not fit neatly into human experience. Absence of disease, or minimization of the impact of it, does not directly equate to well-being. We are complex creatures and there is an interplay between what happens in our minds, our social environment, and in our relationships that feeds directly into well-being. This interplay is not limited to mental events but has physiological, biochemical, hormonal, and immunological impacts. Simply focusing on harm reduction is not enough to enhance well-being. To provide the highest quality of care, professionals have to focus on what makes a good life.

The shift in the conceptual mindset needed to provide the highest quality of care requires professionals to move from a deficit-based model to consideration of well-being in the context of people's lives. Health and disease do not happen in isolation to an individual. We are the most social of animals and well-being relates directly to what matters most to us in our lives. For professionals, providing the best care through improving well-being requires an understanding of what living well means for the people they serve. Even short-term illness has a direct impact on the people surrounding the patient. Long-term illness, whether this is terminal or not, stretches the resilience of caring networks. The unit of care includes the networks of family, friends, neighbours, work colleagues, and community members. In the palliative care setting, through a process of discovery, goals can be formulated around making the most of life remaining, not just for the person with the illness but also for the close networks of relationships that surround them.

The problem for palliative care, both specialist and generalist, lies in discovering what is important to people undergoing the experiences of death, dying, loss, and caregiving, over and above minimizing harm. There is sparse evidence of what matters most to people in making a good life in the palliative care research literature. Kellehear, in his book *The Inner Life of the Dying Person* (Kellehear, 2014), in his chapter on 'Hope and Love—Connection' (chapter 7), examines a variety of themes on the positive experiences of end of life care for patient, family, and friends. He draws upon narrative accounts from patients and family members who have experienced terminal illness or caring, as well as references to these experiences in the humanities.

Well-being in the palliative care setting

While the literature on well-being is extensive, its definition is elusive (Dodge et al., 2012; Huppert, 2017). The concept of well-being can be used flexibly depending on a theoretical or practical perspective. The range of definitions varies from dynamic equilibrium (Headey and Wearing, 1989) to psychological perspectives (Huppert, 2017) among many others. Well-being in palliative care, however, remains largely unexplored.

Recognition of the multidimensional domains involved in well-being can be found in the United Nations 1948 Universal

Declaration of Human Rights (United Nations General Assembly, 1948). Well-being is specifically mentioned in article 25:

> Everyone has the right to a standard of living, adequate, for, the health and well-being of himself and of his family, including food, clothing, housing and medical care and necessary social services, and the right to security in the event of unemployment, sickness, disability, widowhood, old age or other lack of livelihood in circumstances beyond his control.

Other articles related to well-being include freedom of thought, expression, movement, education, and freedom from oppression. The World Health Organization directed its attention to health and well-being in the Ottawa Charter for Health Promotion (World Health Organization, 1986). The five domains for action are:

1. Building healthy public policy.
2. Creating supportive environments.
3. Strengthening community action.
4. Developing personal skills.
5. Reorienting healthcare services towards prevention of illness and promotion of health.

The charter recognizes that health and well-being is intertwined with relationships of people and place. The Shanghai declaration on promoting health in the 2030 Agenda for Sustainable Development (World Health Organization, 2017) built on the Ottawa Charter, recognizing that sustainable development needs to be part of consideration of health and well-being. Furthermore, good political governance is a necessary requirement if these policies are to be put in place and enacted.

These principles were used by Kellehear (2015) to formulate the Compassionate City Charter. The 13 areas for social action focus on places and relationships, all of which relate to well-being. Furthermore, this focus is not solely on the person with the illness, but engages everyone on a societal level, whether this be in schools, churches and temples, workplaces, trade unions, museums and galleries, and others. As Kellehear (2013) says, end of life care is everyone's responsibility.

Social ecological models

Attention to people and place is central to social ecology. The roots of social ecological models are to be found in the 1970s, with increasing development over time. Urie Bronfenbrenner's (1977) ecological framework for human development outlined its use in the field of childhood development. Bronfenbrenner postulated that human development is affected by the environment in which we live. This can be conceptualized as microsystems, the direct contact with the world in which we live; mesosystems, the connections between the microsystems and the community; and macrosystems, the culture, values, customs, and laws of any society (Paquette and Ryan, 2001). Further development of these ideas includes chronosystems, impact of genetics, environment, and public policy (Golden and Earp, 2012). These models have been absorbed into the field of health promotion, giving theoretical, experimental, and practical guidance on where and how to develop interventions.

In their report entitled *End of Life Care at Home: Co-creating an Ecology of Care*, Horsfall and colleagues (2015) describe the experiences of being involved in a caring network for someone who has a terminal illness. They summarize what the ecological model means in the palliative setting:

> We found that the dying person and their caring networks exist within a complex web of social-environmental relationships where knowledge, skills, values, attitudes and beliefs of network members are influenced by factors such as: existing relationships with people and place; formal and informal organisations and groups to which they already belong; the nature of the communities in which they live; social norms and expectations of the groups and cultures with which they identify; experiences and knowledge of health services and other social support organisation. (Horsfall et al., 2015, p. 61)

Home sits squarely in the centre of place in the context of social ecology in the palliative setting. Historically, the main focus for this has been place of death, rather than place of living well up until the end (Hoare et al., 2015). A variety of factors are given as to why patients and relatives choose home as the place to die: freedom from pain, management of difficult symptoms, fear, control, privacy, and dignity (Steinhauser et al., 2000; Agar et al., 2008). The interpretation of these choices can be categorized as a form of harm reduction rather than improving well-being. Other factors, directly related to the positive aspects of improving well-being, are also mentioned, including sharing time with family, friends, and pets. People and places in this context can be summed up as the people we know and love in the places we know and love:

> An ecological view also asks that we see 'home' not as an isolated place where a dying person and their carer may live, but as a place which exists with/in a larger environment: the block or garden, the street, the village, the neighbourhood. These are dynamic and inhabited with people, trees, flowers, creatures, sounds, smells, and sensations such as the sun on your skin. These places are not passive. (Horsfall et al., 2015, p. 63)

Relationships are primarily important in human health and well-being

The studies of the impact of relationships on health and well-being show it to be a primary factor. High-quality relationships are associated with living a longer, happier, and healthier life. The epigraphs at the beginning of this chapter are about or from two leaders of the Harvard Grant Study of Adult Development (Vaillant, 2012; Waldinger, 2015). This US study tracked the lives of a cohort of men who attended Harvard University from 1938 onwards, using the physical and psychological methods of the day to trace their progress through life's ups and downs. The Glueck Study of Juvenile Delinquency began in 1940, following the lives of children who came from underprivileged backgrounds in the Boston area in the US (Glueck and Glueck, 1950). From 1970 onwards, the analysis of these two groups have been combined, which continue into the present day. Second- and third-generation people are now enrolled. Robert Waldinger is the fourth study lead. Quoting from his TED Talk (Waldinger, 2015) he summarized the findings.

> It turns out that people who are more socially connected to family, to friends, to community, are happier, they're physically healthier, and they live longer than people who are less well connected. And the experience of loneliness turns out to be toxic. People who are

> more isolated than they want to be from others find that they are less happy, their health declines earlier in midlife, their brain functioning declines sooner and they live shorter lives than people who are not lonely.
>
> Once we had followed our men all the way into their 80s, we wanted to look back at them at midlife and to see if we could predict who was going to grow into a happy, healthy octogenarian and who wasn't. And when we gathered together everything we knew about them at age 50, it wasn't their middle age cholesterol levels that predicted how they were going to grow old. It was how satisfied they were in their relationships. The people who were the most satisfied in their relationships at age 50 were the healthiest at age 80. And good, close relationships seem to buffer us from some of the slings and arrows of getting old. Our most happily partnered men and women reported, in their 80s, that on the days when they had more physical pain, their mood stayed just as happy. But the people who were in unhappy relationships, on the days when they reported more physical pain, it was magnified by more emotional pain.

Julianne Holt-Lunstad and colleagues' study on the impact of relationships and mortality found that those with adequate social relationships had 50% greater likelihood of survival compared to those with poor or insufficient social relationships. The impact was at least as large as giving up smoking and more effective than giving up alcohol, improving diet, reducing weight, taking up exercise, drug treatment of hypertension, and others (Holt-Lunstad et al., 2010). In a further meta-analysis looking at the impact of loneliness and social isolation, Holt-Lunstad and colleagues (2015) found that, after accounting for multiple covariates, the increased likelihood of death was 26% for reported loneliness, 29% for social isolation, and 32% for living alone.

The large impact of social relationships on health and well-being goes beyond the effect on the psyche alone. The primary hormone associated with socialization is oxytocin. Its presence is ubiquitous in vertebrates, including fish and amphibians (Knobloch and Grinevich, 2014). It has reproductive and prosocial behaviour functions. Its presence, from an evolutionary perspective, indicates that social behaviour is fundamentally important for survival. This is particularly the case in human beings, who are the most social of animals. Herbert Spencer (1820–1903) was a philosopher who coined the inadequate term 'survival of the fittest', developing the ideas of social Darwinism. Survival of the fittest suggests that those who are physically the strongest and the most sexually attractive have the characteristics that are needed for successful adaptation and evolution. Darwin had a different view of human evolution, seeing compassion as a primary requirement for survival (Darwin, 1902; Ekman, 2010). There is increasing recent interest in compassion being a vital part of human survival, with good anthropological evidence that humans looked after each other in times of illness, disability, and need (Spikins, 2015). The ubiquitous presence of oxytocin indicates its importance as an evolutionary pressure. Social relationships are not just a nice thing to have, they are a necessary part of our survival. The health-giving benefits of oxytocin and associated hormones are well documented, opposing the impacts of long-term stress both physiological and biochemically. Compassionate behaviour is the basis of social connectedness (Seppala et al., 2013). Establishing meaningful relationships of love, laughter, and friendship is difficult without compassion as a foundation. If the person you are talking to does not care about your welfare, developing trust is difficult.

In summary, social relations and connectedness are integral to human health and well-being. They are a primary driver for us at all stages of our life, from the cradle to the grave (Pinker, 2015). This is as true for all patients and their caring networks in the palliative setting as it is in life when we are well. Furthermore, recognition of this importance provides a keen focus of intervention in the palliative setting.

Circles of care–naturally occurring networks

One of the challenges for palliative care professionals is how to focus on what matters most to people undergoing the experiences of death, dying, loss, and caregiving and what can be done to enable this. For the majority of people, social relationships are the most important part of their lives. As Robert Waldinger indicates in his findings from the Harvard Grant and Glueck studies, the quality of their relationships determines what a meaningful life is (Waldinger, 2015). An understanding of what naturally occurring networks of social relationships are and how they function is a starting point for conceptualizing how these networks can be enhanced and how palliative care services can relate to them on an equal footing and as a fundamentally important as part of care.

The circles of care model (Fig. 7.1) (Abel et al., 2013) is similar in structure to Bronfenbrenner's social ecological model (Bronfenbrenner, 1977).

The circles of care diagram is a naturalistic description of how social connections manifest. The evidence base for it in the palliative setting has been elucidated through network analysis (Rosenberg et al., 2015). While the diagram depicts discreet circles, there is a degree of flexibility with no clear boundaries between different circles. The key to understanding the diagram is to see the circles as being descriptive of relationships. The quality of relationships will determine where someone is placed in the diagram.

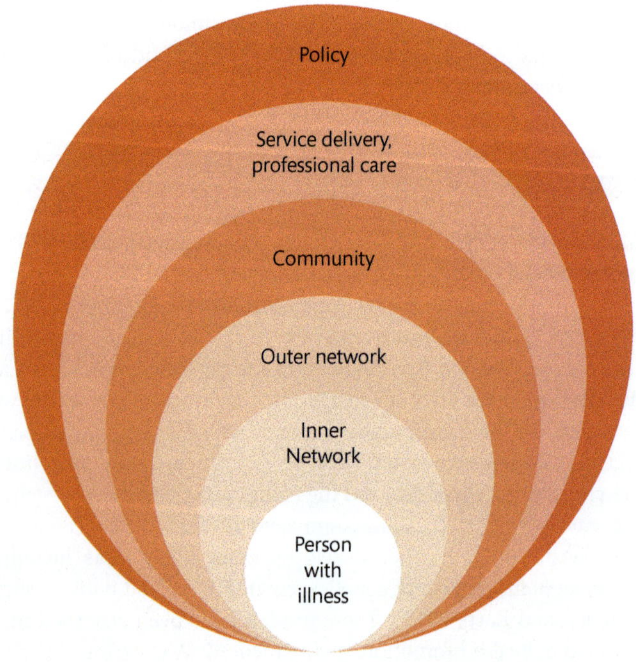

Fig. 7.1 Circles of care.

Reproduced with permission from Abel, J., et al. (2013). Circles of care: should community development redefine the practice of palliative care? *BMJ supportive & palliative care*, 3(4), 383–388.

Relationships vary over time and in accordance with circumstances. For example, someone who may be considered to be in the outer network or in the community might become a close friend during the course of the illness. Likewise, difficulties can arise with someone who might be in the inner network, resulting in them not being considered to be part of the supportive network at all. Furthermore, health and social care professionals might well become part of the outer or inner networks, depending on closeness of relationships.

Confusion can arise when considering who is in each of the circles. Professionals in particular may mistake the ability to perform tasks of care with closeness of relationship. However, as we shall see, compassion, love, laughter, and friendship, not just between the person with the illness but between network members, form the basis of who sits where. The ability or willingness to perform tasks of care are part of being in a close network but not a necessity. People may not even want close family members and friends to perform these tasks but nevertheless they may still have very close, valued relationships and be part of the inner network.

Inner network

The circles start with the person with the illness. Rather than describing them as a patient, from a well-being perspective, someone may have a serious, life-limiting illness, but still fully express themselves and are valued humans with a meaningful existence. This is in keeping with taking a health and well-being promotion approach.

The inner network, surrounding the person with the illness, is made up from people who are close to them and who generally see them on a regular basis. Even this description requires some flexibility. For example, a child or grandchild might well live away from home and only rarely visit. Nevertheless, they can be considered to be part of the inner network. Electronic face-to-face communication can help to keep relationships close. Typical members of the inner network can include spouse or partner, children, close friends, and work colleagues. The size of the inner network varies, dependent on the circumstances and personalities of the people involved. Inner networks may be as small as two and as large as 20. Having a larger network is not necessarily better than having a smaller one—the quality of relationships is more important.

Outer network

The closeness and strengths of relationships in the outer network can vary from very close to remote. For example, a close friend or family member may not be part of the inner network but nevertheless be an important part of the variety of social relationships. In addition, people in the outer network may not be close to the person with the illness or even see them at all. They may be a close friend or family member of someone in the inner network who acts as a support for them.

Many people, when thinking about the outer network, underestimate the numbers of people who play a valued role. Family members and close friends are easy to include when counting. However, social relationships can extend from the close to the very light and occasional. For example, gentle friendships can form while watching children play sports. Equally, regular contact with someone who serves at a much-frequented shop helps to develop a web of positive interactions in the community. Chemists have an important role to play, when they get to know their clients as they collect their regular medication. The list starts to expand when thinking creatively about positive social relationships. Choirs can be helpful in nourishing a sense of well-being among its participants. Sports clubs and special interest groups can do the same. Moving away from a task-orientated perspective when thinking of networks to include compassion, love, laughter, and friendship, as important as tasks, expands the numbers of people involved. This can include friends of children and their parents. Having someone who is happy to look after children and pick them up from school makes them part of the network without necessarily knowing them well. A neighbour may keep an eye on someone they see pass their gate on a regular basis. They may be very sensitive to someone being less well or being seen less frequently.

When taking this inclusive approach to considering the outer network, numbers can expand quite rapidly. Someone who has lived in the same place for a number of years may have built up hundreds of contacts. Typical numbers in the outer network may be between ten and 20 people but this can extend to 200 or more.

Community

In the context of positive relationships, definitions of community can be extensive. Community includes social contact with people other than in the inner or outer network. Examples include a wide variety of community groups. Community building, such as asset-based community development, seeks to bring people together to be part of what Cormac Russell calls 'the associational life' (Russell, 2016; McKnight and Russell, 2018). People are naturally rich in gifts and talents. When they come together there is an abundance of wealth of community, which can used both simply as association or turned towards defining and solving problems their community may face. In addition, groups can be activity related, such as walking or knitting groups, or may be disease specific, such as long-term condition groups. A variety of different groups can spring up through community development centred around primary health centres. Examples from Frome in Somerset, a market town of 28,000 people in the south west of England, include self-management groups, talking cafes for people who just want to chat, pain management groups, and many others that developed in response to the needs of the town's inhabitants. But community means much more than town centres, community halls, or neighbourhoods. Communities build up in workplaces or online. Following sporting teams can result in life-long friendships. Activities in which social interaction takes place arise wherever there are humans. They are a facet of our deeply embedded social nature. They are places where compassion, love, laughter, and friendship can develop. People are drawn to things that naturally interest them. The friendships that happen along the way evolve from common activities. In terms of health and well-being benefits, the moments of companionship are the ones that are important. Each positive social interaction is a small shot of oxytocin and the associated hormonal cascade. Individually, this may be small, but when combined together, people can have not only a sense of belonging and feeling part of the community, they get the health benefits at the same time.

Service delivery and professional care

When asking healthcare professionals where they sit in the circles of care, they generally place themselves in the inner network (Horsfall et al., 2012). This is perhaps a reflection of the closeness of relationships professionals feel they have with the people they care for. This is not negative, but the perception of those in the inner and outer networks of the role and closeness of the healthcare professionals may be different from that of the professionals (Leonard et al., 2020). People in the inner network may consider healthcare professionals to sit on the periphery of their network. The tendency for professionals to place themselves at the heart of the network can lead to a very professional-orientated view of what is important and matters most. This can result in the social networks being ignored or not considered valuable. This can cause harm, worsening the experiences of those involved in the network which persist into bereavement (Rosenberg et al., 2015, 2018). Altering this perception of centrality is a challenge that needs to be overcome by professional health and social care organizations. The rich resources of the inner and outer networks should be considered as the primary unit of care and come before consideration of professional caring services. As discussed, people live in the context of their relationships. Identity is intimately bound to this and loss of relationships leads to loss of meaning and value in life. Carers whose identity becomes subsumed in the caring role can suffer a similar loss of a sense of value as the person with the illness. Professional services cannot take the place of the supportive network and give the same sense of value that comes from close relationships. At the most basic level, professionals are paid to support people in times of need. Even with the best motivation, this is different from the support given freely by the people we know and love. A similar kind of closeness may be felt and appreciated when professionals and volunteers step outside of their statutory role and go beyond what is expected of them. With regard to the placing of professionals and service delivery, they are essential but not central. It is the responsibility of organizations to align their services to make most of the community resource, including the inner and outer networks, and then appropriately fill the gaps where necessary. This requires professionals reducing their sense of ownership of the tasks that go with their jobs. Assessment of symptoms and use of medication may be best done by relatives, who spend prolonged periods of time with the person with the illness. Training the inner network in simple symptom recognition, with some guidelines on management, reduces the reliance on professionals. The same applies to tasks associated with manual handling. Service reorganization based on these principles are discussed elsewhere in subsequent chapters.

Policy

Policy can be used as a way of supporting the rich resources contained in networks of support. Policy is commonly used as a control mechanism for professional activity with risk aversion and fear of litigation being high on the list of priorities. This defensive form of the practice of caregiving causes harm. It may reduce the risk of litigation but at the same time can result in ignoring the strengths of supportive networks. Training caregivers in manual handling is a good example. Organizations may avoid training carers on how to move people safely, for fear that they injure themselves and then sue the trainers. Caregivers then remain untrained and are more at risk of injuring both themselves and the person with the illness. The reality of terminal illness is that the vast majority of people will need some form of physical support for movement. Not routinely training caregivers in how to do this safely, or even providing information so that people can find out how to do this themselves, is a serious, harmful omission.

In the context of health and well-being, policy makers using the public health approach to palliative and end of life care will need to shift their focus to seeking the natural wealth of communities and supportive networks. Policy can act to work with them rather than against or even not taking them into account. Bronfenbrenner's social ecological model is a good way of developing an overview of how policy can support people and communities at micro, meso, and macro levels. Thinking about people and places, particularly focused on good relationships with both, helps to focus on the different ways of supporting what matters most at the end of life.

On a micro level, supportive communities should be seen at the centre of palliative care professional services and policy should reflect this. The starting point of consideration is to fully understand what matters most to health and well-being and then consider how policy can focus on helping develop this as much as possible. This would, for example, overcome the difficulties some palliative care organizations have in training people in manual handling, identifying this as being a high priority and then working out ways in which training can be given safely. The same argument applies to carers giving subcutaneous medication for symptom control. It is extremely distressing for relatives watching their loved ones suffer when symptom-relieving medication is in the house and cannot be given for hours, waiting until a busy health professional arrives. In resource-poor areas, health professionals may not be available at all and there is no choice other than to train and trust relatives in symptom relief. There are many examples of how perceptions of policy makers could change through considering what matters most to the person with the illness *and* their caring network as the primary priority.

At a meso level, local commissioning bodies, including local councils or administrative areas, can focus in a similar way on what matters most for the caring unit at end of life. Setting palliative care strategies to include the public health approach, rather than focusing on harm reduction interventions, can shift how palliative care services develop their organizations. Supporting local voluntary organizations who provide care, such as befrienders, can help. Local amenities, such as parks and other leisure activities, can be part of the enjoyment of life, and should be considered to be part of the full range of well-being considerations. Further overviews and examples are discussed in the respective chapters of the textbook.

In the same way, national policymaking can shift its attention to embedding communities at the heart of palliative care. This process began in the UK with the 'Ambitions for Palliative and End of Life Care 2015–2020' (National End of Life Care Partnership, 2015; Abel et al., 2016). Ambition six, 'Each community is prepared to help', has four components:

1. *Compassionate and resilient communities.* Public health approaches to palliative and end of life care need to be accelerated and support given to people and communities who can provide practical help and compassion.
2. *Public awareness.* Those who share our ambition should work to improve public awareness of the difficulties people face and create a better understanding of the help that is available.
3. *Practical support.* Local health, care, and voluntary organizations should find new ways to give the practical support, information,

and training that enable families, neighbours, and community organizations to help.

4. *Volunteers*. To achieve our ambition more should be done locally and nationally to recruit, train, value, and connect volunteers into a more integrated effort to help support people, their families, and their communities (National End of Life Care Partnership, 2015).

A national policy such as this places a requirement for health and social care organizations to implement it. This in turn creates the opportunity to review plans to see whether progress is being made against the policy. Commissioning bodies can seek evidence of progress as part of an agreement for continuation of funding on a contract.

Kellehear's Compassionate City Charter takes a population-based approach as to how this can be applied across multiple settings, extending into all areas of life, from communities to churches and temples, from workplaces to museums and galleries (Kellehear, 2015). The need for support for anyone undergoing the experiences of death, dying, loss, and caregiving is present wherever they are. Given that all of our lives are impermanent, and that the vast majority of us will be part of an inner network multiple times in our lives, there is a simple need to support others undergoing these experiences in a compassionate way. Having an organized focus such as the Compassionate City Charter helps to create a programme of change that can extend into different areas as it progresses.

Enhancing naturally occurring networks

Enhancing naturally occurring networks is at the centre of improving health and well-being, not just for the person with the illness but for the caring network as a whole. The two main ways in which these networks can help are, firstly, compassion, love, laughter, and friendship and, secondly, practical tasks:

1. *Compassion, love, laughter, and friendship*. As discussed, relationships are at the heart of meaning and value in life. A primary experience of ill health is loss of identity. People often value and identify themselves through what they do, such as their ability to earn money, to help with domestic chores, to drive, and many others. These tasks are lost with the fatigue of progressive illness, resulting in a loss of identity (Charmaz, 1983). The positive impact of good relationships can help to make people feel valued despite these losses. The experiences of fatigue and loss of identity happen in the caring networks as well as for the person with the illness. When caring falls upon a single person or a small number of people, they may become fatigued and overwhelmed by the physical and emotional demands of this role, resulting in loneliness and isolation (Broady, 2017). Good relationships, not task orientated but simple friendship, where the normal things of life can be discussed and shared, help to alleviate some of these difficulties. Enjoying an evening out with a friend can be restorative. Recognition of the importance of relationships, both for the person with the illness and for individuals within the supportive network, helps to develop interventions that strengthen these relationships as a priority.
2. *Practical tasks*. The focus of practical tasks is not limited to hands-on care of the person with the illness, an assumption often made by healthcare professionals. The many tasks of daily life, such as shopping, cooking, cleaning, gardening, walking pets, and providing lifts, all continue in addition to the role of being a carer. When these tasks fall on a small number of people, it can feel overwhelming; shared out among a network of support means that different individuals can contribute in a manageable way through taking on a small task, but together they can make an enormous difference.

Building and helping people to enhance naturally occurring networks is a clinical skill that should be part of the routine care for people who use palliative care services. To help understand its central role, health and social care professionals can discover the role of these networks in their own lives. This can be done as an exercise in which each person explores their own networks, not thinking about whether the people they know are prepared to help or not, but simply recalling the people they know and where they sit in the inner and outer networks. This exercise can be extended to look at the different ways in which people help. The phrase compassion, love, laughter, and friendship arose from a training session run by the author of this chapter, when asking about the different ways in which support can be given. We appreciate the people we know and love for the compassion, love, laughter, and friendship they share with us. Sometimes this is expressed through giving practical help and sometimes it is companionship. Both are appreciated and both enhance a sense of meaning and value.

Working with the caring unit to enhance and build networks of support can prove to be challenging. There are many reasons why people are reluctant to build them. This includes not wanting to be a burden, maintaining a sense of dignity and privacy, not wanting to disturb people who have busy lives, not wanting to hear someone say no to a request for support, and many others. Building networks requires an understanding of where the obstacles lie and where the strengths in each network are. Exploring networks should become a routine part of clinical care, looking at ways in which they can be enhanced. An ecomap can be given to the caring unit so that they can fill it out with the people involved. An example, developed in Frome in Somerset, is given in Fig. 7.2.

The main carer is not necessarily best placed to be a network organizer. They may be reluctant to ask for support from those around them, even if there is a desire to give help. Sometimes, a good network organizer can be a child or grandchild. It is possible to organize networks from remote places through the use of electronic communication, such as email, Skype, or Zoom or use of apps such as WhatsApp, Jointly, or Gather My Crew. These latter two apps have been developed for carers, specifically for organizing networks of support. One of the advantages of using apps like these is that it is possible to keep people updated in real time, as well as being able to ask a crowd for support. Someone in the network is likely to say yes to a request, for example, for a lift or cooking a meal. This helps to create a positive supportive environment in which people can fit in as suits their schedules.

As clinicians become more skilled and accustomed to helping to enhance naturally occurring networks, they will discover for themselves what works and how obstacles are best addressed. While there are general solutions, such as just say yes when someone offers to help, explaining that caring is a marathon not a sprint, or seeing the value of not excluding close family to caring for the person they love, judicious application of these solutions is needed to address

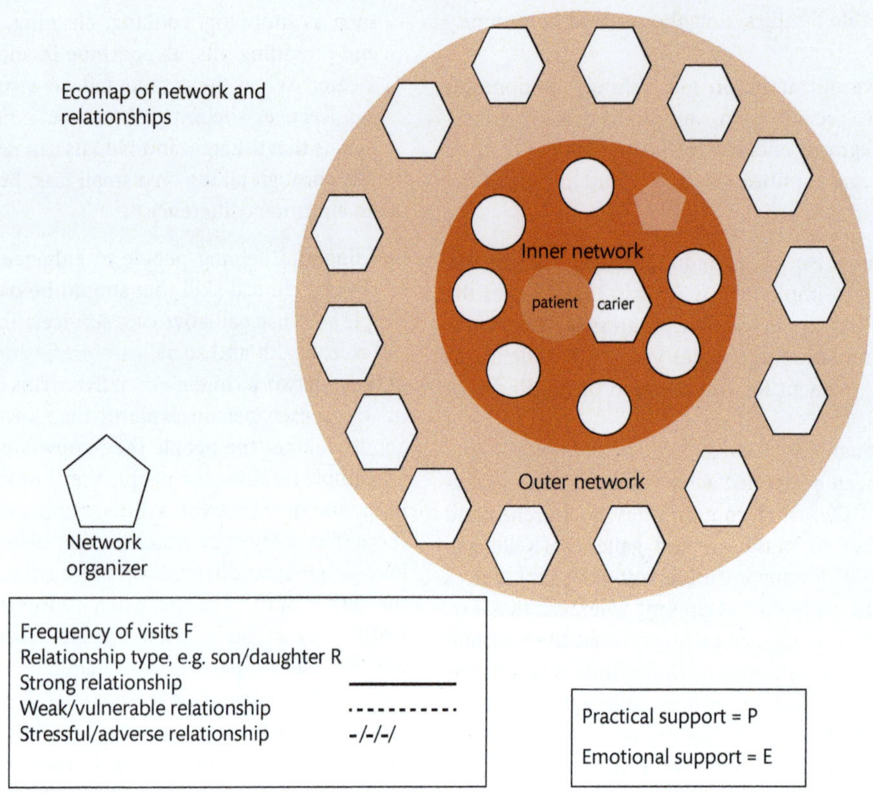

Fig. 7.2 Ecomap of network and relationships.

the specific problems each individual will have. Furthermore, there is likely to be a variety of different obstacles from within the same family. For example, the person with the illness may not want to see more people but at the same time be happy for their partner or spouse to receive support. The spouse may have different reasons for not involving others.

Social networks in the isolated and disenfranchised

Network mapping is particularly important for those people who may seem to be isolated. This includes immigrant communities, the homeless, prison populations, LGBQT+ people, and care homes among others. Sometimes the perceptions of health and social care professionals as to what constitutes networks of support is quite different from the perceptions of people in those networks. In addition, the process of network mapping can help people see where their support lies. Exploring existing social relationships highlights where they exist, and also makes it clear where there are gaps. The social networks of the homeless are reduced but nevertheless present (Nooe and Patterson, 2010). It is particularly important to discover where people get support from, not only to try and mobilize this support in a time of need but also because unless professionals are aware of the gaps, providing extra support may be inappropriate and difficult. In addition, institutions may interact either occasionally or on a regular basis with these groups. Lack of understanding of the structure of existing networks, unconscious biases, and lack of engagement contribute to poor understanding of the networks that are present (Nooe and Patterson, 2010).

Social support and social relationships are even more important in health and well-being for those people who suffer from a lack of them. The communities in which they live may be well placed to give support, and this support can sometimes be powerful. There are many historical examples of how peer support has been a cornerstone of treatment programmes on an international scale, particularly recent examples of HIV/AIDS (Grimsrud et al., 2020) and the Ebola epidemic in West Africa (Barker et al., 2020). Knowledge and understanding of deficiency of social networks places the emphasis of the necessity of health and social care services to have programmes of mobilization of communities of support, as indicated in the Compassionate City Charter. Social networks and relationships in prisons (Barker et al., 2020) can be used to develop communities of care at the end of life (Maull, 1998).

Networks as a routine part of clinical care

As well as improving health and well-being for all involved, there are some simple practical reasons as to why networks are so centrally important. When considering the size of networks, the numbers quickly multiply and an enormous resource of support can become available. Discovery and mapping of these networks might uncover 50 people who are prepared to help. The findings from Horsfall and her colleagues in the studies of the University of Western Sydney suggest that a typical network will include 16 people who are prepared to help in multiple practical ways (Horsfall et al., 2017). Studies of social network size have produced a wide range of numbers, from 250 to 5000. Hill and Dunbar (2003) found that positive interactive social networks typically number 150 people. The ways these networks can help are many more than can be managed by professional services, even in resource-rich nations. Not only are they better placed to help in terms of meaning and value, practical considerations make it reasonable to use them prior to sharing out the precious and limited resources of professional caring services.

Conclusion: living well

The central priority for those people undergoing the experiences of death, dying, loss, and caregiving is how to live well, making the most of precious time remaining. This is true in both health and illness, as it is for the person with the illness and their caring networks of support. Well-being is found in people and places and palliative care definitions and intervention planning should include both of these. Palliative care services can contribute in a structured and positive way through participating with communities, as broadly defined in the Compassionate City Charter, to enhance quality of life. Freedom from fear, whether physical, social, psychological, or spiritual, is part of palliative care but not to the exclusion of a positive focus on well-being. The failure of the research literature to understand the basis of what well-being means in the palliative setting is a significant omission that has hampered the ways in which it can be enhanced. The positive focus on improving well-being opens new doors for palliative and end of life care, seeking ways to make it everyone's responsibility.

REFERENCES

Abel, J., Sallnow, L., Murray, S., and Kerin, M. 2016. *Each Community is Prepared to Help: Community Development in End of Life Care—Guidance on Ambition Six*. London: National Council for Palliative Care.

Abel, J., Walter, T., Carey, L. B., Rosenberg, J., Noonan, K., Horsfall, D., et al. 2013. Circles of care: should community development redefine the practice of palliative care? *BMJ Supportive & Palliative Care*, **3**, 383–388.

Agar, M., Currow, D. C., Shelby-James, T. M., Plummer, J., Sanderson, C., and Abernethy, A. P. 2008. Preference for place of care and place of death in palliative care: are these different questions? *Palliative Medicine*, **22**, 787–795.

Barker, K. M., Ling, E. J., Fallah, M., Vandebogert, B., Kodl, Y., Macauley, R. J., et al. 2020. Community engagement for health system resilience: evidence from Liberia's Ebola epidemic. *Health Policy and Planning*, **35**, 416–423.

Broady, T. R. 2017. Carers' experiences of end-of-life care: a scoping review and application of personal construct psychology. *Australian Psychologist*, **52**, 372–380.

Bronfenbrenner, U. 1977. Toward an experimental ecology of human development. *American Psychologist*, **32**, 513–531.

Charmaz, K. 1983. Loss of self: a fundamental form of suffering in the chronically ill. *Sociology of Health & Illness*, **5**, 168–195.

Darwin, C. 1902. *The Descent of Man*, Volume 1. New York: American Home Library.

Dodge, R., Daly, A. P., Huyton, J., and Sanders, L. D. 2012. The challenge of defining wellbeing. *International Journal of Wellbeing*, **2**, 222–235.

Ekman, P. 2010. Darwin's compassionate view of human nature. *JAMA*, **303**, 557–558.

Glueck, S. and Glueck, E. 1950. Unraveling juvenile delinquency. *Juvenile Court Judges Journal*, **2**, 32.

Golden, S. D. and Earp, J. A. L. 2012. Social ecological approaches to individuals and their contexts: twenty years of health education & behavior health promotion interventions. *Health Education & Behavior*, **39**, 364–372.

Grimsrud, A. T., Pike, C., and Bekker, L.-G. 2020. The power of peers and community in the continuum of HIV care. *Lancet Global Health*, **8**, e167–e168.

Headey, B. and Wearing, A. 1989. Personality, life events, and subjective well-being: toward a dynamic equilibrium model. *Journal of Personality and Social Psychology*, **57**, 731–739.

Hill, R. A. and Dunbar, R. I. 2003. Social network size in humans. *Human Nature*, **14**, 53–72.

Hoare, S., Morris, Z. S., Kelly, M. P., Kuhn, I., and Barclay, S. 2015. Do patients want to die at home? A systematic review of the UK literature, focused on missing preferences for place of death. *PLoS One*, **10**, e0142723.

Holt-Lunstad, J., Smith, T. B., Baker, M., Harris, T., and Stephenson, D. 2015. Loneliness and social isolation as risk factors for mortality: a meta-analytic review. *Perspectives on Psychological Science*, **10**, 227–237.

Holt-Lunstad, J., Smith, T. B., and Layton, J. B. 2010. Social relationships and mortality risk: a meta-analytic review. *PLoS Medicine*, **7**, e1000316.

Horsfall, D., Leonard, R., Rosenberg, J. P., and Noonan, K. 2017. Home as a place of caring and wellbeing? A qualitative study of informal carers and caring networks lived experiences of providing in-home end-of-life care. *Health & Place*, **46**, 58–64.

Horsfall, D., Noonan, K., and Leonard, R. 2012. *Bringing Our Dying Home: Creating Community at End of Life*. Research Report. Sydney: University of Western Sydney.

Horsfall, D., Yardley, A., Leonard, R., Noonan, K., and Rosenberg, J. P. 2015. *End of Life at Home: Co-Creating an Ecology of Care*. Research Report. Sydney: University of Western Sydney.

Huppert, F. A. 2017. Challenges in defining and measuring well-being and their implications for policy. *Future Directions in Well-Being*. New York: Springer.

Kellehear, A. 2013. Compassionate communities: end-of-life care as everyone's responsibility. *QJM: An International Journal of Medicine*, **106**, 1071–1075.

Kellehear, A. 2014. *The Inner Life of the Dying Person*. New York: Columbia University Press.

Kellehear, A. 2015. *The Compassionate City Charter*. Abingdon: Routledge.

Knobloch, H. S. and Grinevich, V. 2014. Evolution of oxytocin pathways in the brain of vertebrates. *Frontiers in Behavioral Neuroscience*, **8**, 31.

Leonard, R., Horsfall, D., Rosenberg, J., and Noonan, K. 2020. Carer experience of end-of-life service provision: a social network analysis. *BMJ Supportive & Palliative Care*, **10**, e20.

Maull, F. W. 1998. Issues in prison hospice: toward a model for the delivery of hospice care in a correctional setting. *The Hospice Journal*, **13**, 57–82.

McKnight, J. L. and Russell, C. 2018. *The Four Essential Elements of an Asset-Based Community Development Process: What is Distinctive about an Asset-Based Community Process?* Chicago, IL: Asset-Based Community Development Institute, DePaul University.

Mineo, L. 2017. Good genes are nice, but joy is better. *The Harvard Gazette*, 11 April. [Online] Available at: https://news.harvard.edu/gazette/story/2017/04/over-nearly-80-years-harvard-study-has-been-showing-how-to-live-a-healthy-and-happy-life/

National End of Life Care Partnership. 2015. *Ambitions for Palliative and End of Life Care: A National Framework for Local Action 2015–2020*. London: National Palliative and End of Life Care Partnership.

Nooe, R. M. and Patterson, D. A. 2010. The ecology of homelessness. *Journal of Human Behavior in the Social Environment*, **20**, 105–152.

Paquette, D. and Ryan, J. 2001. Bronfenbrenner's ecological systems theory. [Online] Available at: http://dropoutprevention.org/wp-content/uploads/2015/07/paquetteryanwebquest_20091110.pdf

Pinker, S. 2015. *The Village Effect: How Face-to-Face Contact Can Make Us Healthier and Happier*. Toronto: Vintage Canada.

Rosenberg, J. P., Horsfall, D., Leonard, R., and Noonan, K. 2015. Informal caring networks for people at end of life: building social capital in Australian communities. *Health Sociology Review*, **24**, 29–37.

Rosenberg, J. P., Horsfall, D., Leonard, R., and Noonan, K. 2018. Informal care networks' views of palliative care services: help or hindrance? *Death Studies*, **6**, 362–370.

Russell, C. 2016. Sustainable community development: from what's wrong to what's strong. Lecture, TEDx Exeter, Exeter, UK. 16 May. [Online] Available at: https://www.youtube.com/watch?v=a5xR4QB1ADw&ab_channel=TEDxTalks

Seppala, E., Rossomando, T., and Doty, J. R. 2013. Social connection and compassion: Important predictors of health and well-being. *Social Research*, **80**, 411–430.

Spikins, P. A. 2015. *How Compassion made us Human: The Evolutionary Origins of Tenderness, Trust and Morality*. Barnsley: Pen and Sword.

Steinhauser, K. E., Christakis, N. A., Clipp, E. C., McNeilly, M., McIntyre, L., and Tulsky, J. A. 2000. Factors considered important at the end of life by patients, family, physicians, and other care providers. *JAMA*, **284**, 2476–2482.

United Nations General Assembly. 1948. *Universal Declaration of Human Rights*. Paris: United Nations.

Vaillant, G. E. 2012. *Triumphs of Experience*. Cambridge, MA: Harvard University Press.

Waldinger, R. 2015. What makes a good life? Lessons from the longest study on happiness. TED Conferences. 25 January. [Online] Available at: https://youtu.be/8KkKuTCFvzI

World Health Organization. 1986. *The Ottawa Charter for Health Promotion: First International Conference on Health Promotion, Ottawa, 21 November 1986*. Geneva: World Health Organization.

World Health Organization. 2017. Shanghai declaration on promoting health in the 2030 Agenda for Sustainable Development. *Health Promotion International*, **32**, 7–8.

8

Prevention and harm reduction

Libby Sallnow

Introduction

Public health is a broad and diverse field focused on disease prevention, promotion of health and well-being, and the prolongation of life (Acheson, 1988). It sits as distinct from clinical services, provided to individual patients, due to its explicit attention to populations, whether those populations are local neighbourhoods, groups in society, or entire countries. This distinction between clinical services offered at the level of the individual and public health interventions offered at the level of a population is fundamental to understanding public health approaches to palliative care. Fig. 8.1 illustrates this distinction further. The focus of a public health intervention is an entire population, which could mean all those facing a life-limiting illness, all carers, or indeed the full population of a town or country. This means any interventions should have an impact on the whole population, not just on selected individuals within it. This is represented as the full grey shaded area in the top left graph. Healthcare service interventions by contrast focus only on individuals or patients with a certain condition or identified biopsychosocial risk, and tailor management plans to their specific conditions, represented by the shaded area at the extreme of the top right graph. Successful public health interventions shift an entire population's likelihood of developing a condition or complications (bottom left graph). Impacts are seen for all. Healthcare service interventions, again by contrast, see outcomes only for those individuals or patients under the care of the service or the focus of the intervention. While these may be significant for individuals, the broader population remains unaffected.

Interventions in public health

The field of public health employs a number of approaches to prevent disease, promote health and well-being, and prolong life. The three tenets of public health action are prevention, early intervention, and harm reduction (Table 8.1).

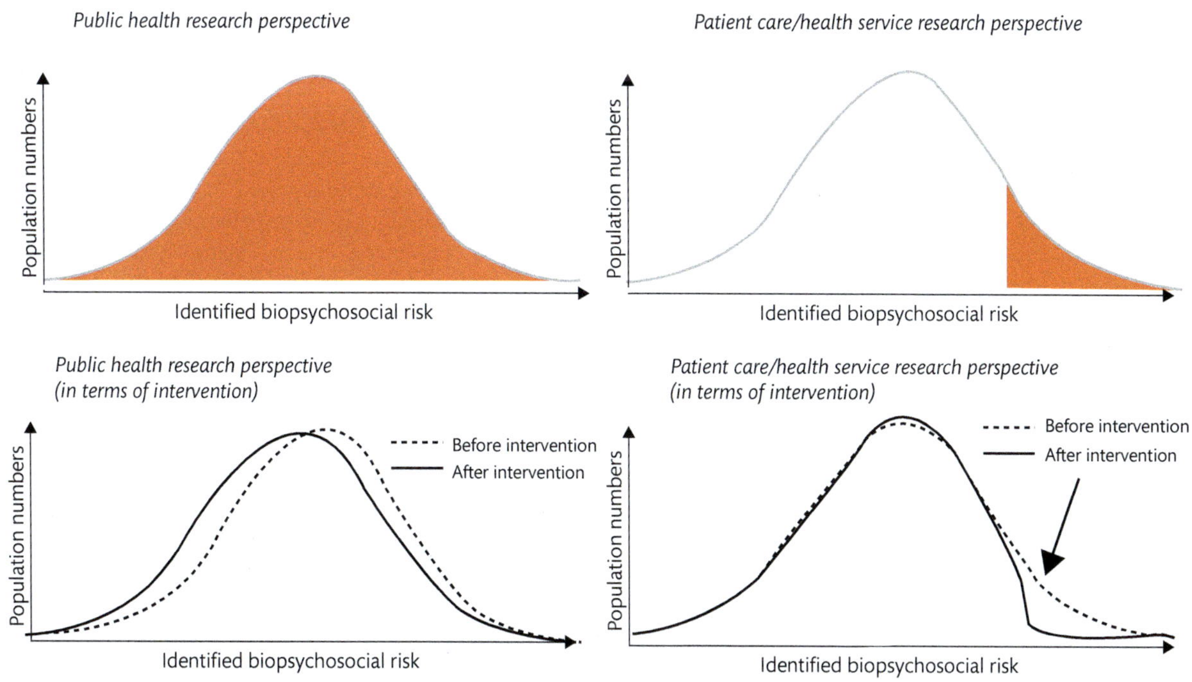

Fig. 8.1 A public health research perspective versus a patient care/health service perspective in end of life care research.

Table 8.1 The three levels of interventions in public health

Level of prevention	Intervention	Definition	Examples
Primary prevention	Prevention	To avoid the development of a disease or disability in healthy individuals	Fluoride in toothpaste, vaccinations for communicable disease, healthy eating advice, seat belts in vehicles
Secondary prevention	Early intervention	Early disease detection and screening to prevent worsening of the disease and the emergence of symptoms, or to minimize complications and limit disability or mortality	Screening for cancer, e.g. breast and cervical cancer, screening for gestational diabetes, public campaigns to recognize the signs of meningitis or a stroke, needle exchange programmes for users of injectable drugs
Tertiary prevention	Harm reduction	To reduce the negative or long-term impacts of an already established disease or condition by restoring function and reducing further complications	Rehabilitation after a stroke, opioid substitution programmes, supervised injection facilities, disability- or dementia-friendly policies and environments

Prevention efforts aim to stop a disease, condition, or state from occurring. Many well-known public health activities fall under this categorization and actions may include the provision of information, direct interventions, or mandating standards or requirements. The labelling of alcoholic drinks, cigarettes, or food with high fat or sugar content focuses on the giving of information to populations to enable healthier choices to be made. Interventions such as the addition of fluoride to toothpaste or the addition of iodine to manufactured bread aim to prevent dental caries or hypothyroidism through the direct provision of the compound to a population. The imposition of speed limits or the legal requirement to wear a seat belt or motorcycle helmet are examples of legally enforceable rules set by governments to prevent mortality or morbidity as a result of road traffic accidents. Prevention efforts are seen throughout society with national governments, education services, manufacturing businesses, healthcare services, local councils, community groups, individuals, and others assuming responsibility.

Early intervention or secondary prevention efforts aim to diagnose a disease or recognize a condition early in its course, such that progression can be halted or slowed, or severe complications can be avoided. Screening populations for conditions such as diabetes, hypertension, or some cancers are forms of early intervention. Public awareness campaigns on the signs and symptoms of serious conditions such as a stroke, myocardial infarction, or meningitis are also examples of early intervention initiatives, designed to allow conditions to be recognized and treated early, reducing the likelihood of disability or death. In addition to reducing physical complications of conditions, initiatives to support people coming back to work after a period of ill health or prolonged absence such as maternity leave also fall into this category through the prevention of job loss or related social consequences of serious illness or absence from work.

Harm reduction or tertiary prevention efforts focus on people or communities who have an established condition or disease and aim to mitigate and reduce the impact of that condition on their lives. Interventions may relate to clinical aspects of the disease such as the setting of glycaemic control targets for people with established diabetes mellitus, or providing safer opioid substitution programmes for people with opioid addictions, or on functional aspects such as rehabilitation for people to regain strength and function following a stroke or a fracture. Interventions may also include environmental changes such as adaptations to workplaces for disabled employees or making public transport accessible. The recent 'dementia friendly communities' movement (Buckner et al., 2019) contains elements of a harm reduction approach by supporting people living with dementia to continue to shop, go to pharmacies, or use public transport despite living with dementia.

Interventions at these different levels are essential in managing diseases such as diabetes mellitus, hypertension, and coronavirus disease 2019 (COVID-19) but also complex or 'wicked' problems such as addiction or obesity (Willett et al., 2019). Interventions must take place across these three domains in order to achieve meaningful impacts. For example, efforts to reduce mortality and morbidity due to heart disease must not only focus on cardiac rehabilitation following an extensive myocardial infarction. Messages about healthy eating must be part of education in primary schools, accompanied by labelling of unhealthy food and national screening programmes for hypertension. Further to this, questions must be asked of the structures in societies that either empower or disempower people to make choices about their lives. Structures such as racism, gender inequalities, discrimination on the basis of ethnicity, age, sexuality, or disability, poverty, or access to education all influence the power or agency people possess to engage with public health interventions. This chapter will review the principles of prevention and harm reduction and how they are applied to death, dying, loss, and care. Chapter 9 will focus on strategies for early intervention.

Understanding prevention

The arrival of COVID-19 and the global pandemic that ensued have placed public health prevention methods at the heart of billions of people's lives around the world. Primary prevention techniques such as social distancing, frequent handwashing, the wearing of face masks, quarantine, and mass vaccination programmes have become the pillars of the response to contain and control the spread of the virus. Campaigns based on similar principles were witnessed at the end of the last century to contain the HIV pandemic with abstinence from sexual contact and other measures forming an important part of the response (Merson et al., 2008).

Prevention forms the backbone of public health approaches and is an essential component of all public health initiatives. Box 8.1 describes the 'river parable', a story often used to illustrate the futility and unsustainable nature of early intervention or harm reduction efforts without an underlying prevention strategy.

This parable illustrates the differences between harm reduction and prevention, and of the importance of 'upstream' interventions. To elaborate the parable further, in addition to the preventative approach of tackling the issue of people being 'pushed off the bridge',

Box 8.1 The river parable

Irving Zola relates the story of a physician trying to explain the dilemmas of the modern practice of medicine:

> 'You know,' he said, 'sometimes it feels like this. There I am standing by the shore of a swiftly flowing river and I hear the cry of a drowning man. So I jump into the river, put my arms around him, pull him to shore and apply artificial respiration. Just when he begins to breathe, there is another cry for help. So I jump into the river, reach him, pull him to shore, apply artificial respiration, and then just as he begins to breathe, another cry for help. So back in the river again, reaching, pulling, applying, breathing and then another yell. Again and again, without end, goes the sequence. You know, I am so busy jumping in, pulling them to shore, applying artificial respiration, that I have no time to see who the hell is upstream pushing them all in.' (McKinlay, 1979, p. 9)

a broader human rights-based approach (HRBA) may ask why it is certain groups of people are more likely to be on the bridge at all, and whether interventions are needed to address these deeper, structural factors.

A significant evidence base underpins primary prevention and a number of examples demonstrate the impact these measures can have. In the early 1980s, as the HIV/AIDS pandemic was gaining ground, one of the most globally recognized primary prevention approaches emerged. As governments scrambled to accept or understand the disease, a number of community activist groups, many composed of people living with HIV/AIDS, devised the 'safe sex' message for prevention of HIV infection. These early community efforts predated and informed the national and global efforts that followed. The 'Denver Principles', drafted by a number of people living with HIV/AIDS in the US are widely understood as representing the foundation of the AIDS activist prevention movement, recognizing the central role people living with the disease played in prevention (Merson et al., 2008).

HIV prevention today is understood to involve a range of approaches across the spectrum. Condom use, a cornerstone of the safe sex prevention message, has been shown to reduce transmission by 80% in heterosexual intercourse (Weller and Davis-Beaty, 2002) and by 70% in men who have sex with men (Smith et al., 2015). Medical male circumcision has been demonstrated to reduce the transmission of HIV from women to men by 60% (Weiss et al., 2010). Series of interventions have dramatically reduced rates of transmission from mother to child during pregnancy (European Collaborative Study, 2005). These approaches are understood to rely on government action, community engagement, access to appropriate health and social care services and treatment, and social and cultural change.

In 1999, a 10-year strategy was introduced in England to tackle the historically high rates of teenage pregnancy, substantially higher than in many other European countries. Teenage pregnancy was acknowledged as a public health issue, both influenced by inequality and a driver of inequality (Hadley et al., 2016). The prevention aspect of the strategy focused on improved access to contraception, high-quality relationships and sex education in school curricula, and a national communication campaign, alongside the harm reduction intervention of increased support for teenage parents. Though the strategy was developed and funded by the government, it was implemented and adapted locally. The aim of the strategy had been to halve the rate of pregnancies in under 18s over a 10-year period and by 2018 the rate had dropped by 64% (Hadley, 2020). Evaluations have cited the reasons for success as including:

> Research evidence on what works needs translating into clear guidance for local areas, with all agencies and practitioners understanding their role in preventing teenage pregnancy. Good data and use of local intelligence from service providers are essential for monitoring and improving local performance. Senior, visible leadership at national and local level is critical for prioritising action. A hub and spoke structure is important for supporting local areas and maintaining momentum. The key to success however is translating the evidence into a multi-agency whole system approach. (Hadley, 2014, p. S35)

Understanding harm reduction

Harm reduction principles are most well known in their application in the substance misuse field, particularly with regard to alcohol, tobacco, or illicit drug use. Harm reduction approaches in illicit drug use aim to reduce the negative impacts that can come from drug use, rather than reduce drug use itself. Needle exchange programmes have been shown to reduce the transmission of HIV or other blood-borne pathogens and supervised injection facilities can reduce overdose incidence, address risk behaviours, transmission of blood-borne viruses, and harms associated with discarded syringes or litter (Ritter and Cameron, 2006). A programme combining overdose education for people at risk of opioid overdose and bystanders, alongside distribution of naloxone syringes, demonstrated a significant reduction in opioid-overdose related deaths (Walley et al., 2013).

Gambling and sex work have both been the focus of harm reduction strategies in recent years. A systematic review of public health interventions in gambling in the US in 2017 demonstrated the efficacy of a range of measures such as self-appraisal pop-up messages, $1 maximum bets, removal of large note acceptors and ATMs, reduced operating hours, and smoking bans in reducing expenditure and time spent gambling (Tanner et al., 2017). Harm reduction approaches for sex workers have often focused on the importance of self-determination, autonomy, and control over situations. Successful initiatives have built negotiating skills, access to and use of condoms, training to recognize and escape from violent situations, and safe houses (Rekart, 2005).

Returning to the HIV/AIDS pandemic, harm reduction approaches have focused on the access and availability of antiretroviral therapies to prevent the progression of HIV into AIDS and reduce morbidity and mortality associated with the virus. Initiatives such as 'treatment to prevent' utilize this harm reduction strategy as a primary prevention measure, as people living with HIV with an undetectable viral load have a greatly reduced risk of transmission of the virus. These measures are now being considered alongside other primary prevention approaches as part of a concerted approach (Chang et al., 2013).

A concerted approach is essential in tackling public health challenges and threats. Utilizing only a harm reduction approach without primary prevention or early intervention measures will not succeed in addressing the complex roots and drivers of many contemporary public health challenges. Further to these approaches is a broader appreciation of the underlying structures in societies that determine the power or control people have over their lives, the opportunities they have to engage with public health measures, and their abilities to make choices for themselves. This broader perspective will be discussed in the next section.

A human rights-based approach

A HRBA gained recognition in the early 2000s as a means of placing the principles of international human rights at the heart of development work (Uvin, 2007). Organizations around the world adopted 'The Human Rights Based Approach to Development Cooperation' which set out the principles of this approach (United Nations Sustainable Development Group, 2003). A HRBA focuses on the most marginalized, excluded, or discriminated against in a society. People are understood to be active participants in addressing challenges that face them, not passive recipients of services. A distinction was drawn between needs and rights with initiatives focused on protecting, advocating for, and fulfilling the rights of people rather than provision of services to meet their needs. When rights are discussed instead of need, there is a corresponding responsibility or obligation. The HRBA sets out the dual requirements on rights holders (individuals, communities) and duty bearers (governments, statutory services). The HBRA asserts that provision of services or mandating behaviour through policy action does not address the structures in society that create vulnerability, discrimination, or marginalization. People are often unable to access or make use of such opportunities. An example of this is in gender and reproductive rights. Some women may lack access to information to make choices about the number or spacing of children or services to access contraception while others face discrimination, coercion, or violence as they attempt to exercise these rights. The provision of further information or services will not address these structural issues of power, gender inequality, and discrimination.

New public health approaches share a great deal with a HRBA, with their shared focus on social justice, equity, and empowerment. Participation is seen as both a means and an end and the processes that take place in both new public health approaches and HRBA are just as important as the outcomes that may result. The Sustainable Development Goals and the movement to address the social determinants of health similarly draw heavily on the principles and methods of a HRBA (Sachs, 2012). It builds on the agency of vulnerable groups and places the rights and actions of the vulnerable alongside obligations of the state (London, 2008).

Social epidemiology and the social determinants of health

Social epidemiology is the study of how social structures, institutions, and relationships influence health (Berkman et al., 2014). It describes how the social world shapes patterns of disease, health, and mortality. Although social epidemiology is a relatively new field, the recognition that the social environment affects mortality and patterns of disease is not. Thinkers such as Chadwick (Hamlin, 1994), Virchow (Waitzkin, 2006), and Villermé (Porter, 1999) began the early collection of mortality rates for different geographical areas and observed their association with social deprivation and wealth. Durkheim explored the relationship between different societal structures and suicide rates (Durkheim, 1897). These patterns of disease or death continue today to be associated with aspects of people's lives such as socioeconomic status, gender, age, or ethnicity and this was once again demonstrated during the COVID-19 pandemic (Ahmed et al., 2020).

Research, advocacy, and action in this field have led to a renewed focus on the social determinants of health over the past 30 years. The World Health Organization (WHO) convened the Commission on the Social Determinants of Health in 2005, with the aim of understanding how health equity can be promoted and to foster a global movement to achieve it (WHO, 2008). The social determinants of health have become a common term in health, development, and policy discourse and can be seen in programmes and initiatives such as the Sustainable Development Goals (Sachs, 2012). While the literature and evidence base relating to the social determinants of health has continued to grow (Marmot and Wilkinson, 2005), Marmot (WHO, 2008) summed up the evidence succinctly when he stated 'poorer people live shorter lives'.

The impact of social determinants on health are manifest throughout the life course, from birth to death. High perinatal and maternal mortality are linked to poverty, access to clean water and healthcare services, and education and empowerment. Gender equality, access to education, and ability to control decisions around marriage, reproduction, and contraception determine the lives and deaths of women around the world. Safe environments, from the impacts of conflict and displacement to air pollution or rising sea levels are a major determinant of health and discrimination, structural violence, and lack of agency are at the heart of much ill health and inequity today (WHO, 2008). Differences in life expectancy and premature mortality from avoidable causes determine how and why people die and the experiences and memories of those deaths influences the lives and health of those surviving them.

Returning to the example of HIV/AIDS once again, it provides a model through which the impact of social factors on disease can be recognized and appreciated. It allows social impacts to be considered as risk factors in their own right, instead of being dismissed as confounding variables to be controlled for. Poundstone and colleagues (2004) describe a series of social-level factors and structural-level factors that have been shown to influence and account for significant differences in HIV transmission across different communities, contexts, and countries (Fig. 8.2). Social networks, the positions people occupy or play within them, and the social relationships they participate in are associated with differing rates of HIV transmission (Friedman et al., 1997). The influence of peer behaviour and social norms have been demonstrated to exert a significant effect on practices and behaviours such as condom use or drug taking and therefore impact on transmission (Rice et al., 2005; Bhattacharjee et al., 2013). Place-based influences also play a significant role, beyond the effect of social networks. The segregation of communities within certain neighbourhoods increases residents' exposure to certain risks and limits their access to resources that may help them. Determinants such as poverty, income, access to education, physical environment, and safety have been shown to influence rates of transmission of infectious disease (Barr et al., 2001; Cohen et al., 2007).

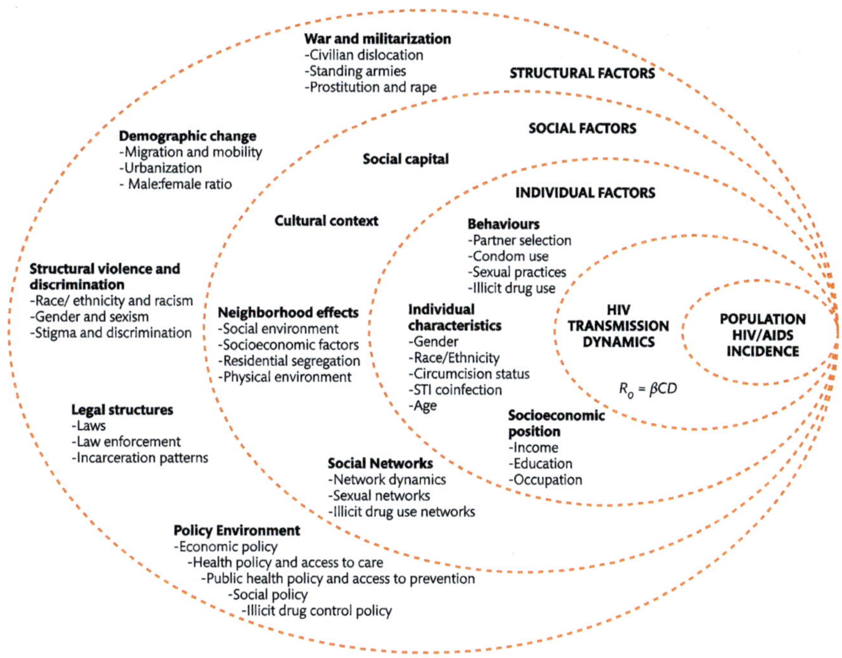

Fig. 8.2 A heuristic framework for the social epidemiology of HIV/AIDS. The dotted lines separating the levels illustrate the porous nature of the distinctions between levels of analysis. In reality, there are extensive linkages between factors at all levels that give rise to observed epidemic patterns. STI, sexually transmitted infection.

Reproduced with permission from Poundstone, K.E., Strathdee, S.A. and Celentano, D.D., 2004. The social epidemiology of human immunodeficiency virus/acquired immunodeficiency syndrome. *Epidemiologic reviews*, 26(1), pp. 22–35.

Finally, Poundstone and colleagues (2004) describe the structural-level determinants of HIV transmission, looking at structural violence and discrimination including race/ethnicity and racism, gender, sexism, and stigma, legal structures, demographic changes, the policy and legal environment, and war and militarization (Fig. 8.2). It is essential to understand these structural determinants of health and to shift the focus from individual-level risk factors or determinants to community- or societal-level risk factors or determinants. Understanding how risk can be shifted on a population level is essential in accounting for and addressing these disparities. They cannot be addressed on an individual basis.

The social epidemiology of death, dying, and bereavement

Death, dying, and loss are universal human events and experiences; they affect everyone within in a population. While death is seen as the end point and in many ways the ultimate failure of public health interventions, experiences relating to death, dying, and loss can themselves be the focus of prevention, early intervention, harm reduction, and HRBA interventions.

Bereavement is an intensely painful emotional experience, but in addition to the strong affective component, bereavement can impact significantly on mental, physical, and social well-being (Stroebe et al., 2007). It can increase a bereaved person's risk of dying, including through suicide, meaning there is a mortality risk associated with bereavement (Latham and Prigerson, 2004). It increases the risk of cardiovascular disease (Prigerson et al., 1997) hospitalization and medication use (Stroebe et al., 2007), and of mental health issues such as depression (Tateno et al., 2011). Bereavement can also lead to adverse social challenges. Studies suggest that, in many circumstances, bereavement can lead to a disintegration of social ties and networks as friends, neighbours, or co-workers do not know what to say or how to offer support, meaning the bereaved person becomes progressively isolated. This is particularly true when a death has been sudden, violent, or stigmatizing or when a child dies. A study exploring the changes in social networks and support for people bereaved through road traffic accidents suggested these deaths can be particularly stigmatizing and social networks can retract. A quote from a woman whose daughter died in car crash illustrates this poignantly (Breen and O'Connor, 2011):

> People find the loss of a child more confronting than the loss of a spouse. Having lost two spouses I've noticed the difference. When my first husband died, people would come up to me in the street, pat me on the shoulder and say 'how are you?'. When Mary-Anne died … I felt as if I'd been caught doing something I shouldn't have been doing … and this was the difference. When you've lost a child, people will cross the road if they see you coming, it's as if it's contagious, and it could happen to them. (pp. 110–111)

In many cultures around the world, a woman's social standing and support may come as a part of (heterosexual) marriage. When a woman's husband dies, she may lose these assets or social support structures, leading to discrimination, poverty for her and her children, or the need to undergo damaging rituals. Widows and orphans are among the most vulnerable populations in the world (Loomba Foundation, 2016) and widowhood in other settings such as the US can predispose to socioeconomic consequences and loss of health insurance (Weir, 2003). Further social consequences of bereavement may be prolonged absence from work, lost employment, and economic consequences (Fox et al., 2014).

Dying itself can lead to a series of adverse outcomes, aside from the fact of the impending mortality. People can become isolated, stigmatized, or withdraw from social ties and connection following a terminal diagnosis. People may experience severe pain or other physical symptoms which are unrelieved, leading to serious health-related suffering (Knaul et al., 2018) and significant distress to those caring for or close to the dying person. Serious health-related suffering is predicted to rise in all regions with the largest proportional rise in low-income countries (Sleeman et al., 2019). Inequity in access to opioids for pain when dying has been labelled one of the most significant global inequities of our time (Knaul et al., 2018). Difficult or traumatic deaths are acknowledged to adversely affect caregivers in their bereavement, potentially leading to complicated grief (Kaltman and Bonanno, 2003).

People dying can suffer with existential, spiritual, or religious distress (Boston et al., 2011). A loss of faith, a fear that god is issuing punishment, or deep guilt or regret at actions in one's life can cause extreme anguish that make the dying process distressing for the person and those close to them (Tedeschi and Calhoun, 2006).

The social epidemiology associated with death, dying, and bereavement can be significant and while it represents an urgent consideration for public health, it is important to note that for many people dying is a peaceful, intimate, or even creative process. People dying speak of a heightening of sensation and feelings, as Dennis Potter famously described as he was dying of cancer:

> I see it is the whitest, frothiest, blossomest blossom that there ever could be, and I can see it. The nowness of everything is absolutely wondrous, and if people could see that, you know. There's no way of telling you; you have to experience it, but the glory of it, if you like, the comfort of it, the reassurance. (Potter, 1994)

Similarly, the majority of bereaved people adapt to their loss and are able to continue with their lives without significant impairment. The loss and the person who died are incorporated into their lives and their story and they are able to look to the future. Grief has led to the creation of some of the most poignant poetry, music, or literature and led to many architectural achievements, or funds set up in memory of those who have died. The important question is not how we can minimize or reduce death and bereavement, these are significant and essential parts of all our lives, but rather how we can face them with equity, understanding, and care, such that the preventable negative impacts on lives are diminished.

Inequities in the social epidemiology of death, dying, and bereavement

While death, dying, and bereavement may be universal experiences, they are not evenly distributed within societies or across the world. Stark differences in avoidable mortality, such as perinatal deaths, maternal deaths, or deaths through accident are seen both between countries and within countries. There is almost a 20-year difference in the life expectancy for someone living in the UK or Malawi while the probability of dying prematurely, aged 15–60 years is 27.9 per 100,000 in Malawi and 6.8 in the UK (United Nations, 2019). These gradients in life expectancy, likelihood of dying before 60 years old, or dying of a preventable cause are due to the inequities rife in societies globally, the social determinants of death. These significant inequities affect not only those dying but those close to them and equate to significant inequities in bereavement and grief. Families, communities, neighbourhoods, or countries with high numbers of early or preventable deaths mean families and social networks are more likely to face multiple, early, and potentially traumatic deaths of family members, friends, and neighbours. Conservative estimates of the impact of a death suggest that two or three people are affected by each death, with other estimates suggesting closer to six people, meaning that as death and bereavement are distributed unequally across society, so too are the mental, physical, and social sequalae.

Studies of racial disparities in the US have demonstrated that black communities die earlier and sicker than their other American counterparts. Umberson and colleagues (2017) estimated racial differences in exposure to family member deaths with data from two national datasets and found that black Americans were more likely than white Americans to have experienced the death of a mother, a father, or a sibling from childhood through midlife. Black Americans were at twice the risk of losing a mother and at about 50% greater risk of losing a father by age 20. They highlight how previous studies of the impact of bereavement have focused on single bereavements only, rather than the effect of frequent and multiple losses, as experienced by many in their study. They suggest that this is a distinctive stressor and an important contributor to the cumulative disadvantage faced by black communities in the US.

Studies of childhood bereavement have shown that it is not the fact of bereavement per se that is damaging for the child, but rather the context and circumstances of the death and the presence or absence of stable and supportive relationships surrounding the child (Akerman et al., 2011). The field of adverse childhood experiences (ACEs) has grown rapidly in recent years (Boullier and Blair, 2018) and offers insights into the long-term impacts of traumatic events in childhood. The loss of a parent is a destabilizing and highly distressing event in a child's life but the presence of stable and supportive networks around the child can mitigate or harm reduce these long-term impacts. Children who are bereaved who lack supportive networks, or children who are bereaved following violent or traumatic deaths or suicide, are much more likely to experience issues into adulthood. ACEs include a range of experiences beyond bereavement such as abuse, neglect or violence, substance misuse, or mental illness in the home. ACEs are correlated with a range of issues in adulthood such as poor physical and mental health with an increased incidence of cardiovascular disease, diabetes, depression or cancer, behaviours such as smoking, alcohol or drug use, and difficulty forming stable relationships, and lost opportunities in education and employment (Felitti et al., 1998; Brown et al., 2009; Liu et al., 2013). It is the high prevalence of ACEs in population and the preventable nature of many of these experiences that has led to significant national efforts on the part of many countries to tackle the root causes and determinants of ACEs (Centers for Disease Control and Prevention, 2019; NHS Health Scotland, 2019).

Death, dying, and bereavement as both consequences and drivers of inequity

Death, dying, and bereavement are natural and unavoidable human events. Dying of preventable conditions, early in life, under traumatic circumstances or with unrelieved pain are not unavoidable. Indeed, in many settings around the world, people are living longer, healthier lives and dying what would be perceived as a 'good death' in later life. But as we have seen, these experiences are not

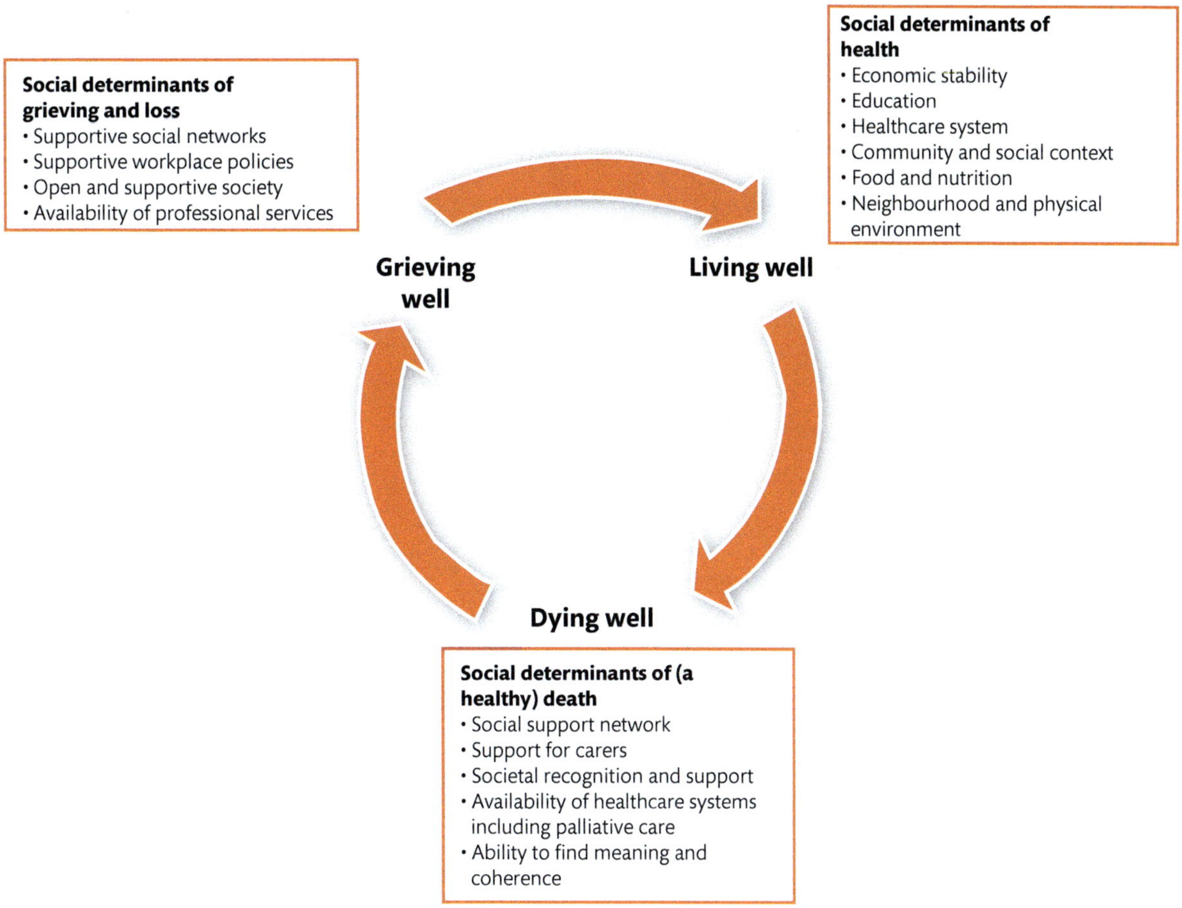

Fig. 8.3 The social determinants of dying, living, and grieving.

equitably distributed throughout the world, leaving some communities bearing the brunt of both avoidable and high rates of mortality alongside the complex and long-term impacts of multiple losses and bereavement. Premature death, dying, and multiple or traumatic bereavement can be understood as being both the consequence of inequity but also a driver for inequity. This is a crucial point. Fig. 8.3 illustrates the cyclical nature of life, death, and grief and how damaging or positive experiences at each point are reinforcing and go on to influence subsequent experiences. How we live, die, and grieve are interconnected and the conditions for living well, dying well, and grieving well draw on common roots.

Prevention and harm reduction approaches in death, dying, and bereavement

One of the most well-known harm reduction interventions in death and dying is the field of palliative care. Palliative care services are harm reduction services by definition, as they manage, mitigate, and 'cloak' the symptoms and impacts of advanced and incurable illness. Palliative care has been recognized as a component of universal health coverage (WHO, 2014) and services have been demonstrated to improve symptom relief and quality of life (Gomes et al., 2013) and outcomes for carers (Grande et al., 2017), reduce inappropriate health service utilization, and increase the likelihood of care concordant with people's wishes (Gomes et al., 2013). Recent studies have explored the role of palliative care as an early intervention approach in serious or incurable illness and have demonstrated important benefits for people and those close to them (Temel et al., 2010, 2017).

Despite evidence of effectiveness and continued calls for access to palliative care for all (WHO, 2018), access remains disappointingly skewed along the traditional lines of discrimination, marginalization, and structural vulnerability (see Chapter 20). The shocking inequity in access to oral morphine, used as a proxy for access to palliative care services, represents this lack of access on a global scale (Fig. 8.4).

Even within the inflated countries such as the US, Canada, Australia, and some counties in Europe, steep gradients in access exist for marginalized communities (Dixon et al., 2015; Griggs, 2020). It is often the communities facing the most complex needs around death, dying, and bereavement that have the poorest access to support, following the inverse care law seen throughout healthcare (Tudor-Hart, 1971). Initiatives that tackle these entrenched patterns of lack of access, care, and support are urgently needed.

Returning now to Fig. 8.1 at the start of the chapter and the graphs representing the differences between a health services approach and a public health approach, palliative care provided to patients and families can be understood as a health service response to individuals rather than populations. Efforts to address inequities in access to services or opioids are public health approaches, aiming

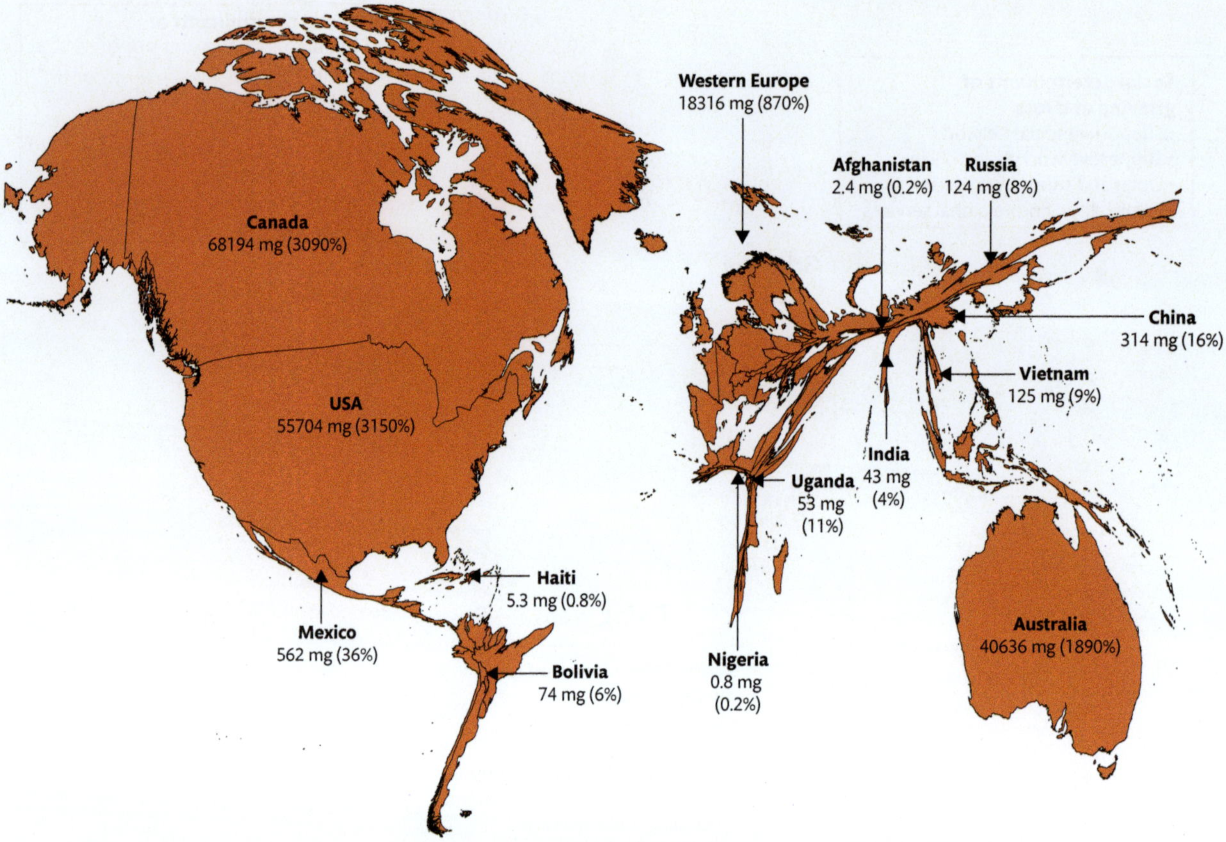

Fig. 8.4 Distributed opioid morphine equivalent (morphine in mg/patient in need of palliative care 2010–2013), and estimated percentages of need that is met for the health conditions with serious health-related suffering.

Reproduced with permission from Knaul, F.M. et al. (2018) Alleviating the access abyss in palliative care and pain relief—an imperative of universal health coverage: The Lancet commission report. ***The Lancet***, 391(10128), pp. 1391–1454.

to address the needs of a population and while essential, they still represent a limited, reactive, harm reduction approach. Moving beyond these service-based, harm reduction approaches of palliative care services, what primary prevention or HRBA interventions exist for death, dying, and bereavement? What are the equivalents to vaccination programmes, screening for cancer or healthy eating campaigns?

Over the past 20 years, these questions have been asked by many around the world. The result has been the emergence of the fields of a new public health approach to palliative care, health-promoting palliative care, public education, social network and community development initiatives, compassionate communities, and compassionate cities approaches. They all represent different means of responding to this challenge.

Many such initiatives are combinations of prevention, early intervention, and harm reduction, depending on your position within a project or your place on your life course. Interventions designed to foster supportive networks for people at the end of life and their carers may act as early intervention or harm reduction initiatives for those dying and caring, but as primary prevention interventions for people who may be well but who are learning how to build networks and understand the place dying and caring has in all our lives.

We now consider the range of initiatives around the world that have responded to the question of 'What public health interventions exist within death, dying, and bereavement?' Many are described in detail in other chapters in this book. The evidence base informing and emerging from these approaches is explored in Chapter 22.

Public awareness, national events, or festivals

A number of countries hold public awareness days or weeks, festivals, or run national programmes to bring issues of death, dying, and bereavement to a national audience. These initiatives prompt people to reflect on, discuss, or take action around these issues. Examples include Dying Matters Week (Dying Matters, 2021), Good Grief Festival (Good Grief Festival, 2021) and Good Life, Good Death, Good Grief (Good Life, Good Death, Good Grief, 2021) in the UK; Dying to Know Day in Australia (https://www.thegroundswellproject.com/dying-to-know-day); Life Before Death in Singapore (Lien Foundation, 2021); and the Curios festival in Kerala (Institute of Palliative Medicine, 2021), India.

Initiatives such as these fall broadly under the prevention category. By asking whole populations, the majority of whom are not dying, caring, or grieving at that time, to consider their own mortality or that of their families and friends, it is hoped that people will feel more comfortable discussing these issues. This may reduce issues at the end of life that stem from a lack of communication or awareness of wishes and may address the stigma prevalent in many cultures in discussing these issues.

Public education programmes

Some initiatives take a step further and move from prompting conversations or providing a space to exploring issues relating to death, dying, and loss, to the provision of education to the general public. These educational initiatives are distinct from educational programmes provided for healthcare professionals or volunteers who are delivering care and support to individuals. Initiatives such as Last Aid (Bollig and Heller, 2016) teach members of the public about how to care for someone as they die, the changes that take place as someone dies, and how to support someone grieving. Some initiatives focus on children in schools and put age-appropriate discussions on death, dying, and bereavement into the personal and social education curriculum (Paul et al., 2019). Again, these interventions to provide education to all children of a certain age are distinct from discussions or sessions provided to teachers or children when a child in the school dies or is bereaved. Interventions such as these broadly fall into the prevention category, as people have the opportunity to reflect on these issues and learn certain skills or build networks before they face them in their own lives.

Community action

On a more local level, some communities have taken action themselves to support people dying or grieving among them. The death doula movement aims to support people and their families deal with the practical, emotional, and spiritual issues that emerge when faced with a terminal illness (Rawlings et al., 2019). They often act as a bridge or link between lay or family networks and professional networks of care and aim to fulfil a role that is missing for many people. In Australia, a project was designed to link people who had previously cared for a family member or a friend dying at home with someone currently undertaking that role, to facilitate the sharing of skills and knowledge within a community (Leonard et al., 2010). Again, depending on the point at which such connections are made, initiatives such as these can be early interventions or harm reduction approaches for the person dying and those caring for them.

Some local action has expanded to influence at the national level. In the southwestern Indian state of Kerala, the Neighbourhood Network in Palliative Care was a community response to poorly accessible and professionalized end of life care (Kumar, 2007). What started as a grassroots response, mobilizing volunteers and fostering supportive social networks to care for people with incurable illnesses, led to demonstrations, media campaigns, and a national policy which stipulates that care for the dying must include community participation (Paleri, 2008). This initiative was built not only in response to the poor care that existed for people as they died, but on ideological grounds, that communities have a right and a responsibility to support people living with life-limiting illnesses, caring, and grieving and that processes should be put in place that allow and facilitate this. The programme focuses on the building of these skills in communities, independently of the care provided to patients and families (Kumar, 2020).

There is a subtle distinction between initiatives intending to improve the care for people dying and their carers on a population level, through the process of community action and others aiming to improve the skills and capacity of general populations, independently of the need to provide care and support for people. This is the difference between community engagement, which harnesses the resources and skills of communities to provide better care and services for people, and community development in which the primary aim is to foster new skills and confidence in people, quite aside from any outcomes that may result for those using services or needing care. Again, depending on where you are positioned in these projects, community action initiatives may be prevention, early intervention, or harm reduction initiatives.

Environmental and civic action

The places people live, play, and work exert a significant influence over their health and well-being and a number of initiatives have worked historically to harness this place-based influence (Kelly, 2014). Universities, workplaces, or civic bodies such as local councils can influence how people experience dying, caring, or grieving through early intervention or harm reduction approaches such as compassionate leave policies or carers or bereavement support groups (Chapter on compassionate cities/universities). But further to this, through comprehensive approaches such as the compassionate cities movement, cities, towns, or villages can integrate human rights-based and prevention approaches to death, dying, and loss alongside early intervention and harm reduction approaches. Placing issues of inequity, discrimination, and poverty as central to how a society cares for those dying is a cornerstone of a HRBA to death, dying, and bereavement. Compassionate cities crucially take issues of death and dying out of the professional frame of reference and into the everyday spheres of work, rest, and play. By making these issues part of everyday, civic life and not ones that you only stumble upon in a crisis, populations are able to learn about them, discuss them with those close to them, and prepare for them.

Policies

Supportive policies are an essential strand of any comprehensive public health approach. The staggering inequity of global access to morphine and the international efforts to ensure access for all to essential medications at the end of life is an example of a harm reduction policy in the field of death and dying (Knaul et al., 2018). Other examples include policies that mandate paid bereavement leave or paid carers or compassionate leave. A number of countries such as Australia, China, France, and Brazil have statutory, paid bereavement leave enshrined in legislation, but the US and Canada do not. Open and supportive attitudes to bereavement and grief cannot be cultivated if they are not acknowledged and provided for by policies and legislation. In the UK, a new law came into effect in 2020 allowing for parents whose child has died while under the age of 18 to take 2 weeks paid bereavement leave (Department for Business, Energy & Industrial Strategy, 2020). This makes it one of the most supportive paid bereavement policies in the world. Policies such as these are important harm reduction approaches in this field.

Human rights-based approaches

Over recent years there has been significant discussion about palliative care as a human right. This often focuses on the role of pain relief in the right to be free from inhumane or degrading treatment and other key aspects of the human rights charter (Gwyther et al., 2009; Lohman et al., 2010). The duty on the part of governments and statutory services is to ensure appropriate and accessible palliative care services are available to all in a population. A HRBA goes beyond the provision of palliative care services, bringing issues of disadvantage and discrimination to the fore. In the UK, the charity Sue Ryder and the British Institute of Human Rights developed a joint initiative focusing on the fulfilment of human rights at the end of life. This included a guide for staff and a series of workshops to develop awareness of this an issue in care (British Institute of Human Rights, 2016). Moving beyond educational programmes, a number of national initiatives have developed in the UK. The Care Quality Commission, the regulator for care and health institutions, has adopted a HRBA (Care Quality Commission, 2019) aiming to create a culture of fairness, equity, and inclusion for staff and to place these issues at the centre of their assessments of institutions. In Scotland, the principles of a HRBA have been used to create a Charter of Rights for people living with dementia and their carers, aiming to tackle the cultural, social, and economic barriers they often face in fulfilling their rights (Alzheimer Scotland, 2009).

In Canada, there has been focused attention on the role of structural inequities at the end of life. Studies understanding how structural inequities affect people while caring, dying, or grieving (Stadujhar et al., 2020; Schneider and Dosani, 2021) help to inform initiatives such as Equity in Palliative Approaches to Care (ePAC) (ePAC, 2021) and Palliative Care Education and Care for the Homeless (PEACH; McGill Council on Palliative Care, 2021) (see Chapter 20).

Finally, there has been caution issued in the assumptions made and language used when advocating for palliative care services or compassionate community projects. Gott and colleagues (2020) argue, through the lens of gender, that much 'community' care falls on the shoulders of women and that this is broadly unacknowledged, undervalued, and expected. She argues for a paradigm shift in research, practice, and policy in end of life care and for an intersectional approach to be adopted by all.

Conclusion

Comprehensive public health measures are essential to protect and improve the health and well-being of populations and this applies throughout the life course. Prevention, harm reduction, and early intervention approaches are essential in reducing the prevalence of obesity or smoking, adverse childhood events, depression, or loss of social networks following a bereavement, carer isolation and burnout, or dying with unrelieved pain or symptoms.

The provision of clinical palliative care services is an established and important harm reduction intervention, but it is not sufficient to address the complex social epidemiology of death, dying, and bereavement. A comprehensive approach will move beyond this, understanding how experiences of death, dying, and bereavement intersect with structural issues such as race, gender, sexuality, or poverty to perpetuate cycles of loss, despair, and disadvantage.

These comprehensive public health interventions must sit within a broader approach that recognizes the power and agency people have to engage with public health provisions and how inequity, discrimination, and disadvantage shapes how people live, die, and grieve. New public health approaches blend prevention, harm reduction, and early intervention approaches with a HRBA that recognizes the rights and responsibilities that exist throughout society. These must be respected and fulfilled in order for these critical but natural events in people's lives to be experienced as peaceful, dignified, and timely rather than as damaging and harmful events.

REFERENCES

Acheson, S. D. 1998. *Independent Inquiry into Inequalities in Health Report*. London: Stationery Office.

Ahmed, F., Ahmed, N. E., Pissarides, C., and Stiglitz, J. 2020. Why inequality could spread COVID-19. *Lancet Public Health*, **5**, e240.

Akerman, R. and Statham, J. 2011. *Childhood Bereavement: A Rapid Literature Review*. London: Child Wellbeing Research Centre.

Alzheimer Scotland. 2009. *A Charter of Rights for People with Dementia and their Carers in Scotland*. Edinburgh: Alzheimer Scotland.

Barr, R. G., Diez-Roux, A. V., Knirsch, C. A., and Pablos-Méndez, A. 2001. Neighborhood poverty and the resurgence of tuberculosis in New York City, 1984–1992. *American Journal of Public Health*, **91**, 1487–1493.

Berkman, L. F., Kawachi, I., and Glymour, M. M. (eds.) 2014. *Social Epidemiology*. Oxford: Oxford University Press.

Bhattacharjee, P., Prakash, R., Pillai, P., Isac, S., Haranahalli, M., Blanchard, A., et al. 2013. Understanding the role of peer group membership in reducing HIV-related risk and vulnerability among female sex workers in Karnataka, India. *AIDS Care*, **25**, S46–S54.

Bollig, G. and Heller, A. 2016. The last aid course – a simple and effective concept to teach the public about palliative care and to enhance the public discussion about death and dying. *Austin Palliative Care*, **1**, 1010.

Boston, P., Bruce, A., and Schreiber, R. 2011. Existential suffering in the palliative care setting: an integrated literature review. *Journal of Pain and Symptom Management*, **41**, 604–618.

Boullier, M. and Blair, M. 2018. Adverse childhood experiences. *Paediatrics and Child Health*, **28**, 132–137.

Breen, L. J. and O'Connor, M. 2011. Family and social networks after bereavement: experiences of support, change and isolation. *Journal of Family Therapy*, **33**, 98–120.

British Institute of Human Rights. 2016. *End of Life Care and Human Rights: A Practitioner's Guide*. London: British Institute of Human Rights and Sue Ryder.

Brown, D. W., Anda, R. F., Tiemeier, H., Felitti, V. J., Edwards, V. J., Croft, J. B., et al. 2009. Adverse childhood experiences and the risk of premature mortality. *American Journal of Preventive Medicine*, **37**, 389–396.

Buckner, S., Darlington, N., Woodward, M., Buswell, M., Mathie, E., Arthur, A., et al. 2019. Dementia friendly communities in England: a scoping study. *International Journal of Geriatric Psychiatry*, **34**, 1235–1243.

Care Quality Commission. 2019. *Our Human Rights Approach for How We Regulate Health and Social Care Services: February 2019*. London: Care Quality Commission.

Centers for Disease Control and Prevention. 2019. *Preventing Adverse Childhood Experiences: Leveraging the Best Available Evidence*. Atlanta, GA: National Center for Injury Prevention and Control, Centers for Disease Control and Prevention.

Chang, L. W., Serwadda, D., Quinn, T. C., Wawer, M. J., Gray, R. H., and Reynolds, S. J. 2013. Combination implementation for HIV prevention: moving from clinical trial evidence to population-level effects. *Lancet Infectious Diseases*, **13**, 65–76.

Cohen, J. M., Wilson, M. L., and Aiello, A. E. 2007. Analysis of social epidemiology research on infectious diseases: historical patterns and future opportunities. *Journal of Epidemiology & Community Health*, **61**, 1021–1027.

Department for Business, Energy & Industrial Strategy. 2020. UK set to introduce 'Jack's Law' – new legal right to paid parental bereavement leave. 23 January. [Online] Available at: https://www.gov.uk/government/news/uk-set-to-introduce-jacks-law-new-legal-right-to-paid-parental-bereavement-leave

Dixon, J., King, D., Matosevic, T., Clark, M., and Knapp, M. 2015. *Equity in the Provision of Palliative Care in the UK: Review of Evidence*. London: Personal Social Services Research Unit, London School of Economics and Political Science.

Durkheim, E. 1897. *Suicide: A Study of Sociology*. Paris: Félix Alcan.

Dying Matters. 2021. Awareness week. [Online] Available at: https://www.dyingmatters.org/AwarenessWeek

ePAC. 2021. Equity in palliative approaches to care. [Online] Available at: https://www.equityinpalliativecare.com/

European Collaborative Study. 2005. Mother-to-child transmission of HIV infection in the era of highly active antiretroviral therapy. *Clinical Infectious Diseases*, **40**, 458–465.

Felitti, V. J., Anda, R. F., Nordenberg, D., Williamson, D. F., Spitz, A. M., Edwards, V., et al. 1998. Relationship of childhood abuse and household dysfunction to many of the leading causes of death in adults: the Adverse Childhood Experiences (ACE) Study. *American Journal of Preventive Medicine*, **14**, 245–258.

Fox, M., Cacciatore, J., and Lacasse, J. R. 2014. Child death in the United States: productivity and the economic burden of parental grief. *Death Studies*, **38**, 597–602.

Friedman, S. R., Neaigus, A., Jose, B., Curtis, R., Goldstein, M., Ildefonso, G., et al. 1997. Sociometric risk networks and risk for HIV infection. *American Journal of Public Health*, **87**, 1289–1296.

Gomes, B., Calanzani, N., Curiale, V., McCrone, P., and Higginson, I. J. 2013. Effectiveness and cost-effectiveness of home palliative care services for adults with advanced illness and their caregivers. *Cochrane Database of Systematic Reviews*, **6**, CD007760.

Good Grief Festival. 2021. Good grief: a virtual festival of love & loss. [Online] Available at: https://goodgrieffest.com/

Good Life, Good Death, Good Grief. 2021. Demystifying death week. [Online] Available at: https://www.goodlifedeathgrief.org.uk/

Gott, M., Morgan, T., and Williams, L. 2020. Gender and palliative care: a call to arms. *Palliative Care and Social Practice*, **14**, 1–15.

Grande, G. E., Austin, L., Ewing, G., O'Leary, N., and Roberts, C. 2017. Assessing the impact of a Carer Support Needs Assessment Tool (CSNAT) intervention in palliative home care: a stepped wedge cluster trial. *BMJ Supportive & Palliative Care*, **7**, 326–334.

Griggs, J. J. 2020. Disparities in palliative care in patients with cancer. *Journal of Clinical Oncology*, **38**, 974–979.

Gwyther, L., Brennan, F., and Harding, R. 2009. Advancing palliative care as a human right. *Journal of Pain and Symptom Management*, **38**, 767–774.

Hadley, A. 2014. Reducing teenage pregnancy: lessons learned from the UK Government's teenage pregnancy strategy for England. *Journal of Adolescent Health*, **54**(2), S35.

Hadley, A., Ingham, R., and Chandra-Mouli, V. 2016. Implementing the United Kingdom's ten-year teenage pregnancy strategy for England (1999–2010): how was this done and what did it achieve? *Reproductive Health*, **13**, 1–11.

Hadley, A. 2020. Teenage pregnancy: strategies for prevention. *Obstetrics, Gynaecology & Reproductive Medicine*, **30**, 387–339.

Hamlin, C. 1994. State medicine in Great Britain. In: Porter, D. (ed.) *The History of Public Health and the Modern State*, pp. 132–164. Amsterdam: Rodopi.

Hart, J. T. 1971. The inverse care law. *Lancet*, **297**, 405–412.

Institute of Palliative Medicine. 2021. Kerala Curios Festival. [Online] Available at: https://www.instituteofpalliativemedicine.org/eventdetail.php

Kaltman, S. and Bonanno, G. A. 2003. Trauma and bereavement: examining the impact of sudden and violent deaths. *Journal of Anxiety Disorders*, **17**, 131–147.

Kelly, M. 2014. *Healthy Cities. Research and Practice*. London: Taylor and Francis.

Knaul, F. M., Farmer, P. E., Krakauer, E. L., De Lima, L., Bhadelia, A., Kwete, X. J., et al. 2018. Alleviating the access abyss in palliative care and pain relief—an imperative of universal health coverage: The Lancet commission report. *Lancet*, **391**, 1391–1454.

Kumar, S. 2020. Community participation in palliative care: reflections from the ground. *Progress in Palliative Care*, **28**, 83–88.

Kumar, S. K. 2007. Kerala, India: a regional community-based palliative care model. *Journal of Pain and Symptom Management*, **33**, 623–627.

Latham, A. E. and Prigerson, H. G. 2004. Suicidality and bereavement: complicated grief as psychiatric disorder presenting greatest risk for suicidality. *Suicide and Life-Threatening Behavior*, **34**, 350–362.

Leonard, R., Horsfall, D., and Noonan, K. 2010. Models of caring from India and Australia and their relationship to social capital. *Nepalese Journal of Public Policy and Governance*, **xxvi**, 15–25.

Lien Foundation. 2021. Life before death. [Online] Available at: http://lifebeforedeath.com/about-us/

Liu, Y., Croft, J. B., Chapman, D. P., Perry, G. S., Greenlund, K. J., Zhao, G., et al. 2013. Relationship between adverse childhood experiences and unemployment among adults from five US states. *Social Psychiatry and Psychiatric Epidemiology*, **48**, 357–369.

Lohman, D., Schleifer, R., and Amon, J. J. 2010. Access to pain treatment as a human right. *BMC Medicine*, **8**, 1–9.

London, L. 2008. What is a human-rights based approach to health and does it matter? *Health and Human Rights*, **10**, 65–80.

Loomba Foundation. 2016. *World Widows Report*. London: Loomba Foundation.

Marmot, M. and Wilkinson, R. (eds.) 2005. *Social Determinants of Health*. Oxford: Oxford University Press.

McGill Council on Palliative Care. 2021. PEACH – Palliative Education and Care for the Homeless. [Online] Available at: https://www.mcgill.ca/council-on-palliative-care/article/peach-palliative-education-and-care-homeless

McKinlay, J. B. 1979. A case for refocusing upstream: the political economy of illness. In: Enelow, J. D. and Henderson, J. B. (eds.) *Patients, Physicians and Illness: A Sourcebook in Behavioral Science and Health*, pp. 9–25. Dallas, TX: American Heart Association.

Merson, M. H., O'Malley, J., Serwadda, D., and Apisuk, C. 2008. The history and challenge of HIV prevention. *Lancet*, **372**, 475–488.

NHS Health Scotland. 2019. *Adverse Childhood Experiences in Context*. Edinburgh: NHS Health Scotland.

Paleri, A. K. 2008. Showing the way forward: pain and palliative care policy of the government of Kerala. *Indian Journal of Palliative Care*, **14**, 51–54.

Paul, S., Cree, V. E., and Murray, S. A. 2019. Integrating palliative care into the community: the role of hospices and schools. *BMJ Supportive & Palliative Care*, **9**, e31.

Potter, D. 1994. Interviewed by Melvyn Bragg for Channel 4 'Without Walls', broadcast 5 April.

Prigerson, H. G., Bierhals, A. J., Kasl, S. V., Reynolds, C. F., Shear, M. K., Day, N., et al. 1997. Traumatic grief as a risk factor for mental and physical morbidity. *American Journal of Psychiatry*, **154**, 616–623.

Rawlings, D., Tieman, J., Miller-Lewis, L. and Swetenham, K. 2019. What role do death doulas play in end-of-life care? A systematic review. *Health & Social Care in the Community*, **27**, e82–e94.

Rekart, M. L. 2005. Sex-work harm reduction. *Lancet*, **366**, 2123–2134.

Rice, E., Milburn, N. G., Rotheram-Borus, M. J., Mallett, S., and Rosenthal, D. 2005. The effects of peer group network properties on drug use among homeless youth. *American Behavioral Scientist*, **48**, 1102–1123.

Ritter, A. and Cameron, J. 2006. A review of the efficacy and effectiveness of harm reduction strategies for alcohol, tobacco and illicit drugs. *Drug and Alcohol Review*, **25**, 611–624.

Sachs, J. D. 2012. From millennium development goals to sustainable development goals. *Lancet*, **379**, 2206–2211.

Sallnow, L., Tishelman, C., Lindqvist, O., Richardson, H., and Cohen, J. 2016. Research in public health and end-of-life care—building on the past and developing the new. *Progress in Palliative Care*, **24**, 25–30.

Schneider, E. and Dosani, N. 2021. A retrospective study of a Toronto-based palliative care program for individuals experiencing homelessness. *Journal of Palliative Medicine*, **24**, 1232–1235.

Sleeman, K. E., de Brito, M., Etkind, S., Nkhoma, K., Guo, P., Higginson, I. J., et al. 2019. The escalating global burden of serious health-related suffering: projections to 2060 by world regions, age groups, and health conditions. *Lancet Global Health*, **7**, e883–e892.

Smith, D. K., Herbst, J. H., Zhang, X., and Rose, C. E. 2015. Condom effectiveness for HIV prevention by consistency of use among men who have sex with men in the United States. *Journal of Acquired Immune Deficiency Syndromes*, **68**, 337–344.

Stajduhar, K. I., Giesbrecht, M., Mollison, A., Dosani, N., and McNeil, R. 2020. Caregiving at the margins: an ethnographic exploration of family caregivers experiences providing care for structurally vulnerable populations at the end-of-life. *Palliative Medicine*, **34**, 946–953.

Stroebe, M., Schut, H., and Stroebe, W. 2007. Health outcomes of bereavement. *Lancet*, **370**, 1960–1973.

Porter, D. 1999. *The Greatest Benefit to Mankind: A Medical History of Humanity from Antiquity to the Present*. London: Fontana Press.

Poundstone, K. E., Strathdee, S. A., and Celentano, D. D. 2004. The social epidemiology of human immunodeficiency virus/acquired immunodeficiency syndrome. *Epidemiologic Reviews*, **26**, 22–35.

Prigerson, H. G., Bierhals, A. J., Kasl, S. V., Reynolds, C. F., Shear, M. K., Day, N., et al. 1997. Traumatic grief as a risk factor for mental and physical morbidity. *American Journal of Psychiatry*, **154**, 616–623.

Tanner, J., Drawson, A. S., Mushquash, C. J., Mushquash, A. R., and Mazmanian, D. 2017. Harm reduction in gambling: a systematic review of industry strategies. *Addiction Research & Theory*, **25**, 485–494.

Tateno, J., Yamase, H., and Yamase, Y. 2011. Kokunaigai niokeru Izoku Kenkyuu no Doukou to Kongo no Kadai [Motivations and challenges in studying the bereaved]. *Nihon Kango Kenkyu Gakkai Zasshi*, **34**, 161–170.

Tedeschi, R. G. and Calhoun, L. G. 2006. Time of change? The spiritual challenges of bereavement and loss. *OMEGA*, **53**, 105–116.

Temel, J. S., Greer, J. A., El-Jawahri, A., Pirl, W. F., Park, E. R., Jackson, V. A., et al. 2017. Effects of early integrated palliative care in patients with lung and GI cancer: a randomized clinical trial. *Journal of Clinical Oncology*, **35**, 834–841.

Temel, J. S., Greer, J. A., Muzikansky, A., Gallagher, E. R., Admane, S., Jackson, V. A., et al. 2010. Early palliative care for patients with metastatic non–small-cell lung cancer. *New England Journal of Medicine*, **363**, 733–742.

Umberson, D., Olson, J. S., Crosnoe, R., Liu, H., Pudrovska, T., and Donnelly, R. 2017. Death of family members as an overlooked source of racial disadvantage in the United States. *Proceedings of the National Academy of Sciences of the United States of America*, **114**, 915–920.

United Nations. 2019. World mortality 2019: data booklet. [Online] Available at: https://www.un.org/en/development/desa/population/publications/pdf/mortality/WMR2019/WorldMortality2019DataBooklet.pdf

United Nations Sustainable Development Group. 2003. *The Human Rights Based Approach to Development Cooperation: Towards a Common Understanding Among UN Agencies*. New York: United Nations.

Uvin, P. 2007. From the right to development to the rights-based approach: how 'human rights' entered development. *Development in Practice*, **17**, 597–606.

Walley, A. Y., Xuan, Z., Hackman, H. H., Quinn, E., Doe-Simkins, M., Sorensen-Alawad, A., et al. 2013. Opioid overdose rates and implementation of overdose education and nasal naloxone distribution in Massachusetts: interrupted time series analysis. *BMJ*, **346**, f174.

Waitzkin, H. 2006. One and a half centuries of forgetting and rediscovering: Virchow's lasting contributions to social medicine. *Social Medicine*, **1**, 5–10.

Weir, D. and Willis, R. 2003. Widowhood, divorce, and loss of health insurance among near elderly women: evidence from the health and retirement study. Michigan Retirement Research Center Research Paper No. WP 2003-040. [Online] Available at: https://ssrn.com/abstract=1090894

Weiss, H. A., Dickson, K. E., Agot, K., and Hankins, C. A. 2010. Male circumcision for HIV prevention: current research and programmatic issues. *AIDS (London, England)*, **24**, S61.

Weller, S. C. and Davis-Beaty, K. 2002. Condom effectiveness in reducing heterosexual HIV transmission. *Cochrane Database of Systematic Reviews*, **1**, CD003255.

Willett, W., Rockström, J., Loken, B., Springmann, M., Lang, T., Vermeulen, S., et al. 2019. Food in the Anthropocene: the EAT–Lancet Commission on healthy diets from sustainable food systems. *Lancet*, **393**, 447–492.

World Health Organization. 2008. *Closing the Gap in a Generation: Health Equity Through Action on the Social Determinants of Health. Final Report of the Commission on Social Determinants of Health*. Geneva: World Health Organization. Available at: https://www.who.int/social_determinants/final_report/csdh_finalreport_2008.pdf

World Health Organization. 2014. *WHO Strengthening of Palliative Care as a Component of Comprehensive Care Throughout the Life Course*. Geneva: World Health Organization. Available at: http://apps.who.int/gb/ebwha/pdf_files/wha67/a67_r19-en.pdf

World Health Organization. 2018. *Declaration of Astana*. Geneva: World Health Organization. Available at: https://www.who.int/primary-health/conference-phc/declaration

9

Early intervention

John P. Rosenberg

Introduction

> Care at the end of life is not simply a professional or services matter, nor is it a matter of good fortune or serendipity, but rather a conscious, planned and deliberate political and social set of actions taken by the key players in any community to enhance the support and wellbeing of everyone affected by ageing, dying, death, loss and caregiving. (Wegleitner et al., 2016, p. xiv)

Public health palliative care (PHPC) early intervention (Box 9.1) strategies are the pre-emptive approaches taken to mitigate or eliminate the known impacts of ageing, dying, death, bereavement, and caregiving on the health and well-being of individuals and communities. It is the 'set of actions' put in place to influence these experiences in healthy ways. PHPC aims to make organized efforts to alleviate risks, improve health and well-being, and restore economic productivity (Karapliagou et al., 2018). These aims reflect the key action areas of the Ottawa Charter for Health Promotion (World Health Organization, 1986) (Box 9.2) and underpin Kellehear's ground-breaking text *Health Promoting Palliative Care* (Kellehear, 1999). Despite early misgivings about the 'fit' of the Ottawa Charter's key action areas to palliative and end of life care, its conceptual congruence has been explored and there is an increasing number of reports of its successful application to PHPC (Rosenberg and Yates, 2010; Sallnow and Paul, 2015). But what are the impacts early intervention are trying to influence?

The experiences of ageing, dying, death, bereavement, and caregiving have broad impacts. Individuals who have a life-limiting illness, are caregiving, or are bereaved can experience enormous personal and family disruption. In addition to the impact of these on individuals, families can be placed under enormous and often unfamiliar stress; there can be disruption to—or loss of—employment, with resulting financial strain. Social isolation can become a normal part of the lives of caregivers as days become crowded with care and energies wane. Where children are affected, there can be behavioural challenges at home and at school. These disruptions can extend to the life and operation of communities and civic organizations.

But early intervention in PHPC is not simply a problem-based, reactive approach to the constellation of impacts experienced at this time. With an intentional focus on existing relationships and community partnerships, early intervention strategies can minimize social disruption (Aoun, 2020), reduce the number of avoidable hospital admissions, improve symptom control, ease caregiver fatigue and stress, and lessen complicated grieving (Aoun et al., 2012). This intentionality—conscious, planned, and deliberate—and the embrace of the participatory nature of health promotion are key to PHPC. Careful, integrated planning is the hallmark of early intervention. PHPC early interventions that target the different impacts of ageing, dying, death, bereavement, and caregiving should enhance strategic directions, promote health and well-being, and evaluate their effectiveness (Parker and Baldwin, 2019).

If dying is everyone's business, who is 'everyone'?

It is integral to PHPC that *dying is everyone's business*. It follows then that the strategies used to promote health must embrace the specialist and generalist services, community, and civic elements of palliative and end of life care addressed by Abel, Kellehear, and Karapliagou in their important article 'Palliative care—the new essentials' (Abel et al., 2018a). In this article, the positioning of these elements in the social context helps understand who *everyone* might be; this understanding underpins this chapter as it explores early interventions in communities, civic society, and health services. Crucially, of course, people living with life-limiting illnesses, their families, carers, and social networks are the unit of care

Box 9.1 Defining early intervention

PHPC early intervention strategies are the pre-emptive approaches taken to mitigate or eliminate the known impacts of ageing, dying, death, bereavement, and caregiving on the health and well-being of individuals and communities.

Box 9.2 Health promotion key action areas

Key action areas in health promotion:

- Build public policies.
- Create supportive environments.
- Strengthen community action.
- Develop personal skills.
- Reorient health services.

Source: data from World Health Organization, 1986, Ottawa Charter.

around which these elements operate; this will be the starting point in this chapter.

Early interventions for caregiving of people in families and networks

> The patient-centred model of care has limitations when there is a fundamental lack of integrated community policy, development and resourcing. ... we propose a model of care which identifies a person with an illness at the centre of a network which includes inner and outer networks, communities and service delivery organisations. (Abel et al., 2013, p. 383)

Why not begin with the person with life-limiting illness? Many contemporary definitions of palliative and end of life care describe 'person- and family-centred care'. Yet in the quote at the start of this section, Abel and his colleagues propose a refocusing of this approach not because it is without merit, but because it falls short of recognizing the complexities of what it is to be a 'family', how the caregiving role is positioned, and the nature of the broader social contexts within which people with a life-limiting illnesses live, die, and are grieved.

Firstly, *not all families are the same* in terms of their configuration or kinship; for example, blended families with multiple parental figures, LGBTQI+ families, and kinship groups whose understandings of belonging are not represented in dominant Western perceptions of what it means to be a 'family'. Although it is predominantly used to describe diverse minority groups, the term 'kinship' is a helpful way to understand interpersonal and social connection *as defined by those at the centre of care*. It is not simply a measure of 'blood' or 'non-blood' relations, but a view of connectedness, intimacy, and longevity in relationships (Nelson, 2020). Whether configured in these ways or not, families have differences in the strength of their relationships, with some living with long-standing stress and conflict; the ubiquitous term 'loved one' is problematic for its naïve assumptions about the nature of the relationship between the person with a life-limiting illness and family. A family member with a history of perpetrating domestic violence is not likely to become the 'loved one' just because they are dying. Placing an expectation on carers to 'play happy families' is risky and an avoidable source of stress. With carers predominantly being women, assumptions about family can unnecessarily add to the responsibilities many take on. Genograms are one useful strategy for understanding the nature and strength of bonds in families, and help build a picture of the wider social contexts in which PHPC early interventions are developed.

Secondly, *the term 'carer' describes a role that can be filled by any number of people* who exist in the life of the person with a life-limiting illness, including the kinship group they identify. Within the 'inner network' described as *circles of care*, the role of primary carer can be handed around as needs vary, and energy and availability alter (Abel et al., 2013) (Fig. 9.1). In a PHPC approach, individual reactions to crises in life-limiting illness are understood collectively, and highlight the importance of social support and networks (Karapliagou et al., 2018; Rosenberg et al., 2018) (Box 9.3).

How can these circles of care around those with life-limiting illness be better understood? Social network analysis extends beyond the genograms commonly used in clinical practice and

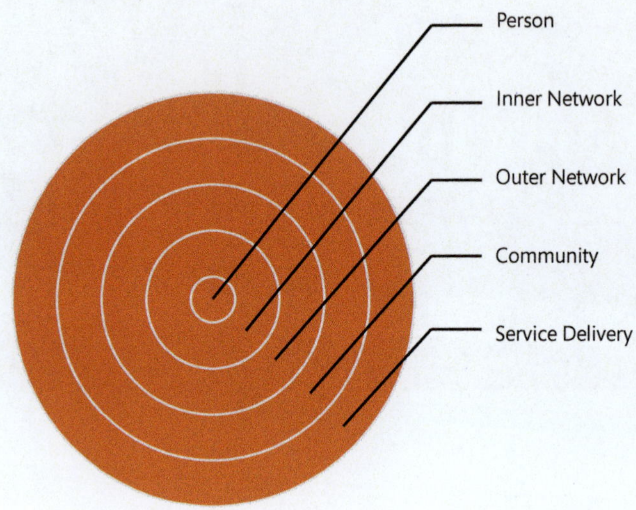

Fig. 9.1 Circles of care.

Adapted with permission from Abel, J., et al. (2013). Circles of care: should community development redefine the practice of palliative care? *BMJ supportive & palliative care*, 3(4), 383–388.

family assessment; it explores the kinship group and wider social context of the dying person to identify existing and potential supporters who can be mobilized to provide care (Leonard et al., 2020; Lindemann et al., 2020). Fig. 9.2 illustrates this, mapping the placement of family, friends, and healthcare professionals around the carer, and noting the strength of these relationships; this information is highly valuable in understanding the collective personal skills surrounding the carer and person with a life-limiting illness. Understanding the configuration of kinship groups and social networks, and assessing their readiness, is a key basis for planning early interventions.

How can social networks be 'ready' to support the living and dying of people with life-limiting illnesses? Early intervention strategies for caregiving focus on the Ottawa Charter's key action area to *develop personal skills* in end of life care. This could include:

- Attending training in the physical tasks of caregiving, for example, through programmes such as *Last Aid* (Bollig et al., 2019; Mills et al., 2020) and a multitude of other face-to-face and online resources.
- Using advance care planning and acting as proxy decision makers (these vary widely between jurisdictions, so it is critical to accurately identify those that apply to specific locations).
- Utilizing different social and welfare supports, including government pensions and allowances, carer's leave provisions in the workplace, income protection, access to superannuation, and more.
- Becoming familiar with local health, palliative care, and social support services, for example, to identify equipment available for home care, and healthcare professionals who can visit at home.

Box 9.3 Collective understanding

In a PHPC approach, individual reactions to crises in life-limiting illness are understood collectively and highlight the importance of social support and networks.

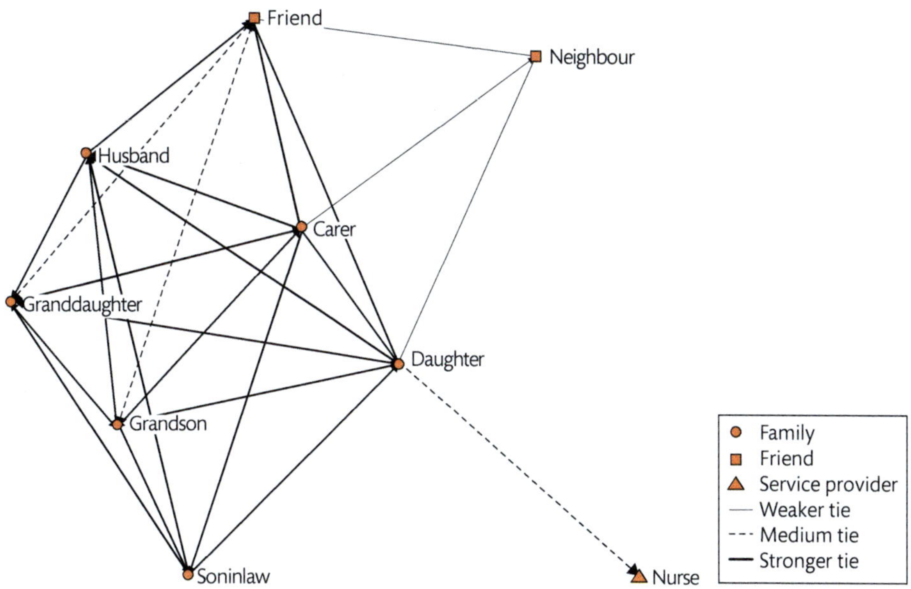

Fig. 9.2 Social network mapping.

Reproduced with permission from Leonard, R., Horsfall, D., Rosenberg, J., & Noonan, K. (2020). Carer experience of end-of-life service provision: a social network analysis. *BMJ supportive & palliative care*, 10(2), e20.

- Understanding and planning for funerals, burials, or cremations, according to local requirements and cultural customs.
- Learning more about grief, loss, and bereavement *in advance* in order to support carers and network members.

A study by Aoun (2012) shows that when bereavement support is focused on the capacity of inner networks, it provides valuable scaffolding for the bereaved person while upskilling the network members. These examples demonstrate the promotion of *death literacy*, which is explored in more detail in the next section.

Early interventions in communities

> Death literacy is an outcome of people's engaged experiences of, and learning about, death and dying. People, and communities, with high levels of death literacy have context-specific knowledge and the ability to put that knowledge into practice. Once this happens death literacy becomes a resource that people and communities can use for their own benefit. (Noonan et al., 2016, p. 34)

It really *is* good fortune when a community identifies, mobilizes, and benefits from its social capital. However, as Wegleitner and his colleagues identify in the opening quote of this chapter, this is not accidental, but planned. Early interventions targeting communities are informed by the social network mapping identified in the previous section and built upon an assessment of existing community assets. Death literacy demonstrates not just the elements of knowledge, skills, and experience of communities, but their *readiness* to act upon the anticipated needs when one of its members is dying or grieving (Noonan et al., 2016; Noonan, 2018). This means that the community is in control of identifying the problem and creating priorities for action.

The *ladder of citizen participation* (Arnstein, 1969) predates the Ottawa Charter by nearly 20 years, but still provides valuable insights into understanding the range of approaches to engagement between healthcare organizations and communities. It informed the development of the ladder shown in Fig. 9.3 which enables organizations to plot their early intervention strategies in PHPC (Rosenberg and Sheldrake, 2015). Each 'step' on the ladder is defined; a description of the approach to engagement is provided; and each step builds on the previous one. For many contemporary palliative care services, the first three steps are achievable in their strategic planning, governance, and operation. Critically though, truly *co-created* community engagement moves beyond the first three steps where services and communities are collaborating on *co-production* of early intervention strategies; to reach the steps to collaborate and empower concretely shifts control from services to communities. This approach uses the Ottawa Charter key action areas to *strengthen community action* and *create supportive environments*. It can form an important part of establishing and negotiating partnerships between those parties invested in creating early interventions in PHPC. This is discussed later in this chapter.

When considered at the community level, this can mean that *readiness* can vary highly as community members possess different levels of willingness to participate in PHPC activities. But there is a caution here: it is easy 'to assume that empowerment, participation and self-care are universally beneficial for and welcomed by all individuals' (Stajduhar et al., 2010, p. 221). It is important to remember that in the same way that not all families are the same, so too not all communities are the same. For example, living in the same town doesn't assume consistent attitudes, knowledge, and skills about dying, death, loss, and caregiving among townsfolk; migrant groups from one region of the world cannot be assumed to possess the same perspectives just because they share this background; members of faith communities do not necessarily hold the same views on end of life issues. This can challenge assumptions about empowerment as a way of working with communities and requires careful consideration in the planned approaches to PHPC. Each nation,

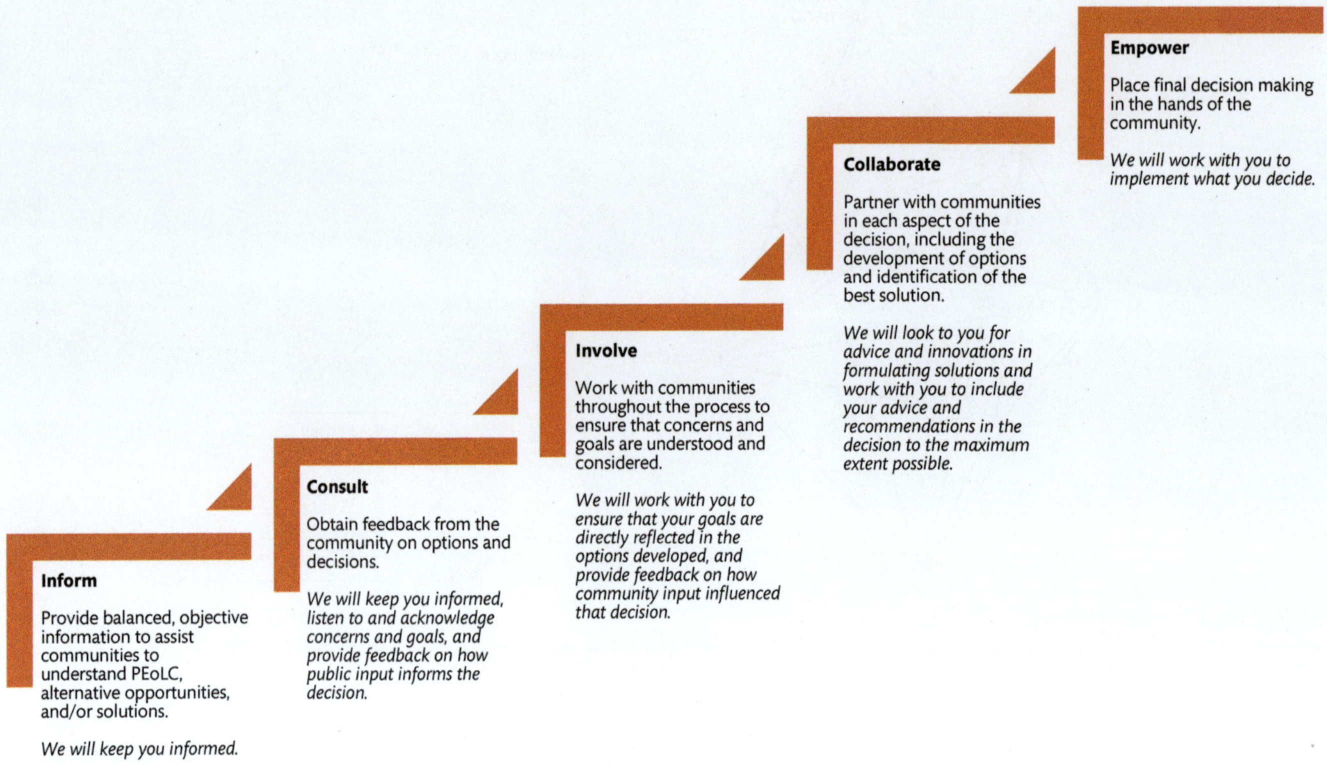

Fig. 9.3 Community engagement ladder. PEoLC, palliative and end of life care.
Reproduced from Rosenberg, J., & Sheldrake, M. (2015). Community engagement strategies: in the too-hard basket? Paper presented at the 13th Australian Palliative Care Conference, Melbourne, Australia.

each region, each city, and each town will possess a different profile of their population.

Nevertheless, early intervention strategies targeting communities are valuable approaches in identifying and strengthening community capacity to create supportive communities. Perhaps one of the better-known methods is found in *compassionate communities*, an approach that promotes and integrates social approaches to dying, death, and bereavement in the everyday lives of individuals and communities. Community awareness of end of life issues and participation in the care and support of people with life-limiting illnesses and their families and carers reflect death literacy. Building networks of care, mobilizing communities to provide practical and emotional support in skilled and informed ways, and developing resilience are all elements of a compassionate community (Box 9.4).

This is well illustrated in the operations of several organizations around the world. *Compassionate Communities UK* (https://www.compassionate-communitiesuk.co.uk/) emphasizes the components of a compassionate communities approach to make the most of the inner and outer networks that already exist, build these networks to provide support in 'ordinary life', and link to broader community activities to reduce loneliness and enhance a sense of belonging, with all of the social and health benefits of these social connections (Abel et al., 2018b). Still in the UK, the highly-regarded *Compassionate Neighbours* project is an example of how local communities can organize and be ready for supporting those at the end of life and their carers at home (Sallnow and Paul, 2018). Recruitment takes place through open days, training is provided to those selected, identification of appropriate roles is jointly determined by the participant and organizers, and matching of the participant to a family takes place as the need arises; ongoing meetings enable the participants to reflect upon their role and practices within these arrangement. The establishment of *Compassionate Neighbours* places control in the hands of a compassionate community, pre-emptively mobilizing inner and outer networks to support others. In Australia, a *Compassionate Communities Toolkit* (Rankin Smith and Read, 2020) has been developed (https://www.thegroundswellproject.com/compassionate-communities-toolkit-2020) (Box 9.5). Another Australian group of researchers found that a volunteer-led model of social, psychological, and practical support for those living with life-limiting illness, their families, and their carers improves social connectedness and community death literacy, and decreases unmet needs of people with life-limiting illnesses and their carers (Aoun et al., 2020).

It is important to note that these are community approaches, not led by healthcare services, and reflective of the community engagement steps illustrated in Fig. 9.3. However, it is not a matter of choosing between the two—a specific approach to developing partnerships between services and communities is explored later in this chapter.

Box 9.4 Compassionate communities

Building networks of care, mobilizing communities to provide practical and emotional support in skilled and informed ways, and developing resilience are all elements of a compassionate community.

Box 9.5 Core elements of compassionate communities

- Building capacity and death literacy through education and shared experiences.
- Value and focus are on existing community strengths and assets.
- Community recognized as the experts on their own life and valued as key stakeholders, not just participants.
- Community identifies needs and is empowered to lead the change.
- There is a focus on equity and inclusion with a broad understanding of health and well-being.
- Sustainability is a core element achieved through partnerships and shared leadership.
- Having a whole-of-community approach, recognizing that palliative care and health services cannot do this alone.
- Thinking beyond individuals to include social and community networks (Compassionate Communities Toolkit; Rankin Smith and Read, 2020, p. 16).

Early interventions in civic societies

> [C]ommunity support cannot offer continuity or quality of care without civic participation and co-operation from public sectors and institutions—schools, workplaces or churches. This is quite simply because these are the key social institutions inhabited by the very neighbours, family members, or friends offering support to the dying or the bereaved. ... neighbourhood caregivers are not faceless social entities but rather actual employees, students, worshipers, shoppers, and club members. The civic component of end-of-life care recognizes this foundational inter-dependency as the very support basis of community care, and mobilises actions that support end-of-life care in public institutions. (Abel et al., 2018a, p. S8)

Clearly, to accomplish PHPC early intervention strategies in civic society, the Ottawa Charter key action area to *build public policies* applies. But this cannot be assumed to be in place. In his 2005 book, *Compassionate Cities*, Kellehear notes that 'both public health and palliative care do not currently share a policy space where end-of-life care is a joint concern' (p. 78). In the years since, has this changed? The answer is 'yes ... and no'. There are several examples, some in this book, that demonstrate successful attempts at the integration of PHPC into civic policy; however, with much of existing PHPC activity being downstream, policy change is not necessarily addressed at this level, despite its crucial role in effecting social change in end of life issues.

Kellehear goes on to present nine 'policy visions' with operational policies within each to provide a platform for policy action. These are illustrated in Fig. 9.4 (for a detailed explanation of each component, see *Compassionate Cities* (Kellehear, 2005, pp. 59–80)). These nine components provide a policy map from which early interventions can be drawn to address issues of ageing, dying, death, bereavement, and caregiving—policy priorities can be identified so that they can be embedded in the strategic direction and governance of a civic society.

Who might be the players in developing public policies for early interventions in PHPC? It is fair to say that 'it depends'. In identifying the policy priorities, so too can the parties with an interest in the particular issue be identified. With the governance of cities, towns, and regions resting typically with local governments, their representatives are obvious key players; similarly, leaders and other representatives of community groups have a role here. This could equally apply to schools or places of worship, and palliative and healthcare services would also provide expertise in issues of dying, death, grief, and caregiving. There are many others, of course, so it becomes essential to carefully scope the selected policies so that all who must be at the table are there.

The 'table' of course refers to working groups whose brief it is to build the policy platform. An excellent example of this is seen in the recent establishment of *Compassionate Brugge* in Belgium (https://www.brugge.be/compassionatebrugge). Through a strong and sustained focus on connections between civic, social, business, health, and other organizations, this city has determined that 'loss, death, grief, situations and serious illness and long-term care are part of the daily life of our city, neighbourhood and community'. They describe the connections between these key groups in their city not only to address existing deficits but to build the capacity of the city to address these issues as they arise in the future.

It is important to note that it is here that a civic society can clearly declare its compassionate intentions. It can be tempting to focus upon the issues experienced by the majority, and while this is worthwhile, there is also an opportunity to establish a clear policy position on the vulnerable and marginalized within the community (Box 9.6). Fig. 9.4 clearly demonstrates this in its consideration of Indigenous and First Nations peoples, those experiencing or at risk of homelessness, and those geographically isolated. Economic, educational, and migratory disadvantage can take many forms and if not addressed at the policy level, leaves a policy platform incomplete.

Equally, diversity is a community asset to be reflected in civic society and its policies regarding issues in dying, death, grief, and caregiving. Indigenous and culturally diverse populations, schools, faith communities, LGBTQI + communities, and many others bring wide-ranging experiences and expectations to the civic life of a community; the policy platform must reflect this diversity, and these policies must be informed by representatives of these diverse groups. This is both a basic human right to self-determination and the path to shared ownership of the activities and outcomes.

Early interventions in health and social services

> Health services providing care to dying people in their homes are present at an interface where the palliative care profession is confronted with the irony of relinquishing its 'ownership' of the business of dying while leading communities to reclaim their principal role in the business of dying. The very services possessing the expertise to lead this shift in control are the same services that would be required to cede that control. (Rosenberg, 2011, p. 24)

Healthcare services—both specialist and generalist—are designed to respond, anticipating known and expected clinical problems. This is equally true of palliative care services and these services can demonstrate high levels of expertise in pain and symptom management, with a multidisciplinary model of care addressing the diverse needs of palliative care people with life-limiting illnesses, their families, and their caregivers. Founded on principles of holistic care, this expertise and approach to care is the legacy of the evolution of care of the dying from the boutique modern hospice movement into the discipline of palliative

1. Has local health policies that recognize compassion as an ethical imperative

- Fosters and supports educational initiative linking health and compassion.
- Fosters and supports compassion in the workplace, school and aged care facility.
- Fosters and supports health-promotion messages to incorporate death and loss.
- Meets the special needs of its aged, those living with life-threating illness and those living with loss.

2. Fosters and supports the community awareness of these special needs

- Fosters and supports positive ageing, positive aspects of chronic illness and posivie aspects of loss.
- Fosters and supports media recognition of their presence and experiences.

3. Has a strong commitment to social and cultural difference

- Fosters and supports anti-racist laws and inclusive policies; discourages religious discrimination based on class, gender, race and sexual preferences.
- Fosters and supports social and cultural differences in public education and school curriculum.
- Fosters and supports practices that recognize social and cultural influences in ageing, serious illness and loss in different groups.
- Any implementation, policy or planning committee must include members chosen for their combination of skills, expertise AND social and cultural diversity.

4. Involves the grief and palliative care services in local government policy and planning

- Any implementation, policy of planning committee should include a member of the local hospice/palliative AND bereavement (sudden death) care team.
- Any implementation, policy or planning committee should include members with direct personal experience of ageing, living with a life-threatening illness or loss.
- Develops a local government policy to address loss and giref matters in the local community.

5. Offers its inhabitants access to a wide variety of supportive experiences, interactions and communication

- Fosters and supports media attempts to compare and contrast experiences of death and loss for its viewers and readers.
- Fosters and supports voluntary social services that assist people to maintain a preferred lifestyle in the face of death and loss.
- Fosters and supports special social support programmes for people in need.

6. Promotes and celebrates reconciliation with indigenous poeples and the memory of other important community losses

- Fosters and supports national, state and local government intitiatives and policies toward indigenous reconciliation.
- Fosters and supports an inclusive approach to Remembrance Days and festivals, including members from ALL sides of former conflicts, and former victims and workers of war.
- Has an annual day of remembrance for death and loss in peace times.

7. Provides easy access to grief and palliative care services

- Promotes and supports a single telephone referral service for loss and palliative care.
- Promotes and supports local grief and palliative care services by facilitating access to schools and workplaces.
- Pomotes and supports public education and awareness campaigns about the existence and nature of these services.
- Promotes and supports community initiatives from these services.

8. Has a recognition and plan to accommodate those disadvantaged by the economy, including rural and remote populations, indigenous peoples and homeless

- Has a research-based understanding of the role of death and loss in the health and illness pattern of these communities.
- Has a plan to address the death and loss issues for these communities.
- Promotes and supports grief and palliative care services for rural and remote areas, indigenous populations and the homeless.
- Involves school, police, churches, workplaces and businesses in the formulation and design of these understandings and plans.

9. Preserves and promotes a community's spiritual traditions and storytellers

- Fosters and supports inclusive religious politics, including ecumenicist and multifaith initiatives, but eschews the proselytization of tribal or medieval prescriptions.
- Fosters and supports 'festivals of the spirit' in an inclusive context, which embraces religions and spiritual traditions both old and new.
- Fosters and supports the role of multifaith chaplaincy, pastoral care and humanist dialogue in their community role of comforting those living with life-threatening illness and loss.
- Fosters and supports the value and importance of spiritual beliefs and meanings in the development and support of health and compassionate lifestyles.

Fig. 9.4 Nine policy visions in PHPC.
Source: data from Kellehear, A. (2005). *Compassionate Cities: Public health and end-of-life care*. London: Routledge, pp. 60–78.

Box 9.6 Vulnerable and marginalized groups

It can be tempting to focus upon the issues experienced by the majority, and while this is worthwhile, there is also an opportunity to establish a clear policy position on the vulnerable and marginalized within the community.

care within mainstream healthcare. However, in advocating for health-promoting approaches to palliative care, the Ottawa Charter names a final key action area, to *reorient health services*. As suggested in the earlier quote, this is because the 'business' of dying goes far beyond what any service—however skilled—can provide. In the same way that regular exercise is not the sole concern of a specialist cardiologist, so too can palliative care services bring their expertise to those living with a life-limiting illness, their families, carers, and communities without attempting to address the whole experience of dying.

When a PHPC approach is utilized, this requires engagement with communities beyond the provision of service. It might be helpful to look again at the *community engagement ladder* in Fig. 9.3. Read from the perspective of a palliative care service provider, it shows how a deeper orientation towards communities brings with it a corresponding relinquishment of control (Box 9.7). This is also explored by Sallnow and Paul (2015) who describe factors that either inhibit or support community capacity and quality of care across a similar spectrum, and the *spectrum of public participation* examined by Noonan and colleagues (2020).

This is important beyond simply a matter of principle. Palliative care services *do* possess both proximity to, and expertise in, issues of dying, death, grief, and caregiving and, as such, are critical to providing a constellation of support to those who live, work, die, and grieve in their own communities. Creating strategies for early interventions target clinical and social support; establishing a network of carers, for example, places a number of people within proximity of the person living with a life-limiting illness who can contribute to the monitoring of issues like comfort, pain control, mobility, anxiety, and so on. Equally, palliative care services can assist in increasing the death literacy and caregiving skillsets of carers and inner network members. At the centre of this exchange is the person and those closest to them, who set the 'ground rules' for the exchange of information about them. The form that these interventions take are co-created within the circles of care (Fig. 9.1).

It is a mistake to assume that this can happen through the power of goodwill. Working together to generate early interventions is more likely to succeed with the application of a partnership development approach. This is explored in the next section.

Box 9.7 Reorienting professional power

Viewing the community as an equal partner in providing quality health care at the end of life, PHPC challenges ingrained hierarchies of professional power; contests established structures of privilege; and provokes services to reorient toward respecting and working with whole communities, whilst urging communities and service providers to build death literacy. (Rosenberg et al., 2020, p. 75)

Using a partnership development approach to early intervention

> [I]nvolvement and active participation by members of the general community ... reflects a public health approach to palliative care where health professionals appreciate and engage with members of the community as equal partners in end-of-life concerns and the provision of social care ... This approach is consistent with calls for health professionals to engage with communities and build collaborative partnerships as part of a public health approach to palliative care. (Mills, 2020, p. 17)

Health promotion and public health is filled with the terminology of collaboration. Whether in the Ottawa Charter, Kellehear's *Health Promoting Palliative Care*, or contemporary examples of the application of PHPC, such as Mills' quoted commentary on the *Ambulance Wish* project, there is a clear need to combine the collective knowledge, skills, and resources of healthcare services *and* communities to support people living with life-limiting illnesses, their families, carers, and social networks. As Mills has rightly noted, PHPC is fundamentally about working as *equal partners*, where the power of the 'expert' service providers is renegotiated to create partnerships that challenge organizational privilege and put services and communities on an equal footing (Rosenberg et al., 2020). As noted, each party brings its own expertise and informs the nature of the relationship (Box 9.8).

How can this be achieved in concrete terms when planning early interventions? Shouldn't it just be a matter of agreeing on well-thought through plans and allocation of responsibilities? These are important components of any collaboration, but not enough to create and sustain an *equal partnership*. This is where *partnership development principles and practices* can offer a valuable approach.

A partnership is an ongoing working relationship where the risks and benefits of the relationship are shared; partnerships aim to achieve much more than individual organizations can achieve on their own (Mundy and Tennyson, 2019). It is the collective power of working in partnerships in the delivery of health promotion that is key to its success. It is worth noting that the word 'partnership' is used freely—but not necessarily accurately—to describe the relationship of palliative care services with communities. For example, recruitment of volunteers, provision of information for the public, and consumer representation on committees each might be described as borne of partnerships with the community. While each has its own merit, they don't *necessarily* constitute a partnership, especially if the power of decision-making rests with the service. These relationships can take many forms and only some of them would meet the PHPC goal of *equal partnerships* upon which to base early intervention strategies. The process of partnership development

Box 9.8 Partnerships for health promotion

Partnerships are an important vehicle for bringing together diverse skills and resources for more effective health promotion outcomes. Partnerships can increase the efficiency of systems that have an impact on health by making the best use of different but complementary resources. Collaborations, joint resourcing, and planned action can also potentially make a bigger impact on health outcomes across diverse sectors. (Victorian Health Promotion Foundation, 2016)

Box 9.9 Partnering principles

Key partnering principles address common challenges:

- Diversity—to address anxiety about difference.
- Equity—to address power imbalance.
- Openness—to address hidden agenda.
- Mutual benefit—to address competitiveness.
- Courage—to address uncertainty.

provides key steps towards an equal partnership. In order to move to the steps of *collaborate* and *empower* in the *community engagement ladder* (Fig. 9.3), services and communities must clearly declare their intentions, realistically assess their capacity, and agree that a partnership approach to their relationship is optimal. Where these elements are missing, any attempt at partnering comes with great risk of failure. Once the parties have identified the agreed level of engagement, they can approach partnership development with this in mind (Box 9.9).

In Fig. 9.5, these steps are spelled out in detail. Notably, the first quarter of the process *precedes* the decision to partner at all—a decision that impacts enormously on the efficient use of resources. This enables the 'conscious, planned and deliberate . . . set of actions' noted at the beginning of this chapter (Wegleitner et al., 2016) to be developed and implemented in the context of equal partnerships between healthcare and communities. Reviewing the early intervention strategies discussed earlier in this chapter through the lens of partnership development can help in determining how they can be effectively implemented. *Compassionate Neighbours*, for example, succeeds because the community members who participate are equally and actively involved in identifying their existing strengths and how best to use them. Their partners in the project provide support for practical training and ongoing personal development (Sallnow and Paul, 2018). Similarly, in Canada, a partnership between rural First Nations communities and palliative care service providers was established to develop local palliative care programmes that align with the cultural traditions of First Nations seniors and their kinship groups (Koski et al., 2017). Through a 'journey mapping' process, they explored both policy and practice approaches to achieve their agreed goal. Communication was key, and the primacy of the voice of First Nations peoples was honoured. These two examples demonstrate clearly that relationship underpins partnership and is critical to success.

Despite many initiatives in the course of its recent history, PHPC remains under-evaluated; this is certainly no less true in evaluating the impacts of early interventions. Notably, the compassionate communities work in the English town of Frome reports both a dramatic decrease in loneliness among townsfolk *and* in emergency service usage—both social and service outcomes that meet the goals of PHPC (Abel et al., 2018b). As noted already, the use of a PHPC approach to support in bereavement was similarly found to improve outcomes for those experiencing loss and grief (Aoun et al., 2012). In their recent systematic review of PHPC, Librada-Flores and colleagues (2020) found little evidence of comprehensive evaluation of the effectiveness of PHPC. This method of partnership development

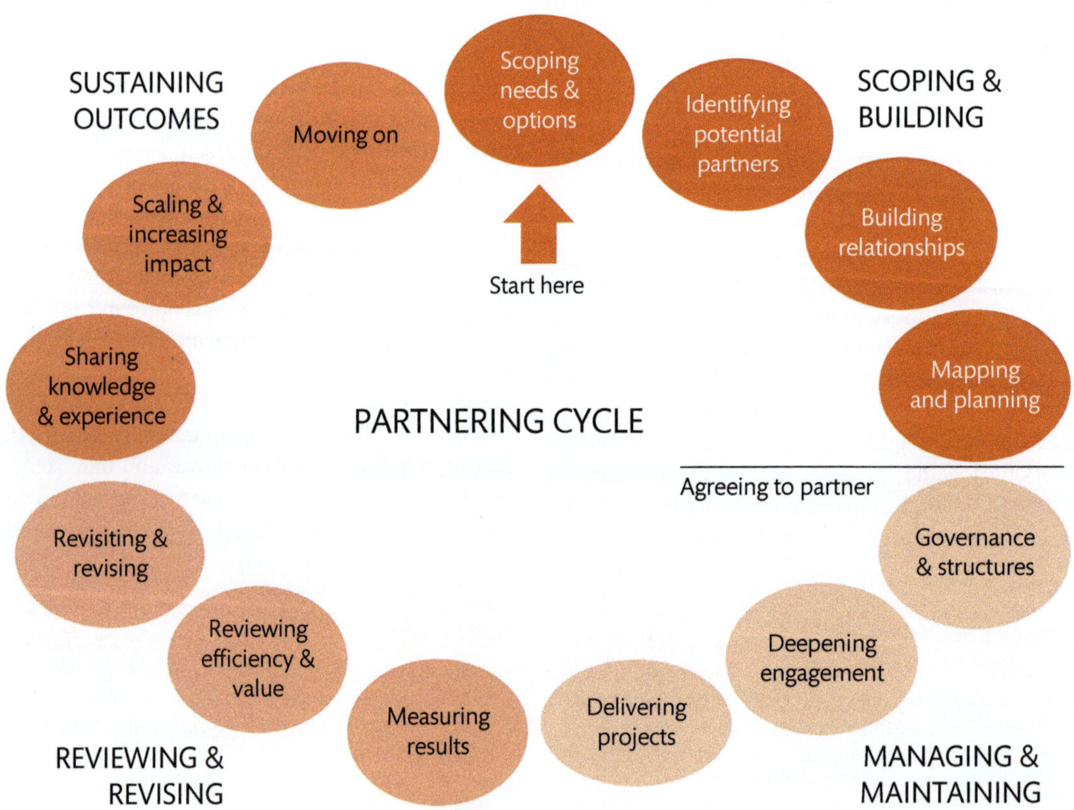

Fig. 9.5 Partnering cycle.
The Partnering Cycle, from 'Brokering Better Partnerships by Investing in the Partnering Process' (p. 9). Reproduced with kind permission of the Partnership Brokers Association.

to develop early interventions might provide for another perspective on evaluation of the effectiveness of PHPC.

Conclusion

> [A]lternative approaches to supporting death, dying, loss and care can offer more holistic, empowering and sustainable models of support. The new public health approach to end-of-life care integrates principles of health promotion, equity, social and environmental responses to ill health and professional/lay power sharing and partnerships. (Sallnow and Paul, 2018, p. 4)

This chapter explores the opportunities for developing and implementing early interventions in the care and support of people living with a life-limiting illness, their families, carers, and networks when a PHPC approach is taken. It is by no means a panacea for the complex, dynamic experiences of those receiving palliative and end of life care, or the communities in which they live. However, a conscious, planned, and deliberate approach that anticipates the known impacts of ageing, dying, death, bereavement, and caregiving can have a significant positive impact on the health and well-being of individuals and communities.

REFERENCES

Abel, J., Kellehear, A., and Karapliagou, A. 2018a. Palliative care—the new essentials. *Annals of Palliative Medicine*, 7, S3–S14.

Abel, J., Kingston, H., Scally, A., Hartnoll, J., Hannam, G., Thomson-Moore, A., et al. 2018b. Reducing emergency hospital admissions: a population health complex intervention of an enhanced model of primary care and compassionate communities. *British Journal of General Practice*, **68**, e803–e810.

Abel, J., Walter, T., Carey, L. B., Rosenberg, J., Noonan, K., Horsfall, D., et al. 2013. Circles of care: should community development redefine the practice of palliative care? *BMJ Supportive & Palliative Care*, **3**, 383–388.

Aoun, S. 2020. Bereavement support: from the poor cousin of palliative care to a core asset of compassionate communities. *Progress in Palliative Care*, **28**, 107–114.

Aoun, S., Breen, L., O'Connor, M., Rumbold, B., and Nordstrom, C. 2012. A public health approach to bereavement support services in palliative care. *Australian and New Zealand Journal of Public Health*, **36**, 14–16.

Arnstein, S. R. 1969. A ladder of citizen participation. *Journal of the American Institute of Planners*, **35**, 216–224.

Bollig, G., Brandt, F., Ciurlionis, M., and Knopf, B. 2019. Last aid course. An education for all citizens and an ingredient of compassionate communities. *Healthcare*, **7**, 19.

Karapliagou, A., Kellehear, A., and Wegleitner, K. 2018. The public health end-of-life care movement: history, principles, and styles of practice. In: Lloyd-Williams, M. (ed.) *Psychosocial Issues in Palliative Care: A Community Based Approach for Life Limiting Illness*, 3rd ed., pp. 1–22. Oxford: Oxford University Press.

Kellehear, A. 1999. *Health Promoting Palliative Care*. Melbourne: Oxford University Press.

Kellehear, A. 2005. *Compassionate Cities: Public Health and End-of-Life Care*. London: Routledge.

Koski, J., Kelley, M. L., Nadin, S., Crow, M., Prince, H., Wiersma, E. C., et al. 2017. An analysis of journey mapping to create a palliative care pathway in a Canadian First Nations community: implications for service integration and policy development. *Palliative Care*, **10**, 1178224217719441.

Leonard, R., Horsfall, D., Rosenberg, J., and Noonan, K. 2020. Carer experience of end-of-life service provision: a social network analysis. *BMJ Supportive & Palliative Care*, **10**, e20.

Librada-Flores, S., Nabal-Vicuña, M., Forero-Vega, D., Muñoz-Mayorga, I., and Guerra-Martín, M. D. 2020. Implementation models of compassionate communities and compassionate cities at the end of life: a systematic review. *International Journal of Environmental Research and Public Health*, **17**, 6271.

Lindemann, D., Borasio, G. D., Führer, M., and Wasner, M. 2020. Visualizing social support in home pediatric palliative care using network maps. *Palliative Medicine*, **34**, 378–386.

Mills, J. 2020. Ambulance wish: an opportunity for public health palliative care partnerships with paramedics and other community members. *Progress in Palliative Care*, **28**, 17–18.

Mills, J., Rosenberg, J. P., Bollig, G., and Haberecht, J. 2020. Last aid and public health palliative care: towards the development of personal skills and strengthened community action. *Progress in Palliative Care*, **28**, 343–345.

Mundy, J. and Tennyson, R. 2019. Brokering better partnerships by investing in the partnering process. [Online] Available at: https://partnershipbrokers.org/

Nelson, M. K. 2020. *Like Family: Narratives of Fictive Kinship*. New Brunswick, NJ: Rutgers University Press.

Noonan, K. 2018. Death literacy—developing a tool to measure the social impact of public health initiatives. *Annals of Palliative Medicine*, **7**, AB007.

Noonan, K., Horsfall, D., Leonard, R., and Rosenberg, J. 2016. Developing death literacy. *Progress in Palliative Care*, **24**, 31–35.

Noonan, K., Sallnow, L., and Richardson, H. 2020. Ten years of public health palliative care conferences: a critical reflection for the next decade. *Progress in Palliative Care*, **28**, 78–82.

Parker, E. and Baldwin, L. 2019. Contemporary practice. In: Fleming, M. L., Parker, E. and Correa-Velez, I. (eds.) *Introduction to Public Health*, 4th ed., pp. 184–196. Chatswood, Australia: Elsevier.

Rankin Smith, H. and Read, N. 2020. *Building Compassionate Communities in Australia: Tools for a Community-Led Approach to End-of-Life Care*. Sydney: The GroundSwell Project.

Rosenberg, J. and Sheldrake, M. 2015. Community engagement strategies: in the too-hard basket? Paper presented at the 13th Australian Palliative Care Conference, 3 September, Melbourne, Australia.

Rosenberg, J. P. 2011. Whose business is dying? Death, the home and palliative care. *Cultural Studies Review*, **17**, 15–30.

Rosenberg, J. P., Horsfall, D., Leonard, R., and Noonan, K. 2018. Informal care networks' views of palliative care services: help or hindrance? *Death Studies*, **42**, 362–370.

Rosenberg, J. P., Horsfall, D., Sallnow, L., and Gott, M. 2020. Power, privilege and provocation: public health palliative care today. *Progress in Palliative Care*, **28**, 75–77.

Rosenberg, J. P. and Yates, P. 2010. Health promotion in palliative care: the case for conceptual congruence. *Critical Public Health*, **20**, 201–210.

Sallnow, L. and Paul, S. 2015. Understanding community engagement in end-of-life care: developing conceptual clarity. *Critical Public Health*, **25**, 231–238.

Sallnow, L. and Paul, S. 2018. New public health approaches to end-of-life care. In: MacLeod, R. D. and Van den Block, L. (eds.) *Textbook of Palliative Care*, pp. 1739–1748. Cham: Springer.

Stajduhar, K., Funk, L., Jakobsson, E., and Öhlén, J. 2010. A critical analysis of health promotion and 'empowerment' in the context of palliative family care-giving. *Journal of Nursing Inquiry*, 17, 221–230.

Victorian Health Promotion Foundation. 2016. *The Partnerships Analysis Tool: A Resource for Establishing, Developing and Maintaining Partnerships for Health Promotion*. Melbourne: VicHealth. Available at: https://www.vichealth.vic.gov.au/media-and-resources/publications/the-partnerships-analysis-tool

Wegleitner, K., Heimerl, K., and Kellehear, A. 2016. Preface. In: Wegleitner, K., Heimerl, K., and Kellehear, A. (eds.) *Compassionate Communities: Case Studies from Britain and Europe*, pp. xii–xvii. Abingdon: Routledge.

World Health Organization. 1986. *The Ottawa Charter for Health Promotion: First International Conference on Health Promotion, Ottawa, 21 November 1986*. Geneva: World Health Organization.

10

Participatory relations

Kerrie Noonan

Introduction

What are participatory relations and participatory relationships? How are participatory relationships similar and different in partnerships and collaborations in the field of public health palliative care? This chapter considers these questions and explores the concept of participatory relations in public health palliative care and some of the practice models of participation.

Public health initiatives depend on participation. Whether it be a grassroots programme led by citizens or a palliative care service delivered to citizens by health professionals, participation—and the way we relate to each other while participating—is important. Relationships and connections between institutions, professionals, and citizens need to be negotiated and nurtured. These reciprocal relationships, however, require that we look at the locus of power and control. Healthcare services need to be aware of both the limits of their contributions and the need to build and support community capacity in end of life care to complement their work (Rosenberg et al., 2016). As such, this chapter will invite you to reflect on your own values and beliefs about participation and participatory relationships (Box 10.1). The first section provides an overview of participatory models, including community engagement, community development, and social networks relating to public health palliative care. The second part of this chapter examines power and empowerment in detail, including the role of participatory relations in public health research methods.

In thinking about the role of participatory relationships in end of life care function, this chapter will also adopt the language 'top-down' and 'bottom-up' to describe public health interventions. This is a simple way to think about participation. Top-down social interventions refer to participation led by institutions. In this sense, 'top-down' refers to health-promoting palliative care approaches (Kellehear, 1999) that usually involve health organizations engaging with the public. 'Bottom-up' is usually associated with community empowerment and initiatives led and implemented by community members (Kellehear, 2005; Sallnow and Paul, 2015).

Box 10.1 Personal reflection 1

What does the term 'participation' mean to you?

What have been your own experiences of 'participating'?

Think broadly about your participation in education about your own healthcare. Were you an active or passive participant? What is the difference? What was it like to participate in that way?

Participation in practice

Public health research and practice is not unlike palliative care, in that it emerged from the belief in 'enabling people to increase control over, and to improve their health' (World Health Organization, 1986, p. 1). The Ottawa Charter (World Health Organization, 1986) was considered the beginning of 'new public health'. It signalled a move away from a narrow view of the biomedical approach to disease prevention. Previous public health strategies had focused on the reduction of mortality and morbidity of communicable diseases and strategies such as better sanitation and nutrition, but did not address social determinants of health (Lupton, 2012; Laverack, 2014). The biomedical model of health focuses on the classification, diagnosis, and treatment of illness and disease in individuals, and concentrates on deficits rather than assets or strengths (Russell, 2020). When limited to thinking about people as a cluster of symptoms or a diagnosis, it is impossible to fully account for the social, cultural, environmental, and political impact on health and well-being (Abel and Kellehear, 2016). Focusing on social determinants, strengths, and capacity requires reciprocity, trust, and the development of relationships provides a broader view of the way that people participate in palliative care.

The World Health Organization (2019), for example, notes that meaningful participation is important so that individuals can participate in the decisions that directly affect them. This includes the design, implementation, and monitoring of health interventions. Public health models view the health and well-being of citizens as a holistic concept that acknowledges the relationship and interplay of human agency and social structures (Yuill et al., 2010). Social models take the view that health can be both enabled and inhibited by the social context of an individual. The effect of participating in adequate social connections has been found to have comparable health effects to stopping smoking (Holt-Lunstad et al., 2010). Social connections are also helpful when caring for people who are dying (Horsfall et al., 2013) and when families are grieving (Aoun et al., 2016). Further participation in social networks also has a role in the self-management of disease, as self-management strategies are most effective when individuals are socially connected (Reeves et al., 2014).

It is also worth acknowledging that for many palliative care services, the primary model of community participation in end of life and bereavement care is volunteering. Volunteers are a significant part of the palliative care workforce, providing a range of services to support the health and medical teams within hospice and palliative care. This can include providing transport, respite for carers, housework and cleaning, and emotional support and counselling. While palliative care volunteering is the predominant model of participation, traditional service models are not always the most satisfactory experience for community members (Gale, 2017). Community members who are death literate (that is, have know-how about how to do end of life and death care), for example, may be experienced and knowledgeable about death, dying, and grief, and want to share this knowledge with other community members, but not want to participate in a formal service delivery model of care (Noonan et al., 2016; Noonan, 2018). Some researchers and practitioners have called for more inclusive and citizen-led community engagement to enhance and acknowledge community participation, which might not even use the term 'volunteering' to describe the role.

Co-design and collaboration models, for example, require renegotiating the relationships between professional services and community networks. Participation in these situations incorporates both the act of negotiation about the 'hows' and 'whys' of the collaboration as well as the direct project work. In this spirit, Russell (2020) offers three key principles for participation:

1. Work with residents to determine whether they can act together to resolve problems using their own community resources.
2. Enhance collective citizen resources by providing supportive municipal assets.
3. Acknowledge there will be some problems that cannot be resolved with citizen resources, even if supported by government assistance. In these cases, the municipality must take full responsibility. (p. 22)

Community engagement and community development

It is important to note that community engagement and community development are terms often used interchangeably, and though related, they are in practice different, especially when considered through the lens of participation and participatory relations. Community engagement usually refers to a palliative care service providing information and consulting with community members (Rosenberg et al., 2016). It exists on a spectrum that extends from informing through to empowering, depending on a range of factors such as the degree of participation from the local community and the intention of the work (Sallnow and Paul, 2015, p. 233).

Within a public health approach, community engagement between palliative care services and the general public is best achieved when working with and for communities. In Fig. 10.1, Sallnow and Paul (2015) have developed a 'spectrum of engagement' in end of life care that is based on Arnstein's (1969) ladder of participation: 'This spectrum is designed to aid professional services and the communities they serve to embark on community engagement projects with an open awareness of the key components underpinning their success' (p. 235). This model provides an overview from low to high levels of engagement with citizens. Low levels of engagement and participation include informing and consulting with the community through leaflets and websites. This is a passive form of engagement and aims to raise awareness rather than involve community members in the 'work' of end of life care. As expected, the other end of the spectrum is 'empower'. Community members are invited to participate in a self-determined way. Often participation in palliative care work is self-organized by community members who design and deliver the work. Although community engagement leading to citizen empowerment is an underdeveloped and under-researched area in relation to public health palliative care, it is important to know it has been applied to other social issues including mental health.

Community development is referred to in a number of ways in the literature. Kellehear (2005, p. 118) defines it as 'any set of initiatives designed to develop the social resources of the community in order to enhance its quality of life'. Public health researchers assert it is a 'process of working with people as they define their own goals, mobilize resources, and develop action plans for addressing problems they collectively have identified' (Minkler, 1991, p. 261, cited in Talbot and Verrinder, 2017). Feminist researchers describe it as 'a political and social process of education and action to achieve self-determination and social justice for marginalised groups' (Emejulu, 2011, p. 379). Further, Ife (2009) states 'Community development can be regarded as a way of thinking, as a philosophy of practice, rather than merely as a process for building stronger communities' (p. 29). The definition, utilized by a programme or practitioner, is

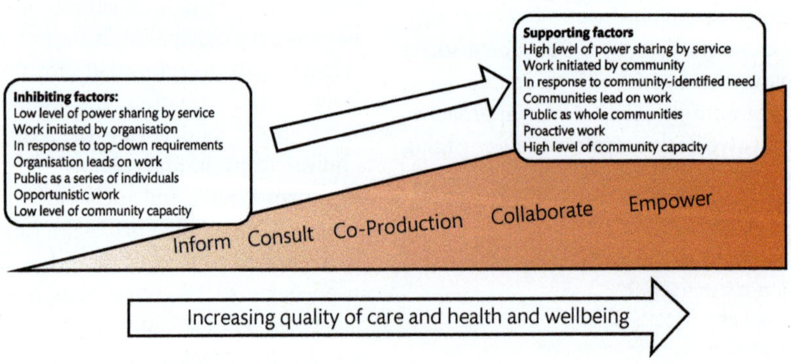

Fig. 10.1 Sallnow and Paul's (2015) spectrum of engagement.

Reproduced with permission from Sallnow, L. and Paul, S. (2015). Understanding community engagement in end-of-life care: developing conceptual clarity', *Critical Public Health*, 25, 231–238.

dependent on whether the approach taken is a top-down/bottom-up approach or a mixture of both (Ife, 2009; Talbot and Verriner, 2017).

Ife (2009) highlights the distinction between bottom-up and top-down approaches to community development. Bottom-up processes are based on the belief that the knowledge and skills of local communities are of central importance and should be 'valued above top-down wisdom and experience' (Ife, 2009, p. 30). Top-down approaches are common in palliative care and are usually designed and implemented by organizations 'for' a community identified as disadvantaged or in need of services. In the top-down approach, organizations must ensure that community participation is not tokenistic, and partnerships are developed with community members. This sounds straightforward enough, but in practice, community development approaches are challenging, especially in the medicalized and bureaucratic models of palliative care.

Social networks

Social networks are the glue that holds families and communities together. Mobilizing and strengthening networks lies at the heart of a social network approach, as does the belief that human experiences, such as loneliness, isolation, grief, and loss, are best supported within communities by family members, friends, and neighbours (Brown and Walter, 2013; Rosenberg et al., 2015). Where this is not possible, professional services have a role in helping to mobilize support (Abel et al., 2013). Traditional end of life organizations tend to address gaps in social networks with services rather than recognizing and supporting the development or growth of caring networks (Horsfall et al., 2013; Rosenberg et al., 2017). Brown and Walter (2013) argue for a social model of care that addresses the issue of professionalization not medicalization, which enables health professionals to rethink how they work with families in a way that enables them to mobilize existing family and social networks and strengthen ties without professionalizing the care needed.

Health practitioners are encouraged to use self-awareness and advocate for the use of social networks to counteract hierarchical and disempowering control in health services. Interestingly, as Brown and Walter (2013) point out, there is limited literature to guide end of life carers on how they can be supported by their social networks. The literature that does exist acknowledges that social networks are mostly hidden from health professionals for two key reasons. First, palliative care typically does not work beyond the patient/carer/family; and second, family meetings in palliative care often focus on clinical issues and tend not to include the social networks of the patient/carer/family (Brown and Walter, 2013; Rosenberg et al., 2017).

In contrast, Abel and colleagues (2013) proposes the 'circles of care' model. This model invites palliative care services to rethink the emphasis on service delivery and use community development approaches to 'restore the ability of families and communities to be able to look after their dying' (Abel et al., 2013, p. 6). Fig. 10.2 illustrates the circles of care model, representing a way of thinking about the types of care and support a dying person has access to. The inner and outer networks are the close family and friends who are likely to provide hands-on care, while the outer circles relate to how services and policy can support the inner networks. This model also provides a way of thinking about participation and the relationships that exist between the 'circles'. For example, policy, at the edge of the circles, has the potential to support the way the other aspects of care relate to each other.

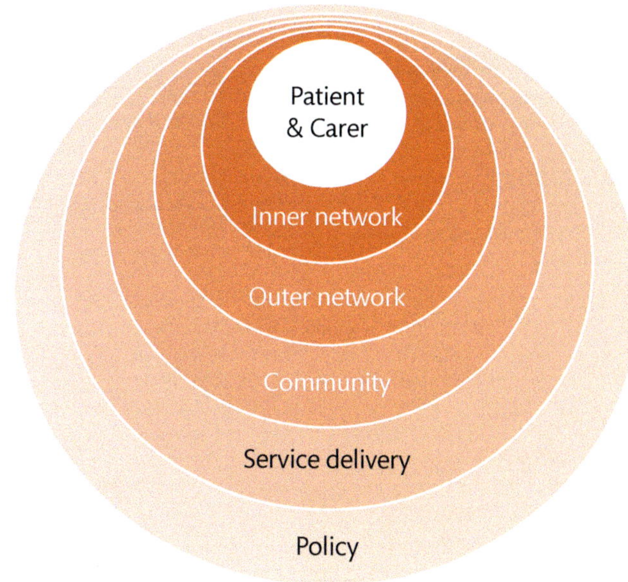

Fig. 10.2 Circles of care.

Adapted with permission from Abel, J., et al. (2013). Circles of care: should community development redefine the practice of palliative care? *BMJ supportive & palliative care*, 3(4), 383–388.

This model is influenced by the Caring at End of Life research project that used participatory research methods (these will be outlined in the next section of the chapter). One insight from this research about participation and participatory relationships suggests that health professionals have a limited role in mobilizing end of life care networks (Rosenberg et al., 2017). Likewise, it highlights that relationships between people in the care networks can strengthen over time (Leonard et al., 2015). Finally, when examining how this is reflected in palliative care policies, it was noted that public health approaches had not always translated in a significant way into palliative care services. This was evidenced by very few health professionals involved in the research referencing social interventions such as community development.

Social network research (Abel et al., 2013; Horsfall et al., 2013; Brown and Walter, 2016) has also provided additional insights about the role that community organizations, such as schools, sporting clubs, service clubs, and places of worship, have in supporting people who are dying and their families. Social network approaches also have a practical application. A recent example in end of life care is the use of advance care planning to initiate social network development in clinical settings (Abel and Kellehear, 2016). This work has shown promise with work in Frome (UK) revealing that increased social support can reduce hospitalizations (Abel, 2018). Another programme is the Healthy End-of-Life Program (HELP), which uses a person-centred collaborative community planning tool to help people to identify their existing social and community resources, to make an end of life plan for care (Grindrod and Rumbold, 2016, p. 2).

Community development is one way to develop social networks and potentially increase participation in end of life care. Leadbeater and Garber (2009), for example, believe that social networks are a key to transforming end of life care in the UK. However, they and other authors argue that not all carers are equipped for their end of life caring role (Abel et al., 2013; Burns et al., 2013), see also Box 10.2. Leadbeater and Garber (2009) note:

Box 10.2 Personal reflection 2

Social innovators such as Leadbeater and Garber (2009) argue that the health promotion strategy to reorient health services towards a social approach will not create the kind of radical and transformational change needed to change end of life care in Western societies. That is, to change end of life care in such a way that it aligns with the wishes of people who are dying and the wishes of their families. Similarly, Russell highlights why transformation is important for community participation when he notes:

> We do not need reform; we need re-function. Institutions, which were once hatched from associational life, have become bloated and arrogant. Their function actually is to do what we cannot do in associational life—no more, no less. Yet they regularly colonize our lives and the lives of our neighbours by trying to manage, regulate, curricularise, and otherwise control free space. Restoring the function of our systems is the work of radicals and, in essence, is an effort toward halting the expansion of the institutional world into the associational world. Another motto of the radical is this: Institutions, know your place. (p. 119)

Take a moment to consider both views expressed here.

What are some of the challenges and benefits of working from within an institution/with institutions?

How will you take this into account while working with community members?

> Our challenge is to help people to achieve what is most important to them at the end of life. That will require the creation of a network of health and social supports so that people can die at and closer to home, with the support of their family and friends, as well as professionals. If we do not create this social network, then in the decades to come many hundreds of thousands of people will experience unnecessarily distressing deaths. We will die badly in places not of our choosing, with services that are often impersonal, in systems that are unyielding, struggling to find meaning in death because we are cut off from the relationships which count most to us.

An example: Compassionate Neighbours (UK)

The 'Compassionate Neighbours' programme at St Joseph's Hospice in London (UK) is a collaboration between a palliative care service and a local community development agency 'Social Action for Health' (Richardson, 2011; Barry and Patel, 2013). Together, the two agencies developed a cross-disciplinary task group and a series of community-led initiatives were designed and undertaken. These initiatives included the development of community hubs where community members address issues about serious illness, death, and bereavement together, and request training and support from the hospice as required (Barry and Patel, 2013). The Compassionate Neighbours programme was initiated and funded by the hospice, using both top-down and bottom-up strategies to address concerns about volunteer autonomy and risk management.

An example: Neighbourhood Networks (India)

The neighbourhood network programme in India has led the way internationally as a programme promoting bottom-up community development in palliative care. Palliative care programmes in many parts of the state of Kerala have developed a highly autonomous and self-reliant model that has local citizens and local communities mobilizing to self-help. Thus the programme has demonstrated how a palliative care service can be led by, and delivered in, partnership with community members and community organizations such as schools, police services, and college students (aged 17–24) (Kumar and Numpeli, 2005).

Volunteering and participation in hospice/palliative care

As previously noted, the predominant model of community participation in palliative care is volunteering. For many health professionals working in palliative care or healthcare, community members participate in palliative care either as a patient/family member or as a volunteer. Both the Compassionate Neighbours and Neighbourhood Networks programmes have engaged with community members who are trained volunteers. Volunteering and volunteer roles in hospice/palliative care have had vital roles in the delivery of end of life care services. These services include fundraising, counselling, bereavement support, and providing respite for family caregivers. Recent research though has argued that the role of palliative care volunteers has been professionalized and the expectation is that they function as an extension of clinical teams (Kellehear, 1999).

It is also worth acknowledging, that for many palliative care services, the primary model of community participation in end of life and bereavement care is volunteering. The volunteers are a significant part of the palliative care workforce, providing a range of services to support the health and medical teams within hospice and palliative care. This can include providing transport, respite for carers, housework and cleaning, and emotional support and counselling. While palliative care volunteering is the dominant model of participation, recent research suggests traditional service models are not always the most satisfactory experience for community members (Gale, 2017).

Community members who are death literate, for example, may be experienced and knowledgeable about death, dying, and grief and want to share this knowledge with other community members and not want to participate in a formal service delivery model of care (Noonan, 2018). Some researchers and practitioners have called for more inclusive and citizen-led models of community engagement to enhance and acknowledge community participation which may or may not even use the term volunteering to describe the role. Co-design and collaboration models, for example, require renegotiating the relationships between professional services and community networks. They also require that health services and health professionals are mindful of how they use their power, their view of empowerment, and self-reliance. These are key concepts to consider when understanding and considering participatory relations in public health palliative care.

Key concepts

Public health palliative care initiatives are aimed at building the knowledge, capacity, and resilience of the whole community in relation to death, dying, and loss (Kellehear and Young, 2011). Community initiatives and research using a social approach emphasize social justice, participation, and well-being (Kellehear,

1999, 2005). The following sections provide an overview of these concepts.

Citizen-centred participation

A third view from asset-based community development is the citizen-centred approach (Russell, 2020). Russell notes:

> Active citizenship begins to retreat in the face of ever-growing professionalism and expertise. People not credentialed by a professional 'guild' become increasingly more dependent on institutional services to do what previously was done by participating in community life. (Russell, 2020, p. 4)

Community development, because of its focus on mobilizing community and capacity building, is considered an important social practice in the field of public health. Health professionals can also work in their traditional nursing or medical roles and have a community development approach (Talbot and Verrinder, 2017). The view of participation is the same, that is, community members and health professionals ought to be equal; however, the mode of delivery can be different. For health services, community development can be a means to an end, for example, promoting palliative care in the community.

The principles of self-reliance and autonomy as applied to communities, not individuals, are key features of community development. It is, however, a significant challenge to the controlling, top-down managerial approach of health services (Kellehear, 2005; Ife, 2009). Bottom-up community development challenges the usual participatory relationships associated with power because it resists the professionalization of caring roles. The question of how community voices and 'lay experts' participate in end of life and bereavement care is central to the issue of participatory relations. Community-led initiatives challenge the idea that volunteering by being recruited, trained, and managed by a hospice or palliative care service is the only legitimate way a citizen, who is not a medical or health professional, can contribute to end of life care. See Box 10.3.

Empowerment

The concept of 'empowerment' is prevalent in healthcare and health promotion. In the literature, empowerment is a complex concept and has been defined in a number of ways, including informed choice, shared decision-making, and patient participation (Piper, 2010). It also has a broader definition referring to the emancipation of individuals through consciousness raising (Laverack, 2013) and 'empowering' people to improve their health (Labonte and Laverack, 2001). Ife and Tesoriero (2006, cited in Talbot and Verrinder, 2017) offer four perspectives on empowerment, the desired end point of community engagement. First, they see empowerment as a process that equalizes because disadvantaged groups can compete more effectively with other interest groups. Second, that empowerment brings an ability to compete with political power. Third, that structural inequality and oppression are major forms of power and empowerment can only be achieved by challenging structural disadvantage through social change. And finally, that power is expressed though discourse. Empowerment is achieved through validating voices other than those currently dominating. See Box 10.4.

It is challenging, but important to note that top-down approaches typically seen in service delivery tend not to promote critical awareness or resistance in community members. As noted by Laverack (2013) 'empowerment implies resistance and struggle to bring about a change in the political order and to challenge the very agencies that often fund and support health programs' (p. 45). As such, empowerment is often pursued rhetorically at the policy and management level of healthcare as opposed to direct care with patients or community members (Stajduhar et al., 2010) or as a set of relations and practices. It is not uncommon for health services to have empowerment as a core value, but to use the term in a tokenistic way that does not address inequality or disadvantage authentically. That is, initiatives 'do to' and 'do for' community members rather than 'do with'. Organizations working within an empowerment model do not aim to 'empower' people, rather they work democratically within the community recognizing that people and communities are the only ones who can empower themselves (Stajduhar et al., 2010; Talbot and Verrinder, 2017).

Box 10.3 Personal reflection 3

What is your view of grassroots-led initiatives and activities that function independently from healthcare services?

Box 10.4 Personal reflection 4

Kellehear (2005) suggests public health approaches to end of life care are 'not new services. They are community members acting toward each other in new and constructive ways to improve their own capacity for end of life care. Any professional rationalisation of these changes into simpler forms of direct service provision is a regressive and important threat to community empowerment' (p. 100).

Empowerment is not given to others. That is, we don't 'empower' others, Empowerment is enabled through validating voices other than those currently dominating.

How are you keeping this in mind?

How are you checking the power and status that comes with your position/role when working with community members?

Power sharing continues to be a sticking point for the public health approach. If power is still viewed as something that the health system 'gives' to people who are dying and their families, this fails to recognize the permeating nature of power.

Power

Health professionals are often working to improve the health of their patients by helping patients change their behaviour through education and motivation (Laverack, 2013). Behaviour change needs systemic support through strong policy and increased participation from community members (Laverack, 2014). This issue of power sharing is central to Sallnow and Paul's (2015) engagement model. Sallnow and Paul (2015) note that the 'degree of power sharing by an organisation and the capacity of the community to mobilise their skills and resources' is key (p. 235). It is not uncommon for community engagement strategies to be 'top-down' (leaflets, education sessions, online videos). Talbot and Verrinder (2017) describe them as 'where organisations with power to direct policy and implement change identify priorities outside the context of the community. Practitioners with expertise and knowledge about a population develop policies and programs aimed at improving the lives of vulnerable groups without necessarily including members of those groups in the decision-making processes' (p. 136).

Traditional structural views of power emphasize the state having control 'over' people, with control being seen as hierarchical (Labonte, 1995). Foucault (1973) uses the single term power/knowledge to bring to awareness that the relationship between power and knowledge is inextricable and inevitable. Experts, such as doctors, have a key role in this power/knowledge structure; however, it is not as simple as the doctor exerting power over patients (as in Labonte's view of power). Foucault instead views power as ubiquitous and in every moment of our social relations each of us enacts power. In this view, power can be both repressive and productive, although never benign. In the case of medicine, power is embodied and enacted in biomedical practices. These practices contribute to the ongoing production, social construction, and dominance of the biomedical discourse. At the same time, the past decade has seen the emergence of non-medical end of life 'experts' who are using their voices to resist and disrupt the dominance of the biomedical model.

Celebrity illnesses and deaths are one example of non-medical experts who live their dying and death in the public sphere. Popular culture and access to information via the internet and mass media provide deeply personal stories and insights into illness, dying, death, and grief. Jade Goody, for example, a UK celebrity who was diagnosed with cervical cancer during her participation on a reality TV programme. Goody's use of social and mainstream media while she was dying provided her with the status of lay expert (Ashton, 2014). Her diagnosis, illness, and death have been examined by a number of academics because they created a significant increase in cervical screening in Britain. This became known as the 'Jade effect' (Kavka and West, 2010; Walter, 2010; Ashton, 2014).

Another example of citizens participating in end of life system are death doulas, or end of life doulas. Death doulas, similar to birth doulas, journey alongside a person with a life-threatening illness and their family providing non-medical support. Some death doulas describe their work as a return to a more 'traditional' view of dying at home, when a trusted and experienced friend or community member might provide support to a person dying and their family. Death doulas also refer to their practice as complementary to palliative care services. There has been a recent emergence of academic literature and research on death doula work providing insights into the biomedical view of the functions of these end of life roles (Rawlings et al., 2019, 2020).

In health systems where the biomedical model regulates the behaviour of dying people and their families, a practice that is wholly outside of that system, and one that doesn't rely on a specialist referral, is disruptive of the normal relations of power. Some authors assert that the growing consumer movement is also changing and challenging medical dominance. For example, Ballard and Elston (2005) argue that consumers of healthcare can both contribute to and resist medicalization and assert that medical dominance and medicalization are not synonymous. They argue that medicalization can also arise through collaboration or collusion between the doctor and patient, suggesting that some patients are 'passively duped into accepting doctor's orders' while others pressure the doctor (Ballard and Alston, 2005, p. 234).

One view is that medicalization can be a process of oscillation between medicalization and demedicalization, or even a process of negotiation between the medical profession and their patients (Ballard and Alston, 2005). There is certainly evidence that advance care planning has, for example, been adopted and embraced by disease-specific groups and advocacy groups as a way people can practise autonomy at the end of their lives. Medical authority and the recent citizen-led movements are also changing power relations (Lupton, 2012). Consider a situation in which a palliative care patient is actively engaged in their care, but is not always compliant with medical advice. When such a person has cultural and social resources to drawn upon, power/knowledge is developed through the strategies used to navigate a path of care (Lupton, 1997).

Health professionals and their patients are seeking to make sense of and interpret each other's motivations and assumptions to create a shared language, and negotiate authority (Lupton, 2012). The question of how the health and medical system manages this authority and power has been examined by health researchers (Broom, 2006; Oudshoorn et al., 2007; Blomqvist et al., 2010). Broom (2006) in particular, notes that very little attention has been paid to understanding the complexity of medical dominance given the current sociocultural context. He notes that applying 'previous structural notions of medical dominance or power' to the contemporary environment overlooks some of the challenges inherent in the lay/expert divide (p. 497). Broom (2006) notes in one study, that oncologists were developing, at least rhetorically, a more holistic model of care based upon patient interest in complementary therapy. The internet was also seen to be playing a role in this citizen/professional interaction in healthcare and in the deathcare industry where information about how to care for people who are dying, how to care for the dead body, and even how to arrange your own funeral is now readily available.

Another example, in Australia, is Flinders University conducting a massive open online course (MOOC) about death and dying (Tieman et al., 2018). There is evidence that some participants in the MOOC have reported feeling more positive and competent in relation to planning for death. This course demonstrates the role internet-based learning can have in the democratization of death and dying knowledge. Further, there is also emerging evidence that palliative care would benefit from separating patient contact that involves education from clinical care (Collins et al., 2017). Collins and colleagues (2017) found that patients wanted palliative care doctors to be more direct and avoid euphemisms. This is an important finding because it challenges the pervasive idea that death is a taboo topic in healthcare. This self-perpetuating idea about the attitudes of citizens, reinforces paternalism and excludes people from fully participating in their healthcare. See Box 10.5 for a personal reflection on power.

Structure/agency

Do you believe change happens because of individual actions or do institutions lead change? The structure/agency concept is also worth acknowledging as it is connected to empowerment, power, and self-determination. The relationship of individual agency to the social structures has long been debated in sociology, but less so in public health or palliative care fields. This basic idea addresses the tension that relates to the source of change—is it individuals or society at large? Howarth's (2007) socio-historical work tracks the social changes within society's changing relationship with death, dying, and loss. She notes the structure/agency debate is also important in how we understand society's view of and relationship

Box 10.5 A personal reflection on power

Whether you are a health professional, policy maker, charity trustee, or a volunteer, understanding the relationship we have with our 'patients' or 'clients', research participants, other healthcare workers, and the general public is deeply important to understanding how we view the concept of participation.

I reflect here as a clinical psychologist with my own experience of working in community development with a programme that supported end of life carers to develop their care networks. The programme had a unique way of harnessing existing community knowledge to complement the palliative care service and enabling community members to be involved in end of life and bereavement care. To do this, community members who had cared for someone to die at home volunteer to mentor and support another caregiver who was also caring. The organization viewed the community mentors as knowledgeable and experienced citizens. While there was supervision and support for mentors, they had relatively autonomous roles within their local community. The mentor training involved learning about community development, communication/mentoring skills, and developing a deeper understanding of their own caring experience and learning. The mentors were death literate community builders and connectors. Unlike traditional palliative care volunteer roles, mentors were viewed as 'knowledgeable friends' and they were network enablers—they normalized carer and care network-led requests for support and organizations of help. They did not do housework or respite, for example, but if there was a need for this kind of practical support, the mentor could act as a sounding board and facilitate the mobilization of the carer's network.

The programme focused on the relationships and networks of the carer, and responsibility and power were shared, reciprocal, and negotiated. As health professionals participating in community building activities, in the words of Cormac Russell (2020), 'we need to be cautious, since community building is not simply referring people to different programs; instead it is about disrupting power with professionals and relocating authority to citizens who are uncredentialled by vested institutional authority and their associations' (p. 110).

There were times when responses to the community development programme were negative and reassurance and education were not helpful. As a health professional, I didn't fully appreciate how disruptive the programme was for my health professional colleagues. As such, when I reflect on the experience I wonder—was it the model of community participation that was so disruptive? Was it the shared power model? Or just simply a fear of a new programme?

Our behaviour and responses to community participation can encourage and discourage collaborations and citizen-led initiatives, so how can those of us working as health professionals be more mindful of our power and own responses when working with community members?

Consider the following:

1. What do you know about the end of life care happening in the diverse community living within walking distance of your service? What about within 10 minutes?
2. Of the communities that access your service too late to fully participate, or if you suspect they are not fully aware of palliative care, what can you do to learn about how these people are currently caring for their dying or bereaved?
3. How do you/does your service respond to new services or programmes that are citizen led? How do you reach out to these new programmes and services? How does you/your service manage anxieties and concerns, and still reach out to community leaders? How might you be relationship focused? (Note: if your reaction to the first question is, we don't know of any services or programmes that are citizen led, how will you find out?)
4. How are existing community capacities to care and community strengths accounted for in the policy and planning undertaken by your service?

with death. Interactionists such as Giddens' (1984) attempt to overcome this duality. His view is that structure and agency both have a role in social change. Social structures are produced and maintained by people, and these structures also restrain and influence how much power an individual can exert on the system.

Self-reliance

The self-reliance of communities is also a central feature of citizen-led community development. Ife (2009) argues that the principles of self-reliance and independence 'become reconstructed within community development as values that need to be applied to communities rather than to individuals' (p. 32). These approaches, within the context of end of life care, can provide a framework to enable palliative care services to expand beyond the provision of clinical services into death education and non-traditional community partnerships that nurture and develop the existing community capacity around death and dying. It is this integration, the normalizing of the connection between life and death, living and dying, that modern medicine and living in a modern society has changed significantly over the past 120 years.

Participatory models in research

This chapter wouldn't be complete without paying attention to the role of participatory methods in public health palliative care research. According to Hampshire and colleagues (2005, p. 341), four ways of participating in research are:

- Contractual: researchers contract local people as subjects of research.
- Consultative: researchers consult local people and ask for their opinions prior to intervention.
- Collaborative: researchers and local people work together on projects designed, initiated, and managed by researchers.
- Collegiate: researchers and local people work together as colleagues with different skills to offer, in a process of mutual learning, where local people have control.

As such, there are many participatory and creative research methods and the chapter author would direct you to the resources at the end of this chapter. The two methods described here, photovoice and digital storytelling, have been used in public health palliative care to examine the role of community knowledge and how this enables or supports participation in end of life and bereavement care.

Photovoice and visual elicitation

Photovoice is defined as 'a process by which people can identify, represent, and enhance their community through a specific photographic technique' (Wang et al., 2000, p. 82). As a community-based participatory research (CBPR) method it has three goals: '(1) to enable people to record and reflect their community's strengths and concerns, (2) to promote critical dialogue and knowledge about important issues through large and small group discussion of photographs, and (3) to reach policymakers' (Wang and Burris, 1997, p. 369).

Horsfall and colleagues (2012, 2017) used photovoice to examine the effects of caring for a dying person at home on their wider community. Initially, this research was seeking to understand more about the benefits of a community development-based intervention. The research methods were developed collaboratively, with a focus on ensuring that caregivers and their care networks had not only a safe space to talk about their experiences, but the methods enabled participants to remain in control of how they tell their stories. End of life carers and their networks were given a camera and a set of questions by the researchers and invited to take photographs of significant events, networks, and relationships that occurred while they were providing end of life care. The carer and their network were then invited to discuss the photos and to analyse the experiences. The community members who participated analysed and interpreted the caring experience for themselves rather than making their lives available for analysis by others. Participants are able to focus on what is important to them, tell stories, and express themselves in their own words. The photos, taken by caregivers, in this sense were a trigger for conversations about end of life caring that traditional interviewing or focus group methods are unable to achieve in the same way.

Digital stories

Digital storytelling is a highly creative participatory method that enables people to develop and produce 3–5-minute visual narratives comprised of images, video, audio recording of music and voice, and text. Digital storytelling is a narrative-based method that has also been used as an education tool and in health promotion (Stewart et al., 2010) and is considered an emergent method in participatory research models (Gulbrium, 2009).

Digital stories, like all storytelling methods, are creative accounts of experiences, where the story takes the central focus (Gubrium, 2009; Lambert, 2009) and it enables 'critical and creative theorizing' (Benmayor, 2008, p. 198). Lambert's (2009) seven-step process is often used to enable people from the general public to construct their own digital stories, and over a number of years he and his team developed and refined this process, resulting in thousands of digital story projects and films being made every year. The seven steps are:

1. Owning your insights.
2. Owning your emotions.
3. Finding the moment.
4. Seeing the story.
5. Hearing the story.
6. Assembling the story.
7. Sharing the story.

These steps are facilitated in a group process consisting of story circles where participants develop their story and script, learning the digital technology skills required to produce the digital story. This process lends itself to both the creative and transformative goals of this research because the participant story remains central to the process. As noted by Gubrium (2009), the story circle process has a similar function to a traditional focus group, enabling participants to openly discuss their shared experiences which naturally facilitates critical self-reflection during the development of the narrative and digital story. Unlike a focus group, however, participants direct the conversation with content from the scripts of their digital stories by seeking feedback and providing feedback to others on their scripts.

One example of digital storytelling in public health palliative care is work done by Moeke-Maxwell and colleagues (2018) with bereaved family members in New Zealand. They state:

> Researchers and participants co-created personalised written stories about the older person and their end-of-life experiences, supported with photographs of family, friends and memorabilia. We aimed to uplift the status of the older person and their family by tangibly reflecting the significance and magnitude of what had been shared and to strengthen our research analysis. (Moeke-Maxwell, 2018, p. 302)

This is an example of collaborative research that is providing deep insights into knowledge and experiences within Indigenous communities. Further, the research process and the outcomes act as a way to transfer intergenerational knowledge about end of life, death care, and bereavement care traditions.

Conclusion

This chapter provided an overview of participatory models including community engagement, community development, and social networks as they relate to public health palliative care, including participatory research methods. A public health framework provides the tools to enable palliative care services to expand the scope of their work into communities and beyond the traditional provision of clinical services. Community engagement and non-traditional community partnerships can provide a way that nurtures and develops existing community capacity around end of life care, caring, and bereavement.

Initiatives influenced by the public health palliative care movement have the potential to initiate a deeper understanding of power and medical control. The field of public health palliative care has yet to grapple with a deeper structural critique of professional power when engaging with the community about dying, death, and loss. As a first step, self-refection is key and this chapter has invited you to reflect on your own values and beliefs about participation and participatory relationships.

Recommended reading

Rekindling Democracy: A Professional's Guide to Working in Citizen Space by Cormac Russell is an excellent place to start when developing your thinking about community participation and reflecting on your role in this work. For people working to do change work from within institutional settings please see chapter 10, 'Rekindling well-being from the inside out: learning from institutional radicals', which provides an overview of highly effective practices of change-makers in institutional settings.

Not everyone identifies with being a radical or a change-maker. Moyer (2001) provides a useful way for people to consider more specifically how they will participate in change work in *Doing Democracy: The MAP Model for Organising Social Movements.* Moyer (2001) has developed a useful way to view the roles and contributions people can have to social change movements; they are citizen, rebel, social change agent, and reformer. Citizens are people who can articulate the vision of the movement. They have a role in ensuring that any attempts to water such approaches down or discredit them are met with evidence or efficacy. The rebel helps put a social issue/movement on the agenda. They turn the heat up and cause tension by highlighting the gap between what is and what should be. They are often empowered to use information from the movement to take action in their own community or contexts. They may be involved in direct action, though are more likely to support and facilitate. The social change agent promotes alternatives and paradigm shifts, and nurtures and develops new cultural practices. A social change agent brings new language and actions into a system. They do this by acting as an 'open system' sharing information and promoting dialogue between the system and the community/public. And finally, reformers change policy, and lead change within institutions by working with powerbrokers and acting as an interface between a social movement and the public. While change-makers are seen as encouraging awareness of a social issue through open dialogue, reformers use their experience and influence to lobby for change in institutions and systems.

REFERENCES

Abel, J., Walter, T., Carey, L. B., Rosenberg, J., Noonan, K., Horsfall, D., et al. 2013. Circles of care: should community development redefine the practice of palliative care? *BMJ Supportive and Palliative Care*, **3**, 383–388.

Abel, J. and Kellehear, A. 2016. Palliative care reimagined: a needed shift. *BMJ Supportive & Palliative Care*, **6**, 21–26.

Aoun, S. M., Breen, L. J., Howting, D. A., Rumbold, B., McNamara, B., and Hegney, D. 2015. Who needs bereavement support? A population based survey of bereavement risk and support need. *PLoS One*, **10**, e0121101.

Arnstein, S. R. 1969. A ladder of citizen participation. *Journal of the American Institute of Planners*, **35**, 216–224.

Ashton, D. 2014. The expertise of illness: celebrity constructions and public understandings. In: Leen Van Brussel, D. and Carpentier, N. (eds.) *The Social Construction of Death*, pp. 114–134. Basingstoke: Palgrave Macmillan.

Ballard, K. and Elston, M. A. 2005. Medicalisation: a multi-dimensional concept. *Social Theory & Health*, **3**, 228–241.

Barry, V. and Patel, P. 2013. *An Overview of Compassionate Communities in England*. London: Murray Hall Community Trust and National Council for Palliative Care.

Benmayor, R. 2008. Digital storytelling as a signature pedagogy for the new humanities. *Arts and Humanities in Higher Education*, 7, 188–204.

Blomqvist, K., Theander, E., and Larsson, V. 2010. What happens when you involve patients as experts? A participatory action research project at a renal failure unit, Nursing *Inquiry*, 17, 317–323.

Broom, A. 2006. Reflections on the centrality of power in medical sociology: an empirical test and theoretical elaboration. *Health Sociology Review*, **15**, 496–505.

Brown, L. and Walter, T. 2013. Towards a social model of end-of-life care. *British Journal of Social Work*, **44**, 2375–2390.

Burns, C. M., Abernethy, A. P., Dal Grande, E., and Currow, D. C. 2013. Uncovering an invisible network of direct caregivers at the end of life: a population study. *Palliative Medicine*, **27**, 608–615.

Collins, A., McLachlan, S., and Philip, J. 2017. How should we talk about palliative care, death and dying? A qualitative study exploring perspectives from caregivers of people with advanced cancer. *Palliative Medicine*. **32**, 861–869.

Emejulu, A. 2011. Re-theorizing feminist community development: towards a radical democratic citizenship. *Community Development Journal*, **46**, 378–390.

Foucault, M. 1973. *The Birth of the Clinic*. London: Tavistock.

Gale, B. 2017. Understanding how belief systems may hinder us in developing compassionate communities. Presented at the 5th International Public Health & Palliative Care Conference, Ottawa, Canada. 20 September.

Giddens, A. 1984. *The Constitution of Society: Outline of a Theory of Structuration*. Cambridge: Polity.

Grindrod, A. and Rumbold, B. 2016. *Healthy End of Life Program (HELP): Offering, Asking for and Accepting Help. Creating an End of Life Collaborative Community Culture*. Melbourne: La Trobe University Palliative Care Unit.

Gubrium, A. 2009. Digital storytelling: an emergent method for health promotion research and practice. *Health Promotion Practice*, **10**, 186–191.

Hampshire, K., Hills, E., and Iqbal, N. 2005. Power relations in participatory research and community development: a case study from Northern England. *Human Organization*, **64**, 340–349.

Howarth, G. 2007. *Death and Dying: A Sociological Introduction*. Cambridge: Polity Press.

Holt-Lunstad, J., Smith, T. B., and Layton, J. B. 2010. Social relationships and mortality risk: a meta-analytic review, *PLoS Medicine*, 7, e1000316.

Horsfall, D., Leonard, R., Noonan, K., and Rosenberg, J. 2013. Working together apart: exploring the relationships between formal and informal care networks for people dying at home. *Progress in Palliative Care*, **21**, 331–336.

Horsfall, D., Leonard, R., Rosenberg, J., and Noonan, K. 2017. Home as a place of caring and wellbeing? A qualitative study of informal carers and caring networks lived experiences of providing in-home end-of-life care. *Health and Place*, **46**, 58–64.

Horsfall, D., Noonan, K., and Leonard, R. 2012. Bringing our dying home: creating community at end of life. *Health Sociology Review*, **21**, 373–382.

Ife, J. 2009. *Human Rights from Below: Achieving Rights Through Community Development*. Cambridge: Cambridge University Press.

Kavka, M. and West, A. 2010. Jade the obscure: celebrity death and the mediatised maiden. *Celebrity Studies*, **1**, 216–230.

Kellehear, A. 1999. *Health Promoting Palliative Care*. Melbourne: Oxford University Press.

Kellehear, A. 2005. *Compassionate Cities: Public Health and End of Life Care*. Abingdon: Routledge.

Kellehear, A. and Young, B. 2007. Resilient communities. In: Monroe, B. and Oliviere, D. (eds.) *Resilience in Palliative Care*, pp. 223–238. Oxford: Oxford University Press.

Kumar, S. and Numpeli, M. 2005. Neighborhood network in palliative care. *Indian Journal of Palliative Care*, **11**, 6.

Labonte, R. 1995. Population health and health promotion: what do they have to say to each other? *Canadian Journal of Public Health*, **86**, 165–168.

Labonte, R. and Laverack, G. 2001. Capacity building in health promotion, part 1: for whom? And for what purpose? *Critical Public Health*, **11**, 125–127.

Lambert, J. 2009. *Digital Storytelling: Capturing Lives, Creating Community*. Berkeley, CA: Digital Diner Press.

Laverack, G. 2013. *Health Activism: Foundations and Strategies*. London: Sage.

Laverack, G. 2014. *A–Z of Health Promotion*. New York: Palgrave Macmillan.

Leadbeater, C. and Garber, J. 2010. *Dying for Change*. London: DEMOS.

Leonard, R., Horsfall, D., and Noonan, K. 2015. Identifying changes in the support networks of end-of-life carers using social network analysis. *BMJ Supportive & Palliative Care*, **5**, 153–159.

Lupton, D. 1995. *The Imperative of Health: Public Health and the Regulated Body*. London: Sage Publications.

Lupton, D. 2012. *Medicine as Culture: Illness Disease and the Body*, 3rd ed. London: Sage Publications.

Moeke-Maxwell, T. H., Wiles, J., Black, S., Williams, L., and Gott, M. 2018. Collaborative story production with bereaved family carers of people who died in advanced age. *Qualitative Research Journal*, **18**, 302–315.

Moyer, B. 2001. *Doing Democracy: The MAP Model for Organising Social Movements*. Gabriola Island, Canada: New Society Publishers.

Noonan, K. 2018. Renegade stories: a study of deathworkers using social approaches to dying, death and loss in Australia (PhD thesis). Western Sydney University.

Noonan, K., Horsfall, D., Leonard, R., and Rosenberg, J. 2016. Developing death literacy. *Progress in Palliative Care*, **24**, 31–35.

Oudshoorn, A., Ward-Griffin, C., and McWilliam, C. 2007. Client-nurse relationships in home-based palliative care: a critical analysis of power relations. *Journal of Clinical Nursing*, **16**, 1435–1443.

Rawlings, D., Tieman, J., Miller-Lewis, L., and Swetenham, K. 2019. What role do death doulas play in end-of-life care? A systematic review. *Health & Social Care in the Community*, **27**, e82–e94.

Rawlings, D., Litster, C., Miller-Lewis, L., Tieman, J., and Swetenham, K. 2020. The voices of death doulas about their role in end-of-life care. *Health & Social Care in the Community*, **28**, 12–21.

Reeves, D., Blickem, C., Vassilev, I., Brooks, H., Kennedy, A., Richardson, G., et al. 2014. The contribution of social networks to the health and self-management of patients with long-term conditions: a longitudinal study, *PLoS One*, **9**, e98340.

Richardson, H. 2011. A public health approach to palliative care in East London: early developments, challenges and plans for the future. In: Sallnow, L., Kumar, S., and Kellehear, A. (eds.) *International Perspectives on Public Health and Palliative Care*, pp. 110–122. Abingdon: Routledge.

Rosenberg, J. P., Horsfall, D., Leonard, R., and Noonan, K. 2015. Informal caring networks for people at end of life: building social capital in Australian communities. *Health Sociology Review*, **24**, 29–37.

Rosenberg, J. P., Horsfall, D., Leonard, R., and Noonan, K. 2017. Informal care networks' views of palliative care services: help or hindrance? *Death Studies*, **5**, 1–9.

Rosenberg, J. P., Mills, J., and Rumbold, B. 2016. Putting the 'public' into public health: community engagement in palliative and end of life care. *Progress in Palliative Care*, **24**, 1–3.

Russell, C. 2020. *Rekindling Democracy: A Professional's Guide to Working in Citizen Space* [Kindle edition]. Cascade Books.

Sallnow, L. and Paul, S. 2015. Understanding community engagement in end-of-life care: developing conceptual clarity. *Critical Public Health*, **25**, 231–238.

Stajduhar, K., Funk, L., Jakobsson, E., and Ohlén, J. 2010. A critical analysis of health promotion and 'empowerment' in the context of palliative family care-giving. *Nursing Inquiry*, **17**, 221–230.

Talbot, L. and Verrinder, G. 2017. *Promoting Health: The Primary Health Care Approach*, 6th ed. Chatwood: Elsevier Australia.

Tieman, J., Miller-Lewis, L., Rawlings, D., Parker, D., and Sanderson, C. 2018. The contribution of a MOOC to community discussions around death and dying. *BMC Palliative Care*, **17**, 31.

Walter, T. 2010. Jade and the journalists: media coverage of a young British celebrity dying of cancer. *Social Science and Medicine*, **71**, 853–860.

Wang, C. and Burris, M.A. 1997. Photovoice: concept, methodology, and use for participatory needs assessment. *Health Education and Behaviour*, **24**, 369–387.

World Health Organization. 1986. *The Ottawa Charter for Health Promotion: First International Conference on Health Promotion, Ottawa, 21 November 1986*. Geneva: World Health Organization.

World Health Organisation (2019) Participation as a driver of health equity. https://apps.who.int/iris/bitstream/handle/10665/324909/9789289054126-eng.pdf?sequence=1&isAllowed=y

Yuill, C., Crinson, I., and Duncan, E. 2010. The social model of health. In: *Key Concepts in Health Studies*, pp. 11–14. London: Sage Publications.

SECTION 3

Basic practice methods

11

Community development

Compassionate communities

Manjula Patel and Kerrie Noonan

Introduction

Before the advances of modern medicine when mortality was higher and life expectancy was much shorter, death and dying was much more part of daily community life. Death was a common social occurrence, more familiar and less fearful as people knew what to do, how to provide care, and it was less socially disruptive (Seale, 1998). Traditionally, religion and cultural knowledge provided a structural framework to death and dying that included rituals and customs, still present in some cultures. However, in secular societies many of these social structures associated with death and dying have been eroded with the professionalism of end of life care. With the medicalization of death, dying moved away from the community and into institutions such as hospitals. In the process, it has isolated the dying person from their community and disempowered the community to provide care. It is within this context that a public health approach to end of life care has emerged.

There are a number of terms and concepts in public health palliative care used to describe the social interventions that make dying, death, grief, and caregiving everyone's business. This chapter focuses on community development in public health palliative care, in particular, compassionate communities, which has come to represent many different initiatives. Compassionate city amplifies the World Health Organization's model of healthy cities to ensure that people living with life-limiting illnesses towards the end of their lives are supported to live well while dying. The aim of the healthy cities model was to create healthier communities and although compassionate cities and compassionate communities operate independently, they are intrinsically linked and strengthen each other. Compassionate communities as part of public health palliative care is a social model of care, caring for people living towards the end of their lives at home. It requires the support of informal networks as well as formal care networks. As a public health approach, it adopts many of the principles of community development which engage individuals within the community-using process rather than a set of instructions. Community development is non-prescriptive so therefore it looks different in every place, region, and continent. Compassionate communities adopts the principles of community development for end of life care and the movement has caught the imagination of many around the world. This chapter provides an outline of community development, compassionate communities, and initiatives in different countries.

Defining community development

There are many ways to describe a community, mostly because communities are no longer constrained to just local areas—people now are virtually connected across the global. The vast majority of us have connections to a community whether that is our neighbourhood, the places where we work, volunteer, worship, and share hobbies and interests, although historically, communities have mostly been thought of as geographical locales where people mutually support each other. The term 'elective belongings' describes how some people choose where they want to belong, unlike those who have a history in a place. One way of understanding community is the interactions of social relationships. The essence of community is the association with solidarity which relates back to the pre-industrial period and pre-dates modernity to a time when communities felt disenfranchised with matters that affected their lives, and collectively came together in solidarity to take social action, to lobby, and to campaign to bring about change. It was in this spirit of people coming together with shared concerns and interests that community groups emerged. From small beginnings, these informal grassroots community groups continue to be the bedrock of community life and many of these have become charities as voluntary associations and organizations with formal structures. At one time, charitable institutions were the extension of faith groups providing support in the community but the charity sector is now diverse and wide ranging and charities of all sizes are to be found in every area of the globe. These charities are referred to as non-government organizations and as part of a voluntary non-profit sector they are community assets that facilitate community development.

The term 'development' can be described as exercising agency to bring about change. Although not exclusively, community development is often (or can be) associated with civic society, formal voluntary organizations, as well as informal community groups. Anyone can engage with community development whether they are paid workers, volunteers, or unpaid members of informal community groups. The origins of community development come from the desire to improve the living conditions for people within the community by the community members themselves. The main purpose of community development is the promotion of solidarity (community) exercising agency (development) (Bhattacharya, 2004). It can be argued that while modernity created many opportunities for some people, it also emphasized the lack of agency for others. As modernity shifted the attention from the collective towards the individual, it eroded the spirit of the community (Bhattacharya, 2004). It is against the background of structural inequalities that have disadvantaged some communities where community development has stimulated the emergence of community associations and organizations. It is in the most deprived areas that community development has been most active and transformative. The value of community development in collectively working with people and groups for positive change to tackle inequalities has been recognized by governments in the UK and other countries. This led to the emergence of state-sponsored community development and hence the term community work is used interchangeably.

Community development is initiated by community members and community organizations at the grassroots level (most desired form), or from a top-down direction of state-sponsored local government agencies; there should always be consensus with the community of the development need. The willingness to genuinely empower a community has to include active community participation at a high level for community ownership to be achieved. This is demonstrated in Arnstein's (1969) ladder of participation; with eight rungs, it is a guide to how power is shared. The first two rungs are 'manipulation' and 'therapy' that aims to heal and educate and are non-participative. The third is the flow of information in one direction of 'informing', the fourth is 'consultation' engaging with people, and the fifth is 'placation' of limiting the involvement of a few; these last three are tokenistic gestures. The sixth rung is 'partnership' involving citizens in decision-making, the seventh is 'delegation' with transfer of power, leading to the last rung of 'citizen control' of empowering the community to manage community programmes. The ladder of participation continues to be widely used as a guide with the aim to graduate to the transfer of power and control.

Although community engagement is integral to community development, it is also distinct and can be undertaken as a process for other purposes, whereas community development is more than just engaging and involving community. As Chapter 10 has covered, participation is crucial in community development. and community members naturally volunteer as they build relationships and bring people together. Community associations and organizations provide the opportunity for people to volunteer in formal and informal roles and they are instrumental within community development. Volunteers are assets within communities; whether they are formal or informal, they are altruistic individuals providing their time for the benefit of others. Voluntary roles are diverse and span the many facets of community life and include roles of project managing as well as befriending and visiting people at home. Whether formal or informal, volunteers offer a unique position of engaging with others and acting as intermediaries within the community between associations, organizations, and other resources.

There is no single way of defining community development as it is multifaceted and pluralistic and there are various ways of describing it. One of the earliest definitions adopted by the United Nations in 1948 was of a movement with active participation for the benefit of the whole community. This ambiguity in the understanding of community development to some extent continues with no agreed universal set of principles but many different versions that nevertheless do include some core principles, such as empowerment, human rights, inclusion, social justice, self-determination, and collective action (Kenny, 2007). It is precisely because people experience social disadvantages that bring them together in solidarity with shared aims of exercising agency for social justice that makes community development so powerful. What is clear is that the process of community development practice is as valuable if not more important than the intended outcomes. In practice, though, community development is a long-term undertaking involving collaboration and inclusive practices which entail people working together and building trusting relationships. This bottom-up approach is emphasized by some as the purest form of community development based on the premise that it is the lived experiences of local people that make them the experts of their lives and their community (Ife, 2009). The approach is organic and involves local community members taking on different roles, to collectively share their knowledge and skills to inform decision-making as they debate and work together, with creative actions to ultimately bring about improvements in the community. Active participation for individuals can be an empowering process as they learn from each other and collectively make decisions, try new activities, build confidence, and increase their self-esteem.

Rather than viewing communities with deficiencies a more positive strength-based approach has been adapted across different countries. The most well-known approach was developed by Kretzmann and McKnight (1993) based on the premise of recognizing that communities have assets and this should be the starting point of community development. Asset-based community development (ABCD) aims to identify and map the assets within the community which include physical space; community members with local knowledge, skills, and networks; local groups/associations/organizations; as well as institutions, statutory organizations, and businesses. The asset-based community development process is defined by three interrelated characteristics: first, to affirm the assets that are present within the community; second, to have an internal focus of starting to seek the skills and knowledge required from within the communities before seeking external support; and third, the process should be relationship driven between local residents, organizations, and institutions (Ketzmann and McKnight, 1993). The relational aspect of the process is the bedrock of community development and community development is the prerequisite of community well-being.

Defining compassionate communities

Compassionate communities have been defined as 'communities that develop social networks, social spaces, social policies and social conduct that support people through the many hours, days, weeks, months and sometimes years of living with a life-threatening or life-limiting illness, ageing, grief and bereavement, and long-term care-giving' (Wegleitner et al., 2016. p. xiv).

A public health approach to palliative and end of life care will influence how individuals with life-limiting illnesses are cared for and supported. It is a social model of care that takes into account the role of social networks and informal carers and provides an important theoretical framework for the development of compassionate communities. The principles of harm reduction and equity begin at a population level to remove barriers that hinder well-being, and seek to empower individuals with agency, control, and the prospect for individuals to live well to the end of their lives. The central concepts of compassionate cities and compassionate communities start with the premise that compassion is an ethical imperative of health, which includes health and well-being even in the presence of disease and disabilities at any stage, including dying, and continues into bereavement living with loss, because compassion is the holistic ecology of care (Kellehear, 2005).

A public health approach is health promoting, builds resilience, and reduces harm. As such, compassionate communities employ the principles of community development (solidarity and agency) to increase the capacity of support and care for people living at home towards the end of their lives. This includes supporting the primary carers as they bear the main responsibility of caring for the dying, and post death, when formal end of life care services ceases, the carers might find themselves alone with their grief. The continued support of informal social networks post bereavement reduces the experience of isolation and loneliness associated with death, dying, and loss. Therefore, compassionate communities are the interactions of social networks surrounding those who are dying in the community and their carers, to support them as they provide the main care. Social networks are composed of those with social identity rather than just local identity. Many of the informal (friends, family) end of life and bereavement care networks are formed naturally independent of formal (service provider) networks of care. Care networks are a combination of both informal and formal carers. The aim of compassionate communities is to enable people who are dying to continue living well at home. The concept is relatively well understood and the response to support this aim has been diverse with many different initiatives being introduced under the banner of compassionate communities. Just as community development is not a prescribed step-by-step approach, so it is true of compassionate communities; instead, it is an organic process of building relationships and social interactions. A systematic review of different models of compassionate communities found there is limited research to date about the development of compassionate communities (Librada-Flores et al., 2020), However, three main models were identified:

- A top-down approach of models from the health services to the community.
- A bottom-up approach of community participation in the promotion of their own health.
- Organization and community participation responding to community needs with solutions.

Arnstein's (1969) original model of community participation has been extended by Sallnow and Paul (2015) as they explored the understanding of community engagement within end of life care and offered conceptual clarity of a spectrum of engagement in end of life care. The spectrum proposes greater involvement is required for higher levels of empowerment which increases levels of health and well-being, as Fig. 11.1 shows.

Sallnow and Paul's (2015) spectrum makes the connection of relating equity of health and well-being with community empowerment. The overall goal of developing compassionate communities is to achieve the transfer of power to 'communities' as the main key actors in end of life care. Community participation is central, especially if the development of compassionate communities is initiated by organizations—it may then begin at a lower level of engagement but the level of community involvement would need to be increased to a collaborative level for empowerment to take place. Each stage of the development can be mapped against the spectrum presented previously.

A scoping review of compassionate communities in England (Barry and Patel, 2013) found there was a range of groups, organizations, and individuals involved with a breadth of approaches that included:

- Public health promotion and death awareness.
- Reconfiguring end of life care.
- Supporting existing networks—community development.
- Establishing formal projects with volunteers.
- Individual acts of compassion with friends and family.

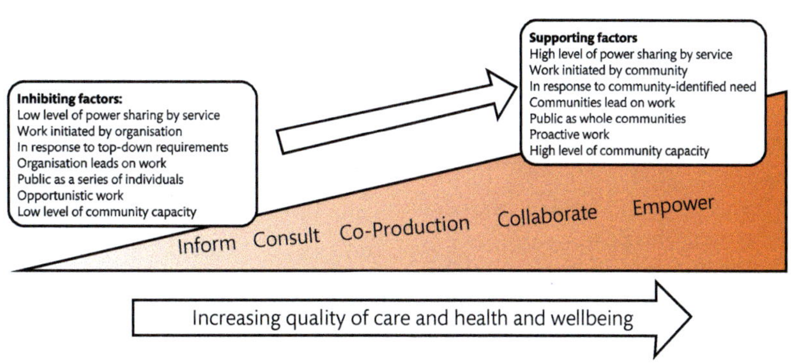

Fig. 11.1 Sallnow and Paul's (2015) spectrum of engagement.

Reproduced with permission from Sallnow, L. and Paul, S. (2015). Understanding community engagement in end-of-life care: developing conceptual clarity. *Critical Public Health*, 25, 231–238.

Raising awareness of death, dying, and loss seems to be an element within compassionate communities but is also an aim in itself. For example, national campaigns such as 'Dying Matters' in the UK is a national awareness week with lots of events taking place locally. Similarly, 'Dying to Know Day' started in Australia is also now in America. Another approach includes 'death cafes' that aims to informally bring people together, sharing refreshments and encouraging conversations about death. Death cafes have been initiated hundreds of times around the globe (https://deathcafe.com/what/).

A public health palliative care practice model has been proposed by Abel and colleagues (2018) called the palliative care new essentials. The model describes how four essential elements would work together to provide continuity of care and support for people living towards the end of their lives at home in the community. The four essential elements include specialist palliative care, generalist palliative care, compassionate communities, and civic end of life care (compassionate city). Compassionate communities as one of the essential elements is positioned to be a bridge between the formal palliative care services and informal community support and civic engagement.

Although limited, the emerging research data have contributed to the conceptual understanding of compassionate communities; for example, Horsfall and colleagues' (2015) research study of co-creating an ecology of care for people dying at home examined natural occurring compassionate communities with bereaved carers. The study highlighted the role of informal carers being more than able to care for people dying at home supported by extensive social networks. Both informal and formal carers are involved in care but do so separately from each other and rarely collaborating; however, both need to work together in co-creating an ecology of care. The findings of this study influenced the conceptual model of 'circles of care' (Abel et al., 2013). The model suggests networks of care surround the dying person with the inner network consisting of a handful of informal carers providing on-hands care; the outer networks also consists of informal carers supporting those in the inner circle; the next circle is of community networks that may also include formal volunteers; and the remaining furthest circle of networks includes formal services and policy. It is perhaps in the 'community' sphere that community development/compassionate communities is ideally positioned to bring together informal and formal networks. The development of compassionate communities around the world is diverse, there are many similarities but also differences between them depending on contexts, culture, environment, and infrastructures that vary. The main elements of these compassionate communities seem to include:

- Providing space and opportunities in the community for discussions about death, dying, and loss.
- Grief, end of life, and death literacy that transforms conversation into community engagement and social actions.
- Formal volunteer programmes to support people who are dying and their carers living at home.
- Increasing the capacity of community members to be the main providers of care and support for people at the end of life.
- Continuation of social relationships post bereavement for those living with loss.

The development of compassionate communities can act to increase the confidence and capacity of community members to actively support people living towards the end of their lives and their carers. The aim of an organizational top-down model of developing compassionate communities may use formal volunteers, which potentially could further create service dependency rather than cultivate active community members. Therefore, it is important to use the spectrum of engagement to map organizational activities (Sallnow and Paul, 2015), especially because, historically, inequity of access to palliative care services has always been challenging. However, within the framework of public health palliative care, compassionate communities has a much wider application. Just as community development is an enabling asset to leverage support, adopting a compassionate communities approach also has the same potential of enabling social networks of community members to be active. Social relationships in the daily acts of spending time with people dying, sharing experiences, making connections, being compassionate, and laughing and crying together are deeply valuable.

The nature of developing compassionate communities with a community development approach is organic as it builds on the unique cultures and assets of communities and precisely why no two will be exactly the same. This may be viewed as a weakness by some but a strength by others. This diversity in approach is highlighted in the overview of the development of compassionate communities in different countries in the following section.

An overview of compassionate communities across the globe

Compassionate communities projects and programmes are now developing across the globe. This section provides an overview of compassionate community initiatives. Given it is a highly evolving field, the initiatives mentioned here have been sourced from grey and published literature. Where possible, we have attempted to provide examples of both local (grassroots) and national initiatives.

UK

There are numerous compassionate communities in the UK that use community development as a guiding principle. Many of the initiatives have been developed by hospices who have dedicated community development and community engagement teams. Some of the larger projects include bereavement cafes and the Compassionate Neighbours programme. The UK has one of the largest hospice networks in the world and much of the compassionate communities work that is occurring is focused on looking beyond the walls of the hospice.

England

In England, it was the End of Life Care Strategy (Department of Health, 2008) that first captured the need to change dominant institutional end of life care to a greater community involvement. There followed the launch of the national 'Dying Matters' campaign to raise the awareness of death, dying, and loss nationally and locally. In 2009, the first compassionate communities projects in England were funded by the NHS West Midlands Strategic Health Authority. A scoping review of compassionate communities (Barry and Patel, 2013) reported on 28 case studies occurring across England. This provided important insights into the breadth of the formative work that included both funded and unfunded projects delivered by organizations and individuals within the communities championing the work. Another scoping study (Paul and Sallnow, 2013) explored the attitudes and involvement of over 220 (hospice) palliative care providers with an online survey. Over 60% of the responses indicated that a public health approach was a priority for their organizations, with most of them working in schools and community groups. They found a broad understanding and interpretation of the terms 'community engagement', 'health-promoting palliative care', and 'compassionate communities'.

In 2015, the National Council of Palliative Care together with Public Health England supported eight pathfinder communities to lead local compassionate communities programmes. Pathfinders were an example of a multipartnership model because of the way projects were led by local authorities, clinical commissioning groups, the NHS, and voluntary sector providers of health and social care. Partnerships development and collaboration has been a strong theme in England. In recent years, hospices have expanded traditional community engagement beyond fundraising and community awareness by introducing community development workers to reach out to communities and co-design work. Community engagement has been well received within the community with many becoming aware of hospices for the first time. Hospices have developed partnerships with other services and community development organizations (Sallnow et al., 2016). These partnerships have led to community development initiatives such as Compassionate Neighbours, and bereavement cafes and help points. The Compassionate Neighbours programme trains volunteers to support people with a life-limiting illness who are isolated and lonely in the community. The model is anchored in community development and other hospices are adapting the model. Another important contribution from England is the work of organizations with people living with intellectual disabilities, who historically have not had good access to end of life care or bereavement support (Allen, 2020).

One of the first community organizations to develop a service with a public health approach was based in the West Midlands in 2001 (Patel, 2016). The service was the result of community members expressing their concern with the lack of support for those living with terminal illness, so together with a community organization they responded with the development of a new supportive care service for people in the last year of life. The service was named by a community member as a metaphor for the service to be a 'bridge' between them as patients and the health and social care systems/professional. The service is an exemplar of a community development approach that is a social model of health that utilizes community support.

A compassionate communities programme known as the Frome model stems from a medical practice that connects people to local charities and community groups. People are referred from the medical practice to local community groups for social connections and support. The model is similar to social prescribing and includes three components to help people to be socially connected:

- Making the most of people's own social networks.
- Building informal social networks to support people with daily living tasks within the community.
- Linking people up to community activities.

Scotland

Scotland has been leading a number of public health initiatives around death, dying, loss, and grief. Most recently, the Scottish Partnership for Palliative Care have developed a compassionate communities initiative. The project works to support local communities across Scotland to improve experiences around death, dying, and bereavement and is called the Truacanta Project. The project is supporting four communities who are working in unique ways to reach the most vulnerable and marginalized people and tackle health inequalities from a grassroots level. The goal is to increase awareness and knowledge of services in local communities, while creating opportunities to discuss death, dying, loss, and care (https://www.goodlifedeathgrief.org.uk/content/thetruacantaproject/).

Another key project in Scotland has been Compassionate Inverclyde, which focused on grassroots community actions. Local community members are encouraged to be involved in a diverse set of activities to support acts of kindness and compassion. The project has five key strands that come together to support the overall movement. The strands of the programme are:

- No One Dies Alone programme.
- High Five school programme.
- Back home boxes.
- Back home visitors.
- Bereavement cafe and support hub.

A recent evaluation of the Compassionate Inverclyde project reported on outcomes that included improved well-being across the domains of personal, relational, and community well-being.

Wales

The compassionate communities movement in Wales began with a pilot project in 2017. As a partnership between the Royal College of General Practitioners, Marie Curie, and Byw Nawr (Live Now) as a Welsh Government-supported initiative with the charity Compassionate Communities UK. The aim of the project was to implement the principles of compassionate communities adapting the Frome model with the Welsh Health Board (Compassionate Communities UK, 2020).

Ireland

The Irish approach to compassionate communities has been a combination of project and policy work. The compassionate communities project at the Milford Care Centre ran for a number of years and was comprehensively evaluated (McLoughlin, 2013). The goals of the project were 'To enrich and support society to live compassionately with death, dying, loss and care and to demonstrate and evaluate the process of developing a compassionate community model in an Irish context' (McLoughlin, 2013, p. 16). The project included the employment of two community development workers who led the delivery of the project's objectives.

'Bill United' was one of the first digital media campaigns used to promote social connections and social networks at the end of life (Milford Care Centre, 2014). Using a series of videos to tell Bill's story, it simply and elegantly described the importance of social connections when people are dying, of caring, and of grieving. Bill's story provided a simple way to describe the way a compassionate community functions and develops.

The Irish Hospice Foundation and All Ireland Institute of Hospice and Palliative Care have conducted a series of consultations and released discussion papers about public health palliative care in Ireland, including compassionate communities. A recent round table consultation has provided a foundation for taking ongoing actions in local communities (Irish Hospice Foundation and All Ireland Institute of Hospice and Palliative Care, 2020).

Europe

Many of the projects across Europe have been supported by research programmes in major universities and strong research programmes and evidence about the compassionate communities approaches are developing. This includes compassionate communities initiatives in Switzerland, Sweden, Belgium, Austria, and Germany. The Last Aid course, established by a working group from Norway, Denmark, and Germany, aims to provide public education as an ingredient of compassionate communities (Bollig et al., 2019). The themes included in the course are care at the end of life, decision-making in advance care plans, symptom management, and cultural aspects of death and bereavement. The course also provides an arena for discussions about death and dying in the community.

The DoBra programme in Sweden is run by an interdisciplinary research team conducting community-based programmes (Kleijberg et al., 2020). The programmes have explored creative ways to facilitate advance care planning conversations and intergenerational arts projects. Another study explores the symbols of Indigenous cultural identity relating to death systems. This Sami community consists of extended family and social networks with systematic socially accepted norms of providing community support in dying, death, and loss (Kroik et al., 2020).

In Austria, a study explored with people the preconditions required for a community end of life care programme (Wegleitner et al., 2018). The study concluded that a web of relationships was involved in the establishment of 'caring communities' as people came together to share their experience and look out for each other. Another study viewed pharmacies as community assets and explored the prospect of them being a base for compassionate communities projects (Plunger et al., 2016).

The Flemish government has emphasized the need for the socialization of care, for the integration of professional care with informal care, between medical healthcare and welfare care. In particular, looking towards a volunteer base to build stronger connections with the community. Vanderstichelen's (2019) study of volunteers within palliative care services in Belgium found formal volunteers experienced the constraints of healthcare legal framework whereas compassionate communities offer the opportunity to work within communities outside of organizational framework.

India

In India, the work of Dr Suresh Kumar and his colleagues at the Institute of Palliative Medicine has demonstrated how palliative care can be led by and delivered in partnership with community members and community organizations such as schools, police services, and college students (Kumar and Numpeli, 2005). The Neighbourhood Network programme in Kerala, India, has led the way internationally as a programme promoting bottom-up community development in palliative care. They have a highly autonomous and self-reliant model that effectively mobilizes local communities to provide support and care of people with life-threatening and chronic illnesses. The Institute of Palliative Medicine, over the course of nearly 30 years, developed a number of compassionate communities initiatives which are led by community members and they are supported by the outpatient clinical teams who are employed by the community volunteer groups.

Taiwan

Taiwan is one of the first countries in the world to adopt compassionate communities at a national level and to support the development of city-wide initiatives. In 2017, the Taiwanese Ministry of Health and Welfare launched a national declaration committing to the principles of health-promoting palliative care. This includes greater partnerships with communities around matters of social support, public education about death and dying (death literacy), and health promotion for end of life care. As a result of this policy work, Taipei City has since developed a compassionate community action agenda that includes the goals to:

1. Improve life literacy, construct community values.
2. Respect the will of good death, promote self-decision making.
3. Integrate with local culture, develop community features.
4. Enhance practical training, cultivate future champions.
5. Share achievement and experience, link up and communicate with the world.

Spain and Latin America

The work of the New Health Foundation in Sevilla, Spain, has provided an integrated model of compassionate communities called 'All With You' (Flores et al., 2018). The model utilized is described as a systemic approach to connect the three arms of the programme: healthcare services, community engagement (compassionate communities or cities), and integrating care (including social services). Compared to other community development approaches discussed in this chapter, the methods utilized within the 'All With You' model is strongly integrated with health service delivery.

Canada and North America

There is a strong emphasis on grassroots community action in Canada. Pallium Canada has been particularly active and was one of the first national organizations to appoint a compassionate communities national lead to grow the compassionate communities movement. They have since developed a toolkit for compassionate communities and the compassionate workplace programme. These two programmes have led to over 200 initiatives across Canada. The Compassionate Workplace Campaign, for example, was designed to ignite a movement across Canada to create supportive environments for the increasing number of employees who are caregiving, grieving, or dealing with a serious illness. The Compassionate Workplace Campaign has developed in conjunction with community expert tools and activities that support workplaces to create a more supportive environment. The goals are:

- Building awareness and understanding of serious illness, caregiving, and grief experiences.
- Decreasing the stigma associated with serious illness, caregiving, and grief.

- Raising awareness of resources and supports.
- Prompting and enabling supportive conversations.
- Empowering people to create a more compassionate culture.

Another end of life care project with Indigenous communities includes a community development participatory action research project (Kelley et al., 2018). The research team in partnership with the First Nations communities worked together to build and/or strengthen local capacity that already existed within the communities. The project included working alongside the community to also develop and establish a culturally appropriate palliative care support.

Australia and New Zealand

The Australian state of Victoria led the way globally with the development of health-promoting palliative care policy and funding for state-wide demonstration projects between 2003 and 2009 (Salau et al., 2007). This work laid the foundation for much of the global research and practice that has followed. Since then, La Trobe University Palliative Care Unit has developed the Healthy End of Life Project (HELP): a framework for compassionate communities. This comprehensive framework is a research-informed and evidence-based public health palliative care resource for communities. The intention of the HELP programme is to shift social norms around offering and accepting help, which are important factors in end of life care. The HELP programme aims to 'identify and build on local values and structures (community capacities) that will form, maintain and sustain a compassionate community' (Grindrod and Rumbold, 2018, p. S78).

In recent years, a number of compassionate communities projects and organizations have started up and are now developing into sustainable projects. This includes both grassroots actions through to more formal service delivery organizations. The Southwest Compassionate Communities Network, for example, has developed a community connector programme providing practical and family support to palliative care patients, carers, and their families (Aoun et al., 2020). The main goal of the project is to have a positive impact on social connectedness, and to understand more about how this has an impact on unplanned hospitalization, advance care planning rates, and caregiver support needs. This initiative was also part of the national network of compassionate communities projects developed by The GroundSwell Project (modelled on the pathfinders project in the UK). This networked and capacity-building approach has also delivered one of the few research reports about the implementation of compassionate communities (Horsfall et al., 2020).

Like the Dying Matters campaign in the UK, Dying to Know Day on 8 August has also been a catalyst for supporting compassionate communities in Australia. The aim of Dying to Know Day is to promote death literacy and to encourage people to 'bring to life' conversations about end of life. Many of the compassionate communities projects in Australia use Dying to Know Day to have community conversations about end of life and palliative care, caregiving, advance care planning, and grief and loss.

There are a number of hospices in New Zealand who are beginning to develop compassionate communities initiatives. This is a growing field in New Zealand and similarly to Europe there is a growing body of research on public health palliative care approaches, including compassionate communities. A recent survey review of compassionate communities projects in New Zealand (Dempers and Gott, 2016) noted the need for policy to support the practices. It also highlighted many of the 'start-up' issues that occur in regard to conceptual clarity. A number of research projects have examined the role of family carers and community, and the significance of family (Gott et al., 2015; Moeke-Maxwell and Gott, 2019; Morgan et al., 2020).

What do compassionate communities look like?

The overview from around the world highlights common themes in the development of compassionate communities which includes the following elements:

- Raising awareness—the starting point and the most dominant theme seems to be raising awareness of death, dying, and loss with the population at large with annual national awareness weeks such as Dying Matters in the UK and, Dying to Know Day in Australia providing a platform for stimulating opportunities.
- Other more local initiatives within community settings include, for example, advance care plans and bereavement cafes.
- Practical support such as a (new) volunteer role to befriend people living towards the end of their lives and their carers in the community.
- Changing the offer and acceptance of support through the HELP project in Australia, encouraging people to accept support.
- Formal end of life care providers engaging with community organizations and groups to be involved in developing compassionate communities.
- Work is happening to improve the integration of formal care with informal care (Spain and Latin America).
- The Neighbourhood Network programme in India is an established example of a community-led end of life care initiative.
- Developing better workplace practice to be more compassionate towards employees caring for a dying family member and those who are bereaved and living with loss.

Practice, research, and evaluation of compassionate communities: what does it tell us?

The initiatives discussed in this chapter have all contributed to the understanding of the roles that community development and compassionate communities have in palliative and end of life care. Although limited, emerging empirical research study findings are contributing to building the evidence base of the development and benefits of compassionate communities in end of life care. The research has extended the understanding of the compassionate communities as a public health approach to end of life care. From the examples of both research and practice we highlight in the following sections some of the benefits and challenges of compassionate communities (please note, this is not an exhaustive list).

Benefits

1. One of the most important benefits of community development is the needs of community members and the community central

to the decision-making process. In other words, the community decides on the actions and 'interventions' taken to address dying, death, loss, grief, and caregiving in their local community.
2. There is a movement in healthcare towards acknowledging health promotion principles, notably that community well-being can be as important as individual well-being. Further, there is a body of evidence that notes individual and community well-being are inextricably linked. That is, an individual's health and well-being is connected to the health and well-being of the community they live in. This is an important aspect of the compassionate communities movement.
3. Improve equity of care and support so that more people can be supported in the community to carry on living at home in the community and reduce the number of people unnecessarily dying in institutions.
4. Informal networks at the end of life and bereavement care are also naturally occurring elements of compassionate communities. The experience of being part of the caring network is life enhancing and affirming.
5. Carers who are supported to care are more able to continue caring to the very end of life as their support network helps bear some of the stress and strain of caring, enabling many carers to fulfil the desire to provide the care required to keep their loved ones at home.
6. People with past experience of providing end of life care are better prepared and more confident to provide care for the dying again. Many of the end of life care volunteers volunteer because of their own experience and they want to use their experiences to support others.
7. With more people caring for the dying at home, the community's ability to share knowledge and skills with others to care for dying family members and friends and their carers is increased.
8. Informal care networks who support carers and family members while they are caring, continue to provide support when bereaved. This reduces the isolation and loneliness that many people who are bereaved and grieving feel.
9. Most importantly, community development methods have been used in some projects to enable care for those who are dying to continue to live well with their family and friends, to the very end of their lives at home within their community if that is their preferred place of care.

Challenges

1. The dichotomy of person-centred care versus a community development approach is reflected in this chapter; we noticed that many of the compassionate communities programmes are being run by health services or institutions. Hospitals, hospices, healthcare organizations, universities, and aged care facilities dominate the landscape.
2. There is always a risk that community development and capacity-building programmes are taken over or rolled out by mainstream health services to control the development of compassionate communities.
3. The challenge of the principles of community development is to empower the community to lead and build capacity and ultimately to control the process of developing compassionate communities. For some, the risk of the transfer of power is maybe a step too far?
4. Funding and ongoing sustainability is often a challenge for compassionate communities initiatives, especially because community development has historically been underfunded and often funding is given to services providing healthcare for individuals rather than conducting projects that enable and support community members to lead projects.
5. Community organizations may themselves perceive death, dying, and loss as the domain of health professionals and may lack the confidence to initiate a compassionate communities project.
6. Gate-keeping and paternalism most notably by healthcare services is experienced by informal carers and citizen-led projects.
7. Professional boundaries and organizational systems make integration of formal and informal care at the end of life challenging.

Conclusion

This chapter began with defining community development, and the core principles that are present in practice, emphasizing the process is equally as important as the outcomes, and the appreciation and understanding of the roots of community development as being *solidarity* and *agency*. Social interactions are at the heart of community development, bringing people together in genuine collaborative partnerships. The underlying principles of community development are integral in developing compassionate communities. We have outlined how the principles of community development are interpreted when developing compassionate communities approaches. The spectrum of engagement (Sallnow and Paul, 2015) provides a spirit level of community participation which is particularly important to pay attention to if the development of compassionate communities is from a top-down model. As the proposed palliative care new essentials model (Abel et al., 2018) highlights, compassionate communities has a pivotal role in embedding a public health approach with palliative care services and end of life care.

This chapter has provided an overview of different compassionate communities approaches and projects from across the globe. It does not include all the local initiatives of developing compassionate communities that are beyond the scope of this chapter. Readers who would like to explore more about compassionate communities are encouraged to follow up on many of the references and links that have been provided. The purpose has not been to give a complete picture of the initiatives—this would indeed be a challenging thing to do given the growth and change in this field. Instead, our aim was to provide the reader with a big-picture overview of some of the key initiatives. It is noticeable that in India, an underdeveloped country, the neighbourhood volunteers are the main providers of end of life care, and the clinical services support the volunteers. While in developed countries, it is often the clinical services or research groups that are leading compassionate communities projects.

While the developments of compassionate communities are being led by formal end of life care organizations, informal care networks do and are capable of caring for the dying. There are common themes across the practices as well as similarities and differences in the practice of community development/compassionate communities. The most pronounced is a top-down approach by healthcare services compared to a community-led bottom-up approach. There is no one way to do community development and this is particularly true for the development of compassionate communities, but what is most definite is the need to include the community is central.

As the whole world lives through the experience of the global coronavirus disease 2019 pandemic, the number of people dying from the virus is unprecedented. The safety measures of social isolation have changed the experience of death, dying, and loss. The risk of spreading the virus and recurring lockdowns of societies have transformed all pre-pandemic normal ways of life. It has changed everything including the normal practice of compassionate communities which was mostly social face-to-face interactions. What is clear is the need for compassionate communities to provide care and support has been amplified and will be crucial when we emerge from this pandemic lockdown and isolation measures.

Questions to ask yourself

See Boxes 11.1 and 11.2 for some reflective questions.

Box 11.1 Questions to ask when thinking about doing compassionate communities/community development work in your community

1. What role might community development have in your organization or community?
2. What do you know about end of life and palliative care in your local community?
3. What are these communities good at? What do they need support with?
4. What are some of the barriers/opportunities for working with community members?
5. What community development organizations, programmes, or workers currently exist that you could work with?
6. Before you assume a community 'needs' something, how will you collaborate and talk with local citizens?
7. What role might community development have in your organization or community?
8. What do you know about end of life and palliative care in your local community?
9. What are these communities good at? What do they need support with?

Box 11.2 Questions to ask about your own approach to community development

1. What are some of the key differences between bottom-up and top-down community development projects?
2. What are some of the reasons for this?
3. Is the overall aim to transfer knowledge and control for the community members and groups to provide care?
4. Is there the will for a transfer of power, for letting go for communities to take control of ownership?
5. If you are part of an organization, what is the overall aim of the organization to develop compassionate communities?
6. What role do end of life care organizations/services have within a compassionate communities approach?

REFERENCES

Abel, J., Kellehear, A., and Karapilagou, A. 2018. Palliative care—the new essentials. *Annuals of Palliative Medicine,* 7, S3–S114.

Abel, J., Walter, T., Carey, L., Rosenberg, J., Noonan, K., Horsfall, D., et al. 2013. Circles of care: should community development redefine the practice of palliative care? *BMJ Supportive & Palliative Care,* **3**, 383–388.

Allen, G. 2020. A creative approach to exploring loss for people with intellectual disabilities. Ehopsice. 31 March. [Online] Available at:https://ehospice.com/uk_posts/a-creative-approach-to-exploring-loss-for-people-with-intellectual-disabilities/

Aoun, S. M., Abel, J., Rumbold, B., Cross, K., Moore, J., Skeers, P., et al. 2020. The Compassionate Communities Connectors model for end-of-life care: a community and health service partnership in Western Australia. *Palliative Care and Social Practice,* **14**, 1–9.

Arnstein, S. R. 1969. Ladder of citizen participation. *Journal of American Planning Association,* **35**, 216–224.

Barry, V. and Patel, M. 2013. *An Overview of Compassionate Communities in England.* London: The Dying Matters Coalition and Murray Hall Community Trust.

Bhattacharya, J. 2004. Theorizing community development. *Journal of the Community Development Society,* **34**, 5–32.

Bollig, G., Brandt, F., Ciurlionis, M., and Knopf, B. 2019. Last aid course. An education for all citizens and an ingredient of compassionate communities. *Healthcare,* **7**, 1–12.

Compassionate Communities UK. 2020. Compassionate Communities UK Wales. [Online] Available at: https://www.compassionate-communitiesuk.co.uk/compassionate-communities-uk-wales

Dempers, C. and Gott, M. 2016. The status of a public health approach to palliative care at New Zealand hospices. *Progress in Palliative Care,* **25**, 75–81.

Department of Health. 2008. *End of Life Care Strategy.* London: Department of Health.

Gott, M., Allen, R., Moeke-Maxwell, T., Gardiner, C., and Robinson, J. 2015. 'No matter what the cost': a qualitative study of the financial costs faced by family and whānau caregivers within a palliative care context. *Palliative Medicine,* **29**, 518–528.

Grindrod, A. and Rumbold, B. 2018. Healthy End of Life Project (HELP): a progress report on implementing community guidance on public health palliative care initiatives in Australia. *Annals of Palliative Medicine,* **7**, S73–S83.

Horsfall, D., Psychogios, H., Rankin-Smith, H., Read, N., and Noonan, K. 2020. *Researching Compassionate Communities in Australia: A Short-Term Longitudinal Study.* Sydney: Western Sydney University.

Horsfall, D., Yardley, A., Leonard, R., Noonan, K., and Rosenberg, J. 2015. End of life at home: co-creating an ecology of care. [Online] Available at: http://researchdirect.uws.edu.au/islandora/object/uws%3A32200

Ife, J. 2009. Principles and dimensions of community development. In: *Human Rights From Below: Achieving Rights Through Community Development,* pp. 29–66. Cambridge: Cambridge University Press.

Irish Hospice Foundation and All Ireland Institute of Hospice and Palliative Care. 2020. Round table on a public health approach to palliative and end of life care on the island of Ireland. Report. [Online] Available at: https://aiihpc.org/wp-content/uploads/2020/06/Round-Table-Report.pdf

Kellehear, A. 2005. *Compassionate Cities: Public Health and End of Life Care.* Abingdon: Routledge.

Kelley, M. L., Prince, H., Nadin, S., Brazil, K., Crow, M., Hanson, G., et al. 2018. Developing palliative care programs in indigenous communities using participatory action research: a Canadian application of the public health approach to palliative care. *Annals of Palliative Medicine,* **7**, S32–S72.

Kenny, S. 2007. *Developing Communities for the Future*, 3rd ed. Melbourne: Cengage Learning.

Ketzmann, J. P. and McKnight, J. L. 1993. *Building Communities from the Inside Out: A Path Towards Finding and Mobilizing a Community's Assets*. Chicago, IL: ACTA Publications.

Kleijberg, M., Ahberg, B., Hilton, R., and Tishelman, C. 2020. Death, loss and community—perspectives from children, their parents and older adults in intergenerational community-based arts initiatives in Sweden. *Health and Social Care in the Community,* **28**, 2025–2036.

Kroik, L., Lindqvist, O., Stoor, K., and Tishelman, C. 2020. The past is present: death systems among the Indigenous Sami in Northern Scandinavia today. *Mortality,* **25**, 470–489.

Kumar, S. and Numpeli, M. 2005. Neighborhood network in palliative care. *Indian Journal of Palliative Care,* **11**, 6.

Librada Flores, S., Herrera Molina, E., Boceta Osuna, J., Mota Vargas, R., and Nabal Vicuña, M. 2018. All with you: a new method for developing compassionate communities—experiences in Spain and Latin-America. *Annals of Palliative Medicine,* **7**, S15–S31.

McLoughlin, K. 2013. *Compassionate Communities Project Evaluation Report.* Limerick: Milford Care Centre.

Milford Care Centre. 2014. Bill's story: let's talk series. [Online] Available at: https://www.youtube.com/watch?v=_5tJGaWjRZk

Moeke-Maxwell, T. and Gott, M. 2019. He taonga tuku iho: indigenous end of life and death care customs of New Zealand Māori. In: Selin, H. and Rakoff, R. M. (eds.) *Death Across Cultures. Science Across Cultures: The History of Non-Western Science*, **Volume 9**, pp. 295–316. Cham: Springer.

Morgan, T., Wiles, J., Moeke-Maxwell, T., Black, S., Park, H., Dewes, O., et al. 2020. 'People haven't got that close connection': meanings of loneliness and social isolation to culturally diverse older people. *Aging & Mental Health,* **24**, 1627–1635.

Patel, M. 2016. Compassionate communities in Sandwell, West Midlands, England. In: Wegleitner, K., Heimerl, K., and Kelleahear, A. (eds.) *Compassionate Communities: Case Studies from Britain and Europe*, pp. 46–59. Abingdon: Routledge.

Paul, S. and Sallnow, L. 2013. Public health approaches to end-of-life care in the UK: an online survey of palliative care services. *BMJ Supportive & Palliative Care,* **3**, 196–199.

Plunger, P., Tatzer, V., Hiemerl, K., and Reitinger, E. 2016. Dementia-friendly pharmacy: a doorway in the community in Vienna and Lower Austria. In: Wegleitner, K., Heimerl, K., and Kelleahear, A. (eds.) *Compassionate Communities: Case Studies from Britain and Europe*, pp. 137–152. Abingdon: Routledge.

Salau, S., Rumbold, B., and Young, B. 2007. From concept to care: enabling community care through a health promoting palliative care approach. *Contemporary Nurse,* **27**, 132–140.

Sallnow, L., Bunnin, A., and Richardson, H. 2016. Community development and hospices: a national UK perspective. In: Wegleitner, K., Heimerl, K., and Kelleahear, A. (eds.) *Compassionate Communities: Case Studies from Britain and Europe*, pp. 1–14. Abingdon: Routledge.

Sallnow, L. and Paul, S. 2015. Understanding community engagement in end-of-life care: developing conceptual clarity. *Critical Public Health,* **25**, 231–238.

Seale, C. 1998. *Constructing Death: The Sociology of Dying and Bereavement*. Cambridge: Cambridge University Press.

Vanderstichelen, S. 2019. *Volunteering in Palliative Care: A Study of Volunteer Task, Support, Roles, Involvement and Collaboration with Professionals in the Flemish Healthcare*. Brussels: Vrije Universiteit Brussel Faculty of Medicine and Pharmacy and Ghent University Faculty of Medicine and Health Services.

Wegleitner, K., Heimerl, K., and Kellehear, A. (eds.) 2016. *Compassionate Communities: Case Studies from Britain and Europe.* Abingdon: Routledge.

Wegleitner, K., Schuchter, P., and Prieth, S. 2018. 'Ingredients' of a supportive web of caring relationships at end of life: findings from a community research project in Austria. *Sociology of Health and Illness,* **42**, 987–1000.

12

Compassionate cities

A social ecology at the end of life

Gail Wilson, Emilio Herrera Molina, Silvia Librada Flores, and Allan Kellehear

Introduction

Social ecology—the interdependent relationships of humans with their immediate physical and social settings—has always held a central place in human discussions about health and safety. It is a field and phrase within the broader study of human ecology as a study of how humans adapt and modify their environments and also describes how environments determine human behaviour and lifestyles. Social ecology places a greater emphasis on that interplay within socially constructed environments such as urban spaces, institutional structures, and cultural environments.

For example, it has long been recognized that living near a heavily wooded area may provide concealment from life-threatening enemies and ready access to food. However, wooded areas are also places that pose a risk of wild fire or attacks from wild animals. In recent historical times, clean water and efficient sewerage systems have been recognized to be essential for good health but also infection control. Living in walled cities helped deter invaders or delayed their attack so as to enable reinforcements, or escape. We have long noticed how the wealthy have outlived the poor, showing us repeatedly how the economic life of inhabitants determines where and how they work, where they live, and, in turn, their life chances in sickness and in health. The ecological system around us—the interdependent physical, social, economic, and political settings—has always been a crucial and ever modifiable *resource and determinant* in making or breaking human life and health.

In the last few decades, modern healthcare systems have come to increasingly recognize this often taken-for-granted power and have sought more deliberately to harness it. In this chapter, we will explain how changing the way we organize our relationship with our everyday settings can enhance health and well-being at the end of life. This remoulding of our everyday world is possible not merely by adding more and more professional 'services', but by altering how the settings themselves are organized to enhance and support our lives. This is called the social ecology approach to health and end of life care and its best examples are found in what are now commonly called 'compassionate cities'.

In this chapter, we will first briefly describe what we mean by the phrase 'social ecology'. We will then show how both healthy cities and compassionate cities are public health descendants of this practice approach. We will then describe and discuss two recent examples of these kinds of cities—one from England and the other from Spain.

What is social ecology?

The key literature on the social ecology approach is often described in terms of a social ecology systems framework. This literature reflects the basic tensions in the more fundamental economic literature that underpins it (Partelow, 2018). The underlying arguments of environmental economics rehearse the concerns of two opposing viewpoints. The first argument asserts that environments are largely subject to self-interest leading to overconsumption with an associated powerless to stop others from doing the same (also known as 'tragedy of the commons'—see Hardin, 1968). The second argument asserts that community cooperation can moderate, even triumph over self-interest by mobilizing community assets and public goods to solve social and political dilemmas including those of public health (also known as 'governing of the commons' see Ostrom, 1990). The social ecology systems framework approach has mainly examined the dynamic interdependency of the socioeconomic system (industrial, farming, or fishing practices) alongside the consequences and impact of the physical or geographical systems (e.g. climates, seas, land resource, air quality, etc.) (Herrero-Jauregui et al., 2018), exploring cooperation as a way the two systems can work alongside each other (or not) to the benefit (or not) of each.

The idea that cooperation as a social framework can solve problems related to self-interest and scarce resources has a number of ongoing challenges in both methodological (evaluation/outcomes) research and in actual field implementation. Nevertheless, this broad principle of the centrality of cooperation has been a cornerstone of all major public health practice approaches since the 1960s, especially for general health promotion and community development as well as for its efforts in social ecology. In public health, the emphasis on changing social, physical, and political environments to improve health outcomes is known more simply as the 'social ecological model of health' (Early, 2016).

The social ecology model of health has been described in a general fashion as the interactive characteristics between individuals and their institutional environments. This model emphasizes the *interdependence* of environment and individual behaviour—both are crucial influences on each other. Furthermore, a social ecology approach has opened up possibilities for deliberate manipulation or management of environmental factors that have been identified as shaping and changing behaviours. This type of 'systems' thinking about the influential—and malleable—nature of environments has led to many useful innovations from environmental waste management, business and marketing, building, transport, and recreational design, to urban planning and crowd control.

However, despite the definitional emphases on physical, social, and political changes to environments, most traditional public health research continues to place its change emphasis on individual and interpersonal characteristics within the health service ('health services research'). In health promotion work the major exceptions to this have been in health-promoting schools and in the World Health Organization (WHO) Healthy Cities programmes (Golden and Earp, 2012). Notwithstanding the popularity of interpersonal intervention work, the evidence for the power and effectiveness of ecological principles in promoting health has been consistently strong (see O'Mara-Eves et al., 2013).

The early work of Stokols (1996) has summarized the crucial role of environmental change in changing health outcomes. Stokols argued that physical and social environments can:

- Serve as a medium for disease transmission and control.
- Operate as a stressor affecting mood and performance.
- Function as a source of safety or danger.
- Enable health or exposure to risk.
- Serve as a resource for information, support, and care.

How each of these dimensions determine 'health-promoting' or health-eroding' outcomes is dependent on how each is shaped or constructed by the very people working and living in that environment, that ecosystem so to speak. If self-interest by sectional groups pursue solely non-health goals and are permitted to dominate, health outcomes may be affected negatively. For optimal health to be achieved in any single area, all sectional interests in a defined environment must share a common goal of promoting health and well-being in addition to their other (economic, political, or social) goals. Without this broad-based cooperation, people in areas like villages, towns, or cities may likely live and work in unsafe and unhealthy environments with only their health services to rescue them during crises and need. Prevention and harm reduction activities will have little to no presence in these kinds of communities.

On the other hand, when all sectors do take some responsibility for their own health and well-being, the 'public' health is optimized. For examples, when car manufacturers or the housing sector design for safety, when workplaces and restaurants have a health-promoting policy about drug and alcohol consumption, or when schools and local governments create policies or by-laws to deter violence, local environments—or in other words the 'social ecology'—becomes health-promoting. When these activities are coordinated efforts based on a common vision of health and well-being, these places are commonly called 'healthy cities'.

From healthy cities to compassionate cities

Healthy cities are mostly large-scale urban developments where whole towns and cities are asked to work together cooperatively, at a population level, to influence the social determinants of health. The aim is to promote health and well-being and to address the morbidities and mortality profile of the community in which we all live, work, and play. The formal programme of 'Healthy Cities' was developed in the 1980s by the WHO, commencing in Lisbon with an initial 21 cities. In 1987, Healthy Cities became a formal policy programme of WHO's European Regional Office (Kellehear, 2005).

Although most people live in towns and cities in the twenty-first century, the principles of asking all major social sectors of a community to participate in health promotion is not confined to merely towns and cities. In this context, the term 'city' here refers not merely to urban settlements but to all basic servicing centres for populations—including villages, parishes, or suburbs—where people regularly congregate to meet their employment, educational, cultural, religious, and legal and civic needs. The term 'city' here is closely bound up with the idea of citizenship, both drawing on allied French terms such as 'citoyen' and 'cite' which refer to assemblies of citizens who enjoy limited rights within the city. This idea of citizenship or cities of people unbounded by traditional limitations of tribe, caste, or ethnic origins became the modern idea behind the importance of social solidarity that transcended self-interest and tribal allegiances (Turner, 1993).

The WHO Healthy Cities movement had many democratic and public health strengths as a social ecological idea. It gave global prominence to the idea of the interdependency of health and sickness with physical, social, and political environments, breaking us away from the idea that a caring society was not merely one that provided health and social care services for its citizens but was one where the *whole immediate environment was designed for health and safety*. Health was everyone's responsibility. Workplaces and schools should have a role as well as local governments, cultural organizations, and design teams for housing, roads, transport, or town planning. Your doctor could advise you to stop smoking or moderate your alcohol intake but workplaces and restaurants could play an important role in prevention and harm reduction too.

Furthermore, legislation about pricing of alcohol or tobacco and the promotion of fun runs in cities could all play a role in moderating and influencing individual health conduct and outcomes. Health was a positive thing to be pursued by all sectors of a village, town, or city. However, this 'new' public health emphasis on healthy cities did not include experiences of living with life-limiting illness, advanced ageing, long-term caregiving, and grief and bereavement. Death, dying, caregiving, and loss were omitted in the academic and policy storylines about 'health'.

In this context then, compassionate cities (Kellehear, 2005) were created as a policy and practice corrective. Compassionate cities are designed to integrate these experiences of ageing, dying, loss, and caregiving. After all, these are universal experiences that had been excluded in the twentieth-century grand narratives of public health except insofar as they appeared to signal a failure of that public health approach. Twentieth-century public health viewed these more as events that took days or weeks to occur, and not lifestyles that were years in the making and consequence. Public health observations commonly overlooked the social epidemiology of ageing, dying, loss, and caregiving by viewing these experiences as one-dimensional. For example, grief was seen largely as an emotional reaction to loss, or dying was viewed as the final physical or medical descent towards death. This one-dimensional and short-term view of the end of life permitted the social epidemiology created and accompanying them in their wake to be well hidden and overlooked—the anxieties, depression, sexual acting out, loneliness and social isolation, stigma and rejection, lost work or school days, and even the suicides and sudden deaths. Compassionate cities aimed to recognize these social experiences and to promote health and well-being inside them by bringing greater information, support, and insight into our efforts to prevent or harm reduce the impacts of these consequences.

In the past 10 years or so, compassionate cities were organized largely by colleagues from the hospice and palliative care services. One of the first compassionate cities in the world was the one established in Kerala in India. But other compassionate cities have been created by groups of volunteer citizens or local government departments of public health. Most have in common an action plan more or less following the Compassionate City Charter (CCC). The CCC outlines initial actions to be done in partnerships with workplaces, schools, local government, cultural organizations, faith groups, and local neighbourhoods. There are also exhortations for a civic incentives scheme, cultural programmes, and festivals. It is a 13-point plan. A full copy of the latest edition of the CCC is available in Appendix A of this volume.

The CCC is both a guide and a map of the central sectors of any city anywhere in the world. It is designed to alert new public health activists to the first places to seek out other important civic actors that are the major influencers and shapers of quality of life in any city. Here are the first doorsteps to appear upon, the first targets for phone calls or emails, and the first major organizations to enlist to help create the compassionate city. Here too are the first areas of action needed to plan and initiate.

The CCC is not an exclusive or exhaustive list of key sectors but the initial and politically important allies that need to be enlisted. For example, not all cities or towns will have a prison or a significant homeless population. But attention to the marginalized and easily overlooked is highlighted by the prompt to develop policies for prison or homeless populations mentioned in the Charter. Not all places of worship are best described as churches or temples (mosques, for example) but that part of the CCC serves to remind its readers of the importance of being inclusive of religious/faith organizations. In these ways, the CCC has worked as a list of important civic locations *and* intellectual prompts to begin the work of creating a compassionate city as a social ecology of health and well-being.

Plymouth, UK: a compassionate city

Plymouth is a port city situated on the south coast of Devon, England. It is 230 miles away from London. Plymouth describes itself as 'Britain's Ocean City' as it is nestled between the historic 'Plymouth Sound', which is one of the world's largest natural harbours and the outstanding beauty of Dartmoor Natural Park. The city's industries are advanced engineering, marine technology, and defence-related nuclear expertise as well as emerging specialisms in the health and life sciences. It has a large naval bases, a ferry port, a large fishing industry, and marine research industries. Tourism is a major contributor to the city's economy. The city is home to three universities.

Plymouth's population size is 263,070. There are 7530 resident UK Armed Forces personnel. In the last census, 93% of the population described themselves as White British. Healthy life expectancy in Plymouth is significantly lower than the England average, for both males and females. The working age population (15–64 years) accounts for 65% of the population with 18% of the population being over 65 years.

Creating a compassionate city: a forward-thinking hospice

The idea of Plymouth becoming a compassionate city was instigated by St Luke's Hospice Plymouth. The hospice supports those who are dying in the city and those who live in the outer rural areas of East Cornwall and South and West Devon, serving a total catchment population of 450,000. It is a large hospice that has several clinical teams working in the community, the acute hospital, and the hospice's own 12-bed inpatient unit. The hospice like many others was aware of the rising elderly demographics. However, with constrained resources and increasing demand, the hospice has always sought to create ways of working in partnership with the local communities it serves.

The hospice views education as key enabler in engaging with the community and educating others is a key strategic objective. It has one of the largest education teams among the hospices in the South West, who deliver education to the health and social care sectors. The hospice has an outreach approach and is committed to partnership working. However, at that time the hospice did not have a community development vision.

Following attendance at the fourth International Public Health Palliative Care conference in Bristol, a presentation was delivered by the one of the chapter authors (GW) to the St Luke's Hospice Plymouth senior management team, and introduced the public health approach to palliative care and the CCC. The publication of 'Ambitions for Palliative Care and End of life Care' (2015) by the NHS also provided another strategic driver to deliver a public health approach. The senior management team agreed to support a community development strand to the hospice vision and appointed another public health nurse as a community development lead.

The first aim agreed was to raise awareness about the public health palliative care approach among the clinicians in the hospice as this concept was totally new to them. Hospices are regarded as the experts in end of life and palliative care and are naturally well placed to coordinate the development of a compassionate city. However, the time taken to change cultural attitudes within the hospice itself should not be underestimated—this took 12 months to achieve and is ongoing.

Creating a compassionate city: walking the walk

The second aim was to raise awareness of the needs of those who were affected by dying, loss, and bereavement across the city.

This was achieved by reaching out to the other voluntary groups. In this phase, one of the chapter authors (GW) joined Plymouth Octopus Project—a network of approximately 250 small charities in Plymouth and also became a trustee of this group. This appointment gave a valuable opportunity to engage with the wider voluntary sector within the city in addition to talking to existing stakeholders in the health and social care sectors. It was very apparent that while people did not understand this new approach, they wanted to know more.

So, in 2016 the hospice provided a free conference called 'The Big Conversation' which was open to all sectors. The conference introduced the CCC, provided an opportunity to talk about the needs of those affected by dying, loss, and bereavement, and, importantly, the gap in provision. The conference was oversubscribed and was very well evaluated. People commented on how effective it had been and how everyone needed to talk more about death, dying, and loss. Enthusiasm for another conference was evident.

Next, the hospice needed to 'walk the walk'—to lead by example. Following the success of the first conference in raising the city's awareness of the compassionate city, the hospice was keen to spend the next 18 months creating small pilot projects to progress the CCC objectives. This would create a showcase for some practical progress, demonstrating that it could be done. Nothing sells a concept more than hearing from those who have lived experience. The hospice was successful in gaining grants from Health Education England and the Burdett Nursing Trust to start a number of 'baby steps' projects. The following are a brief description of the three projects that 'seeded' our CCC and shared learning.

Homeless project

This project sought to deliver education and service improvements to the homeless community to enable those who were homeless and those who had substance and alcohol addictions, to have equitable access to end of life and palliative care. The education team, a clinical nurse specialist, and a social worker from the hospice delivered workshops to 55 end of life ambassadors, who ranged from soup-run volunteers and street pastors to drug and alcohol addiction nurses. All reported increasing confidence and skills in holding supportive end of life conversations and signposting to other services. This increased referrals to palliative care and a weekly outreach clinic, with a dedicated palliative care clinical nurse specialist, was set up.

Creating compassionate networks

This project sought to empower individuals at the end of life and their supportive networks, so their care was truly personalized, and patient centred. It sought to challenge the traditional paternalistic attitudes of the formal professional network, so that nurses understood the importance of co-production and raised their awareness of the needs of informal support networks. The project worked with six informal caring networks.

This small pilot demonstrated that ordinary people are willing and can help to support people to stay at home, with a little support and training from formal carers/nurses. As demands for services increase with the rising elderly demographics and a move to focus on home-based care, community services will need to ensure that identifying 'supportive care networks' becomes part of the nursing assessment. This will enable informal networks to be recognized as a vital part of the patient's care and support plan.

Box 12.1 LEND acronym

Listen—help people to actively listen and not to shy away or close people down when they wanted to talk.
Empathy—how to show an empathic approach.
Notice—how to notice when things are not right.
Do—do something, offer to help.

Creating compassionate friends

The concept for creating compassionate friends came from the experience of one of the chapter authors (GW) of being a 'dementia friend'. Dementia, similar to death, was a taboo subject. The St Luke's education team manager designed a 2-hour workshop and created the acronym LEND (Box 12.1).

At the end of the workshop, people could make a personal pledge (something they would do for family) or an active community pledge (something they would do in their community or workplace). The pilot was a great success as judged by the positive feedback. Those who took part stated it should be more widely rolled out.

Enabling end of life choice in prisons

This project saw the hospice's specialist nurses working with Dartmoor Prison nurses and staff, to raise awareness of end of life and how to refer into the hospice. This led to the hospice providing monthly clinics in the prison. This in turn increased skills in the prison staff in recognizing and planning for end of life care, with hospice referrals from the prison population increasing. Due to the success of these pilots, the hospice committed to having 1.2 WTE community development workers to work closely with the education team (across all CCC goals), to support the delivery of a compassionate city. Having experienced community development workers who are used to co-production with diverse communities has really helped drive and deliver the CCC.

Creating a compassionate city: a call to action

In May 2018, the hospice organized a conference called 'Plymouth: A Compassionate City … What Can You Do?' This conference was a call to action. It was important that this conference was a city-owned conference, so it was vital to enlist keynote speakers from city leaders. St Luke's leadership met with Plymouth City Council strategic director for people. While the Council had a very proactive approach to public health and addressing health and social inequalities, there was no real strategy for end of life. The director was very supportive and connected us with the director of public health, the lead for the school's quality mark, and the city lead for healthy employers. In addition, a city councillor who chaired the Health and Wellbeing Board, was extremely supportive and further promoted CCC within the city.

The chief executive officer of the hospice met with local members of parliament and system leaders, who were all very supportive and many offered to speak at the conference and encouraged their staff to attend. The leaders of the city could see the benefits of having a compassionate city and embraced the structure of the CCC. It was also important that this conference had meaningful outcomes and that it could be used as a vehicle to get firm commitment from those present to have an end of life network in the city, with all sectors of the city to work towards achieving the CCC objectives. The keynote speaker was Professor Allan Kellehear whose inspiring presentation challenged all those present to act and commit to the CCC. There were also presentations from those who had been part of the first CCC objectives projects. Attendees could really see the impact on people's lives this collective work was having and there was an infectious enthusiasm within the conference.

In the afternoon, attendees signed up to the CCC objectives they were interested in progressing via CCC breakout groups. They discussed actions they could take and signed up to the various CCC objectives task groups. In the final plenary session those present voted on and agreed the following compassionate city vision for Plymouth:

> Plymouth will not shy away from the taboo subject of death, but talks openly about it, in order to create a city that is truly informed and compassionate towards those facing end of life, or experiencing loss and bereavement.

The conference was a great success. It was a highly effective and coordinated team effort between the hospice's education and community development team and the hospice communication and IT team. Support from system leads was pivotal to making it all happen. Delegates were really inspired by those who had worked on the 'baby steps' CCC pilot projects, who clearly demonstrated what can be achieved by people working together. The CCC had provided a clear framework for action, clear objectives, and gives real purpose and direction to a city 'asking what can they do' to make a difference to all those who are affected dying, loss, and bereavement.

Compassionate Plymouth: where are we now?

Following the 2018 'What Can You Do?' conference, all those who stated they wanted to be involved were contacted and subgroups were created. The hospice community development team and the education department coordinate these subgroups and provide administration, marketing, and facilitation. In time, as the groups become more independent, it is envisaged that the coordination role can be shared. In addition to the 13 CCC objectives, Plymouth has created an objective 14th. This commits to developing compassionate networks across the city, where compassionate friends will do the small things for those in need that make such a big difference (Box 12.2).

It was in November 2019 that the city officially launched Plymouth as a compassionate city and showcased all the subgroups' activities.

Box 12.2 There are eight active compassionate city subgroups working towards the following objectives

- Compassionate schools.
- Compassionate workplaces and trade unions.
- Places of worship.
- Hospices and nursing homes.
- Museums and the arts.
- Compassionate city and social media.
- Creating equality at the end of life for the prison population.
- Compassionate friends.

(For more information about the progress, impact, and activities of Plymouth Compassionate City view the website http://www.plymouthcompassionatecity.co.uk or join the Facebook page 'Plymouth Compassionate City'.)

It was a huge success and many people signed up to work on subgroups and to become compassionate friends. To date, Plymouth has over 697 compassionate friends who have made over 581 action pledges, 13 networks, and ten compassionate cafes.

The seven success factors

1. *The hospice.* Having a hospice management team that believed in the concept and were committed to the vison of community development, and put the resources into developing a compassionate city was pivotal. Hospices are also trusted by the populations they serve and are apolitical and so are ideally placed to coordinate a compassionate city.
2. *A team effort.* Having a dedicated and experienced team to develop and coordinate the compassionate city is key. Gaining funding to 'seed' and trail' the baby steps has also been essential to demonstrate what can be achieved, with small amounts of money, lots of dedication, and big hearts.
3. *The conference.* Gaining support for the CCC was relatively easy, the 'What Can You Do?' conference was the launch pad that moved people to action. Getting people to commit on the day and capturing their interests and details made contacting them after the conference possible. Having an inspirational keynote speaker was another key success factor.
4. *Stakeholder management.* Spending time mapping stakeholders and then meeting them face to face was another key success factor. Ensuring you use your networks to tap into other people's networks is also essential. Don't be shy about asking, just do it. People want to help. Directors of public health are great allies as are local councillors.
5. *Effective branding and communications.* Plymouth Compassionate City has a neutral 'starfish' logo which is not owned by any organization. Every leaflet, every website, every video, and every communication have the starfish logo. Having a symbol that the city can identify the compassionate city with is powerful. Having an effective marketing team and social media presence is key.
6. *Measuring impact.* In order to demonstrate impact and progress you will need to develop both quantitative and qualitative tools to measure impact. Keeping a database of activities, for example, how many compassionate friends have been trained, what pledges have they made, and so on, will help you measure impact. Plymouth Compassionate City uses the starfish tool, a simple Likert scale based around what people say is important to them. It takes about 6 weeks to measure the impact; however, collecting people's stories and showcasing their narrative is powerful and reflective.
7. *Don't duplicate—enhance.* Find out what other organizations are doing. How can you work in partnership to achieve compassionate city aims and what can you do to enhance their offer?

Some unexpected challenges

Professional anxiety

Few of the compassionate friends team were prepared for the level of anxiety that professionals experienced in signposting people or referring people to the compassionate network coordinators for help. Issues of safeguarding, and concerns that people might use the CCC to access 'vulnerable' people, were often used as reasons not to engage. To ameliorate some of these concerns, a safeguarding tool was devised to advise professionals. However, community action is 'community action' citizens do not belong to organizations. If a neighbour wishes to help another neighbour, that is a compassionate act. There are many myths about what citizens can and cannot do for others. If health professionals are to work in partnership with compassionate networks, they need to let go and take considered risks, only then will they learn and understand the power of compassionate citizenship.

People power

Initially it was thought that the city needed a steering board for the compassionate city actions and subgroups. City leaders were invited to be members of the steering group. However, it soon became apparent that what was much more effective, was letting the subgroups decide for themselves, how they would deliver the compassionate city objectives. As with most community development initiatives, the people decide what they want and steer themselves, with limited facilitation.

The Plymouth Compassionate City is thriving. The subgroups remain enthusiastically committed to delivering their compassionate city objectives. The vison is that the subgroups will be self-sustaining in the future. At the 'What can You Do?' conference, a delegate asked Allan Kellehear 'Does this need lots of money?' and he replied, 'No! Just leadership and a willingness to work together for the good of others'. Human beings have great capacity to demonstrate empathy and compassion. When a city uses the CCC as its map, it can create a shared purpose and vision. Ordinary people will do amazing things, and all those affected by dying, loss, and bereavement will no longer feel so alone, but will be wrapped in the warm cloak of compassion.

'Seville with You': a compassionate city in Spain

Seville is the capital of Andalusia, the region located in the south of Spain. With a population of 703,021 inhabitants and a metropolitan area of 1.5 million people, it is the fourth most populous city in Spain. The administration of the city is conducted by the city council and it is divided into 11 very different districts. Every district is organized through a municipal district board with its corresponding delegate, administrative offices, and representatives of the neighbourhood associations in each area.

Inspired by the international movement of 'compassionate communities' and under the conceptual umbrella of the CCC (Kellehear 2016), 'Seville with You, Compassionate City', has been a demonstration project promoted by the New Health Foundation. The New Health Foundation is a not-for-profit organization that seeks to promote and foster a new health model to improve the quality of life of people with advanced chronic disease, high dependency, and those in the last stages of life. Its mission is to help build a committed society that provides care and support to people at the end of their lives. This model is based on the integration of health, social, and community services in palliative care.

The aims of the project were to:

- Identify people with advanced disease and create social awareness of their multiple needs.
- Inspire and promote social involvement towards a more compassionate and caring society.
- Develop a method that could be replicated to other organizations and communities, municipalities, cities, or countries to promote compassionate cities.
- Help to create a social movement with a growing network of associations and organizations aligned by the call of caring.
- Activate, train, and support caregivers and community networks that help people who face the end of their lives.
- Improve the effectiveness and efficiency of healthcare and social care services, using well-coordinated palliative care team networks, that through supporting communities, provide direct care to advanced and terminal patients.
- Evaluate and research the outputs, outcomes, and impact that the project generates.

The New Health Foundation's 'All with You®' method of creating a compassionate city

In 2015, the Foundation designed its own methodology (All with You® method) (Librada et al., 2018a) after an extensive review of the literature (Librada et al., 2020). The aim was to help develop compassionate communities and cities through social innovation. The overall method was implemented gradually by eight phases.

The vision (or the metaphor) underlying the method, viewed the different civic institutions as part of a potential shared and beautiful 'symphony'. The guiding 'sheet music' proposed different roles for every kind of organization, and promoting cooperation between each of them so as to achieve a final, inspired, skilled, and empowered community, partnered with a supportive and integrated health and social care service. As the process developed, a consecutive series of social awareness activities, training sessions, implementation, and evaluation stages were carried out in order to facilitate the emergence of new networks of care.

With this vision in mind, the methods were as follows:

1. *Networking with the city council and the first promoting organizations.* After getting initial commitments through several memorandum of agreements with every public and private organizations, a Constitutional Act for Seville to become a compassionate city was signed by the mayor of the city, in the presence of the social care services' delegates. The main city's media attended the meeting as well, in order to publicize the event and its aims to the general public.
2. *Identify an independent team who could lead*, inspire, facilitate, monitor, and evaluate the project's advances. The New Health Foundation, who had initially designed and led the initiative, was designated for this task.
3. *Establish a board* with the initial public and private promoters, to specify and develop a list of basic activities to be carried out. After several board meetings, those activities evolved into annual action plans. Since the beginning, tem strategic board meetings have been held to ensure the project's progress in the city.
4. *Promote agreements with a growing group of collaborating organizations*: private companies, foundations, official professional associations, scientific societies, brotherhoods, churches, and culture centres. Forty-eight organizations have so far committed to the project in order to promote social awareness and carry out

training actions. These organizations also developed their own strategies to become compassionate organizations towards their own professionals and their families.

5. *Identify beneficiary organizations*: residential care centres, patient associations, hospitals, primary health care centres, and specialized palliative care services, whose patients could require the help of members from the community at some point in the future. Sixteen beneficiary organizations belong to the Seville network.
6. *Promote the engagement of universities and schools*. There are three main universities in the city: University of Seville, Pablo de Olavide University, and Loyola University. All of them, especially from their health sciences colleges, participate in the project through conferences and training cycles on compassionate communities. Eleven primary schools and nine secondary schools in the main intervention areas of the city have joined the initiative of creating the network: '*compassionate schools*'.
7. *Connect with organizations of volunteers*. The six organizations that have volunteers in the city participating in the Seville with You network have followed some special courses to train some volunteers, especially in end of life care, to provide special care and support.
8. *Link and involve professionals who are experts in advanced and end of life care* to participate in raising awareness and teaching in training initiatives and courses. Twenty-nine professionals from the health and social care sectors participate in the network and support the network community management when required.
9. *Prepare and update a map* of current and potential centres and organizations who have or might join the growing network.

Raising social awareness: public media, social networks, public parades, and other interventions

A graphic design, logo, and motto were designed to represent this project: 'Seville with You, Compassionate City'. A website was also created where more than 300 public events developed by the city have been shown. It also contains promotional material and educational resources for citizens, such as visual educational guides, manuals, and flyers with tips for caring, links, and related videos. More than 30 awareness activities per year for a total of 147 awareness-raising actions have been carried out, reaching more than 25,000 people.

Squares, parks, public spaces, and cultural centres have been the best stages for exhibitions, photography contests, and collective mural drawing about how to improve the care for others. Books about care and compassion have been launched and concerts and sports events have taken place. Every year, the World Palliative Care Day has been celebrated in the city. The project has also been promoted through scientific congresses and death coffee sessions around the city.

The project's diffusion in the media has been impactful: 'Seville with You' has had 180 news items in the press, ten on the radio, and four on TV per year. Social networks and YouTube channels got more than 30,000 views a year, spreading the message beyond the city of Seville. Several recognitions and awards for the development of this initiative have been received: Andalusia's Excellence and Solidarity Award (2016), Garra de León Award (2017), and the Janssen Affective Award (2020). The project 'Seville with You, Compassionate City' has been also presented in 27 national and international congresses as a reference model.

Skilling the people, empowering the community: training sessions and courses

Besides sensitizing citizens about the importance of caring, 'Seville with You' focused on creating tools for training those citizens who could need the knowledge to take care of their loved ones in caring skills. A long list of activities was carried out:

- Two-hour workshops for families and caregivers of people with advanced or end of life stage of disease: 50 workshops have been developed for a total of 550 families and caregivers who have received sessions in listening skills, art therapy, music therapy, understanding grief, and networking and looking for help.
- An 'advanced programme in the development of compassionate communities': 550 hours (online) for both professionals and volunteers. There have been 13 editions of this programme, and it has trained more than 200 professionals who currently work in the network.
- A 30-hour course on 'care, compassion, and community' by the city council, directed to train volunteers and health promoters.
- A beautiful programme for schools: 'Caregiver Children, for a future world full of compassion'. In this course, children, parents, and teachers in primary and middle schools received training from professionals to learn techniques in care, with a special emphasis on emotional care and compassion. This promoted intergenerational exchanges as well, through visits to assisted living facilities. Twenty training programmes with 8-hour teaching sessions have been carried out. In fact, some schools in the city have incorporated these sessions into the teaching programmes of the centre, becoming 'compassionate schools'.
- Awareness and training programmes in the three main universities of the city (faculties of health sciences, medicine, nursing, social work, and psychology) within the framework of the development of 'compassionate universities'. Topics on care, compassion, and community development were incorporated.
- Webinars for emotional care and the practice of compassion: eight 1-hour sessions for families and caregivers that have reached more than 900 people.
- One course per year on 'learning to cultivate compassion' directed to health, social care, and community professionals. A special 8-week programme called 'CTT' (compassion cultivation training), with the collaboration of Stanford University, was designed to develop the qualities of compassion, empathy, and love. Three CCT programmes have been carried out, skilling 75 professionals to become trainers in compassion cultivation. As a global summary, an average of 40 training actions are carried out per year, more than 124 training actions from the beginning, having reached more than 5100 people trained.

Spreading the methodology beyond Seville

The National Health Foundation met with various leaders who wanted to be involved in the development of compassionate communities movements to discuss the elements of the method, establish alliances, and extend the initiative within other organizations. Alliances were established with Public Health and Palliative Care

International (PHPCI), the Institute of Palliative Medicine in Kerala (India), the Milford Care Centre in Limerick (Ireland), the Pallium Latin America Institute in Buenos Aires (Argentina), the Pallium Canada and the Societies of Palliative Care of Spain (SECPAL), and the Colombian Society of Palliative Care (ASOCUPAC). As a result, the 'All with You®' method has been tailored to many other cities in Spain and Latin America. Agreements have been signed, and some other leading organizations (promoting institutions) have been designated to spread the model in different cities and countries (Librada et al., 2018b).

A further demonstration project has also taken place in Colombia, where organizations from various communities in the country launched the Declaration of Medellín. This public manifesto called all Colombians to action to by joining a network of cities under the meaningful purpose to become a compassionate country. Helping this shared initiative, several local heroes have developed wonderful project such as 'Bogotá with You', 'Ibagué with You', 'Manizales with You', and 'Santa Marta with You' from the Keralty Foundation and 'Fusagasugá with You' from the Pallium Foundation. The initiative is spearheading efforts to grow and sustain a national network of volunteers eager to provide care and support those at the end of their lives.

Implementing 'Seville with You, Compassionate City' as a felt community reality

To enlighten and activate the community assets to provide care 'from the community to the community' is a goal that would require time to become a tangible reality. The organizations responsible for the project realized that neighbourhoods needed to feel that the networks of care were becoming a reality, and were able to provide direct help when their families required it. To demonstrate that the project was bringing real generation of networks of care was at the same time a demanded necessity from citizens and a challenge for the leaders of the programme.

In order to assess the outcomes of the initiative, two areas of the city, San Pablo-Santa Justa District (60,734 inhabitants) and Macarena District (74,576 inhabitants), were selected by the Seville City Council. A series of actions were established derived from the 'All with You®' methodology:

1. *Activation of the key agents' network*. Organizations that were working bottom-up, should mobilize the community.
2. *Constitution of community connecting commissions*. Dynamic teams were created with some professionals working within the districts, from the Health Promotion and Social Services department of the Seville City Council, primary healthcare teams from the regional health service, and some third sector entities.
3. *The role of community promoters was created*. This group developed the care coordination for patients in need by helping and activating the relatives' networks around every patient. When more promoters were needed, they resorted to community networks, local organizations, and volunteers.
4. *Development of community health connectors*, made up of neighbourhood groups, volunteer organizations, and other groups. This team contributed by identifying community needs, and by supporting and accompanying families.
5. *Systematic sessions in the designated districts for continued awareness and training actions in the 'triple C' (care, compassion and community)*. At the same time that professionals and neighbours were providing care, the training had to continue in order to expand the number of people with the skills and attitude necessary to care for others.
6. *Constitution of community, social care, and healthcare committees*, in which professionals from every sector, palliative care experts, health connectors, and community promoters could meet to identify new cases, keep track of those in need, and, collectively, look for solutions.
7. *Monitoring and evaluation of the project*. This is a continuous and central process of the project that works with a set of indicators of structure, process, and results that have been defined and agreed upon (Librada et al., 2018a) for awareness, training actions, and to measure the outcomes of direct interventions. The evaluation of the project aims to analyse how the development of compassionate communities impacts health and how compassion, care, and community can improve the care at the end of life (Brito and Librada2018). The evaluation is designed to assess four dimensions of experience: (a) the improvement of patients' experience, (b) the improvement of the health in the population, (c) the improvement of the professional experience, and (d) the cost-effectiveness of the organizations.

The evaluation of the improvement in patients and their families is analysed through the improvement of quality of life, reduction of loneliness, decrease of anxiety and depression, decrease of caregiver burden, and increase of care networks. Data collection is procedural and centralized in the foundation's technical office, thus facilitating exhaustive monitoring of progress and achieved results. In the first years, around 120 patients and 400 families/year were identified and supported. Some highlights of the evaluations include that:

- 93.6% of the program's beneficiaries have seen their needs fully covered.
- 64.7% improved their loneliness.
- 100% of the beneficiaries felt more accompanied.
- Anxiety and depression improved clearly by more than 13 percentage points.
- 84.5% of the people could be taken care of at home.
- The involvement of care networks increased by 36%.
- The network of caregivers per person, doubled from three to six people on average.
- 57.9% of the caregivers decreased their physical and emotional overload.
- 97.3% of the programme beneficiaries felt satisfied with the performance of the community promoters.

Barriers and challenges

Social movements need time to develop and their outcomes to be publicly observable and measurable. To influence the social context in order to activate compassion in human communities is a lifelong, multigenerational process. To inspire compassionate communities as a worthwhile social act for any person who enjoys helping others is relatively easy. However, to do the same for a cross-section of public institutions, generating collective improvement within a rather narcissist society is a seriously complex and daunting task.

Modern organizations are more predisposed to compete than to collaborate. It takes a while to understand everyone's aims and to orchestrate them as a whole. In our case, the New Health Foundation had to take the role of neutral central coordinator and to use the tool of strategic alliances and a number of memorandums of agreement to clarify and guarantee everyone's priorities. Such a role raises two important challenges: first, it is not easy to find an independent, not-for-profit organization to devote to a mission like this. Second, to create a method and stick to it can conflict with the bottom-up vision of community development movements that might view ecological transformations as merely top-down initiatives, reflecting power and self-interest. While both kinds of processes are crucial to social change, community activists and cooperation can be suspicious of and resistant to institutionally inspired change.

Additionally, from the point of view of social care and healthcare services, it can be difficult to identify people with advanced diseases and/or at the end of life in a timely manner. Thus, any interventions may be constrained by the time the patient enters the programme. Finally, although it is true that recruiting caring people and charitable organizations willing to help others can require minimal funding, the facts are that training citizens, engaging professionals, creating publicity, and hiring people like community promoters does require basic levels of funding. In our case, the project has been financed to a large extent by New Health Foundation, with some financial support in different phases and periods of the project from the Seville City Council and the participation of different companies in the city. In the end, arguments about funding priorities are always linked to care priorities and the 'Seville with You' project has created a strong, valuable. and ongoing public debate about the balance of professional services-based care with that of civic approaches to the end of life.

Conclusion

The idea of the compassionate city has been built on the foundational public health idea of the social ecology of health. However, the compassionate city is a corrective to an earlier death-denying idea of the healthy city, one that excluded dying, bereavement, and caregiving in its vision of health and well-being. Moving beyond the historical limitations of that culture-bound idea of health, the compassionate city represents a renewed commitment to the broader and deeper truth that health and healthcare are more than merely the provision of professional services—health and well-being are experiences inextricably bound to the social and physical environments in which we live, work, play, and pray.

Compassionate cities aim to create and optimize changes to the civic environment that promote health and well-being, not only as we live, and but also as we age, die, grieve, and care for one another in those environments. The idea and actions of the compassionate city remind each of us who reside in those spaces that support and education for ageing, dying, death, grieving, and long-term caregiving must be firmly rooted in all aspects of our civic life if that care is not to remain, or be reduced to, episodic professional care. Indeed, the success of any future vision of quality and continuity of care at the end of life will crucially depend on that very civic foundation.

REFERENCES

Brito, G. and Librada, S. 2018. Compassion in palliative care: a review. *Current Opinion in Supportive and Palliative Care,* **12**, 472–479.

Early, J. 2016. Health is more than healthcare: it's time for a social ecological approach. *Journal of Nursing and Health Studies,* **1**, 1–2.

Golden, S. D. and Earp, J. A. L. 2012. Social ecological approaches to individuals and their contexts: twenty years of Health Education and Behavior health promotion interventions. *Health Education and Behavior,* **39**, 364–372.

Hardin, G. 1968. The tragedy of the commons. *Science,* **162**, 1243–1248.

Herrero-Jauregui, C., Arnaiz-Schmitz, C., Fernanda-Reyes, M., Telesnicki, M., Agramonte, I., Easdale, MH., et al. 2018. What do we talk about when we talk about social ecological systems? A literature review. *Sustainability,* **10**, 2950.

Kellehear, A. 2005. *Compassionate Cities: Public Health and End of Life Care*. London: Routledge.

Kellehear, A. 2016. The Compassionate City Charter: inviting the cultural and social sectors into end-of-life care. In: Wegleitner, K., Heimerl, K., and Kellehear, A. (eds.) *Compassionate Communities: Case Studies from Britain and Europe*, pp. 76–87. Abingdon: Routledge.

Librada, S. and Donado, I. 2020. *Cómo abordar las comunidades compasivas en nuestra sociedad. En Monografía SECPAL. Comunidades Compasivas al final de la vida.* Madrid: SECPAL.

Librada, S., Herrera, E., Boceta, J., Mota, R., and Nabal-, M. 2018a. All with You: a new method for developing compassionate communities and cities at the end of life. Experiences in Spain and Latin-America. *Annals of Palliative Medicine,* **7**, S15–S31.

Librada, S., Herrera, E., Díaz F., Redondo, M. J., Castillo, C., McLoughlin, K., et al. 2018b. REDCUIDA development and management of networks of care at the end of life (the REDCUIDA Intervention): protocol for a nonrandomized controlled trial. *JMIR Research Protocols,* **7**, e10515.

Librada, S., Nabal, M., Forero, D., Muñoz, I., and Guerra-Martín, M. D. 2020. Implementation models of compassionate communities and compassionate cities at the end of life: a systematic review. *International Journal of Environmental Research and Public Health,* **17**, 6271.

O'Mara-Eves, A., Brunton, G., McDaid, D., Oliver, S., Kavanagh, J., Jamal, F., et al. 2013. Community engagement to reduce inequalities in health: a systematic review, meta-analysis and economic analysis. *Public Health Research,* **1**, 4.

Ostrom, E. 1990. *Governing the Commons: The Evolution of Institutions for Collective Action.* Cambridge: Cambridge University Press.

Partelow, S. 2018. A review of the social-ecological systems framework: applications, methods, modifications, and challenges. *Ecology & Society,* **23**, 36.

Stokols, D. 1996. Translating social ecological theory into guide- lines for community health promotion. *American Journal of Health Promotion,* **10**, 282–298.

Turner, B. S. (ed.) 1993. *Citizenship and Social Theory.* London: Sage.

13

Developing end of life literacy through public education

Rebecca M. Patterson and Mark A. Hazelwood

Defining end of life literacy

This chapter explores the concept of end of life literacy within public health approaches to palliative care, focusing particularly on the role public education can play in supporting the development of end of life literacy among the general public. The chapter is written from a materially wealthy and culturally 'Western' social perspective and the authors acknowledge this limitation. Most but not all of the practice examples and references share this perspective.

Health literacy

Within this chapter we use the term 'end of life' literacy as a broad term to encompass the emerging concepts of 'death literacy' and 'grief literacy' and other related ideas. However, understanding these concepts should be grounded in an awareness of the broader and more widely used idea of 'health literacy'. Health literacy is about the extent to which a person can access, comprehend, and effectively use health information and services. It is influenced by factors such as an individual's skills, knowledge, and motivation, as well as the wider healthcare policies, structures, resources, and processes of the society in which they are operating (Di Fiore, 2020).

Nutbeam (2000) points out that the concept of health literacy can be discussed in terms of three different levels of literacy, defined in terms of what it is that literacy enables someone to do:

- *Basic/functional literacy*—sufficient basic skills in reading and writing to be able to function effectively in everyday situations.
- *Communicative/interactive literacy*—more advanced cognitive and literacy skills which, together with social skills, can be used to actively participate in everyday activities, to extract information and derive meaning from different forms of communication, and to apply new information to changing circumstances.
- *Critical literacy*—more advanced cognitive skills which, together with social skills, can be applied to critically analyse information, and to use this information to exert greater control over life events and situations. (pp. 263–264)

The ideas of 'interactive' and 'critical' literacy are fundamental to the World Health Organization (WHO) definition of health literacy:

> Health literacy implies the achievement of a level of knowledge, personal skills and confidence to take action to improve personal and community health by changing personal lifestyles and living conditions. Thus, health literacy means more than being able to read pamphlets and make appointments. By improving people's access to health information, and their capacity to use it effectively, health literacy is critical to empowerment. (WHO, 1998, p. 10)

According to the WHO, improving health literacy within a population is about enabling citizens not just to play an active role in improving their own health, but also to engage in community action to encourage governments to meet their responsibilities in addressing health and health equity. They emphasize the role of governments in leading the development and implementation of health literacy promoting policies and empowering vulnerable populations.

Death literacy

Attempts to define a specific concept of 'death literacy' emerged from Australian research into social and caring networks, which found that caring for someone towards the end of their life is a catalyst for learning about how to provide care, and how to navigate the health system and the 'death system'. The outcome of this learning process was labelled 'death literacy' (Leonard et al., 2020):

> Death literacy is … the knowledge and skills that people need to make it possible to gain access to, understand, and make informed choices about end of life and death care options. People and communities with high levels of death literacy have context specific knowledge about the death system and the ability to put that knowledge into practice. (p. iv)

The death literacy model has been influenced by the notion of critical health literacy, in particular the idea that health literacy is a repackaging of the relationship between health education and empowerment. Central to this model of death literacy are genuine community development and engagement practices, and this model highlights experiential learning as a key component. It is also suggested that providing informal care at home at the end of life can provide deeper understanding and contribute to changes in attitudes and social actions around death and dying (Noonan et al., 2016).

Efforts have been made to create a tool, the Death Literacy Index (DLI), to measure death literacy within populations. The DLI questionnaire gathers information about four key areas: practical knowledge, experiential knowledge, factual knowledge, and community knowledge.

The hope of researchers is that the DLI can be used to inform targeting of future interventions to address gaps in death literacy, measure the impact of interventions, and to make comparisons across different communities (Leonard et al., 2020).

Grief literacy

Breen and colleagues (2020) suggest a model of 'grief literacy' to augment the concept of death literacy. They provide a helpful series of vignettes to illustrate what grief literacy could look like in practical terms, and propose the following definition of grief literacy:

> - The capacity to access, process, and use knowledge regarding the experience of loss.
> - This capacity is multidimensional: it comprises knowledge to facilitate understanding and reflection, skills to enable action, and values to inspire compassion and care.
> - These dimensions connect and integrate via the interdependence of individuals within socio-cultural contexts.
>
> Our definition of grief literacy integrates the three components of knowledge, skills, and values. Their connection and integration means that grief literacy is greater than the sum of its parts. In addition, we envision that grief literacy is embedded in an inclusive, nurturing community that involves the interdependence of individuals within sociocultural contexts. Thus, grief literacy extends beyond the individual person; instead, it is a broader concept that reflects the capacity and values of a community and society. (Breen et al., p. 3)

End of life literacy

The concepts of 'grief literacy' and 'death literacy' have emerged relatively recently, and it will take time for their specific definitions to become embedded in common usage. Within this chapter we use the term 'end of life literacy' to provide freedom from existing definitions to explore the related concepts of death literacy and grief literacy as defined previously, alongside relevant aspects that are not explicitly explored within these models.

For the purposes of this chapter, we use the term 'end of life literacy' as an umbrella term to refer broadly to the collection of knowledge, skills, experiences, attitudes, opportunities, and behaviours that enable an individual to plan for, deal with, and support others through the difficult times that can come with dying, death, loss, and care.

As explored earlier, various elements are of significance when considering an individual's ability to cope with and offer support through deteriorating health, dying, or bereavement, including:

- *Knowledge* about the issues that can arise towards the end of life and in bereavement, about different people and services that can help, and about where to find out more information.
- *Information* that can be accessed when needed.
- *Practical skills* to provide help and support to friends, family, and community members when they need it.
- *Experience* of caring for others that takes knowledge and skills beyond the theoretical.
- *Values* that inspire compassion and care.
- *Empowerment* so that people have the confidence and opportunities to seek knowledge, skills, and experience, act on their values, to question current norms, and seek better conditions for their community.
- *Communities* that expect and enable their members to care and offer practical help.
- *Action* putting knowledge, skills, and experience to use to help others at the end of life and through bereavement, being part of a community and empowering others to be end of life literate.

Why is end of life literacy important?

Family, friends, and communities have an important role to play in providing informal support when someone is faced with deteriorating health, caring responsibilities, death, or bereavement (Abel et al., 2011; Aoun et al., 2015). However, unless individuals and communities have a certain level of end of life literacy, they will lack the confidence, skills and/or opportunities to offer this support.

> It is ... now hard to reach adulthood unaware that people die or without having posted an online condolence. What is lacking, however, is first-hand knowledge of what happens physically to a dying or dead body, the spiritual pain of dying, caring for a dying family member, how to arrange a funeral, or the searing pain of grief. We can only be thankful that most twenty-first century children are spared such experiences, but it does leave today's citizens with a legacy of ignorance about death, sometimes lasting until late middle age when eventually one's own parents die. (Walter, 2017, p. 11)

Various problems are caused because people are unprepared for the experiences of death, dying, and bereavement (The GroundSwell Project, 2020a; Dying Matters, 2020), communities are disempowered from providing support to people who are dying or bereaved (Abel et al., 2011) and health and social care professionals, individuals, and families are unprepared for death-related discussions (All Ireland Institute for Hospice and Palliative Care, 2019a). For example:

- People who are dying or bereaved can experience isolation because people don't know what to say or how to act towards them.
- People may die without wills, leaving complicated situations for their families and friends.
- Healthcare professionals often struggle to have conversations with their patients about what care or treatments they want as they approach death. This makes it hard to plan the care that a person really wants.
- If the fact that someone is dying is not acknowledged then opportunities to resolve issues and say goodbye may be missed.
- People may be afraid of some aspects of care, dying, or loss because they are unaware of what is likely to happen and/or ways in which difficult experiences can be commonly avoided or ameliorated.

A lack of end of life literacy can contribute to attitudes, systems, and processes that have an impact at individual, organizational, and policy levels, for instance:

- Health and social care policies and strategies often fail to mention death, dying, and bereavement.
- Organizations providing services for older people or for those with life-limiting long-term conditions often fail to acknowledge

explicitly that they support people for whom uncertainty and the possibility of death are strong influences in their lives.
- Individuals and/or their families are often reluctant to discuss or formulate preferences and to plan for end of life care. This may be for various reasons: because the potential benefit is not understood; because of a lack of information about choices and options; because it is not perceived as something people 'normally' do; or because suitable opportunity is not provided. (Though for some people disavowal of dying may be part of their coping strategy which must be respected.)

Increasing end of life literacy within populations is important because:

- Low levels of knowledge limit capacity for self-management and provision of informal support.
- Where families know little, it is harder for health and social care professionals to discuss relevant matters with individuals and families.
- An awareness of the natural dying process can enable a focus on care not cure when end of life is imminent and inevitable and empower family and friends to advocate for the needs of someone who is dying.
- Understanding what is happening when someone is very unwell and might be dying enables families to manage their situation as well as possible.
- People who are end of life literate will be better able to access information and support (Patterson et al., 2018).

Increasing end of life literacy

Having established that end of life literacy has an important influence over people's experiences of death, dying, and bereavement, we now consider the question—how can end of life literacy be increased within communities, organizations, and populations?

Learning from health literacy

The WHO outlines the following various stakeholder roles in advancing health literacy that are worth considering with reference to advancing end of life literacy (WHO, 2020):

- Governments develop policies and plans on health literacy promotion.
- Civil societies work together to bring different expertise, experiences, and capacities for community-based communication and health literacy efforts in all kinds of settings throughout the life course.
- Media (including social media) serve as a critical platform for health literacy messaging.
- Community leaders provide risk communication, particularly during times of crisis.
- Research and academic institutions develop and improve methods to measure health literacy, collate and distribute examples of best practice in health literacy intervention development, and provide evidence of what works, in which contexts, and why.

Public health approaches to palliative care

If the aim of a public health approach to end of life care is to improve health and well-being at the end of life (Karapliagkou and Kellehear, n.d.), then increasing end of life literacy is implicit in that aim. Indeed, though 'end of life literacy' is perhaps not yet a widely used term, many projects and initiatives in the field of public health palliative care aim to support or increase end of life literacy in some way:

- *Building healthy public policy*: various organizations work to influence national and/or local public policy to make provisions for death/dying/bereavement and acknowledge and support the role of communities in death, dying, loss, and care (Scottish Partnership for Palliative Care, 2015; Patterson et al., 2018; All Ireland Institute for Hospice and Palliative Care, 2019b).
- *Creating supportive environments*: compassionate cities work aims to create environments that will support initiatives to nurture neighbourliness, reduce social isolation and increase social networks, and there are a growing number of specific initiatives to encourage supportive workplaces and schools (All Ireland Institute for Hospice and Palliative Care, 2019b; Hospice UK, 2019; Public Health Palliative Care International, 2019; Scottish Partnership for Palliative Care, 2019; The GroundSwell Project, 2020b).
- *Strengthening community action*: community development approaches are key to the compassionate communities movement, with the aim of empowering communities to undertake the change that they want to see (The GroundSwell Project, 2020c; Compassionate Inverclyde, 2020; Pallium Canada, 2020; Strathcarron Hospice, 2020; The Truacanta Project, 2020).
- *Developing personal skills and knowledge*: public education, including courses, information, and public awareness campaigns have been used to try to increase individual skills and knowledge about various aspects of death, dying, and bereavement. Compassionate community initiatives can build skills and knowledge through experience and participation in care networks.
- *Reorientating healthcare services*: formal healthcare services whose traditional role has been the provision of specialist palliative care continue to reorientate efforts towards health-promoting palliative care initiatives such as public education and engaging with the public around death, dying, and bereavement.

Clearly, each of these domains doesn't exist in isolation, and different factors influence and reinforce each other. For example, community action can lead to an increase in individual skills and knowledge, which can in turn lead to further community action. Those who have knowledge and skills can work towards creating supportive environments where others can increase their knowledge, and so on.

Development of the DLI included asking people questions about where they obtained their knowledge about death and dying, and results indicated that personal experience and family connections were most important, then cultural sources such as books and films, and finally formal organizations such as churches, schools, and workplaces.

Leonard and colleagues (2020) suggest various interventions that could be explored as ways to improve various aspects of death literacy, including community education programmes; experiential enquiry; expert consultation; formal programmes about navigating the health and death systems; mentors; providing opportunities for people to learn about providing practical hands-on support; increasing cultural experiences around end of life; and death literacy education in schools. They suggest that the DLI will be helpful in measuring the impact of these interventions.

Public education

As mentioned previously, public education is one example of a public health approach to palliative care that has been used to develop individual skills and knowledge about various aspects of death, dying, and bereavement. Public education about death, dying, loss, and care is vast in scope, both in terms of the potential target audiences and in the subject matter relevant to 'death, dying, loss, and care.' In the following sections we explore how public education can influence end of life literacy, primarily focusing on the role it can play in increasing individual knowledge and skills.

Target audience

In its broadest sense, the target audience for 'public education' is the 'general public', which is one way of saying 'everyone'! Indeed, death is one of very few issues that is of universal relevance. However, education projects often define more specific 'target audiences' based around specific characteristics, for example, 'volunteers', 'healthcare professionals,' or 'carers', or demographic characteristics such as 'children', 'older people', or 'vulnerable communities'.

Subject matter

Death or end of life education has the potential to encompass a huge variety of issues and circumstances. Within the broad term 'death education' there is the scope to explore a wide range of issues relating to practical, financial, legal, emotional, physical, and spiritual matters; issues relating to caring, dying, and grieving; issues relating to palliative care, funerals, and bereavement care; and issues relating to providing support, receiving support, and accessing support. Education could focus on a particular age group—preterm infants, babies, children, young people, or young, middle-aged, old, or very old adults. Or it might explore a particular cause or causes of death, for example, cancer, organ failure, neurological condition, sudden death, traumatic death, miscarriage, suicide, frailty, dementia, or old age.

Aims

Various initiatives have taken place with the broad aim of educating the public about death, dying, and bereavement. The specific aims of such education are not always clearly defined, and links between the aims and intended outcomes aren't always made clear. However, we suggest that the aims of these activities can be categorized under one or more of five broad headings:

- Raising awareness, changing attitudes, and encouraging people to talk about death.
- Increasing knowledge about palliative and end of life care.
- Preparing people with knowledge and skills to support practical responses to serious illness, dying, and bereavement.
- Encouraging people to plan ahead for future ill health or dying.
- Encouraging social action.

Raising awareness, changing attitudes, and encouraging people to talk about death

Much work in this field is in some way aimed at encouraging people to talk about death, and this is tied up with the idea that talking can help to change attitudes to and/or raise awareness of issues relating to death, dying, and bereavement.

For example, in England, the Dying Matters coalition 'to create an open culture in which we're comfortable talking about death, dying and bereavement.' (Dying Matters, 2020). The aim of the death cafe movement is to 'increase awareness of death to help people make the most of their (finite) lives' (Death Cafe, 2020). A key review (Paul and Sallnow, 2013) highlighted 'supporting community dialogue', 'engaging pupils in conversations on palliative care, death, dying and bereavement', and 'promoting Dying Matters week' as some of the most common activities being undertaken by palliative care services as part of their public health approach to palliative care in the UK in 2012.

Tony Walter characterizes this approach as based on the belief that 'breaking the so-called death taboo will enable people to talk about death and thus change their attitudes and actions'. Within *What Death Means Now*, Walter (2017) provides a powerful critique of this idea, pointing to a lack of evidence to support the assumption that talking has a meaningful impact on attitudes and actions. He suggests some potential limitations and downsides to efforts to get people talking about death. Walter additionally questions some of the assumptions that the 'death awareness movement' is based on—that death is unfamiliar, that death is 'taboo', and that death is denied.

Though it is arguable whether 'talking about death' is an end in itself, 'talking' can be seen as helpful as part of a wider approach. For instance, talking about wishes and preferences is an essential part of the process of making a care plan, but the plan then needs to be documented, reviewed, and accessed when needed. Compassionate community initiatives can begin by bringing people together to talk as a first step, which then leads to the growth of networks, greater support, and shared learning.

Helping people to understand what palliative care is and what palliative care services they can access

Research indicates that many people have poor knowledge and misconceptions about palliative care, and that this has a negative impact on their ability and desire to access palliative care services (McIlfatrick et al., 2014; Collins et al., 2020; Patel and Lyons, 2020). Educating the general public about palliative care is therefore seen as an important part of enabling people to access care from which they could benefit, particularly earlier on in their illness.

Various efforts have been made to educate and raise awareness among the general public about palliative care. For example, one of the aims of World Hospice and Palliative Care Day, initiated by the Worldwide Hospice and Palliative Care Alliance, is 'To raise awareness and understanding of the needs—medical, social, practical, spiritual—of people living with a life limiting illness and their families' (Worldwide Hospice and Palliative Care Alliance, 2020). The All Ireland Institute of Hospice and Palliative Care runs Palliative Care week in September each year 'to raise awareness of the difference palliative care can make to people with life-limiting conditions, carers and families throughout the island of Ireland' (The All Ireland Institute of Hospice and Palliative Care, 2020).

Many specialist palliative care services, including hospices, see engaging with communities as part of their role, and public education as an element of this. Paul and Sallnow (2013) found that 'awareness raising' was one of the key categories arising from their review, with examples including raising awareness of 'the hospice', 'health issues such as cancer', and 'end of life care issues'. They also found that 'fundraising was described in its ability to both raise the profile of hospice within the community but also give "people an opportunity to come and talk about death and dying"', and it is worth noting that the boundaries between fundraising and awareness raising sometimes become blurred.

Preparing people with knowledge and skills to support practical responses to serious illness, dying, and bereavement

In recent years, there has been a growing recognition of the need to equip non-professionals with knowledge and skills about caring, dying, and grieving.

This can take place with a specific purpose or situation in mind, for example, educating existing carers with skills that will help them in their immediate role (Corrêa, 2018), or educating interested community members who wish to volunteer to provide support within their own community, such as the training of people to be part of Neighbourhood Networks in Kerala (Kumar, 2007), or Compassionate Neighbours in London (Hospice UK, 2020).

Other initiatives aim to provide upstream education, providing more general education about aspects of dying, caring, and grieving to the general public so that people are better equipped to respond and support others should the need arise (Bollig and Heller, 2016; Patterson et al., 2020).

Encouraging people to plan ahead for future ill health or dying

Several education initiatives are grounded in the conviction that planning ahead for deteriorating health and dying makes it more likely that someone will get the care they would choose, and also reduces stress for their family and carers. Planning ahead in this context can include legal aspects (e.g. making a will, power of attorney, advance directive), healthcare aspects (such as treatment and care preferences), personal priorities (such as walking the dog, seeing grandchildren), and spiritual aspects (such as religious matters, meaning making, and social fulfilment).

Various initiatives therefore aim to educate people about the importance of considering their options, talking to the people important to them, and making plans relating to legal, practical, and medical issues. For example, The GroundSwell Project in Australia has developed 'Ten things to know before you go', an online workshop designed to empower people with the knowledge and resources they need to plan well for the final stages of life (The GroundSwell Project, 2020d). The Irish Hospice Foundation runs 'Putting the House in Order' events that explore wills, enduring power of attorney, care preferences, and other issues (Irish Hospice Foundation, 2020). In England, Gentle Dusk is a socially minded partnership that works with communities and the workforce to raise awareness of the importance of end of life care planning. It delivers training programmes, events, and workshops to staff, volunteers, and the public, helping them overcome barriers to talking about the end of life and increasing their knowledge of end of life planning. The Speak Up Canada initiative includes workshops for the public as part of an integrated approach to promoting advance care planning (Speak Up Canada, 2020).

Encouraging social action

Social actions can be individual, for example, offering practical support to a dying family member, or calling in on a neighbour who has been bereaved. Social actions can also be more collective—for example, bringing people together to improve supportive networks within a community. As discussed earlier, the concepts of community empowerment and social action are central to notions of health, death, and grief literacy, and therefore encouraging social action is an important aim of some public education work in this area.

For example, in Australia, Dying to Know Day is 'an annual day of action dedicated to activating conversations and community actions around death, dying and bereavement'. Education can have more than one aim, and education that increases knowledge and skills can have the overarching aim of encouraging social action. For example, by supporting people to develop skills, confidence, and networks, the Kerala model and the Compassionate Neighbours initiative encourage people to use their skills within their local communities.

Modes of public education

We now turn our attention to explore some of the different ways in which people have tried to educate the general public about death, dying, and bereavement.

Public awareness campaigns

As discussed earlier, many countries now have a day or days dedicated to raising awareness and/or action around death or grief, and there are several examples of one-off or ongoing public awareness campaigns on some aspect of death, grief, or forward planning. Public campaigns in this area vary vastly in terms of aims (and how clearly the aims are defined), budget, length, scale, geography, key issues, and target audience.

What can public awareness campaigns achieve?

Media campaigns have the potential to disseminate well-defined messages to large audiences repeatedly, over time, in an incidental manner, and at a low cost per head. The contribution made by a campaign will depend on various factors, but broadly speaking, public awareness campaigns have the potential to:

- Provide information.
- Signpost to key information sources.
- Explain to people why it is a good idea to become informed about death, dying, loss, and care.
- Help to remove barriers to discussion of these issues, where the barriers are attitudinal or cultural.
- Bring issues to people's attention and create a talking point.
- Raise the profile and/or understanding of an issue among public policy makers and those working in health and social care.
- Help to create a culture where being informed about these matters is seen as important.
- Encourage people to undertake or avoid a specific action.

However, there are also a number of risks to running a media campaign, for example:

- Campaign messages can fall short or backfire.
- Exposure of audiences may not meet expectations, due to inadequate funding.
- Increasingly fractured/cluttered media environment.
- Inappropriate or poorly researched format (e.g. material unsuitable for children).
- Homogeneous messages might not persuade heterogeneous audiences.
- Audiences may lack the resources to change the behaviours being targeted (e.g. making a will).
- The system may be unprepared to respond to/cope with new behaviours.

How effective are public awareness campaigns?

Though little has been published evaluating the effectiveness of public awareness campaigns relating to death, dying, and bereavement, there is evidence from other spheres that media campaigns can be effective in changing attitudes and behaviour, at an individual level and by changing social norms (Wakefield et al., 2010).

Clearly not all public awareness campaigns will be equally successful—much is dependent on the campaign design and surrounding factors. For example, there are indications that campaigns are more effective when linked to broader activity (Levin et al., 2017)—for instance, smoking prevalence has been reduced when mass media campaigns have been combined with, for example, tobacco taxation measures (Wakefield et al., 2010).

Without more published evaluation, it is speculation to attempt to judge whether public awareness campaigns relating to death, dying, and bereavement are being successful. There are difficulties associated with measuring the impact of certain campaigns—for example, where a campaign aims to 'raise awareness', consideration needs to be given to *how* 'awareness' can be measured, and what expense might be associated with this. Additionally, even if a difference can be measured, it can be hard to attribute causality to a particular campaign.

What can we learn from public awareness campaigns in the area of death, dying, and bereavement?

Work in Scotland by Good Life, Good Death, Good Grief explored what can be learnt from existing public awareness campaigns relating to death, dying, and bereavement, and concluded that before embarking on a public awareness campaign relating to death, dying, and loss, appropriate consideration should be given to:

- The problem or issue that is being addressed.
- The potential of a media campaign as the best or most appropriate way to address that issue, or whether a similar amount of money spent in a different way might have more impact.
- What stakeholders should be involved to ensure work is informed by adequate understanding of the issues involved.
- The potential challenges of a media campaign in that area.
- The potential benefits of a media campaign in that area, including the potential for financial benefits for individuals or savings for public services, and of improvements to well-being.
- What other complementary initiatives might be required to enable the campaign's success—for example, if encouraging the public to take a particular action such as making a power of attorney, what barriers will they face and can these also be addressed?
- What resources would be required to genuinely make a sustained impact, and whether sufficient resources are available.
- How the impact of the campaign can be evaluated.
- Health inequalities issues—will the campaign be of most benefit to those who are most disadvantaged (Patterson et al., 2018)?

Formal courses/training

There are several examples of education courses that focus on some element of serious illness, caregiving, dying, or loss that are designed for the general public. Courses vary in terms of topic, length, delivery method, and target audience. Table 13.1 provides some illustrative examples.

Though by no means a comprehensive list, Table 13.1 illustrates some of the different approaches that can be taken to provision of education courses, and a detailed scoping would likely reveal many more courses either in use or under development.

It is clear that there is an appetite for education courses on this subject matter. The University of Glasgow's Future Learn course attracted 3600 learners from 132 countries when it was initially launched (Clark, 2020). By 2017, more than 1200 people had completed the Last Aid Course (Bollig and Bachman, 2017), and each year Gentle Dusk has ample participants to run several workshops in the Islington area of London alone (Gentle Dusk, 2018).

People's personal relationships to the subject matter mean that running a course of this kind takes sensitivity and care. People engage in different ways, challenging course designers to structure in flexibility and develop courses that appeal to a variety of learning styles. Nevertheless, feedback from those who have participated in or developed courses indicates that subject matter relating to ill health, dying, and bereavement is not in itself a barrier to people finding courses useful, engaging, interesting, and even enjoyable (Clark, 2020; Patterson et al., 2020).

Though it is the hope of course organizers that such courses will result in individuals and populations becoming more prepared for end of life care experiences, it cannot be assumed that education alone leads to action. Gentle Dusk complements its planning workshops with an advice and planning service whereby people can request a one-to-one appointment with a volunteer to support them to put a plan in place. In 2017/2018 they delivered a total of 20 community engagement events: nine workshops, six death cafes, three information stalls, one theatre event, and one discussion group. These community events reached 463 members of the public, 26 of whom requested a follow-up appointment/information. In the advice and planning service, 117 one-to-one appointments were delivered to 91 different service users. As a result of the one-to-one appointments with a volunteer, 52 plans were put in place (Gentle Dusk, 2018). This gives an indication that, even when concerted efforts are made to provide free, tailored support, many people do not follow up their education with action.

So far there is little information available about the long-term impact on individuals and societies of citizens undertaking this type of course, and a number of questions therefore remain to be answered. Are courses limited to the theoretical, or do they also

Table 13.1 Examples of education courses

Title	Subjects covered	Duration and mode of delivery	Delivered by	Local, national, or international?	Target audience
Hospital-based group education programme	What is palliative care?; the typical role of a family carer; support services available to carers; preparing for the future; self-care strategies to promote optimal well-being	Face-to-face; approximately 2 hours	A health professional who is both experienced in facilitation of adult education sessions and palliative care service delivery	Information about running the course freely available on the website of the Centre for Palliative Care, Melbourne, Australia	Primary family carers of patients receiving palliative care in an in-patient hospital or hospice setting
Public health approaches to death, dying, and bereavement	Theory and practice relating to public health palliative care	Online, 4-week part-time module	University of Edinburgh	International	Masters students in public health
Future Learn: End of Life Care—Challenges and Innovation	Dying and palliative care practice around the world; new trends and ideas surrounding end of life care issues	Online, 4 hours per week for 3 weeks	University of Glasgow	International	People interested in or engaged in matters relating to death, dying, bereavement, and palliative and end of life care
End of Life Aid Skills for Everyone	Providing practical and emotional support to people who are dying or bereaved; planning ahead; navigating the health and social care system; growing more comfortable and confident to provide support	Online or face-to-face: 2–3 hours per week for 4 weeks	Local volunteer facilitators	Local groups across Scotland	General public. The level of content was explicitly designed to be widely accessible
Future Matters	Advance care planning, recording funeral wishes, wills, and lasting powers of attorney	Face-to-face workshops	Gentle Dusk	Mainly Islington, London, England, but can go elsewhere	Groups of adults of any age, for example: community and voluntary groups; carers groups; Faith groups; expert patient programmes
The Omega Course (The Omega Course, 2020)	Planning for the future; talking to ill or bereaved friends or neighbours; decreased fear of the unknown	Face-to-face, four 2-hour workshops plus a full day session, health education and role play	The Omega Course	Local to Warwickshire, England	General public
Last Aid (Bollig and Heller, 2016)	Care at the end of life; advance care planning and decision-making; symptom management; cultural aspects of death and bereavement	Face-to-face, 3 hours plus a 30-minute break	Trained Last Aid facilitators with professional knowledge of palliative care	Local courses delivered in several European countries	General public
10 things to know before you go	End of life planning	Online, 2 hours	The GroundSwell Project	National across Australia (delivered in small group settings)	General public

provide people with practical skills to provide help and support to friends, family, and community members? Do people progress from learning about making plans to actually making their own end of life plans? Do such courses go beyond providing knowledge and information, and contribute towards empowerment and social action? Who participates in courses such as these and do such courses cater for people with a diversity of backgrounds and experiences?

Additionally, work in this area should consider potential unintended consequences of formal education programmes. Noonan and colleagues (2016) point out that 'because death education programmes are typically not designed to mobilize networks or create social action they may actually promote compliance with the dominant medical approach by reinforcing the primacy of professional knowledge. As such these traditional models of education rarely recognize, mobilize or develop the existing knowledge within communities' (p. 34). Consideration should therefore be given to how courses can be designed to support the development of social networks and sharing of learning and experiences between participants, and avoid presenting professionals as the sole repository of expertise in this area.

Experiential learning

'You can't do things for somebody and then expect them to know ... They've got to be able to do it. If they're hands on it's a different kettle of fish.' (Horsfall et al., 2015, p. 42)

Not all the education that people receive about serious illness, caregiving, dying, and bereavement is directed or intentional; people learn about death, dying, loss, and care through their own experience over the course of their lifetime. Health and social care professionals routinely contribute to this education by sharing with individuals and their carers specific information or skills that will help them in their personal situation. Finding themselves in the position of being, or caring for someone who is, seriously ill, people might also seek out condition-specific support groups, and gain education through those.

The role of experiential learning was explored by Horsfall and colleagues (2015) in the Caring at End of Life Study, which looked at how ordinary people supported each other to care for someone dying at home. They observed that when caring for someone who is dying at home, carers and their networks are engaged in learning about how to provide care and navigate the surrounding formal health and care systems.

People described how the experience of caring for someone at the end of life had changed their attitudes, behaviour, and perspectives as they became more able to focus on meaningful moments and discovered within themselves new depths of resilience and compassion. Through caring at home for someone at the end of life, people learned about how a society 'does death', and changed their own attitudes, actions, and beliefs about death.

Through their caring role, people learned how to provide practical support and emotional support to someone towards the end of life, and also skills in how to ask for support and make arrangements for care. People who had cared before recognized that they were better equipped for end of life care and they felt they were able to re-engage with social networks if, and when, required. Social networks themselves transformed as social relations and networks were mobilized to support and help with caregiving, and members of these networks learn from each other (Horsfall et al., 2015). The death literacy model therefore emphasizes experiential learning as integral to increasing death literacy (Noonan et al., 2016).

Tony Walter (2017) highlights that there is evidence from other public health initiatives such as smoking cessation and environmental initiatives that 'attitudes can change behaviour, but also that behaviour can change attitudes':

> A teenage girl offers to walk a dying neighbour's dog after school each day. Each time she visits the house to collect and return the dog, she learns about dying; she does not need to talk about death in order to walk the dog (she just needs to like dogs), but walking the dog will teach her about death. (p. 54)

It is therefore clear that experience has an important role to play in educating people about death and dying. Though education might help to prepare people for such experiences, it seems unlikely that other modes of learning could replace the learning that comes from experience. However, efforts can be made to create more opportunities for people to actively engage in caring networks, for example, through 'compassionate communities' initiatives to grow caring networks.

Incorporating death, dying, and bereavement into existing formal mainstream education

Death and loss are key themes throughout art and literature; the life cycle and the biology of disease is part of our scientific understanding of the world; studying history and geography can teach about causes of and attitudes to death at a societal level; and religious and moral education is an opportunity to explore culture, rituals, and existential aspects relating to death and dying. Therefore, it is clear that people can learn about death, dying, loss, and care through formal education on a variety of subjects.

For example, work within Scottish primary schools identified several opportunities to explore aspects of death and dying within the existing national school curriculum, and has had some success introducing these subjects within mainstream education on a local level. Children were supportive of school staff talking to them about, and educating them on, death, dying, and bereavement and had a number of related questions they felt their teachers might be able to answer (Paul, 2015). Efforts have been made to produce resources that can support schools to introduce these subjects (Irish Childhood Bereavement Network, n.d.; Patterson et al., 2015). However, barriers have also been identified in relation to bringing these subjects into primary schools, in the form of the training and confidence of teachers, perceived parental concerns, and the lack of policy focus on death, dying, and bereavement (Paul, 2015).

The area where efforts to incorporate death, dying, and bereavement into existing curriculums have been best documented is probably within medical and nursing undergraduate curriculums (Walker et al., 2016; White et al, 2019; McMahon and Wee, 2019). However, given that everyone will at some stage deal with these issues, there is an argument for introducing education about death and dying more broadly into other education courses, including primary and secondary school education, and college/university courses, particularly those for public-facing professions such as teachers, police officers, and social workers.

It is clear that there is scope to incorporate death, dying, and bereavement into a variety of existing education courses, both at school and further education level. It would be informative to scope the extent to which this is already being done—to what extent do educators exploit or ignore opportunities to explore aspects of death, dying, and bereavement within their courses?

Peer education

Peer education takes place when people educate others who share with them an element of common identity that is important to them—for example, social background, age, ethnicity, or another area of life experience. Peer education can be structured, for example, through the delivery of a specific education course, or take place more informally through chatting within more informal social situations. Peer educators are often volunteers.

Commonly associated with projects involving young people, peer education has been shown to be effective in achieving positive change in various areas of health including smoking, sexual health, HIV, and drugs. However, peer education has also been used to encourage discussion and planning ahead relating to end of life issues, with some success particularly if the peer educators are already embedded within an existing community group (Seymour et al., 2011).

In addition to formally organized peer education projects, peer education can take place fairly informally, for example, through church groups, rotary clubs, or community groups organizing talks and workshops and sharing knowledge between members. In this context, there is the potential for some overlap with 'experiential learning' as discussed previously, where people learn from others within their caring networks.

Citizen-led self-education

People learn about death and dying passively throughout the course of their lives, for example, through the social media, television, and films they are exposed to. But not all learning is passive—people also actively seek out information and learning about matters they perceive as important. There is the potential for individuals to educate themselves about death, dying, and bereavement by accessing information via books, films, leaflets, and websites.

This is only possible if comprehensive good quality information is freely available and accessible to people. Internationally, statutory organizations and charitable bodies provide information about various aspects of planning, palliative care, illness, care, dying, and bereavement on their websites. Some hospices, hospitals, care homes, and general practitioners make available public information leaflets, and initiatives such as palliative care awareness days attempt to raise awareness of the information that is available. Increasing amounts of information are available through blogs, social media, and films that have been made by people with personal experience of illness, care, or bereavement.

However, though perhaps more information is now available than ever before, it is important to note that information is *not* education in itself. We know that people's ability to access, understand, evaluate, use, and navigate health and social care information and services is related to their overall health literacy level. It is also recognized that an individual's health literacy tends to be related to their social circumstances, with educational attainment being a predictor of good health literacy, and people with limited financial and social resources more likely to have lower health literacy (Public Health England, 2015).

In other words, not everyone will be able to, or choose to, access information, and those who do access information will differ in their ability to understand, evaluate, and use the information provided. Therefore, though it is important that good-quality information is available for people, we cannot assume that this is sufficient to enable most people to educate themselves about matters relating to death, dying, loss, and care.

Consideration should also be given to the quality and accuracy of information relating to death, dying, and bereavement. Many people gain information from informal sources such as soap operas, documentaries, social media, and newspaper articles. Though this can result in greater awareness of issues, it can also result in the spread of myths, biases, and misunderstandings. For example, valid concerns relating to 'Do Not Attempt (Cardiopulmonary) Resuscitation' documentation and the Liverpool Care Pathway have been simplified by some media outlets in a way that has contributed to misunderstandings and fear among members of the public (Seymour and Clark, 2018; Reid, 2020).

The comprehensiveness and presentation style of information is also an important consideration. Too often, the provision of public-facing information about serious illness and dying is overly guided by a desire to protect members of the public from anxiety, and this can result in the use of indirect language, euphemistic content, and omitting information that might be perceived as bad news. Such information is often generated by healthcare professionals for whom it can be very difficult to fully escape professional perspectives and terminology.

Learning that someone will not get better, or that the ideal support services are not available, or that the end of life is close, will likely always be difficult. Yet, without honest information, individuals and families are ill-equipped to make decisions. In addition to the moral argument that important information should not be withheld, there is also an argument that for many people the facts may be less worrying than whatever they are imagining (BBC Ideas, 2018).

The variances and uncertainties involved in predicting an individual's illness journey can present a challenge to the provision of comprehensive information, but acknowledging and exploring these uncertainties within public-facing information is possible and worthwhile. Communicating sensitively is always important when providing potentially unwelcome information, but this is not the same as limiting exposure or sugar-coating facts. It is possible to provide comprehensive, accurate information that acknowledges uncertainties, while maintaining a tone of kindness, empathy, and respect for the reader.

Conclusion

Within this chapter we have used the term 'end of life literacy' to describe an individual's ability to cope with and offer support through serious illness, caring, dying, and bereavement. End of life literacy is influenced by a complex interaction of information, knowledge, skills, experiences, values, community, empowerment, and action, and can be improved by work in various interacting domains as set out within the Ottawa Charter.

Moving on to focus specifically on the role that public education can play in increasing end of life literacy, we have focused primarily on how education affects individual knowledge and skills relating to death, dying, loss, and care. Increased knowledge and skills can also influence individual and community values, empowerment, experiences, and action, but this is not explored in depth in this chapter.

It is clear that education relevant to the field of public health palliative care encompasses a wide range of subjects, target audiences, aims, and modes. Before embarking on a new education initiative, it is important to consider the intended impact of that activity—what are the aims of education, are they in line with the intended outcomes, and what mode of education would best achieve these aims?

More work is needed to explore questions relating to the effectiveness and long-term impact of different modes of public education in this area, and the potential role of incorporating matters relating to death, dying, loss, and care into mainstream education curriculums.

Education can occur as a by-product or secondary aim of other activities, for example, work to build social networks in a community relating to death and dying will increase knowledge and skills in that community, and experiential learning is an important form of education. Enabling people to feel more able to play an active role in their community and caring networks can equally be a primary aim of education. Information is necessary to enable education, but information on its own is not education.

Education can also have unintended consequences—educators need to take care to avoid reinforcing the idea that professionals are the sole repository of expertise in this area. Educators should also work to tackle rather than increase health inequalities by concerted efforts to bring education to the individuals and communities who most need it, not just those who are easiest to access.

REFERENCES

Abel, J., Bowra, J., Walter, T., and Howarth, G. 2011. Compassionate community networks: supporting home dying. *BMJ Supportive & Palliative Care*, **1**, 129–133.

All Ireland Institute of Hospice and Palliative Care. 2019a. Better public understanding of palliative care required to improve care for end of life patients. [Online] Available at: https://aiihpc.org/9906-2/

All Ireland Institute of Hospice and Palliative Care. 2019b. Round Table on a Public Health Approach to Palliative and End of Life Care on the island of Ireland. [Online] Available at: https://aiihpc.org/wp-content/uploads/2020/06/Round-Table-Report.pdf

All Ireland Institute of Hospice and Palliative Care. 2020. Palliative care week. [Online] Available at: https://thepalliativehub.com/palliative-care-week-2021/

Aoun, S. M., Breen, L. J., Howting, D. A., Rumbold, B., McNamara, B., and Hegney, D. 2015. Who needs bereavement support? A population based survey of bereavement risk and support need. *PLoS One*, **10**, e0121101.

BBC Ideas. 2018. Dying is not as bad as you think, with Dr Kathryn Mannix. [Online] Available at: https://www.bbc.co.uk/ideas/videos/dying-is-not-as-bad-as-you-think/p062m0xt

Bollig, G. and Heller, A. 2016. The last aid course – a simple and effective concept to teach the public about palliative care and to enhance the public discussion about death and dying. *Austin Palliative Care*, **1**, 1010.

Bollig, G. and Bachman, K. 2017. The Last Aid Course—an international project to educate the public about death and dying. Poster presented at the 15th World Congress of the European Association for Palliative Care Progressing Palliative Care, Madrid, Spain, 18–20 May.

Breen, L., Kawashima, D., Joy, K., Cadell, S., Roth, D., Chow, A., et al. 2020. Grief literacy: a call to action for compassionate communities. *Death Studies*, 1–9. Advance online publication. https://doi.org/10.1080/07481187.2020.1739780

Clark, D. 2020. Online learning about the end of life. University of Glasgow. 17 February. [Online] Available at: http://endoflifestudies.academicblogs.co.uk/online-learning-about-the-end-of-life/17

Collins, A., McLachlan, S. A., and Philip, J. 2020. Community knowledge of and attitudes to palliative care: a descriptive study. *Palliative Medicine*, **34**, 245–252.

Compassionate Inverclyde. 2020. Compassionate Inverclyde: capturing moments that matter. [Online] Available at: https://ardgowanhospice.org.uk/how-we-can-help/compassionate-inverclyde/

Corrêa, S. 2018. Proposal of a new public health end of life approach for Brazil: how the Project EstaraoSeuLado-Primary Palliative Care is working and how it can help. *Annals of Palliative Medicine*, 7, AB009.

Death Cafe. 2020. What is death café? [Online] Available at: https://deathcafe.com/what/

Di Fiore, D. 2020. End of life literacy. Developing a measure of capacity to seek, understand and use end-of-life health information within an aged care setting. Research Notes: Palliative Care. 26 March. Available at: https://blogs.flinders.edu.au/research-notes-palliative-care/2020/03/26/end-of-life-literacy-developing-a-measure-of-capacity-to-seek-understand-and-use-end-of-life-health-information-within-an-aged-care-setting/

Dying Matters. 2020. Homepage [Online] Available at: https://www.dyingmatters.org/overview/about-us

Gentle Dusk. 2018. Future matters: empowering communities to plan for the end of life. [Online] Available at: http://www.gentledusk.org.uk/future-matters_in-detail.html

Horsfall, D., Yardley, A., Leonard, R., Noonan, K., and Rosenberg, J. 2015. End of life at home: co-creating an ecology of care. University of Western Sydney & Cancer Council of NSW. [Online] Available at: https://researchdirect.westernsydney.edu.au/islandora/object/uws:32200

Hospice UK. 2019. Compassionate employers. [Online] Available at: https://www.hospiceuk.org/what-we-offer/compassionate-employers

Hospice UK. 2020. Compassionate neighbours. [Online] Available at: https://professionals.hospiceuk.org/what-we-offer/community-volunteering-hub/case-studies/compassionate-neighbours

Irish Hospice Foundation. 2020. Putting the house in order Limerick. [Online] Available at: https://hospicefoundation.ie/public-engagement/putting-the-house-in-order-limerick/

Karapliagkou, A. and Kellehear, A. n.d. Public health approaches to end of life care: a toolkit. Public Health England and the National Council for Palliative Care. [Online] Available at: https://pdf4pro.com/view/public-health-approaches-to-end-of-life-care-ncpc-521897.html

Kumar, S. K. 2007. Kerala, India: a regional community-based palliative care model. *Journal of Pain and Symptom Management*, **33**, 623–627.

Leonard, R., Noonan, K., Horsfall, D., Psychogios, H., Kelly, M., Rosenberg, J. P., et al. 2020. *Death Literacy Index: A Report on its Development and Implementation*. Sydney: Western Sydney University. Available at: https://doi.org/10.26183/5eb8d3adb20b0

Levin, K., Carson, J., and Crighton, E. 2017. Measuring the impact of a public awareness campaign to increase Welfare Power of Attorney registrations in Scotland. *Age and Ageing*, **46**, 659–664.

McIlfatrick, S., et al. 2014. How well do the general public understand palliative care? A mixed methods study. *BMJ Supportive & Palliative Care*, **4**, A2.

McMahon, D. and Wee, B. 2019. Medical undergraduate palliative care education (UPCE). *BMJ Supportive & Palliative Care*, **11**, 4–6.

Noonan, K., Horsfall, D., Leonard, R., and Rosenberg, J. P. 2016. Developing death literacy. *Progress in Palliative Care*, **24**, 31–35.

Nutbeam, D. 2000. Health literacy as a public health goal: a challenge for contemporary health education and communication strategies into the 21st century. *Health Promotion International*, **15**, 259–267.

Pallium Canada. 2020. Compassionate communities. [Online] Available at: https://www.pallium.ca/compassionate-communities/

Patel, P. and Lyons, L. 2020. Examining the knowledge, awareness, and perceptions of palliative care in the general public over time: a scoping literature review. *American Journal of Hospice and Palliative Medicine*, **37**, 481–487.

Patterson, R. M., Gibb, C., and Hazelwood, M. A. 2020. End of life aid skills for everyone: a public education course. [Online] Available at: https://www.palliativecarescotland.org.uk/content/publications/18-End-of-Life-Aid-Skills-for-Everyone.pdf

Patterson, R. M., Peacock, R., and Hazelwood, M. A. 2018. *A Road Less Lonely*. Edinburgh: Scottish Partnership for Palliative Care.

Paul, S. 2015. Advancing education and support around death, dying and bereavement: in schools, hospices, schools and health promoting palliative care. Doctoral thesis. University of Edinburgh.

Paul, S. and Sallnow, L. 2013. Public health approaches to end-of-life care in the UK: an online survey of palliative care services. *BMJ Supportive & Palliative Care*, **3**, 196–199.

Public Health England. 2015. Local action on health inequalities improving health literacy to reduce health inequalities. [Online] Available at: https://assets.publishing.service.gov.uk/government/uploads/system/uploads/attachment_data/file/460709/4a_Health_Literacy-Full.pdf

Public Health Palliative Care International. 2019. Overview of tools and resources for building compassionate communities. [Online] Available at: https://phpci.info/tools

Reid, S. 2020. Condemned by a 'care pathway'... again: elderly patients are still given 'Do Not Resuscitate' orders against their or their families' wishes. *Daily Mail*, 27 November. [Online] Available at: https://www.dailymail.co.uk/news/article-8995229/Elderly-patients-given-Not-Resuscitate-orders-against-families-wishes.html

Scottish Partnership for Palliative Care. 2015. Grasping the nettle: what action can we take to improve palliative and end of life care in Scotland? [Online] Available at: https://www.palliativecarescotland.org.uk/content/publications/Grasping-the-Nettle---final-copy.pdf

Scottish Partnership for Palliative Care. 2019. Compassionate communities toolkit. [Online] Available at: https://www.goodlifedeathgrief.org.uk/content/toolkit_homepage/

Seymour, J. E., Almack, K., Kennedy, S., and Froggatt, K. 2013. Peer education for advance care planning: volunteers' perspectives on training and community engagement activities. *Health Expectations*, **16**, 43–55.

Seymour, J. and Clark, D. 2018. The Liverpool Care Pathway for the Dying Patient: a critical analysis of its rise, demise and legacy in England [version 2; peer review: 2 approved]. *Wellcome Open Research*, **3**, 15.

Speak Up Canada. 2020. Introduction to advance care planning. [Online] Available at: https://www.advancecareplanning.ca/news/advance-care-planning-workshop-december-1-8-2020/

Strathcarron Hospice. 2020. Compassionate communities. [Online] Available at: https://www.strathcarronhospice.net/listing/category/compassionate-communities

The GroundSwell Project. 2020a. What we do. [Online] Available at: https://www.thegroundswellproject.com/what-we-do

The GroundSwell Project. 2020b. The compassionate workplace. [Online] Available at: https://www.thegroundswellproject.com/compassion-at-work

The GroundSwell Project. 2020c. Compassionate communities. [Online] Available at: https://www.thegroundswellproject.com/compassionate-communities

The GroundSwell Project. 2020d. Ten things. [Online] Available at: https://www.thegroundswellproject.com/10-things-workshops

The Irish Childhood Bereavement Network. n.d. Teachers & schools. [Online] Available at: https://www.childhoodbereavement.ie/schools/

The Omega Course. 2020. The Omega Course. [Online] Available at: https://www.facebook.com/theomegacourse/

The Truacanta Project. 2020. Homepage. [Online] Available at: https://www.goodlifedeathgrief.org.uk/content/thetruacantaproject/

Wakefield, M. A., Loken, B., and Hornik, R. C. 2010. Use of mass media campaigns to change health behaviour. *Lancet*, **376**, 1261–1271.

Walker, S., Gibbins, J., Barclay, S., Adams, A., Paes, P., Chandratilake, M., et al. Progress and divergence in palliative care education for medical students: a comparative survey of UK course structure, content, delivery, contact with patients and assessment of learning. *Palliative Medicine*, **30**, 834–842.

Walter, T. 2017. *What Death Means Now: Thinking Critically About Dying and Grieving*. Bristol: Policy Press.

White, N., Oostendorp, L. J., Minton, O., Yardley, S., and Stone, P. 2019. Palliative care training in undergraduate medical, nursing and allied health: a survey. *BMJ Supportive & Palliative Care*, bmjspcare-2019-002025. Advance online publication. https://doi.org/10.1136/bmjspcare-2019-002025

World Health Organization. 1998. *Health Promotion Glossary*. Geneva: World Health Organization.

World Health Organization. 2020. Health literacy. [Online] Available at: https://www.who.int/healthpromotion/health-literacy/en/

Worldwide Hospice Palliative Care Alliance. 2020. World hospice and palliative care day. [Online] Available at: https://www.thewhpca.org/world-hospice-and-palliative-care-day

14

Health Policy

The imperative of palliative care advocacy

Katherine Pettus and Pati Dzotsenidze

Introduction

Palliative care advocacy is the 'back-office' work with public officials and civil servants that ensures the development of legal frameworks and budgets to support delivery of services for all who need them. More precisely, evidence-based advocacy for integration of palliative care into primary healthcare for services at the community level is essential to support the development of funded palliative care *policies* in countries where those services are randomly distributed, inequitable, or non-existent. Home-based services will struggle to sustain themselves without some degree of public funding and will be unable to deliver appropriate clinical care without access to essential palliative care medicines for patients who need them. Adequate access to affordable essential palliative care medicines is a limiting factor for service development in many countries because procurement is an officially mediated—government—function, often involving meticulous coordination between several different ministries and service delivery systems. Since governments are the legally mandated gatekeepers for access to medicines subject to international control, only coordinated, evidence-based advocacy at all levels of governance (local, municipal, national, regional, and international) can begin to improve access to the essential palliative care medicines that remain unavailable, unaffordable, and inaccessible to patients and providers in the vast majority of low- and middle-income countries (LMICs). (Pettus KI and De Lima L 2020).

The International Association for Hospice and Palliative Care (IAHPC) advocates at the international level, through the United Nations (UN) organizations, and supports members in their home countries (the UN member states) to hold their governments accountable for their commitments under international law and multilateral resolutions, such as those adopted by the World Health Organization (WHO). The basic assumptions underlying the IAHPC advocacy theory of change are that (1) palliative care is an element of the right to health, *not a privilege*, and that (2) since rights, by definition, are entitlements, respecting and protecting them entails the development of public policy. As most palliative care services, where they exist, are private, philanthropically funded, and only randomly available, advocacy is required for the explicit inclusion of palliative care in *public* policies and norms to ensure that 'no person is left behind' to echo the tagline of the UN 2030 Agenda for Sustainable Development (UN General Assembly, 2015).

This chapter presents the principles and nuts and bolts of advocacy to illustrate how this form of active citizenship can lay the groundwork for sustainable compassionate communities in countries where integration of palliative care into primary healthcare, and access to essential palliative care medicines (International Narcotics Control Board, 2018), is low to non-existent (WHO, 2020). Part I discusses these principles, and the *praxis* of palliative care advocacy and Part II relates how global advocacy has exposed, and works to end, the 'pandemic of untreated [. . .] pain' (European Society for Medical Oncology, 2013). Such advocacy requires at least a nodding acquaintance with the international law governing access to palliative care and essential palliative care medicines, the institutional landscape of the UN organizations, and a working knowledge of palliative care delivery in a variety of settings. Palliative care advocacy at all levels of governance generates a synergistic feedback loop between patients and practitioners at the bedside (the private sphere) and the advocates, policy makers, and researchers in the academy and the halls of power (the public sphere). Part III, by co-author Dr Pati Dzotsenidze, presents the challenges of advocating for basic palliative care development in the Republic of Georgia, a former Soviet republic.

Part I

Key definitions and basic principles of palliative care advocacy

The noun 'advocacy' and the verb 'to advocate' are derived from the Latin '*voc*', which is related to 'speech'. Etymologically, the term 'advocate' has been associated with courtrooms and judicial processes. Advocacy for health policy is defined as the processes by which the actions of individuals or groups attempt to bring about social and/or organization change on behalf of a particular health goal, programme, interest, or population. Health advocacy includes educating policy makers and the public about evidence-based policy

(Petttus, 2020). Palliative care advocacy at the UN organizations refers to principles of international law and consensus language adopted by UN member states, and therefore relies on traditions of precedence and legal rationality (Habermas, 1989). Because palliative care is a relatively new discipline in the public and global health pantheons, it has been, by definition, missing from the received narrative (precedence), which currently lists government obligations as disease prevention and health promotion, treatment, and rehabilitation (WHO, 1978). Palliative care advocacy seeks to expand that narrative to include attention to serious health-related suffering, data and evidence for which have been absent until very recently. We have had quite a few successes at the global level in the last decade, successes that can be leveraged by palliative care advocates at the regional, national, municipal, and local levels of governance.

Palliative care is the active holistic care of individuals across all ages with serious health-related suffering[1] due to severe illness,[2] and especially of those near the end of life. It aims to improve the quality of life of patients, their families, and their caregivers.

Palliative care:

- Includes prevention, early identification, comprehensive assessment, and management of physical issues, including pain and other distressing symptoms, psychological distress, spiritual distress, and social needs. Whenever possible, these interventions must be evidence based.
- Provides support to help patients live as fully as possible until death by facilitating effective communication, helping them and their families determine goals of care.
- Is applicable throughout the course of an illness, according to the patient's needs.
- Is provided in conjunction with disease-modifying therapies whenever needed.
- May positively influence the course of illness.
- Intends neither to hasten nor postpone death, affirms life, and recognizes dying as a natural process.
- Provides support to the family and the caregivers during the patient's illness, and in their own bereavement.
- Is delivered recognizing and respecting the cultural values and beliefs of the patient and the family.
- Is applicable throughout all healthcare settings (place of residence and institutions) and in all levels (primary to tertiary).
- Can be provided by professionals with basic palliative care training.
- Requires specialist palliative care with a multiprofessional team for referral of complex cases.

The five interrelated principles of palliative care advocacy, discussed briefly in what follows, are solidarity, participation, rights and obligations, subsidiarity, and proximity. This list is by no means exhaustive and can be supplemented or replaced by advocates engaging in their own visioning and strategic planning processes. Palliative care advocacy at all levels of governance, grounded in the principles enumerated, can stay the course when things get rough, as they inevitably will, given the setbacks and tensions that inevitably accompany paradigm shifts. The paradigm shift at stake here is transformation of the current system of neoliberal social service and healthcare 'delivery systems' that prioritize cure and profitability, leaving many patients and communities behind, into equitable systems that prioritize attention to the needs of the most underserved: the chronically ill, differently abled, older persons, and the bereaved—to name only a few groups on the peripheries. Worldwide, over 56.8 million people are estimated to require palliative care every year including 31.1 million prior to and 25.7 million near the end of life. The majority (67.1%) are adults over 50 years old and at least 7% are children. The majority (54.2%) are non-decedents who need palliative care prior to their last year of life (Worldwide Hospice Palliative Care Alliance, 2020).

Solidarity

The palliative care advocacy principle of solidarity aligns with the central palliative care ethical principle of non-abandonment. Palliative care advocates are committed to not abandoning any populations with unmet palliative care needs. This commitment brings palliative care advocacy into the political arena where it might otherwise have stayed in the academy, or within the halls of power of healthcare institutions. Evidence-based advocacy for patients with unmet palliative care is political because it calls on *governments* to be accountable for the welfare of their populations (citizens and non-citizens alike) throughout the life course, including through death, dying, and bereavement. Advocacy's political nature, or preoccupation with what is public, common, and general,[3] is an overt expression of solidarity with those left furthest behind by existing health systems. Solidarity, by definition, entails active citizenship, in the sense of informed participation in the political arena—through constructive engagement with relevant lawmakers, diplomats and civil servants. Solidarity expresses recognition of our inherent common mortality and interrelatedness based on the intrinsic equality and dignity of persons, overcoming barriers of class, ethnicity, language, profession, faith, and so on.

> There is no true solidarity without social participation, without the contribution of intermediary bodies: families, associations, cooperatives, small businesses, and other expressions of society. Everyone needs to contribute, everyone. This type of participation helps to prevent and to correct certain negative aspects of globalization and government action, as also occurs in caring for the people affected by the pandemic. These contributions 'from the bottom' should be encouraged [. . .] This is solidarity and this is the principle of subsidiarity. (Vatican News, 2020)

---

1 'Suffering is health-related when it is associated with illness or injury of any kind. Health-related suffering is serious when it cannot be relieved without professional intervention and when it compromises physical, social, spiritual, and/or emotional functioning.' (http://pallipedia.org/serious-health-related-suffering-shs/)

2 'Severe illness is any acute or chronic illness and/or health condition that carries a high risk of mortality, negatively impacts quality of life and daily function, and/or is burdensome in symptoms, treatments, or caregiver stress.' (https://pallipedia.org/severe-illness/)

3 The 'political' is what Hannah Pitkin (1993), following Sheldon Wolin (1970), calls the 'we', the collectivity, the shared public interest which is developed by means of discourse and requires a plurality of viewpoints.

> The words 'public,' 'common,' and 'general,' Wolin maintains, 'have a long tradition of usage which has made them synonyms for what is political. ... From its very beginnings in Greece, the Western political tradition has looked upon the political order as a common order created to deal with those concerns in which all of the members of society have some interest.' (Pikin, 1993, p. 209, citing Wolin, 1970, p. 9)

Advocacy based on the principle of solidarity breathes life into the rather rarefied concept of intersectionality.[4] Palliative care advocacy is strengthened by our commitment to empower and make visible the palliative care needs of groups that are normally invisible in the medical/charitable/privatized model. This includes, but is not limited to, persons with disabilities, older persons, children and youth, women, incarcerated persons, and undocumented persons.

Participation

The sort of participatory citizenship exercised by advocates for persons experiencing serious health-related suffering transcends the postmodern individualistic citizenship statuses of 'stakeholder', consumer, voter, or bystander. The advocacy of active palliative care citizens in solidarity with patients left behind by contemporary 'healthcare' systems entails participation because it makes palliative care a public issue in the public *sphere*: its provision is a public *good*. The faith-based and philanthropically funded organizations that currently deliver what palliative care there is to underserved populations in the majority of the world's countries, do not need to participate in the public sphere, and can only meet a fraction of population need. This chapter argues that these micro-services are the palliative care seeds needed for publicly funded integration at the population level.

Advocates are patients, families, providers, *and* patients, or legitimate representatives of those impacted populations who engage politically in the public sphere, including in the global public sphere, where international law is shaped and debated. This is very challenging for some, given that their professional realm, and the realm of the seriously ill, is the private sphere—the intimate ambit of the bedside, the clinic, and their professional community—sites of entirely different norms, practices, and rationalities than those that exist in the UN organizations constituted by international law and multilateral agreements. Palliative care advocates participate via institutions: the institutional framework that supports and nourishes this palliative care solidarity consists of duly chartered and registered international, regional, and national non-governmental organizations of palliative care practitioners. Palliative care advocacy requires administrative structures, leadership, vision, strategic planning, and a commitment to the long haul.

Palliative care advocates participate as members of 'civil society'—what the UN defines as the 'third sector' alongside member states and business (UN, n.d.). The category of civil society encompasses professional associations such as palliative care organizations, academia, faith-based organizations, associations of underserved populations such as persons with disabilities and older persons, and community-based associations. The UN system recognizes civil society organizations as 'essential partners' in its work and, following a rigorous programme of evaluation, authorizes applicant organizations to participate in in the meeting of its organizations. Relevant UN organizations that allow civil society participation for global palliative care advocacy are the WHO, the Commission on Narcotic Drugs, the Human Rights Council, the UN General Assembly, and the Open-Ended Working Group on Ageing.

Rights and responsibilities

A rights-based approach to health requires health policy and programmes to prioritize the needs of those furthest behind first towards greater equity, a principle that has been echoed in the recently adopted 2030 Agenda for Sustainable Development and Universal Health Coverage (UN General Assembly, 2015). In the context of palliative care advocacy, those left furthest behind in most countries are the persons experiencing chronic and severe illness and suffering, their caregivers, and the communities lacking integrated palliative care services. Palliative care advocacy uses context-specific data on serious health-related suffering to expose this equity gap and claim violations of the rights to health and freedom from cruel and inhumane treatment (IAHPC, 2019b). The second feature of a rights-based approach is meaningful participation of 'affected communities', discussed previously. Ensuring such participation of those communities as key informants entails including non-governmental organizations in all phases of programming: assessment, analysis, planning, implementation, monitoring, and evaluation (WHO, 2017).

States' obligations to fulfil the right to health means that they must take positive action to facilitate its 'enjoyment'. With regard to palliative care, 'States are under the obligation to respect the right to health by [. . .] refraining from denying or limiting equal access for *all persons*, including prisoners or detainees, minorities, asylum-seekers and illegal immigrants, to preventive, curative *and* palliative health services' (UN Committee on Economic, Social and Cultural Rights, 2000). States *deny* or *limit* equal access through acts of omission, when they fail to support and expand existing services to meet population needs. Palliative care advocacy showcases the work of the existing, usually struggling, palliative care services and presents policy makers with evidence regarding the preventable, serious, health-related suffering[1,2] that governments have undertaken to alleviate through integration of palliative care into primary healthcare (WHO, 2018).

The responsibilities that are the counterparts of their rights, call community members to act in solidarity with those in need in the community, be that the local, national, regional, or global community. Furthermore, it is the state's responsibility to protect the rights of all its people, and particularly those of its members with less material power, those left furthest behind. The state should never abdicate its responsibility to work actively to protect the rights of its most vulnerable and underserved members.

Subsidiarity

Subsidiarity is connected to both solidarity and proximity, discussed later. It focuses on the auxiliary role of government, implying that services should be delivered by those with greatest proximity to the citizen. Implicit in the idea is the assumption that the local power can perform its activities and services just as efficiently as a more distant tier of government, if not more so. The principle of subsidiarity recognizes the appropriate functions of all levels of governance, including the international, with its supra-national human rights and international law framework. The principle of subsidiarity recognizes and celebrates the validity and necessity of

4 'Definition of intersectionality: the complex, cumulative way in which the effects of multiple forms of discrimination (such as racism, sexism, and classism) combine, overlap, or intersect, especially in the experiences of marginalized individuals or groups. [Kimberlé] Crenshaw introduced the theory of intersectionality, the idea that when it comes to thinking about how inequalities persist, categories like gender, race, and class are best understood as overlapping and mutually constitutive rather than isolated and distinct.' (Meriam Webster, 2021)

all levels of service, from the hyperlocal to the cosmopolitan. An argument can be made that the international law governing access to controlled essential palliative care medicines for the patient at the bedside violates this principle of subsidiarity, as it imposes a 'one-size-fits-all' regulatory model on all UN member states, creating inherent disadvantages for those with less developed bureaucracies, no domestic pharmaceutical industry, and fewer resources for health budgets.

Proximity

Proximity is related to subsidiarity in that advocates who are most *proximate* to the populations with unmet palliative care needs know best the context in which they are operating, and the needs of the populations they serve. This proximity is useful for advocacy as it can trigger empathy, itself born of proximity to suffering. Advocates should be close—proximate—to the subject of their advocacy with policy makers in the hope that proximity will draw them into the ad hoc, strategic alliances that will shift the 'healthcare industry' paradigm to one that features a preferential option for the most underserved, including the seriously ill, dying, and bereaved. This is why palliative care practitioners, patients, and caregivers, rather than policy 'experts', make the best advocates: they are proximate to serious health-related suffering of which they speak. That said, nonclinical policy experts can be proximate to the populations they advocate for through volunteering or family caregiving. Proximity ensures that their advocacy is not abstract or disassociated but engaged *praxis*. Advocacy rooted in the principle of proximity is authentic and legitimate, the fruit of lived experience that can be presented as stories, rather than exclusively through data. Although palliative care advocacy should always be evidence based, the principle of proximity counsels that patients, providers, and caregivers can present that evidence as experts in their own right and should be given the floor whenever possible. Proximity unites the head to the heart, ensuring a more powerful message in the public sphere. Palliative care advocates cannot buy seats at the table in the halls of power, they must persuade their way in, using legal arguments, data, connections, and storytelling.

These principles inform the IAHPC's global advocacy for improved access to essential palliative care medicines, discussed in the following section. They are applicable to all levels of governance, from the local and municipal, to the national, regional, and local levels.

Part II

Advocacy for improved access to essential palliative care medicines

Essential palliative care medicines are those medicines and their formulations included in the *WHO Model List of Essential Medicines* (WHO, 2021) The WHO has published the Model List since 1977, updating it every 2 years. The Model List contains the medications considered to be most effective and safe to meet the most important needs in a health system to satisfy the primary healthcare needs of the population. It is based on the scientific evidence of the comparative effectiveness, safety, and cost-effectiveness. Governments, especially of LMICs, often use the Model List to develop their own national lists of essential medicines. Since 2013, the Model List has included a specific list of medications for the management of severe pain, symptoms, and palliative care under Section 2. This signals to WHO member states that they must take the necessary steps to ensure correct estimation of need, adequate procurement, and public availability of the medications needed for the management of pain and palliative care, just as they do for other conditions.

Some of the essential palliative care medicines such as morphine, fentanyl, hydromorphone, oxycodone, and methadone (also called strong opioids) are *also* listed, or 'scheduled' for extra regulatory control under the international drug control conventions.[5] These medications are essential for the treatment of moderate to severe pain and dyspnoea in advanced disease. The latest evidence shows that the majority of the world's people lack access to essential palliative care medicines in large part because of lack of appropriate workforce training and unduly restrictive regulatory barriers arising from their inclusion in the schedules of the international drug control conventions (International Narcotics Control Board, 2018).

The Single Convention on Narcotic Drugs, which has been ratified by 193 UN member states, dates back to the mid-twentieth century before the development of palliative medicine and well before the collection of population level data on serious health-related suffering and the 'pain divide' (Knaul et al., 2015). Because the drug control conventions are not 'self-executing treaties',[6] states must promulgate and enforce their own national drug control laws and regulations, many of which are much stricter than the controls stipulated in the conventions. Such national regulations become unduly restrictive barriers to access to essential palliative care medicines, as is the case in the Republic of Georgia and many other LMICs.

Not only do many national drug control laws mandate harsh punishments for people who use drugs non-medically, they lack positive regulatory frameworks directing states to provide the adequate access to controlled medications stipulated in the conventions (Husain et al., 2014). In other words, the vast majority of *national* drug control laws promulgated to comply with the *international* conventions stipulate no provisions for securing supply chains for essential palliative care medicines or training health workforces in appropriate use. This catastrophic public health failure is yet another casualty of the ongoing global 'war on drugs', inscribed in neocolonial narratives and early twentieth-century legal texts drafted and upheld until very recently by civil servants operating with incomplete information and lack of evidence about 'addiction', treatment, and pain therapies (Pettus, 2019). Global palliative care advocacy is one expression of the movement to 'decolonize' global health structures developed and imposed by the imperial powers on 'their' far-flung empires. Indeed, the global pandemic of untreated

5 Single Convention on Narcotic Drugs 1961 (as amended by the 1972 Protocol) (30 March 1961), UNTS vol. 520 no. 7515 (hereinafter 'Single Convention'); 1971 Convention on Psychotropic Substances (21 February 1971) UNTS vol. 1019 no. 14956 (hereinafter '1971 Convention'); UN Convention against the Illicit Traffic in Narcotic Drugs and Psychotropic Substances (20 December 1988) UNTS vol. 1582 no. 27627.

6 'A self-executing treaty is a treaty that becomes judicially enforceable upon ratification. As opposed to a non- self-executing treaty, which becomes judicially enforceable through the implementation of legislation.' (https://www.law.cornell.edu/wex/self_executing_treaty)

pain maps seamlessly onto the cartographies of saltwater and settler colonialism (Pettus, 2019).

This international legal architecture, or 'drug control machinery' as the UN Office on Drugs and Crime calls it, violates the principle of subsidiarity discussed in Part I.

Global advocates challenge the received 'drug control' narrative

The advocacy principles of participation and solidarity were evident in the process that challenged the entrenched discursive hegemony of drug rhetoric that never considered access to essential medicines a policy priority for UN member states. This global consensus that focused almost exclusively on 'supply control' and ignored the unmet palliative care needs of the majority of the world's people only began to fracture when advocates such as the Pain and Policy Studies Group (Cleary and Maurer, 2018), Human Rights Watch (Ezer et al., 2018), the Union for International Cancer Control, the European Society for Medical Oncology, the IAHPC (2020), the International Drug Policy Consortium, and other academic/civil society collaborations participating in UN meetings began to rewrite the controlled medicines narrative by participating in meetings of the relevant UN organizations.

Civil society advocates now consistently raise the issue of inadequate access to internationally controlled essential palliative care medicines *as a treaty violation*—essentially an error of *omission*, or neglect, rather than *commission* on the part of most member states—at meetings of the Commission on Narcotic Drugs, the WHO, the UN General Assembly, and the International Narcotics Control Board. Now that the peer-reviewed evidence exists to support equitable development and integration of palliative care, as well as evidence-based prevention and treatment programmes for persons with substance use disorder included in 'Model Drug Laws' (Global Commission on Drugs, 2018), member states have no excuse for perpetuating archaic, neocolonial policies and regulations.

States parties to the UN drug control conventions and WHO member states will only be able to change these policies with the collaboration of key informants from duly constituted and registered civil society organizations. Hence the need for advocacy by 'multi-stakeholder collaborations' that establishes a human rights- and public health-based narrative (Pettus, 2018). *Implementation* at the national level of the fruits of advocacy that have resulted in multilateral commitments is quite a different story though. Responses are unique to every member state and are directly related to the degree of advocacy by national and local palliative care associations and municipalities that support integrated service delivery. Multi-stakeholder, culturally specific, intersectional, advocacy strategies that place the well-being of individuals, families, and communities at the centre of national policies are required at *all* levels of governance to ensure the delivery of community and home-based services for all who need them.

It is this 'pharmaceutical' aspect of palliative care—the palliative medicine domain—that is implicated in international law and calls for official engagement, policy development, budgets, and workforce training. Official engagement is directly related to the advocacy generated and expressed at the grassroots level by providers, patients, and civil society organizations in a synergistic feedback loop. Once this engagement reaches the highest levels of national decision-making for public health, education, drug control, and finance, it aligns with the global normative framework, constructed by the foreign affairs ministries of those very same UN member states, which commits them to integrating palliative care and ensuring adequate access to essential medicines.

Nuts and bolts

The IAHPC has chalked up some advocacy wins in recent years as a result of systematic strategic planning combined with relationship building across multiple domains. Through these small victories we inch towards our vision of a world free from health-related suffering. The wins have never been accomplished by this organization alone, but always in partnership with other non-governmental organizations working on the ground. Getting to know key players, doing situation analyses based on data, 'power mapping', and 'spheres of influence' exercises as a core group is essential at the start of an advocacy campaign. A variety of manuals and excellent health advocacy guides have been published including by the WHO (2020), Oxfam (2020), and the Public Health Advocacy Institute of Western Australia (2019).

The process of birthing an advocacy campaign usually begins by convening a core group of local champions and palliative care leaders, including patients and caregivers wherever possible, and engaging in a moderated strategic planning process culminating in consensus mission and vision statements, followed by long- and short-term SMART (Specific, Measurable, Achievable, Relevant and Time-bound) objectives and outcomes (Minnesota Department of Health, 2020). Leadership training is helpful for core group members to learn basic skills in maintaining the vision and shepherding the mission along. This often involves managing the inevitable tensions and stumbling blocks that present themselves on what is usually a long and challenging road. One of these is always lack of sustainable funding for advocacy, as few donors see the cost:benefit ratio when progress is so difficult to see and measure. Another is the temptation to do too much and burn out rather than to delegate and encourage the skills of co-workers and fellow core group members.

These challenges highlight the importance of vision and the leadership called for to maintain it when the going gets rough. A visioning process for palliative care advocacy and service delivery is necessary done in community that includes representatives of all key 'stakeholders'—those who will carry out the work and those most impacted by it. The vision needs to include an ethos not only of self-care but care for one another. The ongoing coronavirus disease (COVID-19) pandemic has highlighted the importance of this need for psycho-spiritual, as well as social support of 'frontliners'. This vision conceives of the global policy advocacy community, the practitioners, and the patients and families we all serve as a 'beloved community'. (MLK Foundation) The vision is not necessarily something that will happen only in the future, but something that already exists. It is codified in international law, in the human rights conventions and the preambular paragraphs of resolutions and high-level political declarations that recognize the inherent dignity of the human person. Many tools and courses are available to support leadership training for palliative care advocacy, including the pioneering Global Leadership Development Initiative initiated by the San Diego Institute for Palliative Medicine (International Palliative Care Resource Center, 2011) (reported by Ferris et al., 2018).

It goes without saying that twenty-first-century advocacy requires competence in the use of social media platforms as well as traditional media outlets to get the message out about the benefits of palliative care and to connect with allies and wider publics. Advocates need digital competence as well as basic training in public speaking and presentation development to hone essential communications skills.

Palliative care advocacy at all levels of governance is an uphill slog as it introduces a new narrative calling for systems change and policy development into the received and lucrative global health narrative that prioritizes saving lives and reducing 'preventable mortality'. The challenge of expanding that narrative to include public health palliative care is to find 'ears that hear' and leaders with the courage to take risks. Tangible rewards along the way can be thin on the ground, so it is important to always keep the patient and family at the centre of concern, celebrate wins, and build productive relationships with both natural allies and 'strange bedfellows'. Palliative care advocates need passion, resilience, and 'fire in the belly' to quote a long-time mentor, Dr Anne Merriman, Founder of Hospice Africa Uganda and a wildly successful advocate for oral morphine, nurse prescribing, and home-based services in one of the poorest countries in the world. Operationalizing the principles discussed in Part I of this chapter has been core to the incremental successes in ensuring inclusion of palliative care and controlled medicines in the global health and 'drug control' narratives. The process of gathering data and measuring serious health-related suffering to build a solid foundation of evidence-based advocacy is ongoing.

Conclusion

Successful integration of palliative care, a relatively new, insurgent specialty, into fragile and under-resourced primary healthcare systems in lower-, middle-, and upper middle-income countries such as the Republic of Georgia, entails advocacy for national policy development and budgeting in the following areas: procurement and regulation of internationally controlled essential palliative care medicines; workforce strengthening and professional education; and improved primary healthcare service delivery and financing. This is because governments are the gatekeepers for access to essential palliative care medicines. They approve procurement quotas and oversee manufacturing, distribution, and consumption of all substances under international control, including opioids. Advocacy is the connective tissue between the international health law framework that includes normative and technical guidance on inclusion of palliative care, and national law and practice that lacks or even undermines those elements. At the time of writing, palliative care services and essential palliative care medicines are available to only a small fraction of the world's population, largely resident in upper-income countries (Knaul et al., 2018; Worldwide Hospice Palliative Care Alliance, 2020). These countries tend to have strong health systems, high political transparency scores, and robust civil society participation rates (Transparency International, 2021). Community- and home-based palliative care, grounded in the principles of solidarity, subsidiarity, and proximity, are the future. To be sustainable and adequately resourced, they must be brought to light by local people working in their own villages, neighbourhoods, and cities, in the context of a legal and regulatory framework that supports appropriate training and access to essential medicines and services.

What follows is a brief reflection written by a palliative care professional and researcher from the Republic of Georgia, who describes the challenges and successes of advocacy in her country for palliative care services. She envisions how a modern compassionate community might take root in this ancient republic that only recently emerged as an independent state from the former USSR.

Part III

Case Study: Introduction

The Republic of Georgia is located in Caucasia with a population of 3.731 million and an area of 69,700 square kilometres. Although the World Bank considers Georgia an upper middle-income country, it has many problems, among them the availability of the palliative care services. About 44,000 people with serious health-related suffering are in need of palliative care in Georgia annually (IAHPC, 2019a).

Citizens within the post-Soviet space find it challenging to discern the boundaries between private and public healthcare services and government responsibilities to ensure availability and accessibility. Although quality of services varied throughout the Soviet Union, healthcare services were available and accessible free of charge for all Soviet citizens. It was possible to stay in hospital even with mild symptoms for months, getting free food and care. Both terminal illnesses and minor health problems were institutionalized during the Soviet era. The medical ethos was paternalistic: the physician was the main decision maker in most cases, usually preferring aggressive interventions. Thus, all responsibilities regarding the health issues of families and communities were handed over to healthcare professionals and institutions. Patients and their families expected aggressive treatment until the end of the life: if they didn't get it, they felt underserved or poorly treated. Since anything associated with religion and spirituality was suspect, patients and families had no non-clinical assistance in the case of an unfavourable prognoses. Patients were not told their diagnoses, as their voices were not considered important. Patients had no right to make decisions and had no right to ask to ask for relief of their pain and suffering.

I (PD) first learned about palliative care through my work in neuro-oncology in the late 1990s. Reading Western medical literature made me think about quality of life and the need to involve patients and families in treatment planning. The misconceptions and attitudes about health on the part of both professionals and the public made me want to run away from the problems. It was clear that providing only disease-focused treatment wasn't enough and that something was necessary to fill the gaps in care and relationships.

While accompanying my husband on assignment in Zambia, I learned how much can be done just by supporting people in need and offering them comfort care. This experience confirmed my suspicion that something was terribly wrong with the system in my country that must be changed. When I returned to Georgia in 2007, I joined the Georgian National Association for Palliative Care and in 2008 became fellow of the Pain Policy Studies Group, based in Madison, Wisconsin. Since that period, I have actively participated in almost all activities concerning palliative care and pain management in Georgia, including the development of national guidelines, palliative care policy work, and improvement of opioid availability and accessibility for incurable patients. Though we have had some success, including changes in legislation (the last was the new definition of palliative and hospice care, which was introduced in the laws of Georgia on Health Care and Patients' Rights in 2019) and working with the high-level health authorities and officials from the ministry, we have seen no tangible results and implementation on the ground. Our success in the various policy domains was the result of continuous work, including advocacy, with all possible interested parties, civil society organizations, and decision makers.

The main reason for the low success rate in policy implementation is lack of public involvement in the process (the principle of participation). The lack of interest and awareness regarding palliative care, added to ongoing stresses such as socioeconomic and political instability, have led to a socially depressed and inactive society. If we really want to succeed, we need to empower public and local communities to make them part of the ongoing process: strengthening their 'we-feeling' (the principle of solidarity) by creating clear examples regarding the benefits of palliative care for families. We have to build the bridge between field experts and the public so government officials hear the voices of their constituents.

Basic situation analysis

Despite the existence of a vertical state programme for palliative care, only 17% of palliative care need is met in the country. There are several reasons for this poor national coverage. Distribution of palliative care services is inequitable: for example, currently almost all inpatient palliative care units are located in Tbilisi and only two-bed unit services are available in three more cities of Georgia (Batumi, Kutaisi, and Zugdidi). Home-based palliative care services are available in only six out of 76 municipalities/cities of Georgia (Tbilisi, Telavi, Kutaisi, Ozurgeti, Gori, and Zugdidi).

The state programme 'Palliative Care for Incurable Patients'[7] covers only terminally ill patients, who need such services only at the end of life. Ambulatory patients can only receive home-based service for 3–6 months. This means that physicians' medical decision-making processes are based solely on prognosis and severity of illness. Their impact on patient quality of life is not considered.

The state programme limits the home-based visits to physician and/or nurse services, though physicians must document all activities. Quality of the care is also a problem because no professional palliative care services are available for home-based care patients. Family doctors are the main providers of palliative care for home-based services and they have no special training. The same goes for nurses. The maximum number of visits allowed per month is eight and the budget is limited, which discourages health professionals' involvement. This makes it impossible to provide quality palliative care and ensure a multidisciplinary approach with holistic care.

Opioids are very strictly regulated in Georgia and can only be prescribed to 'incurable' outpatients in the terminal stage when no other treatment options are left. However, opioids are not always prescribed even to incurable patients to relieve pain and suffering. Like many post-Soviet countries, the strict regulations in Georgia were supported by the approaches of the former Soviet medical education system regarding chronic pain management with opioids, where the issue was almost neglected. Physicians who lack training about management of chronic pain and rational opioid prescribing according to medical need, disdain opioids and don't prescribe them.

A recent study of the issue found that physicians who practise in rural areas and have closer professional connections with the patients and their family/caregivers have more positive attitudes to opioids as a result of their relationships (the principle of proximity). These attitudes are based on their sense of community. Physicians in rural areas who assess patients more thoroughly and perceive their condition more compassionately, demonstrate empathy and exhibit less negativity about prescribing opioids.

The study also showed that, although physicians living in the capital city have more knowledge regarding medical use of opioids, they still consider that non-opioid pain medications are equally effective for treating severe cancer pain. They write new prescription on particular days of the week, rather than prescribing according to the patient's needs, preferring to follow stricter regulations. We attribute this attitude towards pain treatment with opioid analgesics to their infrequent communications with patients, rare assessment of pain, and lack of accurate information about patients' conditions. As opioids are mostly prescribed too late, at the end of life, patients are no longer able to visit physicians themselves. Mostly, after prescribing the morphine, physicians maintain contact only with the family members/caregiver who pick up prescriptions every week.

We concluded from this study that compassion is the power that can overcome and change attitudes, fears, and misconceptions. We asked ourselves, can we awaken innate compassion and channel it for the common good?

Compassionate youth in order to help older people during the COVID-19 epidemic

One recent case during the first months of the COVID-19 pandemic is a good example of compassion. The government was unable to fully respond to the population's needs, and set many restrictions, including mobility limitations for older people. To respond to their needs, young people organized social networks and mobilized volunteers within communities. They identified more vulnerable older persons or persons who lived alone and distributed food, medicines, and other goods. For example, three young woman, the 'three Mariams', were able to mobilize a significant number of compassionate citizens as volunteers in Tbilisi with the aim ' to help elderly'[8] (https://www.facebook.com/groups/483937615824418/about). The compassion of people during the COVID-19 pandemic has shown that a lot of them are ready to support and help others in need, to use their innate compassion and transform it for common interests.

The extended family has been strong in Georgia until recent decades. Even today, families are never left alone during bereavement and grief and are always surrounded and supported by caring relatives and friends. Many families find relief in religious rituals performed during and after funerals. This could be the main explanation for the weak development of a culture of volunteerism in the country: 'For cultural reasons the provision of formal long-term care is limited, as families are expected to care for their elderly or disabled relatives' (Richardson and Berdzuli, 2017, p. 63). However,

7 The state programme 'Palliative Care for Incurable Patients' covers the following components: stationary and home-based services and opioids for outpatients.

8 See https://www.facebook.com/groups/483937615824418/about.

industrialization, urbanization, and a huge migration process (mostly women and youth) have influenced or weakened those relationships. In addition, 'high rates of unemployment and poverty make it very difficult for many families to uphold this tradition' (Richardson and Berdzuli, 2017, p. 63). Currently, in the face of the unmet needs of caring for palliative care patients, the resource of compassionate people can be efficiently used by raising awareness among the community and training volunteers.

The best mini-compassionate community that already exists in Georgia is the Transfiguration Hospice at Mercy Center Tbilisi, Transfiguration Monastery. It is a charitable organization that provides palliative care and spiritual support to patients with incurable diseases at home (in Tbilisi) and in the hospice, free of charge. Mercy Center Tbilisi was established in 2003 and was the first hospice-type facility in Georgia.

Physicians, nurses, caregivers, and volunteers compose the hospice team. The organization has a professional school for caregivers, where any interested person can learn the basics of care according to international standards at no charge. The Mercy learning centre is supported by the Patriarchy of Georgia. Home care and inpatient services are financed by donations. The main aim of the Mercy Center Tbilisi is to support people at difficult and important times of their lives, care for them, and share with the patients the experience of their illness, suffering, and the importance of life and death.

The compassionate staff of the hospice collaborate with the palliative care professionals and the Georgian team for the sustainability of palliative care development[9] with the aim of strengthening the community and community-based palliative care services in Georgia. They believe that already trained, coordinated, and motivated communities will be the best way for the government to improve polices and expand the services in the whole country.

How to plan to help people release their innate compassion and use it in the frame of public health

Palliative care cannot be carried out only by the state programmes: it needs to be coordinated throughout the healthcare system with society, church/faith organizations, non-governmental organizations, media, and community groups. There is a need to raise awareness about palliative care in the general public, and promote volunteerism countrywide by strengthening local communities for self-organization. It is critical to include the community in the development of palliative care, and to facilitate collaborations with the government and community to provide end of life services. There is also a need to improve skills of the healthcare professionals through training, providing specific education, and expanding palliative care services.

The best way to reach all people in need and within their communities is to integrate palliative care services into primary healthcare with the support of organizations within the community groups (principle of proximity). In such cases, the experience of the system of polyclinics widely used in former Soviet countries, the primary healthcare facilities serving patients according to living places throughout the communities and nowadays combined with the system of family doctors in Georgia, can be particularly valuable. But it will be impossible to connect the social, clinical, and community care dots if systemic changes are not enacted through policy. For instance, if the patient is not at the end of life, the physician cannot provide palliative care at the community level and the volunteers from the community without support and feedback from health professionals will not be able to provide enough support to palliative care patients. Thus, the government must establish policies that will enable early interventions for the palliative care patients, where the main supportive force will be community, with the feedback from the primary healthcare professionals.

Takeaways

Advocacy for integrating palliative care in the lower-, middle-, and upper middle-income countries is necessary at all levels of health system governance because:

1. Governments are the legally mandated gatekeepers for access to essential palliative care medicines. The majority of UN member states with low to inadequate access to opioids, unstable political and governmental systems, and low or antagonistic levels of engagement with civil society—including professional medical associations—are ignorant of the benefits of palliative care for their health systems and populations. Practitioners in those countries need the support of the international community and need to know about the global normative framework developed through evidence-based advocacy.
2. Advocacy can overcome the knowledge abyss regarding how international law and non-self-executing treaties allow UN member states to promulgate unduly restrictive regulations that create barriers to essential palliative care medicines. Advocacy can help these legal instruments become fit for twenty-first-century purposes to meet 2030 Agenda 2030 goals and targets.
3. Advocacy reminds governments that they are constituted to produce public goods, such as palliative care, essential for meeting 2030 Agenda goals and targets. Private foundations, charities, and communities can only produce randomized *private* goods for families and patients fortunate enough to fall within their often resource-limited catchment areas. Private insurance, philanthrocapitalism and charity alone cannot fulfil a rights-based, fit for purpose, vision of health for all in the twenty-first century.

REFERENCES

Cleary, J. F. and Maurer, M. A. 2018. Pain and Policy Studies Group: two decades of working to address regulatory barriers to improve opioid availability and accessibility around the world. *Journal of Pain and Symptom Management*, 55, S121–S134.

European Society for Medical Oncology. 2011. Global access to pain relief. [Online] Available at: https://www.esmo.org/content/download/14123/252826/file/Global-Access-to-Pain-Relief-Evidence-for-Action.pdf

European Society for Medical Oncology. 2013. ESMO press release: untreated cancer pain a 'scandal of global proportions,' survey shows. [Online] Available at: https://www.esmo.org/newsroom/press-office/ESMO-Press-Release-Untreated-Cancer-Pain-a-Scandal-of-Global-Proportions-Survey-Shows

9 This team consists of people working in different professional fields, who had together shared the experience of St Christopher's Hospice in 2019 supported by the PACED Foundation and the hospice staff itself, and works in different directions to support sustainable palliative care development in Georgia, including policy, regulatory fields, and awareness. Currently the group members are working on the new palliative care strategy.

Ezer, T., Lohman, D., and de Luca, G. B. 2018. Palliative care and human rights: a decade of evolution in standards. *Journal of Pain and Symptom Management,* 55, S163–S169.

Ferris, F. D., Moore, S. Y., Callaway, M. V., and Foley, K. M. 2018. Leadership development initiative: growing global leaders . . . advancing palliative care. *Journal of Pain and Symptom Management,* 55, S146–S156.

Global Commission on Drugs. 2018. West Africa model drug law. [Online] Available at: https://www.globalcommissionondrugs.org/wp-content/uploads/2018/08/WADC-MDL-EN-WEB.pdf

Habermas, J. 1989. Towards a communication-concept of rational collective will-formation. A thought-experiment. *Ratio Juris,* 2, 144–154.

Husain, S. A., Brown, M. S., and Maurer, M. A. 2014. Do national drug control laws ensure the availability of opioids for medical and scientific purposes? *Bulletin of the World Health Organization,* 10, 108–116.

International Association for Hospice and Palliative Care. 2019a. Global data platform to calculate SHS and palliative care need. [Online] Available at: https://hospicecare.com/what-we-do/resources/global-data-platform-to-calculate-shs-and-palliative-care-need/

International Association for Hospice and Palliative Care. 2019b. Palliative care definition. [Online] Available at: https://hospicecare.com/what-we-do/projects/consensus-based-definition-of-palliative-care/definition/

International Association for Hospice and Palliative Care. 2020. Palliative care advocacy. [Online] Available at: https://hospicecare.com/what-we-do/programs/advocacy-program/

International Narcotics Control Board. 2018. *2018 Annual Report: Supplement.* Vienna: International Narcotics Control Board.

International Palliative Care Resource Center. 2011. Leadership development initiative. [Online] Available at: http://www.ipcrc.net/international-programs-LDI-overview.php

Knaul, F. M., Bhadelia, A., Arreola Ornelas, H., de Lima, L., and del Rocio Sáenz Madrigal, M. 2015. Closing the pain divide: the quest for effective universal health coverage. *Lancet Global Health,* 3, S35.

Knaul, F. M., Farmer, P. E., Krakauer, E. L., De Lima, L., Bhadelia, A., Jiang Kwete, X., et al. 2018. Alleviating the access abyss in palliative care and pain relief—an imperative of universal health coverage: the Lancet Commission report. *Lancet,* 391, 1391–1454.

Meriam Webster. 2021. Definition of intersectionality. [Online] Available at: https://www.merriam-webster.com/dictionary/intersectionality

Minnesota Department of Health, 2020. Smart objectives. [Online] Available at: https://www.health.state.mn.us/communities/practice/resources/phqitoolbox/objectives.html

MLK Foundation. n.d. The King Philosophy – Nonviolence365®. [Online] Available at: https://thekingcenter.org/king-philosophy/

Oxfam. 2020. Influencing for impact guide: how to deliver effective influencing strategies. [Online] Available at: https://www.phaiwa.org.au/the-advocacy-toolkit/

Pettus, K. 2019. Colonial roots of the global pandemic of untreated pain. In: Koram, K. (ed.) *The War on Drugs and the Color Line,* pp. 196–215. London: Pluto.

Pettus, K. 2020. Palliative care and the beloved community. [Online] Available at: https://globalpalliativecare.home.blog/2020/08/02/palliative-care-and-the-beloved-community/

Pettus, K. I. 2018. Improving access to internationally controlled essential medicines in the post-UNGASS, Agenda 2030 framework. In: Klein, A. and Stothard, B. (eds.) *Collapse of the Global Order on Drugs,* pp. 85–100. London: Emerald.

Petttus, K. I. and de Lima, L. 2020. Palliative care advocacy: why does it matter? *Journal of Pain and Symptom Management,* 23, 1009–1012.

Pikin, H. 1993. *Wittgenstein and Justice: On the Significance of Ludwig Wittgenstein for Social and Political Thought.* San Francisco, CA: University of California Press.

Public Health Advocacy Institute of Western Australia. 2019. Advocacy toolkit. [Online] Available at: https://www.phaiwa.org.au/the-advocacy-toolkit/

Richardson, E. and Berdzuli, N. 2017. Georgia: health system review. *Health Systems in Transition,* 19, 1–90.

Transparency International. 2020. Homepage. [Online]. Available at: https://www.transparency.org/en

UN Committee on Economic, Social and Cultural Rights (CESCR), General Comment No. 14: The Right to the Highest Attainable Standard of Health (Art. 12 of the Covenant), 11 August 2000, E/C.12/2000/4, available at: https://www.refworld.org/docid/4538838d0.html [accessed 19 May 2021].

United Nations. n.d. Civil society. [Online] Available at: https://www.un.org/en/civil-society/page/about-us

United Nations General Assembly. 2015. *Transforming Our World: The 2030 Agenda for Sustainable Development. Division for Sustainable Development Goals.* New York: United Nations.

Vatican News. 2020. Catechesis "healing the world": 8. Subsidiarity and virtue of hope. [Online] Available at: http://www.vatican.va/content/francesco/en/audiences/2020/documents/papa-francesco_20200923_udienza-generale.html

Wolin, S. 1970. *Politics and Vision.* New York: Harcourt Brace.

World Health Organization. 1978. *International Conference on Primary Health Care.* Geneva: World Health Organization.

World Health Organization. 2017. Right to health. [Online] Available at: https://www.who.int/news-room/fact-sheets/detail/human-rights-and-health

World Health Organization. 2018. *Astana Congress on Primary Health Care.* Geneva: World Health Organization.

World Health Organization. 2019a. Access to analgesics and to other controlled medications. [Online] Available at: https://www.who.int/medicines/areas/quality_safety/access_Contr_Med/en/

World Health Organization. 2019b. Newsroom/fact sheet/primary health care. [Online] Available at: https://www.who.int/news-room/fact-sheets/detail/primary-health-care

World Health Organization. 2019c. Universal health coverage. [Online] Available at: https://www.who.int/news-room/fact-sheets/detail/universal-health-coverage-(uhc)

World Health Organization 2020. Stop the Global Epidemic of Chronic Disease https://www.who.int/chp/advocacy/chp.manual.EN-webfinal.pdf

World Health Organization. 2020. Chronic diseases and health promotion. [Online] Available at: https://www.who.int/chp/advocacy/en/

World Health Organization. 2021. Model list of essential medicines. [Online] Available at: https://www.who.int/publications/i/item/WHO-MHP-HPS-EML-2021.02

Worldwide Hospice Palliative Care Alliance. 2020. *Global Atlas of Palliative Care,* 2nd ed. London: Worldwide Hospice Palliative Care Alliance.

15

Health promotion and palliative care

Andrea Grindrod

Introduction

Health promotion provides an evidence-based public health intervention framework to guide compassionate cities and communities. It also provides a framework to advocate for our most vulnerable citizens through compassionate policies that redress social inequality.

Health promotion is concerned with health across the life span but despite this has paid little attention to health at the end of life. Palliative care focuses on illness experience at the end of life, but often neglects broader issues of health because of its focus on the signs and symptoms of dying. Both disciplines can contribute to expanding our understanding of end of life experience, but to do so they must look beyond their preferred frameworks and learn to engage each other around people's diverse experiences at the end of their lives. While similarities arguably lie in shared values, differences can emerge depending on who is leading the work, and the fundamental purpose of what each field is designed to achieve. Health promotion uses a public health implementation framework through which complex health and social issues are examined and addressed, while palliative care is grounded in an illness-focused health services perspective. Put simply, health promotion provides the 'how' and palliative care provides the 'what'.

To understand the role of health promotion in palliative care services, we attend to well-being and the social dimensions of the provision of end of life care. To understand illness, dying, and death in the context of health promotion approaches, we focus on the principles and processes that create and maintain citizen choice and control through community participation that determines our sense of well-being at the end of our lives. These perspectives are of course inextricably linked, but the entry points differ. The two disciplines provide alternative lenses through which to view, examine, and understand the subject matter. This chapter argues that the theoretical perspective and practical application of health promotion strategies can improve end of life experiences when used in conjunction with palliative care strategies.

The case for health at the end of life

> 'Seriously ill people ought to be seen as qualifying for health promoting attention ... dying people, are not dead. People who are "dying" – that is, those who live with a terminal or life-threatening illness – are simply people who often know that they will die in a short while.'
>
> (Kellehear, 1999, p. 19)

Understanding and viewing health, within and from a health promotion standpoint, is fundamental to grasping the rationale of a health promotion approach. Health promotion practitioners adopt a broad understanding of health which shapes the strategies employed. The Ottawa Charter for Health Promotion (World Health Organization, 1986) defines health as a resource for everyday life, not the object of living. The emphasis is on social and personal resources. As Maclean (1988) puts it, 'if we are in the business of health promotion in the widest sense we should always remain sensitive to the enormous number of ways of defining health and disease which are held by ordinary people' (p. 43).

Evidence that lay people do not see health in the same way as health professionals (Hughner and Kleine, 2004) reiterates why assumptions about health are to be avoided. If health is so differently defined by diverse individuals and communities, we are likely to get quite different answers to the question, 'Is it possible to be healthy at the end of life?' The paradox of 'healthy dying' is reflected in societal views of death as antithetical to health; in the omission of dying and death from the field of health promotion; and in palliative care services, where a 'good death' is regarded as an aspirational goal, but measured by whose standards—health systems or citizens?

The story of a structured approach to combining health promotion and palliative care began with the seminal work of Allan Kellehear in *Health Promoting Palliative Care* (1999). The broad message of the book was that health promotion offered a framework to privilege the social dimensions and social practice of palliative care, captured in his reflections:

> Why should the prospect of death, an event more certain than illness, exclude anyone from health promotion consideration? ... Dying does not, and should not, disqualify anyone from quality health and social care ... since one of the greatest fears of those with a life-threatening

illness is the prospect of loss of control over their health and their lives more generally, health promotion can be an important source of empowerment and support. (Kellehear, 1999, pp. 15–16)

The rationale is simple. Almost universally, at the end of their lives, citizens wish to remain close to people, places, and possessions that are important to them (Heyland et al., 2006; Gardner and Kramer, 2010), and for the most part, this 'place' isn't a hospital bed. The translation of these wishes into reality brings to the foreground the social dimensions of living and dying with illness, frailty, and disability, bearing in mind the unique and subjective perceptions of health. Additionally, the social practice of caring is substantially met through the role of family, citizens, companions, carers, and community and case workers (social support services) (Horsfall et al., 2015; Rosenberg et al., 2015; Aoun et al., 2018; Ates et al., 2018). While palliative care practitioners provide essential medical, nursing, and allied health services, their expertise should ideally be delivered in the broader social context of living with illness and dying. Health promoters, on the other hand, provide expertise to stimulate citizen and community-driven participation that creates healthy environments for people to die in, according to their preferences and wishes.

If dying and death is viewed as a social event that may not require or receive healthcare intervention, it seems possible, at least from a theoretical and aspirational standpoint, to experience a healthy end of life. In practice, however, the experience can be quite different. The central question of this chapter explores how a sense of health and well-being in the context of illness, dying, death, and bereavement might be achieved. Or, as Kellehear (1999) puts it, 'what would health promotion look like for those whose illness is likely to end in death?' (p. 16). An essential precursor to clarifying this is to examine the driving principles of the health promotion and palliative care fields.

Conceptual clarity: health promotion and palliative care

Palliative care and health promotion use different language. Although this chapter argues for their integration and the subsequent emergent benefits, it's important to recognize that they are different fields of practice, designed to serve different purposes, using different methods. This becomes clear by referring to the evidence-base of whom each field is designed to serve, how this is achieved, and what they are assigned and accredited to do.

The World Health Organization (WHO) offers definitions for palliative care (WHO, 2020) and health promotion (WHO, n.d.). The WHO definition for palliative care discusses care for 'patients and their families', while health promotion refers to those it serves as 'citizens, communities and sectors'. Health promotion embraces enablement, by nurturing self-determination and citizen-driven approaches to redress the factors that harm health and well-being. Palliative and healthcare services, on the other hand, tend to engage with individuals who use their services—who then become patients. In this way palliative care services strive to organize their patients according to their systems, whereas health promotion strives to enable citizens to organize themselves, and the structures that influence their health.

Overview: health promotion

Health promotion is an implementation strategy designed to address complex health and social issues to improve the health and well-being of the public. The Ottawa Charter for Health Promotion (1986) provides an evidence-based practice framework to achieve public health goals at a population and individual level. The following definition of health promotion was developed at the WHO's first International Health Promotion Conference in Ottawa, Canada (1986):

> [Health promotion is] the process of enabling people to increase control over, and to improve, their health. To reach a state of complete physical, mental and social well-being, an individual or group must be able to identify and to realise aspirations, to satisfy needs, and to change or cope with the environment. Health is, therefore, seen as a resource for everyday life, not the object of living. Health is a positive concept emphasising social and personal resources, as well as physical capacities. Therefore, health promotion is not just the responsibility of the health sector, but goes beyond healthy life-styles to well-being. (WHO, 1986)

The Ottawa Charter provides the practice framework to achieve the objectives outlined in the definition of health promotion. Central themes of the definition that are important for its implementation are:

- *Enabling* people to increase control over their health and *well-being*.
- *Enabling* people to *identify* and *meet* their own aspirations and needs.
- Helping people to *change* or cope with the *environment*.
- Health is a *resource* for living, not the object of living.
- Emphasis on *personal* and *social resources*, as well as physical health.
- Health is *not* solely the responsibility of the health sector.

Essential to understanding health promotion is realizing that health and well-being are created outside the health system, where we live, work, learn, and age (WHO, 2008). Health is viewed as both a resource for, and an outcome of, our social circumstances. The healthcare sector provides important services for restoring our health when problems emerge. In the context of the end of life, when physical health can no longer be restored, palliative care services provide important pain and symptom relief, professional care and comfort, within the circumstances of our lives, good or otherwise.

Central value-driven principles reflect these decisive features of a health promotion approach, and underpin practice, policy, and planning in health promotion initiatives and programmes. These include civic participation, citizen and community-driven solutions to identified problems, capacity and capability development to either cope with or change the environmental and social factors damaging health and well-being, inclusivity and social inclusion, social equity and equality, and privileging the voices of diversity and disadvantage.

Three key strategies recommended by the Ottawa Charter uphold these values: enable, mediate, and advocate. To elaborate, these health promotion strategies serve to *enable* others by supporting them to lead and participate; to *mediate* between and on behalf of citizens and key stakeholders to achieve their desired outcomes; and to foster self-advocacy skills, or to *advocate* for vulnerable citizens and communities who are unable to do so themselves. This is achieved by paying attention to the lived experience and voices of those who are often unheard, in order to change social and environmental circumstances harmful to health and well-being.

Although it is not an exact science, health promotion employs strategic interventions and approaches to address a range of health and social issues, using specific principles, practices, and strategies that are particular to the field. That's not to say, however, that it is not evidence-based nor guided by best practice—it is—and this is often a misunderstood and underestimated strength of health promotion. As Baum (2015) explains, public health and public health issues are far too complex to be understood through any single theoretical or practice-based lens:

> Narrow areas of knowledge certainly have their place but public health is, by its very essence, an integrative discipline that hunts and gathers theories and ideas from many other disciplines and professions. Key tasks for the expert public health worker are to be capable of integrating complex areas of knowledge and applying them to public health issues. (p. xxx)

Indeed, the strength of public health approaches and the health promotion framework is their capacity to draw upon, integrate and link multiple theories, principles, disciplines, levels, and practices simultaneously. The Ottawa Charter is designed to attend to the structural and systemic dimensions that influence public health while taking into account the implications, and potential actions, for individuals. Known as the upstream and downstream strategy, this approach recognizes that problems upstream (systems level) such as policy, funding streams, and legislation, often cause issues downstream (community and individual level). This component of health promotion recognizes that individuals are not solely responsible for their health status, and acknowledges, for instance, that simply promoting a healthy lifestyle to those living in poverty fails to take into account the social and environmental circumstances that are not amenable to health, and which fall outside the scope of individual control. It recognizes that no amount of health education targeted at individuals will solve the problem, and that changes need to be made upstream. Furthermore, identifying the location and source of the problem is crucial to developing effective targeted health promotion interventions. In other words, the source of the problem determines the type and location of the intervention required to solve the problem, and most often, multiple strategies at multiple levels are necessary.

As such, the Ottawa Charter for Health Promotion has five areas of action that provide guidance on the range and type of approaches required to achieve public health outcomes. The Charter asserts that in order to achieve population impact, working across all five of these areas is essential. Working in one area alone will not achieve change at a societal or whole-of-community level, or produce sustainable change. This is not to say that working in one or two areas is not valuable, but that it should be undertaken in the knowledge that omitting by design, or excluding through lack of awareness, will not achieve the same population-based outcomes. These five strategic areas of action serve to direct the task of health promotion towards multipronged and multilevel interventions. They are:

- Reorient health services.
- Healthy public policy ('Health in All Policies').
- Strengthen community action.
- Create supportive environments.
- Individual skill development.

Based on the belief that health requires peace, shelter, education, food, income, a stable ecosystem, social justice, and equity (WHO, 2017), the five action areas combined recognize individual, social, societal, and structural levels to promote and protect the health of citizens. The strength of health promotion practitioners, therefore, is their capacity to interrogate public health issues through a range of theoretical constructs, and to apply equally broad solution-focused strategies to address them. Skilled health promotion practitioners (professionally trained or otherwise) will gather evidence at the individual level by mobilizing citizen participatory approaches, and use this to advocate for sustained change in policy and legislation, forcing local issues into local, state, and national policy environments. The central task for successful health promotion practitioners is to assimilate multiple theories, methods, and strategies to unlock, understand, and address complex issues in order to reduce harm and to protect and promote health.

In his seminal book, *Health Promoting Palliative Care* (1999), Kellehear examines how palliative care can become more health promoting, and explores theoretical constructs, benefits, and examples of introducing health promotion to palliative care. Outlining the central concerns for both palliative care and health promotion as it relates to a social model of dying, Kellehear proposes an integrated model that has the potential to address the limitations of each field, in which palliative care recognizes that dying is not solely a medical issue, best supported by professional services alone, and that dying people still deserve health promotion interventions.

Kellehear outlines the goals of *Health Promoting Palliative Care* (1999, p. 28) against the five action areas of the Ottawa Charter for Health Promotion:

1. The provision of education and information for health, dying, and death.
2. The provision of social supports, both personal and community.
3. The encouragement of interpersonal reorientation.
4. The reorientation of palliative care services.
5. The combating of death-denying health policies and attitudes.

To reiterate, health promotion approaches to illness and the end of life assert that health promotion is a 'public health intervention strategy' (the how) and illness, end of life, and palliative care constitute the health and social topic (the what) to be addressed through this strategy. As such, health promotion provides an evidence-based framework with which a range of complex health and social issues can be addressed, and in this case, the end of life.

End of life in the health promotion framework

Bearing in mind the concepts discussed thus far, this next section outlines a health promotion approach to living with life-limiting illness and disability, the end of life, dying, death, bereavement, and palliative care, framed within the five action areas of the Ottawa Charter for Health Promotion. It provides an overview of an integrated approach and outlines a rationale, principles, practice examples, and evidence-based approaches for optimum population impact and sustainability.

Health-promoting palliative care services

Health promotion incorporates health services within its framework but argues for their reorientation towards citizen-focused and community-controlled systems and services that respond to needs identified by communities (WHO, 1986). It calls for a shift of focus from disease intervention to health and well-being. A reorientation towards health-promoting health services encompasses meaningful engagement with the communities they serve and redirecting their services to specifically meet their needs. In the case of palliative care, practice examples are evident internationally, with many hospices and palliative care services recognizing the value in engaging their communities to support or augment the delivery of their services. There are perhaps fewer examples in which community control drives palliative care service delivery. Tension between professionalized services and citizen-controlled initiatives in the ongoing dialogue about custodianship of death is counterproductive to a health promotion approach. Health promotion approaches to palliative care services can be explored to discover how palliative care services may become more health promoting, and how palliative care practitioners can incorporate health promotion approaches into their practice for patients and their families.

Palliative care services can adopt specific measures in line with the evidence base of health promotion approaches. Rather than providing an exhaustive list of all the ways in which palliative care services can become health promoting, key principles of an evidence-based approach are outlined here. The degree to which palliative care services might adopt them will to some extent depend on resources, health promotion expertise, and organizational culture. From a sector/service perspective, activities can be categorized into six main areas of health-promoting strategic action:

1. Providing clarity to patients, families, and carers about what palliative care services do *not* provide, as well as what they do provide.
2. Ensuring palliative care services reach those most in need.
3. Promoting and actively supporting social network enhancement for patients, their families, and their carers.
4. Undertaking capacity-building activities that are not limited to educating others about their services or about palliative care, but supporting genuine capability and capacity in the context of other settings based on their role and strengths.
5. Developing and implementing health promotion policies in palliative care services.
6. Partnering with community and other sectors external to health for an integrated approach.

First, palliative care practitioners are familiar with informing patients and clients of the services they provide. However, it is equally—if not more—important from a health promotion perspective to explain what services will *not* be provided and what care needs will *not* be met. The rationale for this assertion is the need to signal to patients that a citizen-oriented contribution, along with those of their social support networks, is essential for optimal care. Unhelpful assumptions that palliative care will coordinate and attend to all aspects of support is misleading and counterproductive to healthy end of life experiences. Clarifying that the social dimensions of end of life care are primarily met by informal networks of care (Rumbold, 2011) in the context of our community and social lives enhances successful outcomes and avoids setbacks. Concepts and clear messaging at the forefront of this approach include:

- Setting and establishing realistic expectations from the outset.
- Acknowledging and communicating that the informal care network is an integral part of the team, and requires equal attention and coordination to sustain periods of caring.
- Sending clear messages that organizing and preparing for social supports during caring at the end of life is just as important as medical and nursing supports.
- Positioning palliative care as one part of the overall care network.
- Promoting empowerment and citizen-driven involvement by acknowledging their active participation in successful caring, including identifying needs, and how they may lead to meet those needs.
- Promoting the importance of social network enhancement, and making referrals to local community organizations.

Second, a central concern of health promotion is its remit to ensure services reach those who need it. It is fundamental that organizational policies and strategic planning should reach the most disadvantaged and excluded citizens, such as First Nations people, refugees, ethnic minorities, LGBTQI+ communities, and those living with intellectual and physical disabilities, mental health issues, homelessness, and alcohol and drug dependencies. A health promotion approach for palliative care services should attend to the social determinants of health, reflected in the way that those with lower socioeconomic status experience poorer health outcomes, along with poorer end of life care outcomes. Strategically, the best way to incorporate the social determinants of health into service planning is to partner with local government and social services who have existing relationships and services in place to support vulnerable citizens. Health services that don't include strategic planning and policies for deprived populations in their catchment areas are not practising evidence-based health promotion.

Third, palliative care services could include, as part of their suite of resources, social network enhancement tools that support patients to map, unlock, and draw upon the social support networks and social resources available to them to sustain long periods of caring. This means identifying and accessing local community supports with capability and capacity to provide vital assistance that will make end of life care in community settings feasible.

Fourth, viewing the palliative care sector as 'capacity builders' refers to sharing their expertise on all matters concerning life-limiting illness, dying, death, and bereavement with sectors, settings, communities, and citizens outside health systems. The objective of this strategy is for their expertise and custodianship of dying and death to find its way into other settings where it is needed. However, a common mistake made by palliative care services is to reduce this activity to providing palliative care education to others, instead of taking a health promotion approach that builds sustainable capacity using the existing assets and strengths of the environment or sector to tailor the capability required to the setting (Grindrod, 2020). Rather than a stereotyped education programme, services need to ask what strengths exist, what type of capacity needs to be built, for whom, for what purpose, and how might this be sustained? To successfully achieve sustainable capacity, the valuable contribution that others are able to make (public health sectors, communities, and citizens) needs to be acknowledged, along with their expertise, and initiatives designed accordingly. Simply providing education about palliative care is limited in its usefulness if it is not contextualized to the setting in which it's being shared.

Fifth, from a service perspective, health-promoting palliative care policy incorporates health promotion strategies, as outlined previously, into the existing structural, cultural, and practice-based components of the service. Policy that promotes health promotion approaches by removing unhelpful policies that make it difficult for citizens to die according to their wishes is an example of an upstream intervention to influence downstream practices. Health-promoting palliative care policies, though they seek engagement with the communities in their catchment area, retain the lens and governance protocols of a health service perspective, thereby limiting their translation into sectors external to health. Understanding this limitation is essential to clarifying the misnomer that health service-based policy determines population-level health status.

Sixth, the skills of health promotion practitioners are distinctly different to those of clinicians (Abel et al., 2016). Partnering with health promotion practitioners in health-promoting palliative care would strengthen multisectoral and civic partnerships surrounding the hospice or palliative care service. The networks and partnerships inherent to health promotion approaches provide access to, and participatory approaches in, areas not traditionally accessed by health services. Abel and colleagues (2016) recommend that palliative care organizations partner with health promotion and community development organizations, to pool expertise and collaborate on a truly integrated model.

Healthy end of life policy

The first strategy in the Ottawa Charter is building healthy public policy, asserting health as a priority and concern for all policy-makers, in all sectors and at all levels (1986), recognizing that most policies that affect health are located outside the conventional concerns of health agencies, such as in welfare, education, and workplace settings. It refers to the importance of identifying obstacles to health and developing policies so they can be removed to make healthy choices the easiest option for citizens. The development of healthy public policy therefore is of concern to, and the responsibility of, each sector and at every level of government. In the context of end of life policy, this refers to identifying obstacles to dying well and developing policies to remove barriers that contribute to poor end of life outcomes. Kellehear refers to these as the 'combating death-denying health policies and attitudes in the wider society' (Kellehear, 1999, p. 21). Policies, or statements, that articulate a vision for optimal end of life outcomes are useful in sharing aspirational sentiments but limited in efficacy when the impetus for change relies purely on goodwill. Policies are most effective when they redirect a course of action that produces poor outcomes, or when they disrupt existing barriers to quality end of life care, by enforcing protocol or legislative change. Thus, advocating for policy and legislative change to protect disadvantaged citizens from experiencing a disadvantaged death is the most effective and appropriate strategy.

To date, most policy development in the public health palliative care field is situated in palliative care, often calling for the involvement of communities in palliative and end of life care. However, from a public health perspective, it's also important that healthy end of life policies reside in public health settings, such as local government, welfare and disability sectors, social services, the education sector, workplaces, and in the healthy ageing and aged care sector. Policies developed with a health system lens are often unable to transcend their health services framework to encompass meaningful participation outside of the health sector in accordance with the citizen-driven or community-driven lens of health promotion principles.

Policies in the palliative care sector that reflect health promotion ideals often refer to the involvement of communities. The reference to the generic term 'community' in such policies often fails to take into account the social structures and the diverse dimensions of civic participation in all its societal variations. We are only now, for instance, seeing deprived citizens, or 'underserved populations' (as they're referred to from a health service perspective) emerging in palliative care policies (Scottish Government, 2015; The National Palliative and End of Life Care Partnership, 2015; Australian Government, 2018; Health Canada, 2019). Without explicitly developing palliative care policies that attend to barriers to equitable access to services and issues of social inequality, more often than not, such policies allow (or by default, reach) only privileged communities with sufficient social resources to participate, engaging those, who from an equity perspective, need them least.

Central to the challenges of developing healthy end of life policy in public health settings is the way in which matters concerning dying, and death, are funded by governments—that is, through health system-oriented palliative care programmes, thereby creating the policy context. Many sectors, such as public welfare, education, and workforce settings, aren't funded to attend to matters concerning the end of life, making it difficult to embed end of life policies into these settings, beyond (usually minimal) leave entitlements to attend funerals and resolve practical issues that arise when a significant other dies. Despite the fact that citizens will experience caring, illness, death, and grief in these sectors, their lack of recognition and formal arrangements for their contribution to improving the end of life care outcomes of citizens means the policy context (and therefore practice) is absent.

Policy, and therefore practice implications, of dying and death being resourced through healthcare services is that end of life policy rarely shows up in settings external to health. Often, end of life policy found in non-health settings refers to the engagement of palliative care services in that setting, rather than the sector or setting itself developing healthy end of life policy that acknowledges their valuable contribution, based on their expertise and assets, to improve the end of life care outcomes of those citizens with whom they work and engage (Grindrod, 2020). This has implications for the public health palliative care notion that the end of life is everybody's business (Kellehear, 2013).

Strengthening community action and compassionate communities

In the Ottawa Charter, strengthening community action refers to those activities that increase the ability of communities to achieve change in their physical and social environments through collective organization and action (Baum, 2015). The evidence-based practice of community development is largely accepted as the principal framework to progress activities within this pillar of the Charter. In health promotion and palliative care, community development approaches to end of life care and bereavement are increasingly referred to as 'compassionate communities'. Over the last decade, the international compassionate communities movement has progressed significantly in terms of practice, research, and policy.

In the same way that health promotion is an implementation framework used to achieve public health outcomes, the practice of community development is applied to achieve health promotion outcomes. Community developers seek to stimulate, enable, and support citizens with skills and strategies to effect change within their own community. They do this by identifying, valuing, and unlocking the expertise, knowledge, skills, and wisdom of communities (Ife, 2016) to generate local solutions to local problems. Ideally, community developers, whether civic leaders, activists, involved citizens, or professionals, follow the advice of Henderson and Vercseg (2010):

> We can talk about community development only if members of a community themselves, their groups, organisations and institutions, develop their own community. It is not the community development worker who develops the community but the community that develops itself. The community development worker acts as a catalyst and provides professional support in this process. (p. 30)

Although community development practice draws upon a vast range of strategies aimed at building stronger and more resilient local communities, there are two broadly accepted methods of achieving this goal. Minkler and Wallerstein (2012) updated and adapted earlier types of community intervention and developed a needs-based approach that is conceptualized as either consensual (community development) or conflict based (social action). Health promotion will typically have a mixture of both. Further, an asset-based approach to community development recognizes the strength of a community (Mathie and Cunningham, 2003; Haines, 2014), as compared with a deficit model that focuses on problems, and is useful in identifying and mobilizing the existing local assets to progress the community's collective agenda. The approach, which is particularly useful for stigmatized and deprived groups, assumes all people have strengths, assets, or capabilities, aligning with health promotion philosophies supporting civic participation. An asset-based approach is useful, irrespective of whether the community's assets will be used to enhance the conditions influencing local community life, or confront them.

Descriptions of compassionate communities internationally reflect a diversity of community development practice, ranging from linking communities and neighbourhoods with palliative and hospice care, using the arts to facilitate community involvement, leveraging the role of palliative care volunteers in compassionate communities, applying social network enhancement strategies in communities, involving First Nations people in community-based end of life care, building end of life care into existing community networks such as hobby clubs and community hubs, linking primary care with community development organizations, and creating community bereavement spaces. In other words, application of the compassionate communities' concept is limited only by imagination. Any community-led initiatives that brings people together around matters concerning living with illness, dying, death, and bereavement is valuable.

The growing movement of compassionate communities must understand and anticipate the enablers and barriers that will be encountered. This is true of all community development work, not peculiar to compassionate communities. To date, the majority of compassionate communities initiatives are facilitated by those linked with or employed by palliative care. Community development endeavours originating from health-based settings have certain challenges to overcome to build genuine and sustainable citizen-driven initiatives. Those that originate from communities and citizens have a different premise from the outset, and will flourish in different ways based on their assets and needs. Either way, being aware of the challenges is crucial to facilitating, not delivering, successful, and sustainable compassionate community initiatives.

When it comes to practice, a common mistake is the assumption that community development initiatives are easy to facilitate, are not evidence based, and do not require specific skills implemented by targeted strategic action. This misunderstanding can lead to community events and social marketing initiatives being categorized as community development. While they may form a part of a broader community development initiative, in and of themselves they do not constitute community development, and won't necessarily lead to civic-controlled participation nor reach marginalized and vulnerable citizens unless strategic and explicit strategies designed to achieve this are incorporated.

An evidence-based health promotion and asset-based community development framework designed in Australia (Grindrod and Rumbold, 2018) offers guidance to avoid the common mistakes often made in community development practice. Using the acronym LEADERS, it includes:

- Leading from behind (increase community capacity and capability).
- Ensuring broad community participation (inclusive practice of diverse citizens).
- Asset-based approach (identify, map, and unlock community strengths and assets).
- Designing yourself out of a job (stimulate community action and facilitate citizen-led decisions).
- Exit strategy (foster community control by planning an exit strategy from the outset).
- Recognizing community as the expert (identify and promote their expertise and valuable local contribution).
- Sustainability (only start, and invest in, strategies that the community can sustain).

The intention of producing such guidance is to resource communities, and those who support them, with the evidence base necessary to enhance successful and sustainable outcomes, which in turn promotes community uptake, engagement, and most importantly, achievements that can be celebrated to fuel continued inspiration. The relevance of ensuring community investment is matched with successful outcomes (as determined by the community) is to sustain participation and to expand active engagement, which in turn supports the provision of local end of life care. As Kellehear puts it, 'seriously ill people can have periods of positive wellbeing, and as a community, we can be enhancing those times' (1999, p. 15).

Creating supportive environments in which people can die well

Creating supportive environments, in the Ottawa Charter, refers to developing and maintaining environments in which people can realize their full potential as healthy individuals. The Charter recognizes the importance of social, economic, and physical environmental factors in shaping people's experiences of health. When it comes to the end of life, this extends to environments where people live to their full potential in the context of illness, disability, dying, and grief. This approach is outlined in Kellehear's book, *Compassionate Cities: Public Health and End-of-Life Care* (2005) where illness, dying, death, and bereavement are considered in a 'healthy cities' approach (WHO, 1997).

Creating supportive environments links with the 'healthy settings' approach (WHO, 1980), such as health-promoting schools, organizations, institutions, and cities. A settings approach favours the role of the environment, rather than individual behaviours, in creating health, and is therefore the focus of intervention (Kickbusch, 1996). It recognizes that health and well-being are created in the places that we live, work, learn, and age, and these environments provide the structure and resources for health, as well as for illness, dying, death, and bereavement. In this way, settings themselves become the intervention, affording people living with life-limiting illness the same opportunities, and supporting them to live their remaining life to their full potential. Integral to this approach are the values that support civic participation, such as preserving self-determination, supporting caring networks, nurturing compassion, and challenging policies and practices that constrain autonomy and choice.

Healthy settings and supportive environments are a means to implement collaborative and cooperative action. A multisectoral and networked approach is central, comprising strategies that relate to both individuals and structures, and harnessing collective participation through intersectoral partnerships (WHO, n.d.). An integrated plan includes both top-down and bottom-up strategies to enhance healthy end of life approaches, including the participation of all key stakeholders, changing the culture of the setting, planning activities centred around well-being in the context of illness and dying, understanding the relationships of the environment with other settings, and creating more equitable access to resources and services to support people at the end of their lives, their families, and their carers.

Individual skill development (death and end of life literacy, death education)

The development of personal skills acknowledges the role that behaviours play in promoting health, and therefore their role in promoting health for people approaching the end of life and their carers. The skills called for are those that enable people to make healthy choices (WHO, 1986), and again, healthy end of life choices for themselves. This requires knowledge about how to navigate palliative care and end of life services, how to access appropriate support, and the role of citizens and communities in sharing end of life care practice. This has been described as death literacy (Noonan et al., 2016), meaning the practical knowledge and skills, and know-how, of caring for someone at the end of life. The development of personal skills, along with public education programmes, is yet another important feature of a comprehensive health promotion approach to the end of life for those with sufficient personal resources to mobilize and develop these skills.

Within the Ottawa Charter, personal skill development is the predominant focus of health professionals, often to the exclusion of the remaining four recommended areas of action. This is an example of health promotion being misunderstood, viewed narrowly as a behavioural approach for educating individuals to eat well and exercise, and to avoid known threats to health such as smoking, intended to delay illness and death. Targeted health promotion strategies to encourage individuals to change their behaviours include health education and social marketing campaigns to promote the uptake of a healthy lifestyle. Those with sufficient personal resources might respond to these types of health promotion strategies, but those without, such as disadvantaged citizens, are unlikely to, given the behaviours are structurally and socially determined in the first place. In the context of the end of life, this is where the health promotion framework should guide practice in the field, moving beyond 'psychosocial care' to acknowledge that the other four action areas of the Charter compensate for the fact that individuals, especially those who are disadvantaged or deprived, are not solely responsible for their health status, nor for their end of life experience. This is where the structural aspects of health promotion require specific skills to create healthy environments and settings that produce equitable circumstances and enable equitable choices for everyone (Grindrod, 2020).

Conclusion: future directions

This chapter began by noting that most people wish to remain close to people, places, and possessions at the end of their lives, and that this is best achieved when community and social supports integrate effectively with health and palliative care services in order to meet these needs—when people are cared for in their preferred setting as far as possible. Such integration requires broad civic participation in the social dimensions of end of life care that link with its clinical dimensions. This reflects the overall public health palliative care agenda that end of life care is of concern to, and the responsibility of, everyone (Kellehear, 2005, 2013). Health promotion offers an intervention framework for public health goals, providing practical guidance on how this policy aspiration might be translated in practice, across multiple sectors and jurisdictions, and within different settings and constituents of society, in a way that is sustainable. The skills and networks of health promotion and palliative care experts must be balanced to achieve effective and sustainable public health palliative care programmes.

A review of the public health palliative care literature identified that most initiatives are facilitated by the palliative care sector, and can be categorized within the community action (compassionate communities) pillar of the Ottawa Charter. Creating compassionate communities however, in and of itself, does not lead to societal transformation (Karapliagou et al., 2018). In addition, vulnerable citizens and marginalized populations, who are at particular risk of poor end of life care outcomes and experiences (Dixon et al., 2015; Equity in Palliative Approaches to Care, 2019), must be strategically and intentionally included in health promotion and palliative care initiatives if the benefits of everyone's involvement in providing end of life care are to be realized (Correa and Abel, 2018). To move towards this goal, public health palliative care interventions ought to be expanded across all five action areas of the Ottawa Charter for population impact. At the same time, strengthening evidence-based health promotion practice within the field will enhance the penetration and sustainability of public health palliative care approaches.

REFERENCES

Abel, J., Sallnow, L., Murray, S. A., and Kerin, M. 2016. *Each Community is Prepared to Help: Community Development in End of Life Care—Guidance in Ambition Six*. London: National Council for Palliative Care.

Aoun, S., Breen, L., White, I., Rumbold, B., and Kellehear, A. 2018. What sources of bereavement support are perceived helpful by bereaved people and why? Empirical evidence for the compassionate communities approach. *Palliative Medicine*, 32, 1378–1388.

Ates, G., Ebenau, A. F., Busa, C., Csikos, A., Hasselaar, J., Jaspers, B., et al. 2018. 'Never at ease'—family carers within integrated palliative care: a multinational, mixed method study. *BMC Palliative Care*, 17, 39.

Australian Government. 2018. *National Palliative Care Strategy*. Canberra: Australia.

Baum, F. 2015. *The New Public Health*, 4th ed. Melbourne: Oxford University Press.

Correa, S. R. and Abel, J. 2018. Palliative care for all? How can Brazil develop a palliative care service founded on principles of equity and access for all? *Current Opinion in Supportive and Palliative Care*, 12, 504–509.

Dixon, J., King, D., Matosevic, T., Clark, M., and Knapp, M. 2015. *Equity in the Provision of Palliative Care in the UK: Review of Evidence*. London: London School of Economics and Political Science, Personal Social Services Research Unit.

Equity in Palliative Approaches to Care. 2019. Equity in palliative approaches to care. [Online] Available at: https://www.equityinpalliativecare.com/

Gardner, D. S. and Kramer, B. J. 2010. End-of-life concerns and care preferences: congruence among terminally ill elders and their family caregivers. *OMEGA*, 60, 273–297.

Grindrod, A. 2020. Choice depends on options: a public health framework incorporating the social determinants of dying to create options at end of life. *Progress in Palliative Care*, 28, 94–100.

Grindrod, A. and Rumbold, B. 2018. Healthy End of Life Project (HELP): a progress report on implementing community guidance on public health palliative care initiatives in Australia. *Annals of Palliative Medicine*, 7, S73–S83.

Haines, A. 2014. Asset-based community development. In: Phillips, R. and Pittman, R. H. (eds.) *An Introduction to Community Development*, 2nd ed., pp. 45–56. London: Taylor & Francis Group.

Health Canada. 2019. Framework on palliative care in Canada. [Online] Available at: https://www.canada.ca/en/health-canada/services/health-care-system/reports-publications/palliative-care/framework-palliative-care-canada.html#p2.3.4

Henderson, P. and Vercseg, I. 2010. Community development. In: Henderson, P. and Vercseg, I. (eds.) *Community Development and Civil Society: Making Connections in the European Context*, pp. 29–44. Bristol: Bristol University Press.

Heyland, D. K., Dodek, P., Rocker, G., Groll, D., Gafni, A., Pichora, D., et al. 2006. What matters most in end-of-life care: perceptions of seriously ill patients and their family members. *Canadian Medical Association Journal*, 174, 627–633.

Horsfall, D., Yardley, A., Leonard, R., Noonan, K., and Rosenberg, J. P. 2015. *End of Life at Home: Co-Creating an Ecology of Care*. Sydney: Western Sydney University.

Hughner, R. S. and Kleine, S. S. 2004. Views of health in the lay sector: a compilation and review of how individuals think about health. *Health*, 8, 395–422.

Ife, J. W. 2016. *Community Development in an Uncertain World: Vision, Analysis and Practice*, 2nd ed. Port Melbourne: Cambridge University Press.

Karapliagou, A., Kellehear, A., and Wegleitner, K. 2018. The public health end-of-life care movement: history, principles, and styles of practice. In: Lloyd-Williams, M. (ed.) *Psychosocial Issues in Palliative Care: A Community Based Approach for Life Limiting Illness*, 3rd ed., pp. 1–22. Oxford: Oxford University Press.

Kellehear, A. 1999. Health-promoting palliative care: developing a social model for practice. *Mortality*, 4, 75–82.

Kellehear, A. 2005. *Compassionate Cities: Public Health and End-of-Life Care*. London: Routledge.

Kellehear, A. 2013. Compassionate communities: end-of-life care as everyone's responsibility. *QJM: An International Journal of Medicine*, 106, 1071–1075.

Kickbusch, I. 1996. Tribute to Aaron Antonovsky—'What creates health'. *Health Promotion International*, 11, 5–6.

Maclean, U. 1988. *Ethnographic Approaches to Health*. Oxford: Oxford University Press.

Mathie, A. and Cunningham, G. 2003. From clients to citizens: asset-based community development as a strategy for community-driven development. *Development in Practice*, 13, 474–486.

Minkler, M. and Wallerstein, N. 2012. Improving health through community organization and community building: perspectives from health education and social work. In: Minkler, M. (ed.) *Community Organizing and Community Building for Health and Welfare*, 3rd ed., pp. 37–58. New Brunswick, NJ: Rutgers University Press.

Noonan, K., Horsfall, D., Leonard, R., and Rosenberg, J. P. 2016. Developing death literacy. *Progress in Palliative Care*, 24, 31–35.

Rosenberg, J. P., Horsfall, D., Leonard, R., and Noonan, K. 2015. Informal caring networks for people at end of life: building social capital in Australian communities. *Health Sociology Review*, 24, 29–37.

Rumbold, B. 2011. Health promoting palliative care and dying in old age. In: Gott, M. and Ingleton, C. (eds.) *Living with Ageing and Dying: Palliative and End of Life Care for Older People*, pp. 75–89. Oxford: Oxford University Press.

Scottish Government. 2015. Palliative and end of life care: strategic framework for action. [Online] Available at: https://www.gov.scot/publications/strategic-framework-action-palliative-end-life-care/

The National Palliative and End of Life Care Partnership. 2015. Ambitions for palliative and end of life care: a national framework for local action 2015–2020. [Online] Available at: http://endoflifecareambitions.org.uk/

World Health Organization. n.d. Health promotion: healthy settings. [Online] Available at: https://www.who.int/healthpromotion/healthy-settings/en/

World Health Organization. 1980. Introduction to healthy settings. [Online] Available at: http://www.who.int/healthy_settings/about/en/

World Health Organization. 1986. Ottawa Charter for health promotion. [Online] Available at: http://www.who.int/healthpromotion/conferences/previous/ottawa/en/

World Health Organization. 1997. *Twenty Steps for Developing a Healthy Cities Project*, 3rd ed. Copenhagen: World Health

Organization. Available at: https://www.euro.who.int/__data/assets/pdf_file/0011/101009/E56270.pdf
World Health Organization. 2008. Commission on social determinants of health, closing the gap in a generation: health equity through action on the social determinants of health. [Online] Available at: https://apps.who.int/iris/bitstream/handle/10665/43943/9789241563703
World Health Organization. 2017. Health is a fundamental human right. [Online] Available at: https://www.who.int/mediacentre/news/statements/fundamental-human-right/en/
World Health Organization. 2020. WHO definition of palliative care. [Online] Available at: https://www.who.int/cancer/palliative/definition/en/

16

Clinical practice methods combined with community resources

Helen Kingston, Catherine Millington-Sanders, and Julian Abel

'To help you die peacefully, but also to live until you die.'

Dame Cicely Saunders.

Introduction

In this chapter, we will discuss the following:

- *Improving death literacy across society*:
  - Encouraging a culture where citizens can talk openly about what matters most to them in life and in death.
  - Encouraging a society which values the caring role and supports primary carers, valuing of networks of support, and nurturing the connections that matter.
- *Clinical service delivery*:
  - The fundamentals of good clinical care are important to have in place so that care is systematically available to all. This means ensuring that all staff have skills and understanding in public health approaches to end of life care and, crucially, that clinical services encourage this approach through their culture and working practices.
  - The impact on individuals is recognized for all causes of illness, dying, death, and loss, including miscarriage, sudden deaths, and predictable causes of death and other forms of loss including the loss of pets.
  - The Royal College of General Practitioners and Marie Curie UK Daffodil Standards offer a quality improvement approach to enable general practice to consistently deliver end of life care and bereavement support.
- *Systems leadership*:
  - Our societies are complex ecosystems. Each individual matters. Wrapping care around that individual entails the integration of the many components. Health and social care are delivered through multiple organizations. How these organizations work across organizational boundaries is vital and requires good, integrated collaboration. The strengths and assets within families and communities is a fundamental part of this complex picture.
  - Systems leadership is needed to enable strong trust and understanding across organizational boundaries. This enables honest reflection and co-creation of pathways of care that can be adapted. Citizens and communities need to be involved as equal participants and leaders for change. Current accountability frameworks within health and social care can lead to a focus within individual organizations. To enable cross-organizational working, organizations need to raise their gaze to ensure the whole ecosystem functions together. Leaders who understand and support this bigger picture will help the system to move in this direction. Sometimes this takes a leap of faith with decisions that may seem to go against the short-term benefits for an individual organization.
  - Learning organizations are those with continuous improvement from experiential learning. This includes within and across organizations.
  - Systems leaders should embed a culture that gives frontline staff the autonomy to do what is best for the individual at all times, being free to speak up and to advocate for change. Activated empowered citizens who feel a strong sense of belonging to their communities should work alongside professional organizations to develop strategy and working practices.

The chapter is illustrated with examples from two sources, reflecting the experiences of the authors. The first example draws upon the experience of Frome Medical Practice, which set up an enhanced model of primary care combined with a compassionate community programme, initially in the town of Frome, and later expanded across the population of the Mendip area of Somerset, UK, encompassing 115,000 people. The second is the Daffodil Standards for end of life care, developed by one of the authors. Both the model of care in Frome and the Daffodil Standards are intimately connected, with similar values and practice methods.

Improving death literacy across society

Encouraging a culture where citizens can talk openly about what matters most in life and in death

> 'Death isn't a medical failure, it's a biological certainty. But poorly managed death IS a medical failure.'
>
> Kathryn Mannix, 2019.

Knowledge of death is principally through our life experiences. Literature and drama help us to reflect on this, as do discussions with and observations of those around us. The experience of caring for someone who is dying is the most powerful way of understanding what is needed:

> Some of us will not experience death at close hand in our early years and for many of us it may feel uncomfortable talking about death. We can gain some knowledge, however, through witness of the lives of those around us and literature, on social media, films and soap opera characters. Incrementally we build early skills and knowledge through perhaps the death of family pet, PHSE in schools, the death of a distant relative or neighbour's husband or the story line of novel too. These will mould our understanding of the experience of death. (Holmes and Rahe, 1967)

Death literacy is the knowledge and practical skills that help to inform active choices around end of life options:

> [D]espite the medical model, carers have the ability to 'do it their way' and step outside of institutionalized dying. With no prior knowledge or special set of skills, they showed an ability to care for a person at the end of their life at home. Carers demonstrated they could seek out information and learn the complex physical and emotional end-of-life caring skills. . . . The act of end-of-life caregiving provides a deeply personal connection to death and dying and is a catalyst to developing death literacy. In keeping with new public health approaches death literacy draws on a community development framework which suggests that if a community is to develop its capacity to support the caring of those at EOL [end of life], it needs knowledge and experience, a sense of empowerment and supportive social structures. These aspects are reflected in four features of death literacy – knowledge, skills, experiential learning, and social action. (Noonan et al., 2016, p. 32)

Festivals of living and dying help to raise the profile of death literacy. These are events that offer the space and opportunity to talk and discuss end of life issues as individuals and as a society. See Box 16.1.

Reaching out to existing community groups and starting conversations can be achieved through community development work in conjunction with clinical teams. See Box 16.2.

Box 16.1 Case study 1: 'Pushing up the Daisies' festival

The 'Pushing up the Daisies' festival of living and dying took place in Frome in October 2019. The festival brought conversations about death and dying into the community. The Health Connections Team, the community development service within Frome Medical Practice, attended. They helped to recruit nine volunteers including a retired general practitioner (GP) and a palliative care nurse who wanted to get involved in planning ahead conversations in the community. This helped to set up a broader programme of planning ahead connectors to enable community lead advance care planning.

Box 16.2 Case study 2: advance care planning in the community

Through work with Compassionate Communities UK, the Health Connections Mendip service worked to reach out to lunch clubs and community groups across Mendip to promote the idea of advance care planning, thinking about life priorities at all stages of life. Starting the conversation encouraged some lunch club members to take these conversations forwards with family and sowed the seed of thought for these individuals to talk about what mattered most in their lives.

Initiatives such as death cafes help to embed conversations as part of normal everyday life across families, friends, and social networks and to reach out and have these discussions in the usual places where we meet.

Encouraging a society which values the caring role and supports primary carers, valuing of networks of support, and nurturing the connections that matters

Caring for a person who is terminally ill can be very rewarding, bringing people closer together. However, caring can be physically and emotionally exhausting. While many undertake this role willingly for their loved ones, it is important to recognize the impact this might have on them. Carers should be supported to look after themselves. The first port of call for this can be found within networks and communities. Support for those caring is both physical and emotional input. The ability to offer support may require juggling with the day-to-day necessities of existence (Broady, 2015).

It is important for individuals to feel a sense of belonging, which can be provided by family, friends, and informal social networks that arise in hobbies clubs, societies, and work places. This can help people to feel valued and be a source of self-esteem, confidence, and general well-being. Maintaining these links is important for carer well-being and for re-establishing a sense of belonging when the person needing care has died (Leonard et al., 2015). Failure to provide this investment is likely to have significant negative societal implications (Hudson, 2013).

Compassionate employers may be able to support carers through offering flexible hours (Box 16.3). Hospice UK and Dying Matters campaign for compassionate employers and provide a toolkit and support for employers willing to take this step. Governmental support for this approach such as the Canadian care benefit has helped to lessen caregiver burden (Vuksan et al., 2012).

Strengthening existing networks

> 'When you are an adult you belong to yourself but when you are ill you belong to the family.'
>
> Christian Nzitimura, personal communication.

Our relationships include family, neighbours, friends, acquaintances, and those with whom we have casual interactions. It is easy in a busy life to dismiss the strength of some of these associations, but they are crucial to our well-being (Golden et al., 2009). When we are unwell, we might find that those around us who care are more readily visible. Activating support networks across families and across our communities is often about encouraging people to

Box 16.3 Case study 3: compassionate employers

Linda is a 46-year-old marketing manager. She works full time and has done at the same company for 10 years. Sally, her mother, lives in the same town and had breast cancer 7 years ago which recurred 3 months ago and she began chemotherapy. Linda has been supporting her mum through this treatment. Sadly, 6 weeks ago, her mother's scans showed that the cancer was not responding to treatment. They went together to the outpatient review with the oncology team to discuss her mother's options and her mum decided to stop the chemotherapy. She is well currently but Linda naturally wants to spend some time with her while they can enjoy this together and be there for her mum when her condition progresses. Linda enjoys her work and the friendship she has with colleagues but felt overwhelmed. She wondered whether she should take a break from work completely and resign. With her children having left home, she talked with her husband about whether she could afford to reduce her hours to have more time to be with her mother but she was not sure if this would be possible.

She went to talk to her employer about her situation and her request to reduce to 4 days weekly was accepted. Her boss also suggested she might want to consider home working for part of her week and the option of adjusting her hours again if this becomes necessary. Her boss reassured her about their carers leave policy. Linda felt supported and enabled to offer more support to her mum through her illness.

Box 16.4 Case study 4: community connectors

The Health Connections Mendip website contains details of over 400 groups across Mendip. It is linked to the patient electronic clinical record and is available at the fingertips of all consulting clinicians. This ease of access enables a broader exploration of what matters most in consultation. The directory of resources supports those whose principal priority in life might not be a medical intervention. Printable information can be provided and patients can access the website directly.

An army of community connectors—interested citizens aware of the rich resources in our community—now work with us to reach all members of the community to be aware of what is on offer. In the Mendip area of Somerset, with a population of 115,000, at the time of writing there are 1500 community connectors. On average, each has around 20 conversations a year with neighbours, friends, and colleagues, making therefore up to 30,000 conversations across Mendip, helping activate and nudge their fellow citizens towards greater connection and activity within our community. The more people become familiar with how help can be given, the greater the sense of coming together as a community.

recognize those people around in their day-to-day lives who already care and give help. These networks can be strengthened by nurturing or can fade through neglect. This is important for carers of those with long-term health conditions as their caring role evolves, as well as those in the last stages of illness (Vassilev et al., 2013).

Equally important is encouragement to accept help that is offered to actively maintain the network. It is easy to turn down help, discouraging further offers of support. Facilitation of network enhancement can improve outcomes for carers (Greene et al., 2012). Being specific about what help is being offered makes it easier for someone to say yes, as opposed to general offers of help. Examples include asking 'I wondered if you would like me to run the mower over your lawn while I am doing mine?' or 'I am just popping to the supermarket, is there anything that you need?' Practical and emotional assistance may both be required, and different individuals may be able to offer differing aspects. Having someone who is not the primary carer to coordinate the network can take this away from the primary carer (Abel, 2018). Over the coronavirus disease 2020 lockdown, awareness of our interdependency and the day-to-day contacts increased. This helped to increase awareness of those most at risk of physical and social isolation (Vieira et al., 2020).

Engaging communities can lead to improved outcomes for carers, including decreased fatigue or isolation, increase in size of caring networks, and that wider social networks can influence factors such as place of death and involvement of palliative care services (Sallnow et al., 2016). As discussed by Sallnow and colleagues (2010), the Neighbourhood Network in Palliative Care in Kerala, India, trains volunteers to go into the homes of people who are dying to offer basic care and pain relief. The care the volunteers give is very much of another human being sharing their journey on an equal basis (Sallnow et al., 2010).

Each of our communities is unique and the assets and resources within each will differ. Mapping these resources and ensuring that both community members as well as clinical teams have up-to-date knowledge of what is available can ensure that no one need say 'If only I had known'. Neighbourhoods and communities are there for each other.

The support that is available will change over time and so an up-to-date and easily accessible database of resources is needed to be able to signpost to these resources. Proactive sharing of information can occur through word of mouth. Communities of support can be accessed through a trusted recommendation by a friend or clinical encounter, but can also be shared via posters, through social media campaigns, phone lines, information stands, and websites. See Box 16.4.

Clinical service delivery

With general practice facing increased pressures on workload and capacity, it is crucial that every practice is as well prepared as possible to deliver well-planned end of life care to their population. There are 600,000 deaths per annum in the UK, set to increase by 17% by 2030 and 25% by 2040. An estimated 60–75% of these deaths are 'predictable' and therefore there is an opportunity for us to work in partnership with people to help plan their care better.

The Daffodil Standards are the Royal College of General Practitioners and Marie Curie UK's 'General Practice Core Standards for Advanced Serious Illness and End of Life Care' (Millington-Sanders and Noble, 2018). The Standards are free and provide a blend of quality statements with self-assessment guidance, evidence-based tools, reflective learning exercises, and quality improvement steps. They offer a structure to enable general, whatever the starting level, to be proactive organizations in which continuous learning and quality improvement steps are an integral part of caring for people.

They were developed by general practitioners (GPs) and multiprofessionals to make sure the Standards fit into real-life frontline general practice and to enable consistency in the level of care they provide to their entire population.

The standards are based on the Institute for Health Care Improvement principles, enabling all staff to start and improve at their own individual pace and for a practice to build on their learning journey together as a team. The aim is to support a practice to always be ready to ask questions, find new solutions, and continue to make small steps, using testing cycles of change, removing problems and inefficiencies, and refining practice. This lets practices develop a clear, structured approach that is relevant to their practice, staff, and patients.

Creation of high-functioning teams is key to providing high-quality service delivery. This is achieved through developing relationships between team members and across organizational boundaries. Teams that work together on a regular basis develop trust and they have a clear understanding of each other's skills and capability. Coordination and strong communication across different team components is vital to ensure smooth and consistent patient care. Pain control and other symptom management are important, but communication is also important to enable preparation for death, and the opportunity to achieve a sense of completion are important to most people (Steinhauser et al., 2000).

The Standards cover eight core areas:

1. Professional and competent staff.
2. Early identification.
3. Carer support.
4. Seamless, well-planned, and coordinated care.
5. Assessment of unique needs of the patient—'what matters most' conversations and personalized care and support planning.
6. Quality care during the last days of life.
7. Care after death.
8. General practices as hubs within compassionate communities.

Delivering consistent, high-quality care for those living with dying

Training is needed for staff within general practice surgeries with a broader approach to palliative care, including compassionate communities, in order to be able to provide consistent care. Staff need to actively work with families to promote establishment, and maintenance of informal networks (Horsfall et al., 2013). Induction of new staff in this model, with awareness of local pathways and resources, creates a knowledge base for interventions. Ongoing training needs reviews to ensure the right knowledge, skills, and capacity is in the team as a whole to provide consistent care. This a factor in helping to reduce rapid staff turnover. Continual work to ensure that good practice is embedded across a whole team requires continuous active management (Martin et al., 2012). See Boxes 16.5 and 16.6.

In the context of multidisciplinary working, gaps between services are frequently present. Face-to-face working helps to break down barriers of cross-organizational working. Collective voices can have greater strength to make these required changes.

Proactive identification of those whose health is deteriorating and their carers

Anyone who is ill, whether this is short term or long term, may be reliant on support from those around them. This is particularly the case for people who live with chronic conditions, including life-limiting illness. Systems can be set up in primary care to recognize the need for extra support, both for the patient and the caring network.

Box 16.5 Case study 5: compassionate care and simple use of experience feedback

The Daffodil Standards encourage the use of feedback from staff, patients, and caregivers to triangulate with more quantitative diagnostics.

This doesn't need to be cumbersome and can be incorporated into routine practice with the benefit of helping understand people's experience of care delivered.

An example included a simple conversation between the receptionist and practice carers' lead and a patient whose husband died the previous year after a long battle with prostate cancer:

> She told me that her GP had been 'their rock', particularly towards the end. I asked her what stood out about the practice: 'They cared and they listened to my husband and me.'
>
> She went on to say: 'Even though the surgery was busy, [the receptionist] Amy always asked how Alan and I were doing. One time he had a bad urine infection and she promised she'd get the GP to call me back ASAP. I knew I could trust her. And, of course, the GP did call shortly afterwards.'

Transitions and key moments during the course of an illness are a good alert (Abel et al., 2018). Admission to a care home is a life event that often prompts patients and families to reflect on their changing health and future priorities. Recognizing when transitions or crises have occurred can help facilitate timely intervention and proactive conversations (Boyd and Murray, 2010). Discharge letters, ambulance reports, and calls from other health and social care staff may also identify those who need additional support.

The Daffodil Standards offer diagnostic self-assessment and guidance for improvement across the entire general practice population. Over the first year of the Standards being launched, around one in six UK practices signed up. As part of the development process, feedback was encouraged and practices asked for more 'best practice' tools to embed into day-to-day practice that could generate bite-size quality improvement learning, and learning that could focus on different aspects of care and groups of patients. In response to the latter, a variation in the start audit approach evolved to encompass a three-level implementation model. In addition, the Daffodil Standards were aligned to help practices focus real-time learning from urgent care and deaths in older people's care homes.

- Level 1: core essentials—internal general practice systems to enable consistency of care.

Box 16.6 Case study 6: staff induction

Each year a new cohort of registrars begin work in primary care. In the Mendip area of Somerset, the cohort of registrars attend a training morning to understand the role of care coordination and multidisciplinary working at care coordination hubs. They receive training on the holistic approach to patient care and training in templates and systems for those with increased needs. The morning session enables them to develop an understanding of the importance of networks, and of the role of community groups and the community development service Health Connections Mendip. Meeting staff and understanding how they operate from the start of their training helps to embed this way of working when they start in primary care. In a similar way, all new permanent clinical staff attend a MDT meeting and meet the teams as part of their standard induction.

Box 16.7 Case study 7: Frome care coordination hub

Set up in 2015, the care coordination hub acts as a point of first contact for vulnerable patients across a population of 30,000. It began with a core team of a discharge liaison nurse, district nurse, or local social prescribing service team and practice clinical staff and has grown. Patients, families, and district nurses can ring the hub for support.

The team review all admissions to hospital and are proactive in making contact with those who are recently discharged. They take referrals from all clinical teams and from a broad range of other health and social care teams. Their work is integrated closely with that of the community development service Health Connections Mendip. The Frome Medical Practice care coordinator is part of the hub team. Identification and registration of carers is part of an integral role within the hub. Early and proactive contact with patients enables familiarity and building of relationships. The team proactively contact those having chemotherapy or radiotherapy. Regular MDT meetings enable regular updates and proactive care planning for patients. Frailty and multimorbidity are recognized as reasons for enhanced support and care planning.

The hub has a remit for all those with complex needs and has regular contact with social care, housing, specialist nursing services, and community and district general hospital teams. It provides a focus and its staff have built a wealth of knowledge of local pathways and of community resources, charities, and specialist teams for those with complex needs.

The hub team are able to identify many patients who are coming towards the end of their life at an early stage.

The systematic approach to recording of information enables it to be easily found by all in the practice through use of a standard template.

The administration of communication through the Electronic Palliative Care Coordination System is undertaken by the team so that emergency services are updated to changes in patient status or wishes. This enables clinical staff to spend time on conversations about what matters most, secure in the knowledge that there are strong systems in place to record and share this information.

- Level 2: enhanced—improving communication, shared planning, and compassionate care.
- Level 3: advanced—co-production of care and compassionate communities.

See Boxes 16.7 and 16.8 for examples.

Box 16.8 Case study 8: improving carer support

A practice who focused on 'Standard 3: carer support' identified a need to improve the support they gave to carers. They audited their current practice by looking at the last 20 deaths. They realized two things: only 30% of people who died had been recognized by the practice and only 40% of these had a carer or 'important other' noted. Most of these were carers of cancer patients.

This was presented at their next practice team meeting and they agreed on a system to code the patient with an advanced serious illness on their supportive care register and to place this on the 'problem list'. An administrator stepped forward to make sure each person on the supportive care register had been offered the opportunity to record important family members or carers.

The practice also looked at how they supported carers after someone died. They talked with families of people who had died to help create a leaflet with information about grief, funeral planning, and bereavement services available locally. Within 3 months they reported to have significantly improved their processes and practices.

The new role of care navigators at the reception desk of Frome Medical Practice, UK, helps to build links and relationships with carers (Massey, 2015). A carer's champion at the practice helps identify those in need of support, such as through home visits or discussions at multidisciplinary team (MDT) meetings. The carer's champion is also a great point of contact to ensure that these caring relationships are recorded in a systematic way and that identified carers are signposted to community support and offered holistic assessment of their own needs. Having someone with dedicated time to provide this coordination can ensure that the practice carers register remains accurate.

Seamless, well-planned, and coordinated care over the last days of life

At a population level, delivering excellent care to everyone requires these skills to be supported and nurtured across whole teams (Sevin et al., 2009). Communication within the team is crucial (Moorman, 2007). Just as with other medical and surgical teams, the primary and community teams need to consider how to communicate well with each other, with the patient, and with their informal care network. Structured reviews at regular meetings to review recent deaths and highlight any areas for improvement will ensure this is systematic.

For examples of how to put in place structures that help to make care safe and reliable, see Boxes 16.9–16.11.

By acknowledging, discussing, and reflecting on care outcomes and the impact on individuals, healthcare teams can build more functional pathways through frontline experience of what works well. This helps to apply these pathways sensitively and flexibly for individuals needing care.

Care after death

Experiencing the death of a partner is the most stressful life experience we may face and scores highly on the Homes–Rahe stress scale (Holmes and Rahe, 1967). Being able to share and feel supported along this journey is important. A common concern of the dying is to worry about the welfare of those who are left behind (Aldred et al., 2005). Ensuring that their loved ones are supported provides comfort to those experiencing the end of life. Supporting carers to maintain their own networks of support while caring will help them; ensuring as a society we improve our understanding of grief and feel confident to support the bereaved will also help (Stylianos and Vachon, 1993; Somhlaba and Wait, 2008). GPs reaching out to those who have been bereaved helps to identify those who are in need of extra support. Ensuring that practices have a systematic way of contacting those who have been recently bereaved opens the door to asking for further care at a future date if needed. The Sue

Box 16.9 Case study 9: routine reviews of clinical records

In early March 2020, as coronavirus disease 2019 levels began to rise, a review of clinical records highlighted some patients in residential and nursing care who had not documented advanced care planning. Working together, the Frome Medical Practice team were able to ensure that these patients were reviewed ahead of lockdown and had the opportunity with their families to record advanced care plans which aligned at care homes and across clinical systems.

Box 16.10 Case study 10: consistency of coding to enable consultations, multidisciplinary team reviews, and improvement monitoring

Daffodil Standard 4 focuses on internal practice systems such as confirming the expected end of life care coding dataset and this is supported with a practice electronic template aligned with the recommended Daffodil Standards MDT template. This supports all staff to use the same codes which in turn enables a more efficient review process in the MDT and consultations. Reception and non-clinical staff are better informed of flagged patients and caregivers, for example, if they call to make an appointment, or request medications or a home visit.

Ryder report into the experience of bereavement indicated that the GP was the individual that those who are bereaved feel most comfortable in approaching for support (Main, 2000).

It is one of the great privileges of being a GP to be able to walk alongside fellow human beings in their journey through this life. This becomes an important part of our role in bereavement, helping along with the rest of the community to bear witness to the life that has been lost. The anniversaries that follow a death are difficult times. Being part of a shared humanity supports us all.

Daffodil Standard 7 considers 'Care after death' and Standard 8 'General practice as hubs within compassionate communities'. These two connect seamlessly to enable support from the GP and practice team, both to acknowledge the bereaved person's loss and also to offer sign-posting within their community and supportive networks. See Box 16.12.

Learning and improving

Even when systems and processes are in place, regular reviews identify gaps in how fully these have been applied. The ethos of a learning organization is required for the team to adapt and excel (Davie and Nutley, 2000). A high-functioning team shares trust and collaboration when things are not going smoothly, with the ability to take a pragmatic approach to problem-solving, adapting as a situation evolves. It is open to learning from events and critical review of its own performance as a way of ensuring future improvements. A culture of openness and equality enables a way of continually improving pathways. A structure that supports ongoing education, quality improvement, and learning for clinical practice will ensure that opportunities to improve services are not missed (Stilos et al., 2016). See Box 16.13.

Box 16.11 Case study 11: dedicated palliative care nurse practitioner

The district nursing and primary care teams are co-located in Frome Medical Centre. The practice employs a dedicated nurse practitioner for palliative care support who meets the district nursing team formally on Monday mornings to review any issues that have arisen over the weekend and to jointly plan the week's priorities. A MDT meeting to review cases occurs weekly with the local hospice nurse from Dorothy House Hospice. A standardized template based on Daffodils Standards (see text) is used for MDT discussions so that key actions can be coded and recorded in a systematic way. This enables all those involved to be aware of any gaps and crucially to share and update about conversations and wishes of patients and their families.

Box 16.12 Case study 12: post-bereavement support

Elizabeth felt quite lost when she went to her GP after James had died. Caring for him had been all-consuming and she had not really had the time emotionally or physically to think about herself. When James was unwell with dementia, Elizabeth found that her time was no longer her own. Gradually she became more exhausted and she became upset by his truculent unpredictable outbursts when friends called. She stopped going shopping or trying to meet friends. She arranged a supermarket delivery weekly. Then suddenly James became unwell and was rushed to hospital with a chest infection. He died 3 days later. Those years have sapped her self-confidence. She was always a quiet woman and bore her sufferings with discretion and a stiff upper lip.

At first, the suggestion of attending a talking cafe felt daunting. She took the leaflet but left it on the living-room shelf. But when she did get in touch with the health connectors who ran the group, the individual she spoke to was so warm. Knowing she would be there helped Elizabeth to take that first step. She met Sheila, who had been widowed, and instantly felt she had met someone who could understand what she had been through. It surprised her how much talking helped her process what had happened. Sheila is now a firm friend and they meet regularly. Sharing experiences has helped Elizabeth and she has had the confidence to get back in touch with some of the old friends with whom she had lost contact while James was unwell.

Box 16.13 Case study 13: a learning environment

There had been an incident recently where medication had been delayed as it was not immediately available. The team discussed the event at their weekly MDT meeting. Edward had been close to the end of life and the GP had visited to talk to Edward and his daughter about planning for the next phase of his illness. He had arranged for a just-in-case medication prescription. The district nurses were aware and part of the planning. Edwards's daughter called to ask for assistance because he had become more nauseated and had been vomiting. The daughter said that the prescribed drugs had arrived in the afternoon the day before but when the district nurse arrived, she found that the antinausea medication prescribed 2 days earlier was not in there.

The nurse had to return to the practice find out why and then to collect it and make a second visit. It had been upsetting for them all. The team listened and heard both what had happened and its impact on those involved. They agreed to investigate further and look into how this had happened. It was an opportunity to discuss the impact that the incident had had, to acknowledge the knock of confidence it caused Edward and his daughter, and the stress and embarrassment it had caused the nurse. They talked through the knock-on consequences in managing the rest of her case load and the impact of recent team sickness on the team's capacity.

Investigation showed that the particular usual pharmacy for that patient had run out of stock of the drug. Liaison with the medicines management team of the commissioning body for healthcare resulted in a review and clarification of which local pharmacies stocked palliative care drugs. Recommendations were followed on which drugs these pharmacies should stock. A conversation with the pharmacy that had run out of stock resulted in an agreement to keep a quantity in stock for the future.

Calling again to visit the patient, the team were able to apologize and share some of the investigation with Edward's family. This helped to reassure them that the team were responsive and caring and that changes had been made to prevent a recurrence of this problem.

The team's approach to investigation and learning had helped bring them closer and improved their own understanding of how pathways around them worked. The nurse involved felt supported and all involved in the multidisciplinary discussion the following week felt that the time and investment in working together had been worthwhile.

Supporting those employed to provide care

Working in health and social care can be extremely rewarding, and yet care workers experience a high level of burnout. Dysfunctional teams, inflexible work practices, and inadequate time and resources can lead to a crisis of moral distress for compassionate carers (Oliver, 2018). If health and social care professionals are to provide care sustainably for the population, it is important to retain and nurture staff and address burnout (Kumar, 2016).

Schwartz rounds, clinical supervision, and Balint groups are organized structures for debriefing and reflection (Nielsen and Tulinius, 2009). Multidisciplinary team meetings are an opportunity to share treatment dilemmas and to reach a consensus in difficult cases. Time is required for caring for staff and provide them with the space to reflect on their roles. This is not an optional extra but a vital part of supporting them to deliver excellent care and to maintain their own well-being. It will enable honest conversations and prevent burnout and high staff turnover. It helps to ensure that staff remain emotionally present in their work and able to focus on what matters most to the individual needing care. The small practice teams and practice coffee room after surgery has provided a similar but less formal means of sharing and debriefing.

Systems leadership

The experience of living with dying and of caring is an intense experience and how well the individual and their family are supported in the last few days of life is crucial. A well-led team will be empowered to always focus on what is best for the patient rather than be constrained by organizational boundaries. Systems leadership enables this at a locality level and entrusts team members with autonomy to forge these strong relationships and work together. A good culture of leadership enables this (Ballatt and Campling, 2011). See Box 16.14.

Delivering consistent, good-quality compassionate care requires a whole system approach (Edmonstone, 2020). It requires engagement from both whole teams and individuals, not in having a fixed set of right answers but in responding flexibly to the demands placed on clinical services. Quality improvement methodology, combined with frontline enthusiasm and experience, provides the conditions to work our way towards solution. It requires a long-term approach to building strong relationships, recognizing the value of integration and collaboration. It includes working beyond organizational boundaries as a community of equal players, remaining attuned to the individual needs of each patient, and hearing and being fully present with them. Trust in the judgements of those at the frontline helps to enable working alongside individuals to deliver what is best for that individual. Devolved leadership to frontline workers helps to enable this (Martin et al., 2015).

> **Box 16.14** Case study 14: primary care networks—scaling population improvement
>
> Although the Daffodil Standards are designed for individual GP practices, there is also guidance to support implementation across GP primary care networks, clusters, and federations across the UK, typically 30,000–50,000 patients. This allows practices to work together at scale and consider opportunities to share learning and commissioned resources and work in partnership with their local community across combined practice populations. Common themes include improving practice processes such as coding to enable systematic monitoring of outcomes, and staff learning and development programmes to support people in their roles to achieve outcomes.
>
> Sharing learning across practices becomes particularly fruitful when considering shared resources to support connectivity with enhancing community development and therefore strengthening relationships between health and social care teams and our communities and supportive networks.

System leaders can support the frontline in using the art of their caring (Christiansen et al., 2015). This is as important in primary care as in hospital setting (Firth-Cozens and Cornwell, 2009). Working together in the clinical setting overcomes barriers and enhances care. Co-location of services creates a greater understanding of the capabilities and constraints of colleagues working for different organizations. When 'they' become 'we', we are better able to collectively tackle challenges. Partnership working and sharing success and learning across each other's organizations can be celebrated by leaders. Working together investing in relationships will enable sharing of ideas and perspectives. Leaders can share collective responsibility and support others to work through complex problems.

Language is important to help encourage empowerment, personal responsibility, and understanding of each other's perspectives. Development of compassionate workplaces provides the space and infrastructure in which these subjects can be discussed. Development of compassionate organizations requires a ground-up approach, in which the workforce themselves determine how best to support each other. Top-down support from chief executives and human resource directors is a critical component in ensuring the conditions within organizations support this.

Frontline creativity and innovation are needed to design delivery of care in a way that is best for the community. Delivering this care requires a culture of empowerment not centralization. It requires a supportive and enabling environment and care of the caregivers, grounded in the realities of lived experience. Such an approach encourages everyone to take ownership for their part in the optimal functioning of the whole system, with a shared overall vision and purpose. Individuals work hard to develop this across a whole system (Blackmore and Persaud, 2012).

The whole system at a local level can work together to agree medium- and long-term objectives and how to work towards these; with a long-term commitment, organizations can move away from annual funding cycles and short-term goals (Taylor-Robinson et al., 2008). Sensitivity to the understanding of the drivers and demands that are placed on other organizations helps to share these long-term goals (Hajek, 2013).

Conclusion

If our society is going to support all those undergoing the experiences of death, dying, loss, and caregiving, then a public health approach to palliative and end of life care has to be embedded in clinical care. The implications of doing so are profound. Not only is change needed at the individual level of clinical interactions, whole system change is required to support this. Shifting from siloed organizations through joint initiatives and working practices, developing good relationships across organizations, has to be supported by far-sighted and brave leadership. Putting aside the immediate concerns of individual organizations to build a better future is part of this. At the same time, the fundamental unit of care is the family network, embedded in the community in which this network functions. Professional teams and organizations are the servants of these networks, rather than the leaders or determinants of them. The collaboration of clinical services and communities provides access to good palliative care for our whole population. Together we can work towards equitable access to care including for those with frailty and non-cancer diagnoses. Reflection and learning from our experiences help us understand the human and structural factors that can lead to variability in care.

By activating and empowering our communities, health and social care professionals can work together with the communities they serve, and can support the whole community to receive high-quality care.

At the core of all we do is our shared experience of humanity. This is the guiding principle of our work, treating others with the kindness that we would want for ourselves or our family (Hannah, 2014). System leaders need to ensure that this guiding principle overarches the values and objectives of our ecosystem, so that we can create that compassionate workforce and compassionate community which supports us in the last journey of our life (Abel, 2018; Librada Flores et al., 2018).

Contributors include:

Dr Sarah Holmes, Palliative Care Consultant and Marie Curie Medical Director

Dr Dharini Shanmugabavan, Royal College of General Practitioners Medical Director of Clinical Quality

REFERENCES

Abel, J. 2018. Compassionate communities and end-of-life care. *Clinical Medicine*, 18, 6.

Abel, J., Kingston, H., Scally, A., Hartnoll, J., Hannam, G., Thomson-Moore, A., et al. 2018. Reducing emergency hospital admissions: a population health complex intervention of an enhanced model of primary care and compassionate communities. *British Journal of General Practice*, 68, e803–e810.

Aldred, H., Gott, M., and Gariballa, S. 2005. Advanced heart failure: impact on older patients and informal carers. *Journal of Advanced Nursing*, 49, 116–124.

Ballatt, J. and Campling, P. 2011. *Intelligent Kindness: Reforming the Culture of Healthcare*. London: RCPsych publications.

Blackmore, G. and Persaud, D. D. 2012. Diagnosing and improving functioning in interdisciplinary health care teams. *The Health Care Manager*, 31, 195–207.

Boyd, K. and Murray, S. A. 2010. Recognising and managing key transitions in end of life care. *BMJ*, 341, c4863.

Broady, T. 2015. The carer persona: Masking individual identities. *Persona Studies*, 1, 65.

Christiansen, A., O'Brien, M. R., Kirton, J. A., Zubairu, K., and Bray, L. 2015. Delivering compassionate care: the enablers and barriers. *British Journal of Nursing*, 24, 833–837.

Davie, H. T. and Nutley, S. M. 2000. Developing learning organisations in the new NHS. *BMJ*, 320, 998–1001.

Edmonstone, J. D. 2020. Beyond healthcare leadership? The imperative for health and social care systems. *Leadership in Health Services*, 33, 351–363.

Firth-Cozens, J. and Cornwell, J. 2009. *Enabling Compassionate Care in Acute Hospital Settings*. London: The King's Fund.

Golden, J., Conroy, R. M., Bruce, I., Denihan, A., Greene, E., Kirby, M., et al. 2009. Loneliness, social support networks, mood and wellbeing in community-dwelling elderly. *International Journal of Geriatric Psychiatry*, 24, 694–700.

Greene, A., Aranda, S., Tieman, J. J., Fazekas, B., and Currow, D. C. 2012. Can assessing caregiver needs and activating community networks improve caregiver-defined outcomes? A single-blind, quasi-experimental pilot study: community facilitator pilot. *Palliative Medicine*, 26, 917–923.

Hajek, A. M. 2013. Breaking down clinical silos in healthcare. *Frontiers of Health Services Management*, 29, 45–50.

Hannah, M. 2014. *Humanising Healthcare*. Bridport: Triarchy Press.

Holmes, T. H. and Rahe, R. H. 1967. The social readjustment rating scale. *Journal of Psychosomatic Research*, 11, 213–218.

Horsfall, D., Leonard, R., Noonan, K., and Rosenberg, J. 2013. Working together–apart: exploring the relationships between formal and informal care networks for people dying at home. *Progress in Palliative Care*, 21, 331–336.

Hudson, P. 2013. *Improving Support for Family Carers: Key Implications for Research, Policy and Practice*. London: Sage Publications.

Kumar, S. Burnout and doctors: prevalence, prevention and intervention. *Healthcare*, 4, 37.

Leonard, R., Horsfall, D., and Noonan, K. 2015. Identifying changes in the support networks of end-of-life carers using social network analysis. *BMJ Supportive & Palliative Care*, 5, 153–159.

Librada Flores, S. L., Molina, E. H., Osuna, J. B., Vargas, R. M., and Vicuña, M. N. 2018. All with You: a new method for developing compassionate communities—experiences in Spain and Latin-America. *Annals of Palliative Medicine*, 7, S15–S31.

Main, J. 2000. Improving management of bereavement in general practice based on a survey of recently bereaved subjects in a single general practice. *British Journal of General Practice*, 50, 863–866.

Martin, G., Beech, N., Macintosh, R., and Bushfield, S. 2015. Potential challenges facing distributed leadership in health care: evidence from the UK National Health Service. *Sociology of Health & Illness*, 37, 14–29.

Martin, G. P., Weaver, S., Currie, G., Finn, R., and McDonald, R. 2012. Innovation sustainability in challenging health-care contexts: embedding clinically led change in routine practice. *Health Services Management Research*, 25, 190–199.

Massey, M. T. 2015. Every general practice should appoint a carers' champion. *Nursing Standard*, 30, 32.

Millington-Sanders, C., and Noble, B. 2018. New UK general practice core standards for advanced serious illness and end of life care. *British Journal of General Practice*, 68, 114–115.

Moorman, D. W. 2007. Communication, teams, and medical mistakes. *Annals of Surgery*, 245, 173.

Nielsen, H. G. and Tulinius, C. 2009. Preventing burnout among general practitioners: is there a possible route? *Education for Primary Care*, 20, 353–359.

Noonan, K., Horsfall, D., Leonard, R., and Rosenberg, J. 2016. Developing death literacy. *Progress in Palliative Care*, 24, 31–35.

Oliver, D. 2018. David Oliver: moral distress in hospital doctors. *BMJ*, 360, k1333.

Sallnow, L., Kumar, S., and Numpeli, M. 2010. Home-based palliative care in Kerala, India: the neighbourhood network in palliative care. *Progress in Palliative Care*, 18, 14–17.

Sallnow, L., Richardson, H., Murray, S. A., and Kellehear, A. 2016. The impact of a new public health approach to end-of-life care: a systematic review. *Palliative Medicine,* 30, 200–211.

Sevin, C., Moore, G., Shepherd, J., Jacobs, T., and Hupke, C. 2009. Transforming care teams to provide the best possible patient-centered, collaborative care. *Journal of Ambulatory Care Management,* 32, 24–31.

Somhlaba, N. Z. and Wait, J. W. 2008. Psychological adjustment to conjugal bereavement: do social networks aid coping following spousal death? *OMEGA,* 57, 341–366.

Steinhauser, K. E., Christakis, N. A., Clipp, E. C., McNeilly, M., McIntyre, L., and Tulsky, J. A. 2000. Factors considered important at the end of life by patients, family, physicians, and other care providers. *JAMA,* 284, 2476–2482.

Stilos, K., Wynnychuk, L., Dasgupta, T., Lilien, T., and Daines, P. 2016. Improving end-of-life care through quality improvement. *International Journal of Palliative Nursing,* 22, 430–434.

Stylianos, S. K. and Vachon, M. L. 1993. The role of social support in bereavement. In: Stroebe, M. S., Stroebe, W., and Hansson, R. O. (eds.) *Handbook of Bereavement Research: Consequences, Coping, and Care,* pp. 397–410. New York: Cambridge University Press.

Taylor-Robinson, D. C., Milton, B., Lloyd-Williams, F., O'Flaherty, M., and Capewell, S. 2008. Planning ahead in public health? A qualitative study of the time horizons used in public health decision-making. *BMC Public Health,* 8, 1–7.

Vassilev, I., Rogers, A., Blickem, C., Brooks, H., Kapadia, D., Kennedy, A., et al. 2013. Social networks, the 'work' and work force of chronic illness self-management: a survey analysis of personal communities. *PLoS One,* 8, e59723.

Vieira, C. M., Franco, O. H., Restrepo, C. G., and Abel, T. 2020. COVID-19: the forgotten priorities of the pandemic. *Maturitas,* 136, 38–41.

Vuksan, M., Williams, A., and Crooks, V. 2012. Family friendly policies: accommodating end-of-life caregivers in workplaces. *International Journal of Workplace Health Management,* 5, 4–14.

17

Digital technologies in public health palliative care

Jason Mills and Shyla Mills

Introduction

In the digital age, public health and palliative care are practised within a rapidly evolving society. Ongoing advances in technological innovation combine with clinical and community settings where the providers and recipients of care are either 'digital immigrants' adapting to the digital world, or now more commonly, 'digital natives' born into it (Wernhart et al., 2019). Indeed, advances in digital health technologies represent a key tool to address the global population need for palliative and end of life care, projected to increase well beyond current capacity (Bone et al., 2018). Given this societal context and fusion of technology with human caring, there is a growing need to understand the benefits and limitations to the use of digital technologies within social models of care such as public health palliative care.

In seeking to address this need, a number of questions arise. Is the use of technology congruent with or antithetical to the humanistic tenets of palliative care? What technologies have been used in palliative care? How does the use of technology align with public health principles and what can it contribute in practice? What are the key considerations for achieving clinical and community benefits?

This chapter will explore the use of digital technologies in the context of public health palliative care. Through a dual lens of digital public health and thanatechnology, it provides an overview of the digital technologies used in palliative care, outlining their application to the growing field of public health palliative care. It further considers the inherent risks of technological developments in society, alongside potential benefits for public health palliative care in both clinical and community settings. The chapter concludes with consideration of key issues around the need for co-design of digital health interventions, outcome evaluation, and awareness of social inequities to guide practice, education, and research.

Digital technologies in palliative care

Nomenclature

The concept of the digital age comes with the global recognition of an ageing population. That is, younger populations born in the digital era are considered digital natives, whereas older populations born prior to this are considered digital immigrants (Wernhart et al., 2019). For digital natives and digital immigrants alike, there is an array of technological terms and classifications to become familiar with so as to understand the application and potential utility of digital technologies in palliative care. While terminology has evolved over time, broadening to a contemporary and overarching context of *digital health* (to be discussed in detail later), the most common terms to date as relevant to palliative care are outlined in Box 17.1.

In the early 2000s, eHealth was defined as 'an emerging field in the intersection of medical informatics, public health, and business, referring to health services and information delivered or enhanced through the internet and related technologies' (Eysenbach, 2001, p. 1). Thus, in broad terms, eHealth encapsulates the digitalization of public health activities and healthcare service provision through collaborations between multiple sectors of society. Interrelated, yet more specifically, mHealth describes the 'use of mobile and

Box 17.1 Early use and nomenclature of digital technologies in palliative care

- Electronic health (eHealth).
- Electronic health record (EHR).
- Electronic medical record (EMR).
- Electronic patient-recorded outcome (ePRO).
- Gamification.
- Information and communications technology (ICT).
- Internet of things (IoT).
- Mobile application (app).
- Mobile health technology (mHealth).
- Social media.
- Thanatechnology.
- Telehealth.
- Telemedicine.
- Telepalliative care.
- Virtual reality (VR).
- Weblog (blog).
- Wearable technology (wearables).

wireless technologies to support the achievement of health objectives' (World Health Organization (WHO), 2016, p. 127).

Palliative care context

The digitalization of healthcare involves a myriad of information and communication technologies (ICTs) through the development and use of associated software and hardware. In many applications of eHealth, these technologies rely on what is known as the 'internet of things' (IoT), which can be understood as a system of interrelated and connected 'things'—including people and mechanical or digital devices (Xia et al., 2012). With this interconnectivity and the use of unique identifiers, the IoT enables the transfer of data over a network without reliance on human to computer or human-to-human interaction. This could also involve the use of mHealth (a subbranch of eHealth) devices such as hand-held tablets, smartphones, or wearables such as a smartwatch through the use of a mobile app. In this way, clinicians can use the IoT and eHealth/mHealth technologies to facilitate online consultations or provide real-time remote monitoring of patients' health status. For example, mHealth technology and wearables have been used in palliative care for the continuous monitoring of patients to predict deterioration in health status (Pavic et al., 2019, 2020).

Electronic health records (EHRs), also referred to as electronic medical records (EMRs), represent a form of eHealth utilizing ICTs to facilitate clinical data entry/storage/access to record clinical documentation. Electronic records are increasingly used in health services worldwide, with some undergoing transformation to become a wholly digital hospital. Along with ICTs (Allsop et al., 2015; Ostherr et al., 2016), they have been used for patient identification, communication, and clinical support in palliative care (Cox et al., 2017; Bush et al., 2018).

Similarly, electronic patient-reported outcomes (ePROs) are increasingly used in palliative care to improve quality of assessment and care (Karamanidou et al., 2020). An ePRO is a clinical measurement of health status reported electronically and directly by patients—usually via internet-connected mobile or wearable devices—to clinicians without need for clinical assessment or interpretation to capture them. Telehealth and telemedicine are terms used to describe the use of audio/visual telecommunications technology to provide healthcare and medical consultation or treatment for patients outside of healthcare facilities, generally where geographical or physical distance constraints exist. This approach has been used effectively in palliative care contexts for over a decade in metropolitan or rural settings (Slavin-Stewart et al., 2020), including both adult and paediatric populations (Kidd et al., 2010; Bradford et al., 2013).

Similarly, there is emerging uptake of virtual reality (VR) technologies for paediatric and adult populations. Specifically, VR has been used to support advance care planning (Hsieh, 2020) as well as symptom management and quality of life (Kabir et al., 2020) in palliative care patients.

Following development of the internet and world wide web, personal use of various weblog (blog), microblog, and social media platforms has grown tremendously in global society. Evidence of this can be seen in palliative care (Taubert et al., 2014). For example, *Palliverse* (https://www.palliverse.com) is a virtual community of practice created by an Australian and New Zealand network of people involved in palliative care (Collins et al., 2016). *eHospice* (https://ehospice.com), *CareSearch* (https://www.caresearch.com.au), and *Canadian Virtual Hospice* (https://www.virtualhospice.ca) are online palliative care resources made available and widely accessed through a web-based platform.

Gamification, or the use of online gaming and game mechanics (Sardi et al., 2017), can be a useful tool to reach and engage members of the public in end of life discussions in advance—outside of any clinical context of palliative care. For example, the *Dying To Talk* online card game (https://dyingtotalk.org.au/card-game/) was developed for use as a discussion starter to help people reflect and talk about their preferences for care at the end of life.

Thanatechnology is the term coined by thanatologists to describe the use of technology in contexts of death, dying, grief, loss, and serious illness (Sofka et al., 2012). While this term may not be used or known by all working in palliative care, it is helpful to understand this more contextualized use of technology as applied to palliative care practice, research, and education. Thus, the digital technologies discussed here can best be understood within the context of thanatechnology.

Increasing use of thanatechnology

Given the rapid rate of innovative development and implementation of digital technologies in society, there has been a steady growth in professional discourse and use of thanatechnology. In the decade between 2010 and 2020, a broad and increasing international trend is evident in the peer-reviewed palliative care literature. Table 17.1 depicts this growth, providing an overview of studies and articles addressing the use of thanatechnology across the broad landscape of palliative care service provision—throughout the lifespan and encompassing care in hospital, hospice, residential facility, and home-based care settings. A synthesis of the literature reveals the key foci of thanatechnology in palliative care, as outlined in Box 17.2.

Digital technologies and public health palliative care

The use of digital technologies in public health palliative care is situated at the interface of thanatechnology and digital public health. This is illustrated in Fig. 17.1.

Thanatechnology and digital (public) health

Within this context, thanatechnology can be understood and employed as an enabling conduit for anyone living with dying in contemporary society (Sofka et al., 2012; Bassett, 2015; Arnold et al., 2018). Similarly, digital public health can be understood as the use of technology to promote health through the digitization of public health interests and activities through new approaches that transcend traditional health service models (Murray et al., 2020).

The use of thanatechnology and digital public health in palliative care is informed by the contemporary field of digital health. Digital health is defined as 'the field of knowledge and practice associated with the development and use of digital technologies to improve health' (WHO, 2020a, p. 5). As the current and most inclusive term to encapsulate the myriad uses of technology for health, digital health includes but expands from eHealth and mHealth to incorporate a focus on digital consumers, with a wider range of smart and

Table 17.1 The growth and origin of peer-reviewed literature addressing the use of thanatechnology in palliative care services between 2010 and 2020

Author/s (year)	Location	Article title
Kidd et al. (2010)	UK	Telehealth in palliative care in the UK: a review of the evidence
Oliver et al. (2012)	US	A systematic review of the evidence base for telehospice
Bradford et al. (2013)	Australia	The case for home based telehealth in pediatric palliative care: a systematic review
Ngwenya et al. (2013)	UK	The use of weblogs within palliative care: a systematic literature review
Reis et al. (2013)	Portugal	Information and communication technologies in long-term and palliative care
Taubert et al. (2014)	UK	Palliative social media
Allsop et al. (2015)	UK	Information and communication technology for managing pain in palliative care: a review of the literature
Cox et al. (2015)	US	Using technology to create a more humanistic approach to integrating palliative care into the intensive care unit
Dhiliwal and Salins (2015)	India	Smartphone applications in palliative homecare
Collins et al. (2016)	Australia	Virtual communities of practice: a novel tool for increasing palliative care engagement
Ostherr et al. (2016)	US	Death in the digital age: a systematic review of information and communication technologies in end-of-life care
Royackers et al. (2016)	Canada	The eShift model of care: informal caregivers' experience of a new model of home-based palliative care
Tieman et al. (2016)	Australia	Using telehealth to support end of life care in the community: a feasibility study
Cox et al. (2017)	US	Palliative Care Planner: a pilot study to evaluate acceptability and usability of an EHR system-integrated, needs-targeted app platform
Guo et al. (2017)	Canada	Keep in Touch (KIT): feasibility of using internet-based communication and information technology in palliative care
Meghani et al. (2017)	US	Clinician-targeted mobile apps in palliative care: a systematic review
Pinto et al. (2017)	Portugal	e-Health in palliative care: review of literature, Google Play and App Store
Allsop et al. (2018)	UK/Africa	The state of mHealth development and use by palliative care services in sub-Saharan Africa: a systematic review of the literature
Bush et al. (2018)	US	Systematic review of the use of electronic health record for patient identification, communication, & clinical support in palliative care
Greenle et al. (2018)	US	Identifying mobile apps targeting palliative care patients and family members
Nwosu et al. (2018)	UK	Wearable smartwatch technology to monitor symptoms in advanced illness
Phongtankuel et al. (2018)	US	Mobile health technology and home hospice care: promise and pitfalls
Clabburn et al. (2019)	UK	The use of digital legacies with people affected by MND for continuing bonds: an interpretative phenomenological analysis study
Coop and Marlow (2019)	UK	Do we prepare patients for their digital legacy? A survey of palliative care professionals
Hancock et al. (2019)	UK	Telehealth in palliative care is being described but not evaluated: a systematic review
Jess et al. (2019)	Denmark	Video consultations in palliative care: a systematic integrative review
Niki et al. (2019)	Japan	Novel approach using virtual reality for improving symptoms of terminal cancer patients: preliminary prospective, multi-centre study
Pavic et al. (2019)	Switzerland	Mobile health technologies for continuous monitoring of cancer patients in palliative care aiming to predict health status deterioration
Weingarten et al. (2019)	Canada	Virtual reality: endless potential in pediatric palliative care: a case report
Akard et al. (2020)	US	Transforming a face-to-face legacy intervention to a web-based legacy intervention for children with advanced cancer
Andrews et al. (2020)	US	Legacy building in pediatric end-of-life care through innovative use of a digital stethoscope
Bentley et al. (2020)	Australia	Dignity therapy online: piloting an online psychosocial intervention for people with terminal illness
Hsieh (2020)	Taiwan	Virtual reality video promotes effectiveness in advance care planning
Johnson et al. (2020)	US	Virtual reality use for symptom management in palliative care: a pilot study to assess user perceptions
Kabir et al. (2020)	Canada	Pilot study of 'LIFEView' audiovisual technology: virtual travel to support well-being & quality of life in palliative and end-of-life care
Karamanidou et al. (2020)	Europe/UK	Electronic patient-reported outcome-based interventions for palliative cancer care: a systematic and mapping review
Moore et al. (2020)	US	Using telehealth for hospice reauthorization visits: results of a quality improvement analysis
Pavic et al. (2020)	Switzerland	Feasibility and usability aspects of continuous remote monitoring of health status in palliative cancer patients using wearables
Slavin-Stewart et al. (2020)	Canada	A feasibility study of home-based palliative care telemedicine in rural Nova Scotia
Steindal et al. (2020)	Norway	Patients' experiences of telehealth in palliative home care: scoping review
Towsley et al. (2020)	US	Piloting Me and My Wishes – videos of nursing home residents' preferences
Widberg et al. (2020)	Sweden	Patients' experiences of eHealth in palliative care: an integrative review

Box 17.2 Key foci of thanatechnology in palliative care

- Access/storage and input to health records/information.
- Advance care planning/documentation of health directives.
- Clinician–clinician communication.
- Clinician–patient communication/consultation.
- Decision-making support.
- Education.
- Interprofessional collaboration and engagement.
- Psychological, social care, and bereavement support.
- Quality of life.
- Remote monitoring and management of symptoms.

connected devices. Importantly, this represents a paradigm shift from that of simply introducing more technology to healthcare—to one of enabling healthcare in the social context of digital citizens living and dying in digital societies (Mills, 2019).

Digital health encompasses other digital technologies used for health, including advanced computing, big data analytics, artificial intelligence including machine learning, and robotics (WHO, 2020a). Discussion around the use and implications of these digital health technologies has already begun to emerge in palliative care discourse; namely, the use of big data (Nwosu et al., 2017), machine learning (Avati et al., 2018), artificial intelligence (Kamdar et al., 2019), and robotic technologies (Nwosu et al., 2019).

The centrality of digital health to international progress towards universal health coverage and access to high-quality palliative care is evident in emerging policy frameworks such as the WHO (2020a) *Global Strategy on Digital Health 2020–2024* (Mariano, 2020). It is further reflected in multinational settings where the widescale adoption of digital health technologies is transforming how healthcare is provided and experienced (Novillo-Ortiz et al., 2018; Hambleton and Aloizos, 2019). For example, *Australia's National Digital Health Strategy* (Australian Digital Health Agency, 2018), as a civic initiative with an explicit focus on improving end of life care, provided the policy platform to implement the *My Health Record*, an individual's electronic health record that is accessible to patients and clinicians nationwide. It further paved the way for state-based specialist and generalist healthcare services to work in partnership with their communities to develop more localized clinical and consumer digital health charters (Sullivan et al., 2020). In Queensland, the *Digital Health Consumer Charter* (http://www.hcq.org.au/qdhcc-full/) was developed by the non-clinical community to ensure that the voice of everyday citizens is heard and can directly inform the development of digital health policies and design of new programmes or technologies that impact the whole community.

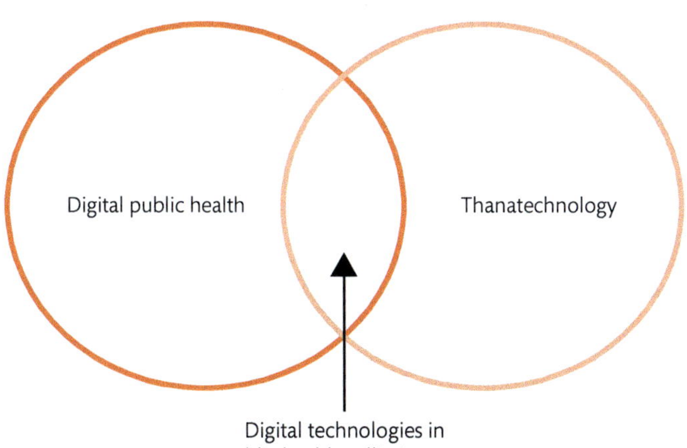

Fig. 17.1 Interface of digital public health and thanatechnology.

In this way, there is a clear thread of continuity and concerted public collaboration between the civic sector, specialist and generalist healthcare services, and everyday citizens in the community to share responsibility for and progress towards digitally enabled models of care. In that context, the combined application of digital public health and thanatology to the health-promoting principles and practice of public health palliative care opens up new and empowering opportunities beyond the bounds of traditional service provision models. That is, opportunities to better promote community engagement, meaningful connection, and participatory action through digitally enabled social partnerships.

Digitally enabled public health palliative care

As core health-promoting features of public health palliative care, social partnerships and participatory action can be enabled by existing or emerging digital technologies. This can best be conceptualized and achieved through the connectivity and combined efforts of the key stakeholders involved in palliative care. The new essentials model of palliative care (Abel et al., 2018) outlines the key stakeholders within its four basic components of palliative and end of life care:

- Specialist palliative care.
- Generalist palliative care.
- Compassionate communities.
- Civic programme for the Compassionate City Charter (Kellehear, 2016).

Given that effective coordination between these components can improve well-being at the end of life for every citizen affected by a life-limiting condition, the use of digital technologies in public health palliative care, then, can be understood as a virtual, enabling chain of connection operating between the civic, compassionate community, specialist, and generalist cogs of palliative care. This is illustrated in Fig. 17.2.

Digital technologies within the new essentials model of palliative care

The new essentials model of palliative care represents a novel approach to integrating the processes and operations of specialist palliative care, generalist palliative care, compassionate communities, and civic end of life care. In introducing this model, Abel and colleagues (2018) outlined a number of change recommendations for each of these domains to enhance palliative and end of life care. By way of example, Table 17.2 indicates the potential use of digital technologies to address and enable at least one of the recommendations in each of the domains.

Drawing from the various advantages of digital technologies, each individual cog, combined as a collective, can realize multiple benefits shared between each sector of society. Those working in generalist palliative care, for example, could benefit from more effective collaboration with others working in specialist palliative care—as

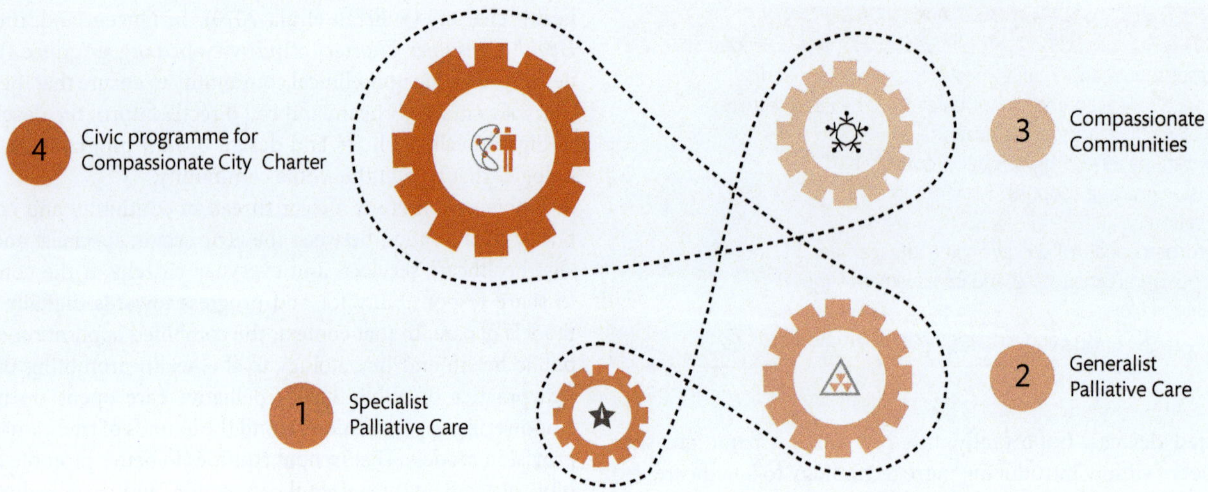

-------- Digital technologies as a virtual and enabling chain of connection

Fig. 17.2 Conceptualizing digital technologies within the new essentials model of palliative care.
Reproduced with permission from Abel, J., Kellehear, A. & Karapliagou, A. 2018. Palliative care—the new essentials. *Annals of Palliative Medicine*, 7, S3–S14.

well as better communication with compassionate communities that are supported by civic initiatives and possess basic knowledge and capacity to support end of life care (Abel et al., 2018). Together, palliative care services and compassionate communities can improve care in the last days, weeks, months, and years of life (Mills and Rosenberg, 2019)—increasing quality of life and the number of deaths at home, where most people would prefer to die.

To be of full benefit, the use of digital technologies within public health palliative care should be approached through the dual lens of thanatechnology/digital public health and must be applied in ways that directly enable the new essentials of palliative care. This is consistent with the public health approach to palliative care as conceptualized by Tziraki and colleagues (2020), whose global model identifies digital technologies as a key enabler to public health palliative care.

Social media and community-based online resources

Helping to put the 'public' into public health (Rosenberg et al., 2016), the use of social media and other online resources in the community can play an important enabling role for participatory action and social partnerships in palliative care. Indeed, these digital technologies are used by individuals and organizations from each sector of society involved in palliative care. Most citizens now own connected devices (smart phones or smart TVs and smart homes), and many have access to high-speed internet/wireless connectivity in private/public settings and use mobile apps as a routine part of daily life. Thus, the use of digital technologies in public health palliative care can be experienced as empowering and enabling, rather than a form of clinical 'intervention'. A wide range of online resources, social media, and social networking sites exist, and their use in palliative care contexts has proliferated over the past decade (Sofka et al., 2012; Taubert et al., 2014).

In particular, online grief support and community-focused education feature in the literature. Massive open online courses (MOOCs) such as the *Dying2Learn* MOOC have provided supportive and accessible opportunities for the community to engage in collaborative discussions about death and dying (Miller-Lewis et al., 2018; Tieman et al., 2018). Other education such as *Last Aid* has

Table 17.2 Enabling technology for the new essentials of palliative care

New essentials component	New essentials change recommendation (Abel et al., 2018)	Potential enabling technologies
Specialist palliative care	'Changing job plans so that specialist palliative care advice and supports available in the community on a 24-hour basis through the use of video technology Participation in starting and supporting compassionate community initiatives, including the Compassionate City Charter'	Telemedicine /telehealth video conferencing platforms Virtual community of practice enabling asynchronous interaction
Generalist palliative care	'Early identification of people at the end of life, irrespective of diagnosis Setting up bereavement peer support groups and linkages to community groups of support and common interest'	Shared access to integrated national EMR/EHR for timely identification/care coordination Online grief communities for peer support interaction via social networking sites
Compassionate communities	'Develop a directory of resources that support end-of-life care in the community, and are available to all citizens—the public and professionals alike … to be regularly updated'	Online directories made freely available via website; mobile apps enabling communities to create neighbourhood support networks to support social care
Civic programme of action	'Regularly engage social media and cultural centres to stimulate death, caregiving and grief and bereavement projects'	Ongoing social media engagement with citizens via YouTube/Facebook/Twitter

been provided online with a focus on capacity building for compassionate communities, in line with the health promotion action areas of developing personal skills and strengthening community action (Mills et al., 2020a). In 2017, Palliative Care Australia developed the mobile app *Allow Me* to support family caregivers and friends of people living with life-limiting illness in creating a connected community of care around them, communicating their needs for social care. Other online alternatives to this include *CaringBridge* (https://www.caringbridge.org/) and *Gather my Crew* (https://www.gathermycrew.org.au/).

Social media and social networking sites such as Facebook have been used in supportive contexts of grief, mourning, and memorialization (Moore et al., 2017; Willis and Ferruci, 2017). Indeed, many online grief networks have been developed by community members to enable peer support for the bereaved, by the bereaved (Hartig and Viola, 2015). Mobile apps such as *MyGrief* (https://youtu.be/MFfwcdmX-Z0) and online games such as *Apart of Me* (https://www.apartofme.app/) have also been used to support healthy grieving in both adults and children internationally. Other online fora such as *Glowwormshome* (https://glowwormshome.org.au/), a palliative care equipment and consumables donation platform, are used for connecting families experiencing loss to build resilience and compassion in the community. Online memorialization sites such as *After Cloud* (https://myaftercloud.com/) and end of life planning resources such as *MyWishes* (https://www.mywishes.co.uk/) also provide innovative forms of support and connection.

Anther novel use of social media is the promotion of death awareness and organ donation in gaming communities. For instance, the *Restart Project* (http://dev.pipedigital.com/restart/en/) was developed in Brazil to target players who have just died (in the game) as well as the developers behind the games to include the software in other games. After installation, when a gamer dies, they are shown the message: 'You are dead, but you can still donate your organs. Be a donor and help someone else to have a new life in the game.' A choice to donate is then shared with an individual's social network and across the gaming community.

Commonly used social media platforms in palliative care are outlined in Box 17.3. Public Health Palliative Care International conference proceedings have been shared in real time via Facebook livestream and later been made available via YouTube (https://www.phpci.org/), which has also been used by palliative care researchers to explore end of life content in online videos (Mitchell et al., 2017). Another online video platform, vimeo, has been used by the *What Matters* conversations movement to promote the *What Matters Most Charter* (https://www.whatmattersconversations.org/2020-charter) and its short film *What Matters to Me* (https://vimeo.com/488130017)—both openly available online to the public. These contemporary resources are increasingly important to the promotion of a public health approach to advance care planning, with a more direct focus on what to do (what matters) rather than what not to do (Abel et al., 2020). In addition to online video platforms, palliative care organizations have used both Facebook and Twitter to extend the social reach of conferences and facilitate community engagement through online dialogue and feedback (Mills and Mills, 2016).

Box 17.3 Common social media platforms and social networking sites

- Facebook.
- Twitter.
- YouTube.

Twitter is widely used in both clinical and social contexts of palliative care. Key to the application of Twitter in palliative care is the use of hashtags (Katz et al., 2019) and tweet chats (Collins et al., 2016). As used in healthcare research, a hashtag is a form of metadata prefixed with # and used as a means of indexing a thread of continuous online discussion content/tweets (Pinho-Costa et al., 2016). A tweet chat is an organized virtual event that uses a predetermined hashtag to facilitate global discussion and sharing of online media/resources in real time via the Twitter platform. By way of example, in 2016 a compassionate communities tweet chat was hosted by Palliverse and Palliative Care Australia (https://palliverse.com/2016/07/21/pallanz-tweetchat-compassionate-communities/), using the hashtag #PallANZ which reflects the Australian and New Zealand palliative care community as intended participants. Commonly used Twitter hashtags used in contexts of digital health and public health palliative care are listed in Box 17.4.

Beyond the use of blogs by professionals and academic institutions, community-focused blogs such as that by Compassionate Communities UK (https://www.compassionate-communitiesuk.co.uk/) share a variety of resources and blog posts, as well as the popular podcast series *Survival of the Kindest*.

Digital responses to the COVID-19 pandemic

The relevance and utility of digital technologies in public health palliative care were highlighted with the emergence of the coronavirus disease 2019 (COVID-19) global pandemic, as it impacted populations and palliative care services across the world (The Lancet, 2020). With the combined impact of increased need for end of life care, together with enforced physical distancing restrictions, there was a rapid adoption of widespread digital technology use (Kuntz et al., 2020; Lau et al., 2020; Sutherland et al., 2020; Wu et al., 2020). A synthesis of the literature published in 2020 alone reveals six key foci, with impacts on and supports for, both clinical and community populations. These are outlined in Box 17.5.

Box 17.4 Common social media hashtags used on Twitter

#advancecareplanning	#endoflifecare
#bereavement	#gooddeath
#comcom	#goodgrief
#compassionatecities	#griefawarenessweek
#compassionatecommunities	#healthpromotingpalliativecare
#communitydevelopment	#hospice
#d2kd	#loss
#deathcafe	#mhealth
#deatheducation	#openuptogrief
#deathliteracy	#palliativecare
#deathoverdinner	#pallicovid
#digitalhealth	#phpc2013
#digitalhealthliteracy	#phpc2015
#digitaldeath	#phpc2017
#dyingtoknowday	#phpci2019
#ehealth	#publichealthpalliativecare
#ehr	#qualityoflife
#emr	#stnicslifesquestions
#endoflife	#thanatechnology

Box 17.5 Key foci of digital technologies during the COVID-19 pandemic

- Telecommunication with patients and families/consultation.
- Patient communication with family and social networks.
- Virtual funerals and online memorialization.
- Social closeness in the clinical context of physical distance.
- Human connection via technology.
- Interprofessional collaboration/engagement.

Palliative care services met the emerging challenges through a combination of online support and sharing of professional resources (Mills et al., 2020b, 2020c), as well as the reinvention of traditional palliative care service provision models through the adoption of digital technologies (Ritchey et al., 2020; Wang et al., 2020). In particular, the use of mobile videoconferencing apps was critical in facilitating real-time communication between patients and families/social networks (Abel and Taubert, 2020; Bettini, 2020). Twitter was also used during the pandemic to connect those working in palliative care and mobilize support. For example, in March 2020, Public Health Palliative Care International held a tweet chat entitled 'Empowering and informing communities in the time of COVID-19: What is the role of compassionate communities in response?' using the hashtags #comcom and #palliCOVID (https://twitter.com/PHPalCare/status/1243119034645663745). In the following month, Palliverse held a tweet chat about Telehealth and working from home—also using the hashtag #palliCOVID (https://twitter.com/palliverse/status/1246914257867829250). Between March and December 2020, there was in excess of 30,000 tweets globally, using #pallicovid—which on average, is around 100 tweets per day around the world (https://www.symplur.com/healthcare-hashtags/PalliCovid/analytics/?hashtag=PalliCovid).

Community members were also met with significant challenges and navigated these through the use of digital technologies, particularly in the areas of grief and loss. For example, private virtual funerals and online memorialization were key priorities to be addressed in the context of public health palliative care (Kohn, 2020; Lowe et al., 2020; Muturi et al., 2020). Other, more public, virtual events included Good Grief, a virtual festival of love and loss (https://goodgrieffest.com/).

The creation of digital legacies is increasingly important to bereavement support for patients and their families/social networks (Akard et al., 2020). As an annual conference that explores death, dying, bereavement, and the internet, gatherings such as the Digital Legacy Conference (https://digitallegacyconference.com/) therefore play a valuable role in promoting professional awareness and building community capacity to enhance bereavement support in these ways. This approach is especially important, given the evidence to suggest that people living with dying are not routinely supported to prepare a digital legacy (Coop and Marlow, 2019). 'PalliCovid & Exploring New Dimensions' was the theme chosen for the (virtual) 2021 Digital Legacy Conference. In this way, there have been clear benefits to the use of digital technologies for both clinicians and compassionate communities alike (Abel and Taubert, 2020; Mills et al., 2020). These benefits must be considered alongside the associated challenges to using digital technologies in public health palliative care.

Key considerations for the development and use of digital technologies

Alongside the various benefits, there are a number of challenges to the use of digital technologies in public health palliative care. Due consideration must be given to each, if the advantages are to outweigh any associated disadvantages. Ensuring cybersecurity can be a challenge. Awareness of potential risks and maintaining transparency for those using digital technologies will be paramount in addressing privacy and security concerns in the digital health era (Filkins et al., 2016). Digital health equity can also be a challenge, particularly for digital health promotion within social contexts of a 'digital divide' and other health inequities that may be exacerbated by social disadvantage or an overreliance on digital technologies to meet basic health needs (Lupton, 2015). Consideration of the digital determinants of health—such as internet access and literacy in the use of mHealth and ICTs—is equally important to addressing other social and cultural determinants of health (Novillo-Ortiz et al., 2018; Azzopardi-Muscat and Sørensen, 2019; Crawford and Serhal, 2020). Similarly, education will be important in the building of digital health literacy for those who might need it, both in the general community and the palliative care workforce (Kuek and Hakkennes, 2019; WHO, 2020b). The financial and logistical resource implications of acquiring and maintaining digital technology infrastructure are also important considerations.

Maintaining the perception and qualities of human connection can be a challenge, even where communication is enabled by technology. This may often be attributed to resistance or other negative attitudes towards the use of technology (Sansom-Daly and Bradford, 2020). Those working in palliative care should understand the large-scale use of digital technologies represents a cultural transformation in traditional healthcare—a transformation towards greater flexibility and access to health information as well as greater control for autonomous decision-making by everyday citizens (Meskó et al., 2017).

But digital health is far from a panacea; while it can prove a valuable tool, its use in public health palliative care must be judicious, with social connection and participatory partnerships maintained as central (Mills, 2019). Challenges in appropriate bedside manner have now shifted towards an awareness of 'webside manner' (Chua et al., 2020). Concerns around maintaining human connection in an increasingly digital society are amplified in the often emotion-charged contexts of palliative and end of life care (Payne et al., 2020). Therefore, care must be taken to ensure that technology is designed and used to enable or enhance the social expression of compassion at the end of life.

While the use of digital health technologies has increased markedly in recent years, the pace of outcome measurement has not kept up with development and implementation. Indeed, many technological innovations in palliative care are being 'described but not evaluated' (Hancock et al., 2019). Moreover, many do not include everyday citizens in their design, development, or testing. Future use of digital technologies in the context of public health palliative care should incorporate co-design with community members as a key stakeholder. This is especially important where specific cultural considerations are important (Rice et al., 2016; Jones et al., 2017). They should also undergo rigorous evaluation to demonstrate their public health impact on health system outcomes and strengthening community action in palliative care (Sallnow et al., 2016; Collins et al., 2021).

The development and implementation of future digital technologies should be guided by key policy frameworks such as the WHO (2020a) *Global Strategy on Digital Health*, national and local digital health strategies where they exist (Mills, 2019), and the *Global Atlas of Palliative Care* (Worldwide Hospice Palliative Care Alliance, 2020) as appropriate. The WHO (2018a) report on the use of appropriate digital technologies for public health, combined with its international classification and recommendations for digital health interventions (WHO, 2018b, 2019) would also assist the development and implementation of future digital technologies. Together, these considerations are key for the areas of practice, education, and research in public health palliative care.

Conclusion

With an ageing population and increased need for end of life care, coupled with limitations to service provision, the use of digital technologies is likely to increase as palliative care services and communities seek to enhance the quality and accessibility of care at the end of life. An awareness of digital public health together with an ability to advocate and influence developments in this area through the lens of thanatechnology are therefore vital. To be of full benefit, the use of digital technologies within public health palliative care should be approached through the dual lens of thanatechnology/digital public health and must be applied in ways that connect and enable the specialist, generalist, compassionate community, and civic components of palliative care.

This chapter has explored the use of digital technologies in the context of public health palliative care. The broad range of digital technologies used in palliative care were outlined, highlighting potential benefits and limitations as applied to the tenets of public health palliative care. The benefits of using technology in both clinical and community contexts must be considered alongside any potential risks. Awareness of social inequities, the co-design of digital health interventions and outcome evaluation, together, represent key considerations for practice, education, and research.

While relatively underutilized in the past, the growing and judicious use of digital technologies can serve to promote social connection in the face of physical isolation, and in this way, has great potential to humanize care rather than de-humanize it. The use of digital technologies in public health palliative care will increasingly transform our approaches to death, dying, grief, and loss—to digitally enable and enhance the ways we provide whole-of-society compassionate care for everyone living with dying.

REFERENCES

Abel, J., Kellehear, A., and Karapliagou, A. 2018. Palliative care—the new essentials. *Annals of Palliative Medicine*, 7, S3–S14.

Abel, J., Kellehear, A., Millington Sanders, C., Taubert, M., and Kingston, H. 2020. Advance care planning re-imagined: a needed shift for COVID times and beyond. *Palliative Care and Social Practice*, 14, 2632352420934491.

Abel, J. and Taubert, M. 2020. Coronavirus pandemic: compassionate communities and information technology. *BMJ Supportive & Palliative Care*, 10, 369–371.

Akard, T. F., Wray, S., Friedman, D. L., Dietrich, M. S., Hendricks-Ferguson, V., Given, B., et al. 2020. Transforming a face-to-face legacy intervention to a web-based legacy intervention for children with advanced cancer. *Journal of Hospice & Palliative Nursing*, 22, 49–60.

Allsop, M., Taylor, S., Mulvey, M., Bennett, M., and Bewick, B. 2015. Information and communication technology for managing pain in palliative care: a review of the literature. *BMJ Supportive & Palliative Care*, 5, 481–489.

Allsop, M. J., Powell, R. A., and Namisango, E. 2018. The state of mHealth development and use by palliative care services in sub-Saharan Africa: a systematic review of the literature. *BMJ Supportive & Palliative Care*, 8, 155–163.

Andrews, E., Hayes, A., Cerulli, L., Miller, E. G., and Slamon, N. 2020. Legacy building in pediatric end-of-life care through innovative use of a digital stethoscope. *Palliative Medicine Reports*, 1, 149–155.

Arnold, M., Gibbs, M., Kohn, T., Meese, J., and Nansen, B. 2018. *Death and Digital Media*. Abingdon: Routledge.

Australian Digital Health Agency. 2018. National Digital Health Strategy. Australian Government. [Online] Available at: https://conversation.digitalhealth.gov.au/sites/default/files/adha-strategy-doc-2ndaug_0_1.pdf

Avati, A., Jung, K., Harman, S., Downing, L., Ng, A., and Shah, N. H. 2018. Improving palliative care with deep learning. *BMC Medical Informatics Decision Making*, 18, 122.

Azzopardi-Muscat, N. and Sørensen, K. 2019. Towards an equitable digital public health era: promoting equity through a health literacy perspective. *European Journal of Public Health*, 29, 13–17.

Bassett, D. J. 2015. Who wants to live forever? Living, dying and grieving in our digital society. *Social Sciences*, 4, 1127–1139.

Bentley, B., O'Connor, M., Williams, A., and Breen, L. J. 2020. Dignity therapy online: piloting an online psychosocial intervention for people with terminal illness. *Digital Health*, 6, 2055207620958527.

Bettini, E. A. 2020. COVID-19 pandemic restrictions and the use of technology for pediatric palliative care in the acute care setting. *Journal of Hospice and Palliative Nursing*, 22, 432–434.

Bone, A. E., Gomes, B., Etkind, S. N., Verne, J., Murtagh, F. E. M., Evans, C. J., et al. 2017. What is the impact of population ageing on the future provision of end-of-life care? Population-based projections of place of death. *Journal of Palliative Medicine*, 32, 329–336.

Bradford, N., Armfield, N. R., Young, J., and Smith, A. C. 2013. The case for home based telehealth in pediatric palliative care: a systematic review. *BMC Palliative Care*, 12, 4.

Bush, R. A., Pérez, A., Baum, T., Etland, C., and Connelly, C. D. 2018. A systematic review of the use of the electronic health record for patient identification, communication, and clinical support in palliative care. *JAMIA Open*, 1, 294–303.

Chua, I. S., Jackson, V., and Kamdar, M. 2020. Webside manner during the COVID-19 pandemic: maintaining human connection during virtual visits. *Journal of Palliative Medicine*, 23, 1507–1509.

Clabburn, O., Knighting, K., Jack, B. A., and O'Brien, M. R. 2019. The use of digital legacies with people affected by motor neurone disease for continuing bonds: an interpretative phenomenological analysis study. *Palliative Medicine*, 33, 812–822.

Collins, A., Brown, J. E. H., Mills, J., and Philip, J. 2021. The impact of public health palliative care interventions on health system outcomes: a systematic review. *Palliative Medicine*, 35, 473–485.

Collins, A., Mills, J., Sinclair, C., Li, C., Campbell, E., Chapman, M., Fullerton, S., and Jap, J. 2016. Virtual communities of practice: a novel tool for increasing palliative care engagement. *European Journal of Palliative Care*, 23, 80–83.

Coop, H. and Marlow, C. 2019. Do we prepare patients for their digital legacy? A survey of palliative care professionals. *Palliative Medicine*, 33, 114–115.

Cox, C. E. and Curtis, J. R. 2015. Using technology to create a more humanistic approach to integrating palliative care into the intensive care unit. *American Journal of Respiratory and Critical Care Medicine*, 193, 242–250.

Cox, C. E., Jones, D. M., Reagan, W., Key, M. D., Chow, V., McFarlin, J., et al. 2017. Palliative Care Planner: a pilot study to evaluate acceptability and usability of an electronic health records system-integrated, needs-targeted app platform. *Annals of the American Thoracic Society*, 15, 59–68.

Crawford, A. and Serhal, E. 2020. Digital health equity and COVID-19: the innovation curve cannot reinforce the social gradient of health. *Journal of Medical Internet Research*, 22, e19361.

Dhiliwal, S. and Salins, N. 2015. Smartphone applications in palliative homecare. *Indian Journal of Palliative Care*, 21, 88–91.

Eysenbach, G. 2001. What is e-health? *Journal of Medical Internet Research*, 3, E20.

Filkins, B. L., Kim, J. Y., Roberts, B., Armstrong, W., Miller, M. A., Hultner, M. L., et al. 2016. Privacy and security in the era of digital health: what should translational researchers know and do about it? *American Journal of Translational Research*, 8, 1560–1580.

Greenle, M. M., Morgan, B., Sayani, S., and Meghani, S. H. 2018. Identifying mobile apps targeting palliative care patients and family members. *Journal of Palliative Medicine*, 21, 1380–1385.

Guo, Q., Cann, B., McClement, S., Thompson, G., and Chochinov, H. M. 2017. Keep in Touch (KIT): feasibility of using internet-based communication and information technology in palliative care. *BMC Palliative Care*, 16, 29.

Hancock, S., Preston, N., Jones, H., and Gadoud, A. 2019. Telehealth in palliative care is being described but not evaluated: a systematic review. *BMC Palliative Care*, 18, 114.

Hartig, J. and Viola, J. 2015. Online grief support communities: therapeutic benefits of membership. *OMEGA*, 73, 29–41.

Hsieh, W.-T. 2020. Virtual reality video promotes effectiveness in advance care planning. *BMC Palliative Care*, 19, 125.

Jess, M., Timm, H., and Dieperink, K. B. 2019. Video consultations in palliative care: a systematic integrative review. *Palliative Medicine*, 33, 942–958.

Johnson, T., Bauler, L., Vos, D., Hifko, A., Garg, P., Ahmed, M., and Raphelson, M. 2020. Virtual reality use for symptom management in palliative care: a pilot study to assess user perceptions. *Journal of Palliative Medicine*, 23, 1233–1238.

Jones, L., Jacklin, K., and O'Connell, M. E. 2017. Development and use of health-related technologies in indigenous communities: critical review. *Journal of Medical Internet Research*, 19, e256.

Kabir, M., Rice, J. L., Bush, S. H., Lawlor, P. G., Webber, C., Grassau, P. A., et al. 2020. A mixed-methods pilot study of 'LIFEView' audio-visual technology: virtual travel to support well-being and quality of life in palliative and end-of-life care patients. *Palliative Medicine*, 34, 954–965.

Kamdar, M., Centi, A. J., Agboola, S., Fischer, N., Rinaldi, S., Strand, J. J., et al. 2019. A randomized controlled trial of a novel artificial intelligence-based smartphone application to optimize the management of cancer-related pain. *Journal of Clinical Oncology*, 37, 11514.

Karamanidou, C., Natsiavas, P., Koumakis, L., Marias, K., Schera, F., Schäfer, M., et al. 2020. Electronic patient-reported outcome-based interventions for palliative cancer care: a systematic and mapping review. *JCO Clinical Cancer Informatics*, 4, 647–656.

Katz, M. S., Anderson, P. F., Thompson, M. A., Salmi, L., Freeman-Daily, J., Utengen, A., et al. 2019. Organizing online health content: developing hashtag collections for healthier internet-based people and communities. *JCO Clinical Cancer Informatics*, 3, 1–10.

Kellehear, A. 2016. The Compassionate City Charter: inviting the cultural and social sectors into end of life care. In: Wegleitner, K., Heimerl, K., and Kellehear, A. (eds.) *Compassionate Communities: Case Studies from Britain and Europe*, pp. 76–87. Abingdon: Routledge.

Kidd, L., Cayless, S., Johnston, B., and Wengstrom, Y. 2010. Telehealth in palliative care in the UK: a review of the evidence. *Journal of Telemedicine and Telecare*, 16, 394–402.

Kohn, T. 2020. Small funerals, online memorials and grieving from afar: the coronavirus is changing how we care for the dead. [Online] Available at: https://theconversation.com/small-funerals-online-memorials-and-grieving-from-afar-the-coronavirus-is-changing-how-we-care-for-the-dead-134647

Kuek, A. and Hakkennes, S. 2019. Healthcare staff digital literacy levels and their attitudes towards information systems. *Health Informatics Journal*, 26, 592–612.

Kuntz, J. G., Kavalieratos, D., Esper, G. J., Ogbu, N., Jr., Mitchell, J., Ellis, C. M., et al. 2020. Feasibility and acceptability of inpatient palliative care e-family meetings during COVID-19 pandemic. *Journal of Pain and Symptom Management*, 60, e28–e32.

Lau, J., Knudsen, J., Jackson, H., Wallach, A. B., Bouton, M., Natsui, S., et al. 2020. Staying connected in the COVID-19 pandemic: telehealth at the largest safety-net system in the United States. *Health Affairs (Millwood)*, 39, 1437–1442.

Lowe, J., Rumbold, B., and Aoun, S. M. 2020. Memorialisation during COVID-19: implications for the bereaved, service providers and policy makers. *Palliative Care and Social Practice*, 14, 2632352420980456.

Lupton, D. 2015. Health promotion in the digital era: a critical commentary. *Health Promotion International*, 30, 174–183.

Lupton, D. 2016. Digitized health promotion: risk and personal responsibility for health and illness in the Web 2.0 era. In: Davis, J. E., and Gonzalez, A. M. (eds.) *To Fix or to Heal: Patient Care, Public Health, and the Limits of Biomedicine*, pp. 152–176. New York: New York University Press.

Mariano, B. 2020. Towards a global strategy on digital health. *Bulletin of the World Health Organization*, 98, 231.

Meghani, S. H., MacKenzie, M. A., Morgan, B., Kang, Y., Wasim, A., and Sayani, S. 2017. Clinician-targeted mobile apps in palliative care: a systematic review. *Journal of Palliative Medicine*, 20, 1139–1147.

Meskó, B., Drobni, Z., Bényei, É., Gergely, B., and Győrffy, Z. 2017. Digital health is a cultural transformation of traditional healthcare. *mHealth*, 3, 38.

Miller-Lewis, L., Tieman, J., Rawlings, D., Parker, D., and Sanderson, C. 2018. Can exposure to online conversations about death and dying influence death competence? an exploratory study within an Australian massive open online course. *OMEGA*, 81, 242–271.

Mills, J. 2019. Digital health technology in palliative care: friend or foe? *Progress in Palliative Care*, 27, 145–146.

Mills, J., Li, C., Fullerton, S., Chapman, M., Jap, J., Sinclair, C., et al. 2020b. Staying connected and informed: online resources and virtual communities of practice supporting palliative care during the novel coronavirus pandemic. *Progress in Palliative Care*, 28, 251–253.

Mills, J., Ramachenderan, J., Chapman, M., Greenland, R., and Agar, M. 2020c. Prioritising workforce wellbeing and resilience: what COVID-19 is reminding us about self-care and staff support. *Palliative Medicine,* 34, 1137–1139.

Mills, J. and Rosenberg, J. P. 2019. Compassionate communities. *International Journal of Palliative Nursing,* 25, 107.

Mills, J., Rosenberg, J. P., Bollig, G., and Haberecht, J. 2020a. Last aid and public health palliative care: towards the development of personal skills and strengthened community action. *Progress in Palliative Care,* 28, 343–345.

Mills, S. and Mills, J. 2016. Future directions for community engagement as a public health approach to palliative care in Australia. *Progress in Palliative Care,* 24, 15–18.

Mitchell, I. A., Schuster, A. L. R., Lynch, T., Smith, K. C., Bridges, J. F. P., and Aslakson, R. A. 2017. Why don't end-of-life conversations go viral? A review of videos on YouTube. *BMJ Supportive & Palliative care,* 7, 197–204.

Moore, S. L., Portz, J. D., Santodomingo, M., Elsbernd, K., McHale, M., and Massone, J. 2020. Using telehealth for hospice reauthorization visits: results of a quality improvement analysis. *Journal of Pain and Symptom Management,* 60, e22–e27.

Moore, J., Magee, S., Gamreklidze, E., and Kowalewski, J. 2017. Social media mourning: using grounded theory to explore how people grieve on social networking sites. *OMEGA,* 79, 231–259.

Murray, C. J. L., Alamro, N. M. S., Hwang, H., and Lee, U. 2020. Digital public health and COVID-19. *Lancet Public Health,* 5, e469–e470.

Muturi, I., Freeman, S., and Banner, D. 2020. Virtual funerals: a feasible and safer option during the COVID-19 pandemic. *Journal of the American Geriatrics Society,* 20, 2472–2473.

Ngwenya, N. B. and Mills, S. 2013. The use of weblogs within palliative care: a systematic literature review. *Health Informatics Journal,* 20, 13–21.

Niki, K., Okamoto, Y., Maeda, I., Mori, I., Ishii, R., Matsuda, Y., et al. 2019. A novel palliative care approach using virtual reality for improving various symptoms of terminal cancer patients: a preliminary prospective, multicenter study. *Journal of Palliative Medicine,* 22, 702–707.

Novillo-Ortiz, D., Dumit, E. M., D'Agostino, M., Becerra-Posada, F., Kelley, E. T., Torrent-Sellens, J., et al. 2018. Digital health in the Americas: advances and challenges in connected health. *BMJ Innovations,* 4, 123–127.

Nwosu, A. C., Collins, B., and Mason, S. 2017. Big data analysis to improve care for people living with serious illness: the potential to use new emerging technology in palliative care. *Palliative Medicine,* 32, 164–166.

Nwosu, A. C., Quinn, C., Samuels, J., Mason, S., and Payne, T. R. 2018. Wearable smartwatch technology to monitor symptoms in advanced illness. *BMJ Supportive & Palliative Care,* 8, 237.

Nwosu, A. C., Sturgeon, B., McGlinchey, T., Goodwin, C. D. G., Behera, A., Mason, S., et al. 2019. Robotic technology for palliative and supportive care: strengths, weaknesses, opportunities and threats. *Palliative Medicine,* 33, 1106–1113.

Oliver, D. P., Demiris, G., Wittenberg-Lyles, E., Washington, K., Day, T., and Novak, H. 2012. A systematic review of the evidence base for telehospice. *Telemedicine Journal and e-Health,* 18, 38–47.

Ostherr, K., Killoran, P., Shegog, R., and Bruera, E. 2016. Death in the digital age: a systematic review of information and communication technologies in end-of-life care. *Journal of Palliative Medicine,* 19, 408–420.

Pavic, M., Klaas, V., Theile, G., Kraft, J., Tröster, G., Blum, D., et al. 2019. Mobile health technologies for continuous monitoring of cancer patients in palliative care aiming to predict health status deterioration: a feasibility study. *Journal of Palliative Medicine,* 23, 678–685.

Pavic, M., Klaas, V., Theile, G., Kraft, J., Tröster, G., and Guckenberger, M. 2020. Feasibility and usability aspects of continuous remote monitoring of health status in palliative cancer patients using wearables. *Oncology,* 98, 386–395.

Payne, S., Tanner, M., and Hughes, S. 2020. Digitisation and the patient–professional relationship in palliative care. *Palliative Medicine,* 34, 441–443.

Phongtankuel, V., Adelman, R. D., and Reid, M. C. 2018. Mobile health technology and home hospice care: promise and pitfalls. *Progress in Palliative Care,* 26, 137–141.

Pinho-Costa, L., Yakubu, K., Hoedebecke, K., Laranjo, L., Reichel, C. P., Colon-Gonzalez, M. D. C., et al. 2016. Healthcare hashtag index development: identifying global impact in social media. *Journal of Biomedical Informatics,* 63, 390–399.

Pinto, S., Caldeira, S., and Martins, J. C. 2017. e-Health in palliative care: review of literature, Google Play and App Store. *International Journal of Palliative Nursing,* 23, 394–401.

Reis, A., Pedrosa, A., Dourado, M., and Reis, C. 2013. Information and communication technologies in long-term and palliative care. *Procedia Technology,* 9, 1303–1312.

Rice, E. S., Haynes, E., Royce, P., and Thompson, S. C. 2016. Social media and digital technology use among Indigenous young people in Australia: a literature review. *International Journal for Equity in Health,* 15, 81.

Ritchey, K. C., Foy, A., McArdel, E., and Gruenewald, D. A. 2020. Reinventing palliative care delivery in the era of COVID-19: how telemedicine can support end of life care. *American Journal of Hospice & Palliative Care,* 37, 992–997.

Rosenberg, J. P., Mills, J., and Rumbold, B. 2016. Putting the 'public' into public health: community engagement in palliative and end of life care. *Progress in Palliative Care,* 24, 1–3.

Royackers, A., Regan, S., and Donelle, L. 2016. The eShift model of care: informal caregivers' experience of a new model of home-based palliative care. *Progress in Palliative Care,* 24, 84–92.

Sallnow, L., Richardson, H., Murray, S. A., and Kellehear, A. 2016. The impact of a new public health approach to end-of-life care: a systematic review. *Palliative Medicine,* 30, 200–211.

Sansom-Daly, U. M. and Bradford, N. 2020. Grappling with the 'human' problem hiding behind the technology: telehealth during and beyond COVID-19. *Psycho-Oncology,* 29, 1404–1408.

Sardi, L., Idri, A., and Fernández-Alemán, J. L. 2017. A systematic review of gamification in e-Health. *Journal of Biomedical Informatics,* 71, 31–48.

Slavin-Stewart, C., Phillips, A., and Horton, R. 2020. A feasibility study of home-based palliative care telemedicine in rural Nova Scotia. *Journal of Palliative Medicine,* 23, 548–551.

Sofka, C. J., Noppe Cupit, I., and Gilbert, K. R. 2012. Thanatechnology as a conduit for living, dying and grieving in contemporary society. In: Sofka, C. J., Gilbert, K. R., and Noppe Cupit, I. (eds.) *Dying, Death, and Grief in an Online Universe,* pp. 3–15. New York: Springer.

Steindal, S. A., Nes, A. A. G., Godskesen, T. E., Dihle, A., Lind, S., Winger, A. et al. 2020. Patients' experiences of telehealth in palliative home care: scoping review. *Journal of Medical Internet Research,* 22, e16218.

Sullivan, C., Staib, A., McNeil, K., Rosengren, D., and Johnson, I. 2020. Queensland Digital Health Clinical Charter: a clinical consensus statement on priorities for digital health in hospitals. *Australian Health Review,* 44, 661–665.

Sutherland, A. E., Stickland, J., and Wee, B. 2020. Can video consultations replace face-to-face interviews? Palliative medicine and the

Covid-19 pandemic: rapid review. *BMJ Supportive & Palliative Care*, 10, 271–275.

Taubert, M., Watts, G., Boland, J., and Radbruch, L. 2014. Palliative social media. *BMJ Supportive & Palliative Care*, 4, 13–18.

The Lancet. 2020. Palliative care and the COVID-19 pandemic. *Lancet*, 395, 1168.

Tieman, J., Miller-Lewis, L., Rawlings, D., Parker, D., and Sanderson, C. 2018. The contribution of a MOOC to community discussions around death and dying. *BMC Palliative Care*, 17, 31.

Tieman, J. J., Swetenham, K., Morgan, D. D., To, T. H., and Currow, D. C. 2016. Using telehealth to support end of life care in the community: a feasibility study. *BMC Palliative Care*, 15, 94.

Towsley, G. L., Wong, B., Mokhtari, T., Hull, W., and Miller, S. C. 2020. Piloting Me and My Wishes – videos of nursing home residents' preferences. *Journal of Pain and Symptom Management*, 59, 609–617.

Tziraki, C., Grimes, C., Ventura, F., O'Caoimh, R., Santana, S., Zavagli, V., et al. 2020. Rethinking palliative care in a public health context: addressing the needs of persons with non-communicable chronic diseases. *Primary Health Care Research & Development*, 21, e32.

Wang, S. S. Y., Teo, W. Z. W., Teo, W. Z. Y., and Chai, Y. W. 2020. Virtual reality as a bridge in palliative care during COVID-19. *Journal of Palliative Medicine*, 23, 756.

Weingarten, K., Macapagal, F., and Parker, D. 2019. Virtual reality: endless potential in pediatric palliative care: a case report. *Journal of Palliative Medicine*, 23, 147–149.

Wernhart, A., Gahbauer, S., and Haluza, D. 2019. eHealth and telemedicine: practices and beliefs among healthcare professionals and medical students at a medical university. *PLoS One*, 14, e0213067.

Widberg, C., Wiklund, B., and Klarare, A. 2020. Patients' experiences of eHealth in palliative care: an integrative review. *BMC Palliative Care*, 19, 158.

Willis, E. and Ferrucci, P. 2017. Mourning and grief on Facebook: an examination of motivations for interacting with the deceased. *OMEGA*, 76, 122–140.

World Health Organization. 2018a. *Use of Appropriate Digital Technologies for Public Health: Report by the Director-General*. Geneva: World Health Organization. [Online] Available at: https://apps.who.int/gb/ebwha/pdf_files/WHA71/A71_20-en.pdf

World Health Organization. 2018b. Classification of digital health interventions v1.0: a shared language to describe the uses of digital technology for health. [Online] Available at: https://apps.who.int/iris/bitstream/handle/10665/260480/WHO-RHR-18.06-eng.pdf?sequence=1&isAllowed=y

World Health Organization. 2019. WHO guideline: recommendations on digital interventions for health system strengthening: evidence and recommendations. [Online] Available at: https://apps.who.int/iris/bitstream/handle/10665/311980/WHO-RHR-19.10-eng.pdf?sequence=1&isAllowed=y

World Health Organization. 2020a. *Global Strategy on Digital Health 2020–2024*. Geneva: World Health Organization. Available at: https://www.who.int/docs/default-source/documents/gs4dhdaa2a9f352b0445bafbc79ca799dce4d.pdf

World Health Organization. 2020b. Digital education for building health workforce capacity. [Online] Available at: https://apps.who.int/iris/bitstream/handle/10665/331524/9789240000476-eng.pdf?sequence=1&isAllowed=y

Worldwide Hospice Palliative Care Alliance. 2020. *Global Atlas of Palliative Care*, 2nd ed. London: Worldwide Hospice Palliative Care Alliance. [Online] Available at: https://www.thewhpca.org/resources/global-atlas-on-end-of-life-care

Wu, Y. R., Chou, T. J., Wang, Y. J., Tsai, J. S., Cheng, S. Y., Yao, C. A., et al. 2020. Smartphone-enabled, telehealth-based family conferences in palliative care during the COVID-19 pandemic: pilot observational study. *JMIR Mhealth Uhealth*, 8, e22069.

Xia, F., Yang, L. T., Wang, L., and Vinel, A. 2012. Internet of things. *International Journal of Communication Systems*, 25, 1101–1102.

SECTION 4

Population-based approaches

18

Health services redesign

Emma Hodges and Nikki Archer

Introduction

The modern hospice movement turned 50 in 2017. Following Dame Cicely Saunders' foundation of St Christopher's Hospice in London, hundreds of hospices emerged across the UK. Hospices arose due to the appalling deficits in care for people with terminal cancer and while there has been some diversification, the majority of people cared for by specialist nurses in the community and in hospice beds have a malignant disease. Hospices have been at a crossroads for a number of years. The increased demand for care and the financial constraints facing UK charitable hospices lead to questions such as 'Who can a hospice afford to care for?' The movement has been subject to criticism that someone without cancer is treated like a 'second class citizen' (Commission into the Future of Hospice Care, 2013, p. 17), or that people with malignant disease are 'singled out for deluxe dying' (Douglas, 1992, cited by Sleeman, 2016).

There has been a concerted effort to challenge hospices to care for wider groups of people such as those dying with dementia or heart failure (Commission into the Future of Hospice Care, 2013; Hospice UK, 2015, 2017a, 2017bi). However, funding has not followed and hospices remain concerned about capacity and resources. One in four people who need hospice care cannot currently access it (Hospice UK, 2017b) yet most hospices only receive about 33% of the money they spend on care from the National Health Service (NHS) (Hospice UK, 2016). During 2020, Hospice UK reported that 80% of hospices were planning on making redundancies as a consequence of the financial challenges associated with COVID-19 (Hospice UK, 2020).

The ethos of hospice care was never to remove or replace the community response to supporting people who are terminally ill. However, for various reasons, arguably this happened, perhaps due in particular the formation of the NHS, which was still very young when hospices emerged and the specialization of palliative care (Clark, 2002, 2016a, 2016b).

The public health approach to palliative care provides an alternative narrative. It argues that some elements of current palliative and hospice care medicalize what is a social issue. The specialization of palliative care in 1987 was criticized by some as separating out care of the dying from everyday practice (Fordham et al., 1998; Clark, 2002), further removing it from communities at a social and a primary care level.

Clark (2002) summarizes the challenges for palliative care as 'The challenge for palliative physicians is no different to that facing their counterparts elsewhere in medicine: how to reconcile high expectations of technical expertise with calls for a humanistic and ethical orientation for which they are largely unselected and only partially trained' (p. 907).

There are now perhaps two narratives for hospices. The first is the specialist palliative care provided for those who require expert care for often acute and complex symptoms. The other is the wider societal question of the impossible acceptance of inequalities of access to palliative care, and improvements in care of the dying for everyone. In the context of UK strategy, bereavement support is an accepted component of palliative care.

Asset-based community development shares its ethos with a public health approach to palliative care and offers a way to reconcile this challenge and possibly create a third way interfacing the need for specialist palliative care with a social response.

This combined approach has provided opportunities for hospices to reach a wider population who are dying or grieving who would not otherwise be able to access services (Sallnow et al., 2012). However, a public health approach is not just a different way of providing care, it is an ethos and a fundamental shift in thinking. As the two case studies will demonstrate, there is a long way to go before these two approaches are truly integrated.

The next section will provide a theoretical framework within which service redesign can be cited. After that, the practical experience of service redesign in the context of a public health approach will be discussed. The theoretical framework will help contextualize the challenges faced.

Theoretical framework

There are many theories, models, and texts relating to organizational change. However, service redesign within the health sector, particularly in the context of the public health approach, is complex; the challenge, or one of them, is organizational institutionalization.

In healthcare, the word 'institution' conjures up images of old-fashioned residential settings such as workhouses. However, it is also used to refer to types of organizations and behaviours. To consider the challenge of service redesign in the health economy, consideration needs to be made to how services and organizations have developed, recognizing 'its history and to the way it has been influenced by the social environment' (Selznick et al., 1957, p. 6). If an organization or service has become institutionalized it is said to 'infuse with value beyond the technical requirements of the task at hand' (Selznick et al., 1957, p. 22). Professions can be institutionalized, not just services or organizations (Muzio et al., 2013). The social value and history of healthcare means that it is very much institutionalized and has been for many years, creating a strong and perhaps stubborn narrative that must be understood for care to be realigned.

The reason this matters is that it is fundamental to understanding service redesign. In itself, redesigning a service is not a difficult task. The challenges are often seen as ones of adequate resources. However, changing an institutional narrative, a cultural shift, is a significant challenge and essential to ensure the benefits of redesign. Change in an institutional setting often requires people to let go of long-held views relating to their role and professional identity. Recognizing that an organization or service is institutionalized helps consider how to approach redesign.

In the context of a public health approach for palliative care, there is a strong argument to suggest that UK hospice care for people with cancer is institutionalized (Hodges and Read, 2018), that is, it is embedded in society and has value beyond the practical elements of care. The value assigned to the institution of hospices include the social value felt by staff, volunteers, supporters, and donors.

Fig. 18.1 describes a possible model of hospice care from an institutional perspective; whether this is through the lens of an organization or an individual it demonstrates how newer areas of hospice activity are not yet part of the institutional narrative (Hodges and Read, 2018).

The point of Fig. 18.1 is to illustrate how elements of hospice care are not yet accepted as the 'norm'; this isn't about how they are structured but how they are accepted as part of hospice narrative. A key concept in organizational institutionalism is one of 'legitimacy', defined as 'a generalised perception or assumption that the actions of an entity are desirable, proper or appropriate within some socially constructed system of norms, values, beliefs and definitions' (Suchman, 1995, p. 574).

This is critical. Is it legitimate, from the perspective of a healthcare professional, to enable people to take a greater degree of control or risk in relation to their health? Is it legitimate for a volunteer to provide bereavement support rather than a counsellor? How does a healthcare professional make sense of these changes from the perspective of their role identity and how do members of the public accept changes in 'who' provides support? The socially constructed norms are that health is a medical matter, that services are required to solve problems such as loneliness, grief, and so on, and along with services comes the requirements of funding, key performance indicators, reports, and structure (Cottam, 2018; Russell, 2020a).

The question of legitimacy within an institutionalized organization or health system must be understood in order to elicit change. This is because to really achieve the sort of change a public health approach advocates, a process of deinstitutionalization is required, ensuring that the norms and beliefs of the institution are no longer believed to have social value over and previously mentioned alternative ways of thinking (Greenwood et al., 2002; Clemente and Roulet, 2015).

Greenwood and colleagues (2002), present a model for institutional change derived from a study relating to the transformation of an institutionalized field, in this case professional associations. Hodges (2019) referenced this model in order to assess the institutional factors impacting change within the English hospice movement in the context of services for people with dementia.

Institutional change starts with a 'jolt' (stage one in the model), something that creates the need to change, that might be social, technological, or regulatory. There have been significant social jolts, coronavirus disease 2019 (COVID-19) being one, but also demographic changes such as the increase in older people and social changes in the make-up of family and society. Society today is not the same as when the welfare state was designed, therefore 'jolts' that are modern-day problems are being 'solved' within a traditional institutionalized framework of behaviour (Cottam, 2018; Russell, 2020a). The next stage is deinstitutionalization, where old ways are questioned by new voices that start to emerge and be heard. This is followed by 'pre-institutionalization' (stage three), where there are new innovations and key elements Greenwood and colleagues (2002) describe as 'technical viability'. Stage four is 'theorization' where the argument starts to form, where there is a 'specification of organizational failing', 'justification of abstract possible solutions', and a moral legitimacy is formed. After this there is a process of 'diffusion', where the new technically viable solutions combined with

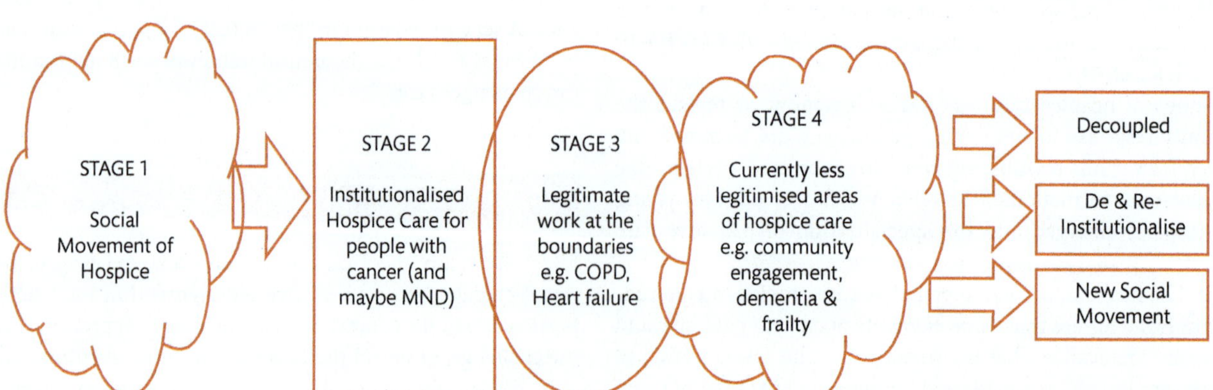

Fig. 18.1 The evolution and current structure of hospice as an institution.

Reproduced with permission from Hodges, E. & Read, S., 2018. How might organisational institutionalism support the challenges of the modern hospice? *The International Journal of Health Planning and Management*, 33(4), pp. 768–774.

moral arguments and solutions start to spread and become an accepted change. Stage six is either that the changes are lost as a 'fad' *or* the process of 'reinstitutionalization' is achieved. Stages four, five, and six move from moral and pragmatic to cognitive legitimacy, that is, a growing voice that things need to be different based on a moral argument, to a general acceptance, to it becoming a new norm. These three stages of legitimacy have to be achieved for a new model to become embedded as the norm (Greenwood et al., 2002).

This model of institutional change helps in understanding why so much change in health and care systems is not achieved. There are no shortage of ideas; however, stages three, four, and five are often not undertaken or are unsuccessful (Hodges and Read, 2018). The issue of legitimacy, particularly from the perspectives of healthcare professionals and the general public, is often not fully explored or understood.

In realigning end of life and palliative care, institutional change applies (Hodges and Reid, 2018). This theoretical framework will be woven into the two case studies to help articulate the challenges faced in redesigning services within two sometimes competing ethoses of specialist palliative care and community development.

St Giles Hospice

St Giles Hospice opened its door for patients in 1983. It is an English, charitable hospice providing specialist palliative care both in an inpatient and community setting to a population of approximately 850,000 in part of the West Midlands.

In addition, St Giles provides bereavement services, well-being activity, and education. The hospice is supported by a workforce of approximately 400 along with 1000 volunteers. Two-thirds of the cost of delivering care is met via voluntary sources (i.e. fundraising, a lottery, and charity shops). The remainder of the cost of care is funded via the NHS.

Like many English hospices, St Giles was founded out of a response to the care of people dying with cancer. The Reverend Paul Brothwell worked alongside general practitioners (GPs) and district nurses in the village of Whittington in Staffordshire just outside Lichfield. He had heard Dame Cicely Saunders, the founder of the modern hospice movement, speak, and that combined with his experience of caring for the dying inspired him to develop St Giles Hospice. Reverend Brothwell was driven by a response to the challenge that 'nothing more could be done' and understood that while that might be the case medically in the context of a cure, it wasn't the case psychologically, socially, physically, or spiritually. He continued to be actively involved in advocating for improvements in palliative and end of life care until his death in 2020.

It became very apparent several years ago that the demographics in the UK would mean that demand for hospice care would outstrip supply (Commission into the Future of Hospice Care, 2013). Part of St Giles' strategic thinking was how to improve end of life care for more people in the local community while not being able to afford to expand services. Part of St Giles' strategy since 2011 included elements of community development and at this early stage of thinking, it was simply a recognition that members of the public needed to have a greater role in how end of life care services were designed and delivered. The public health approach provided an ethos that felt right along with a way to possibly address the criticism of 'deluxe dying' or 'a bit of heaven for the few'. It demonstrated that the solution to the dilemma of 'who to care for' is within our communities and not necessarily about more services (Clark et al., 2005; Sleeman, 2016).

There were several influences during this early strategic thinking including partnership working with Murray Hall Community Trust who were already involved in Compassionate Communities, hearing Libby Sallnow speak, exploring the examples provided by the publication of *International Perspectives on Public Health and Palliative Care* (Sallnow et al., 2012), and being introduced to asset-based community development and Cormac Russell via a housing association colleague. In 2013, St Giles employed its first community engagement officer to move this thinking forward more practically.

At this stage, the involvement was purely 'engagement', linking with many groups, clubs, and societies to talk about issues to do with death and dying. This built confidence in others to feel better able to talk to their members, colleagues, and friends when these matters arise in conversation.

One of the dominant themes was a need to support people in 'understanding loss' and how to be alongside someone who is grieving. From this work the bereavement help point model emerged, which is discussed in detail in case study 1. An additional team member joined in 2015.

In 2017, St Giles was approached by a local group who had secured some lottery funding and wanted to create an end of life care service for their locality. St Giles worked with two other providers to create a 'community hub' which opened in 2018. This was a space where there could be a combination of outreach clinics to provide care closer to home and also a place where local people could establish their own support groups for issues such as death, dying, loss, frailty, and social isolation. This centre, known as 'Uttoxeter Cares', became key in the developing role with primary care that led to the hospice's involvement in social prescribing which is discussed in case study 2.

St Giles describes itself as both a provider of specialist care and as a community development organization. Currently, these two elements coexist rather than being integrated as part of an agreed common purpose across the organization. The future of how these areas work together and interface, alongside the challenges that hospices are facing financially and the changing structure of the health economy, is still emerging.

The two case studies will demonstrate how these early steps into community development have challenged, redesigned, and created new ways of supporting people affected by death, dying or loss.

Case studies: theory in practice

Case study 1: bereavement

Bereavement support provides an interesting example of service redesign and realignment. As the case study will demonstrate, UK hospices supported bereaved relatives of patients as an early response to the grief they were witnessing. The initial response was a more sociological response rather than a formal professionalized approach. However, while this shifted over time with counsellors taking over providing some of the support from volunteers, there were still elements of the sociological response retained. It could be argued that despite this, the approach was still far from being based in a public health or community development ethos. It was support restricted to only those family members of hospice patients and while designed to improve individual well-being, it was not embedding or growing resilience within communities.

A historical narrative review of the bereavement service at St Giles Hospice offers a case study to illustrate 'service redesign', not in the usual context of service redesign, but in the context of how the service, influenced by the social environment, has over time gone through a process of institutional change in reaching its current position of embracing both an 'institutional' service provision and a public health community development offer.

The early days of bereavement care in the UK and at St Giles

Although it has been described as the Cinderella of palliative care, bereavement support has been integral to hospice care since the earliest days of the hospice movement and it remains an important element of hospice care as part of its holistic approach (Hospice UK, 2020).

In 1959, the launch of 'CRUSE clubs' introduced the notion of 'bereavement support' for widows. Margaret Torrie, concerned about the plight of widows during her work as a social worker, saw the impact the loss of a husband often had as a major emotional, social, and economic crisis for many women and their children. The need to do something to help led to the development of the national charity CRUSE bereavement care. The legitimacy for hospices in offering bereavement support as an integral aspect of care quickly became established following the development of bereavement support at St Christopher's Hospice and St Joseph's Hospice under the guidance of the psychiatrist Dr Colin Murray Parkes.

It is interesting that in her recollection of how CRUSE bereavement care began back in 1959, Margaret Torrie' (2009) describes the 'quiet experiment in social care' where a group of widows of all ages came to drink tea and share their experiences', as this was also how bereavement support was introduced at St Giles Hospice. Soon after it opened in 1983, nursing staff and Reverend Brothwell recognized the impact the loss of a family member had and, supported by a team of local people, began inviting bereaved family members of patients who died at the hospice back on a Sunday afternoon for a cup of tea and a chat. This 'informal' peer support approach to bereavement care was born out of compassion and a human response to family distress but soon became more formalized and 'professionalized' within a framework of service delivery.

The formal launch of a bereavement support service at St Giles in 1987 saw the introduction of 'bereavement visitors' and a social support group. People from the local community were trained in bereavement support, and volunteered to visit and support family members at home in the days, weeks, and months after their bereavement. Visits took the format of a listening ear and a helping hand with practical issues where needed. One of the early bereavement visitors recently recalled, 'we would go out to see people at home, often as well as listening and supporting them emotionally we would help them practically. I remember helping one lady by laying some garden slabs'. The original Sunday afternoon family sessions were replaced by 'Monday Club' a monthly social support group organized by hospice staff and bereavement visitors, which provided a programme of social activity for people who were lonely and isolated. Although this early formal bereavement care framework was firmly embedded in a social model of support and ethos of volunteering, it reflects a subtle and significant shift in power and understanding of bereavement as a shared lived experience to one where there are 'experts' who are able to help and support.

Towards professionalization and institutionalization

The 1990s saw the development of a model of 'therapeutic' bereavement support begin to emerge and dominate. Motivated by the work of psychologists such as William Worden (1991), psychiatrists such as Dr Colin Murray Parkes (1986), and researchers such as Margaret Stroebe (1993), understanding of grief began to develop, heavily influenced by a psychological and medical perspective. The dominant narrative and focus was on 'helping' 'at-risk' bereaved people to work through their grief by focusing on the emotional experience of grief. It was against this backdrop that in 1996 St Giles appointed a specialist children's worker and a counsellor to lead the bereavement service. Subsequently, bereavement visitors became bereavement support volunteers and 'Monday Club' was closed as it appeared to be creating a dependency on the hospice and it was not clear how it was helping people in their bereavement. These changes reflected a shift from the social model of help and support to a therapeutic, structured, formal, and more institutionalized approach.

By the early 2000s, bereavement support at St Giles had shifted from a 'shared community response' to promoting a default position of specialist one-to-one support. Bereaved people, of whatever age, would require expert care and should therefore be seen by 'experts' in the field, including trained and specially selected volunteers. Such a narrative reflected growing institutionalization, empowering the purpose of the organization and the role of those who work within it. As a consequence, the role of those within the local community in supporting their fellow citizens was being disempowered, creating greater demands on the service. The bereavement service was facing challenges aligned to those being experienced by the wider hospice movement:

- Increased demand for service based upon the traditional and institutionalized model which had developed.
- Reduced resources, both financial and human, with which to deliver to this increased demand.
- Criticism of a little bit of heaven for the few. Access to bereavement support was dependent upon the patient being known to the hospice. Those who had already received support were able to get more, while those possibly most in need were denied access.

These challenges began to drive the need for change and several key events occurred which reshaped our thinking about the way in which support was being delivered.

Theory and policy

Firstly, understanding and knowledge about the impact and experience of grief expanded significantly, and importantly embraced different perspectives. Among others, Tony Walter's (1999) sociological criticism of the 'grief police', over professionalization, medicalization, and creation of a dependency model for grief and bereavement support, was influential. Secondly, through Alan Kellehear's work (1999), we were introduced to the ideas of community development and public health palliative care. Seeking to bring about social change by developing ideas of supporting and strengthening communities to talk about and support each other when faced with death, dying, and bereavement. One such example being the use of 'dying to talk beer mats' to enhance the ability to support bereaved people as a new approach to bereavement support within the local community.

Alongside the new theoretical understandings which emerged, there were a number of new national policies and frameworks giving legitimacy to the development of a public health approach to palliative care.

1. *The National Institute for Health and Care Excellence (2004) guidance*: this three-component model offers a framework for mapping support to different groups of bereaved people against different levels of need. Level 1 (most people) do not require 'support' as it is available within their networks, information is useful to enhance resilience. Level 2 (some people) need a listening ear or information provided through a volunteer or peer network. Level 3 (few people) need specialist intervention through professional support.
2. *Dying Matters (2009)*: a core aspect of the Department of Health's (2008) End of Life Care Strategy advocates to brings organizations together to develop a culture which is open to talking about death, and where people feel able to listen and support those who are planning for end of life and who have been bereaved.
3. *The 'Ambitions for Palliative and End of Life Care: A National Framework for Local Action 2015–2020'*: ambition six 'Communities are prepared to help' (Abel et al., 2016), endorses public health approaches to end of life care.

Given this focus, we began to explore and question how we were delivering the bereavement service and what, in the light of this new thinking, needed to change. In 2009, the employment of a schools and colleges coordinator to promote and demystify the work of the hospice began to create connections with local schools and opportunities began to arise for conversations about supporting bereaved children within a school environment. This National Institute for Health and Care Excellence (2004) level 1 approach aimed at building staff confidence in being able to support bereaved children within their classes, creating community capacity for bereavement support. After a while, this initial approach to embracing a public health approach stuttered and the role ceased. The work was seen as peripheral and not understood as part of a continuum of a public health model alongside professionalized services.

While policy documents help create an argument for change, they alone cannot create the impetus and momentum for institutional change. Not all decision makers will have read them, or interpret them in the same way. Charities will have a strong sense of purpose that might be challenged by the policy documents. Professionals may have a strong sense of authority or role identity regarding the proposed changes. In essence, people will often behave or create processes to either disrupt or maintain the status quo.

Only upon reflection is the organizational experience at a strategic level of the public health approach and that which was emerging within the bereavement team understood in the context of institutional change. The appetite for, and interest in, the public health approach continued and strengthened within the then senior management and 2013 saw the introduction of a new role of 'community engagement officer'. This not only reignited the hospice's commitment to exploring a public health approach alongside its core institutionalized services but acted as a 'jolt' which has shifted the focus in the way in which bereavement care is delivered; core to this has been building and enabling community capacity and the development of the bereavement help point model.

It was understood that to truly embed public health thinking within St Giles, there needed to be a shift from 'engaging' to 'developing', truly supporting communities to be less dependent on services and more resilient as neighbourhoods in the context of bereavement. The bereavement help point model as part of bereavement support across the hospice's catchment area was a key shift in strategy and philosophy.

The original bereavement help point, was launched in 2012. It developed in response to the challenges which were being faced including managing increased waiting lists for one-to-one support, needing to widen access to bereavement support beyond hospice families, and recognition that the existing support model did not meet the needs of all bereaved people. It was initially embedded within the traditional service provision model as a support group, facilitated by hospice volunteers and provided to the community by the hospice. From 2013, overlaying this development with the influence of public health palliative care thinking has significantly shifted the ethos of the model from the provision of a 'service' for the community to one which facilitates supporting people and local communities to help one another.

The family support and bereavement team and the community engagement team are part of what is known at St Giles as supportive care. While not intentional in the organizational structure, this colocation undoubtedly helped the family support and bereavement team to understand the transition and realignment of bereavement support, that is, to consider the difference between a professional service, a professional model utilizing the skills or volunteers, and a community development approach.

There were the inevitable conversations relating to skill/role deployment, governance, record keeping, evaluation, and training as part of the integration of the teams' thinking. In a recent discussion with other hospices seeking to be involved in a bereavement help point model, it was apparent that the philosophical differences and trying to shift thinking from an institutionalized norm to a new moral legitimacy of community development are not isolated to St Giles!

The design and philosophy of the help points has changed significantly. Rather than working in isolation to provide a service, partnership working and asset development are fundamental principles embedded in the delivery of the help point model. Working in partnership with other local organizations including CRUSE branches, Tesco's community spaces, church groups, and Age UK, bereavement help points provide a space for people to come together within their local community for information and peer support.

The aims of bereavement help points are to:

- Work in partnership with local community 'assets' to widen access to bereavement information and support across the local community.
- Improve the responsiveness and management of referrals into the bereavement service at St Giles Hospice.

- Provide opportunities for people to meet, talk, grieve, and take care of each other in a social rather than therapeutic environment.

People are welcome to come along however long ago they were bereaved and whatever the circumstances of the death, there is no limit to, or requirement for, attendance. The help points are supported by community volunteers, many of whom are existing members of the help points who have undertaken the basic 'understanding bereavement' training. Generally, they welcome anyone coming for the first time, and sit with them before gently introducing them to other people within the group.

Since the first help point opened, the scheme has gradually expanded as we have worked with new partners in different areas. Prior to the coronavirus disease (COVID-19) pandemic, there were 13 different places and times where help points were held during the week with over 1400 attendances per quarter. One of the key moments over the past couple of years, is when members of the community ask for help to start their own group.

> It's a brilliant place to spend time as everyone understands where I am coming from and knows what I've been through. I can be honest, share how I feel and cry if I want to and at the same time I can enjoy a laugh with the group if that's how I feel too. The group has been a lifesaver for me over the last year and I'm so grateful I found it. (KB, Lichfield Help Point)

Building this capacity of communities supporting each other would not have been possible without the ethos of partnership working with communities of people, a key aspect of health-promoting palliative care (Conway, 2012).

This interface between community engagement and bereavement care at St Giles has developed as a fluid and effective partnership reflecting the integration of a public health approach to traditional service delivery. This alternative narrative has enabled the development of the bereavement help point model and has led to the development of peer mentor programmes and bereavement help points within local schools. It has also changed the philosophy of direct service provision from a paternalistic position of addressing 'needs and deficits' to one embedded in a philosophy of exploring partnership approaches. For example, rather than starting from the position of assuming everyone needs one-to-one bereavement support, the team will explore what local community support is available, and how this network can be mobilized to support the person.

It would be dishonest to say that there has been a clearly defined plan and model for the redesign of bereavement care at St Giles which enabled us to get to this point—the vision has been an emerging one. Challenges remain—the interface between the delivery of direct bereavement support and the availability of bereavement help points in the local community does at times create tension between differing philosophical perspectives.

The realignment of bereavement support highlights some key elements that remain a consideration in relation to the balance of both professional and community-led bereavement support:

- It is not an either/or approach, both a direct and public health approach is required.
- Developing a working interface between both aspects is essential in creating legitimacy.
- Understanding and managing the 'role' of volunteers within the two approaches pose challenges. The need to restrain and control volunteers within the traditional institutionalized approach conflicts with the philosophy of empowering community volunteers to lead and facilitate the approach.
- The evaluation and outcome framework requires both a community development and health system approach which have different approaches to what is valued as evidence.
- Funding models need to also be consistent with community-led support and not force institutional behaviour.

Bereavement case study conclusion

This case study has offered a historical perspective of how the hospice community response to supporting bereaved people was initially aligned to an ethos of mutual self-help and peer support but increasingly became institutionalized as the dominating social and research narrative shifted to reflect a medicalization of grief. More recent sociological challenges and the advent of the public health approach to palliative care has shifted the narrative away from one of 'service provision' to embracing both a 'formal service' and a community development model for bereavement care. As the case study has demonstrated, at St Giles there is a growing legitimacy towards a public health and societal approach in the context of bereavement support.

Due to the policy and theoretical context regarding bereavement and the co-location of the family support and bereavement team and community engagement team, this has perhaps been an easier transition than would be experienced in other areas of practice.

Case study 2: social prescribing

This case study will provide insight into how the concept of community development and the implementation of social prescribing created an opportunity and legitimate narrative in which to move the public health model forward. It will also discuss the challenges of institution and ethos.

What is interesting in this case study, similarly to the bereavement example, is that there was already an element of legitimacy to build on. There was widespread acceptance by GPs that there were a cohort of patients that while needing support, did not require a medical appointment (Barker, 2017). The issue was, what was a legitimate alternative that was appropriate for patient care and technically viable both at a practice level and strategically within the NHS?

There were examples such as in Frome, Somerset, where the compassionate communities, public health approach was gaining momentum as a possible solution.

In 2017, as part of our community engagement work, St Giles, hosted a 'compassionate communities' conference where Julian Abel and Cormac Russell both presented their ideas and approaches to developing 'compassionate communities'. The current chief executive officer at St Giles, having heard Cormac Russell speak before, along with several colleagues shared the belief that a community development approach was an essential way of achieving the hospice's strategy of supporting more people. It was the first time that the chief executive officer had heard Julian Abel speak.

Cormac Russell perhaps speaks to what Powell and DiMaggio (1991) might describe as 'old institutionalists', a focus on community, informal structures and values rather than professions, systems, and sectors. 'Old' not being used as a term for outdated, but for a time in our social history where care was embedded in neighbourliness with less welfare dependency. He advocates a need to shift from a system designed around deficits to one focused on community assets without exploiting or trying to institutionalize them; how institutions support communities rather than creating dependency (Russell, 2020a). One experience of COVID-19 in the UK has been the willingness of neighbours to help each other; while there have been attempts by institutions to lead and organize this response, there are many examples of locally led support. Only time will tell whether this community spiritedness will continue.

Julian Abel is a palliative medicine consultant and relates directly to the system and challenges existing norms. He is an institutional entrepreneur (as Dame Cicely Saunders was too)—people who can use power and resources to change an institution, in particular recognizing the role of individual agency which is consistent with Russell's work (Garud et al., 2007). As a clinician, he is seen as a credible voice advocating for colleagues as well as patients.

Abel presented the very practical compassionate communities work in Frome, Somerset, which embedded a community development worker within primary care and recruits volunteer community connectors from within the community. This was presented alongside a diagram demonstrating the need to shift 'activity' from acute care to primary care, from primary care to the community (i.e. charities, clubs, groups and associations), with a need to also grow community knowledge and awareness. He demonstrated that this model would improve the lives of overworked clinicians, create better social connections within people's communities, and grow 'associational life', and presented evidence of the impact of social connections on mortality (Abel, 2017).

What Julian Abel did was translate Cormac's thinking into a healthcare narrative, a model with an emerging evidence base. This model could demonstrate technical viability with a strong moral argument (Abel, 2017; Russell, 2017) and a vision for the organization's direction of travel. The 'cog diagram', as it became known, gained credibility and was adopted internally as a way of expressing the capacity and demand challenges being faced in hospice care. St Giles' chief executive officer talked about the model to several colleagues in the healthcare system and those conversations started to gain some traction. As a consequence, Julian Abel presented to the local system-level end of life care board and several clinical leaders and commissioners on the work in Frome in Somerset (Abel, 2017). In 2018, a proposal was produced by the clinical commissioning group to implement the Frome model locally. While there was support for the concept and an acknowledgement of the benefits it could bring, the funding was not secured and the work did not move forward. In hindsight, there is an argument that the 'jolt' wasn't significant enough, or the issues relating to end of life care had been problematic for so long that they no longer felt like a 'moment for change'. Perhaps the technical viability didn't gain legitimacy because it was from another geographical area—the 'that won't work here' argument. The concept got lost or reframed and fragmented. However, that is not to say that there weren't positives from that experience. Some people who heard the talks at St Giles about community development and/or heard Julian Abel speak, saw and understood both the technical viability and the moral legitimacy. Discussions continued—perhaps waiting for the right 'jolt' at the right time.

In particular, conversations continued with a local GP from Balance Street Health Centre in Uttoxeter, who had been working alongside St Giles at the 'Uttoxeter Cares' hub. The hope was that an opportunity would emerge where the concept of the Frome model could be implemented.

The opportunity (the jolt) came as a result of policy change, and the emergence of primary care networks and social prescribing within the UK in 2018/2019. Primary care networks are groups of GP practices working together to be more proactively involved in the design of care for the local people they care for based on a population of 30,000–50,000 (NHS England, n.d.).

The emergence of the social prescribing strategy, embedded by NHS England as a core aspect of the new policy, created the potential for a legitimate transition from an institutional model of service to a public health approach to care. Social prescribing enables healthcare professionals to refer patients to non-clinical, community support. It recognizes that 'people's health and well-being are determined mostly by a range of social, economic and environmental factors, social prescribing seeks to address people's needs in a holistic way. It also aims to support individuals to take greater control of their own health' (The King's Fund, 2020).

The term 'social prescribing' is contentious and has generated much debate online. Cormac Russell summarizes this debate by suggesting that 'its very name reveals in its most current operational form it is far too transactional and too governed by the health system that created it to be deemed a genuine community alternative to medicine' (Russell, 2020b, pp. 2–3). There is a risk that social prescribing could quickly be institutionalized with community assets being used to support the system, rather than really understanding the nature of communities and connecting the incredible work taking place in many communities to local people who are perhaps disconnected from their neighbourhood, ensuring that social prescribing is growing associational life not services.

The challenge in implementing social prescribing is how to use the statutory narrative but implement it in a way that is consistent with the ethos of a community development approach.

The NHS policy is that a social prescriber would be embedded in each GP practice, one of the key roles within the new primary care workforce (NHS England, 2019). As soon as the policy shift started to emerge, the team at Balance Street started discussions with St Giles to consider how social prescribing could deliver the Frome model—improving care not only for those who are affected by death, dying, or loss but for the wider population, focused on two primary care networks.

Becoming involved in social prescribing was not going to be straightforward for a hospice. It was important to not 'mission creep'—our work is in the area of death, dying, and loss, not the broad range of patient cohorts that would need to be supported by this new workforce (social prescribers). Frome's model which supports the implementation of a public health approach to palliative care is described as population based.

The opportunity to create a societal shift and possibly reduce suffering and isolation for people affected by death, dying, and loss, funded by the NHS, was an important step. Having advocated for the Frome model and the public health approach for some time, it would have been incongruous to not take this opportunity to support this policy shift. Weighing up the risk of mission creep versus the opportunity to advocate for a public health approach and working with partners who understood that dilemma was important. St Giles was able to connect with its existing networks to

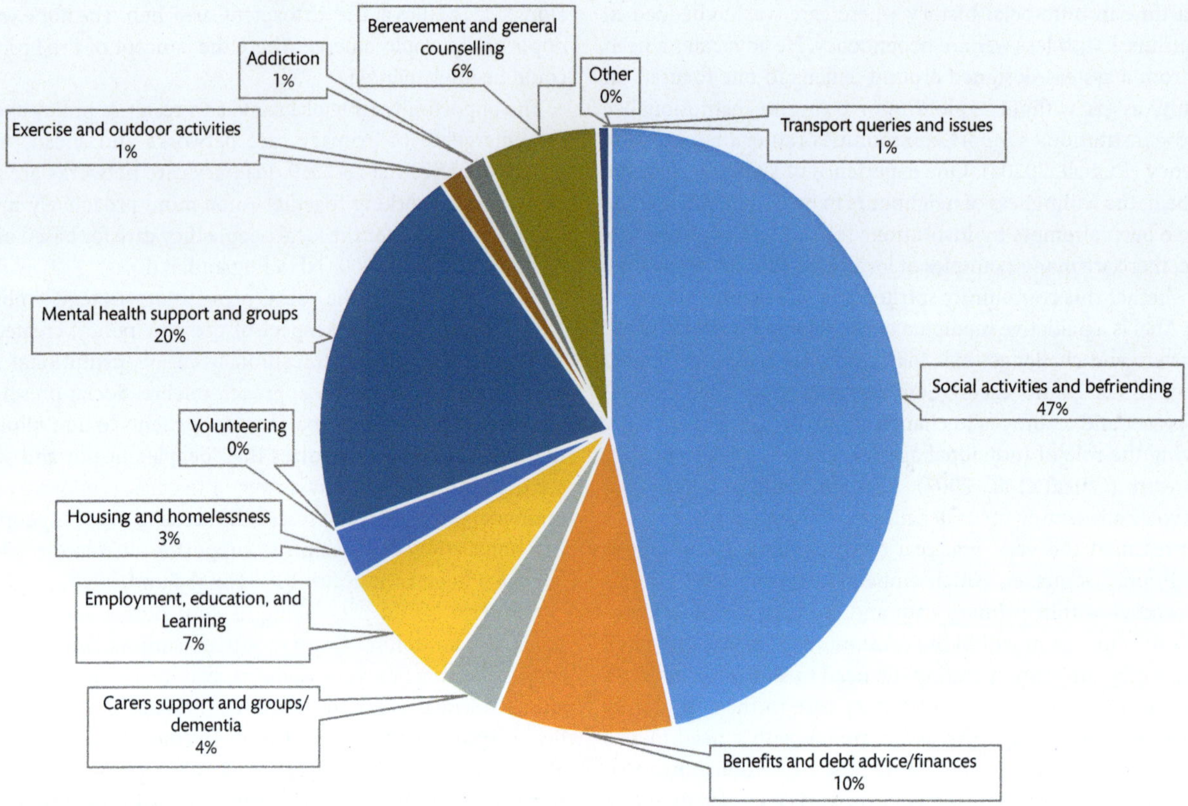

Fig. 18.2 Nature of primary prescription of 246 referrals to social prescribers over first 6 months.
Source: data from East Staffordshire PCN Social Prescribing Report 2019/20.

establish partners in the implementation of social prescribing, particularly around support for older people and mental health.

There are five social prescribing link workers each assigned to a GP practice; the team come from different organizations in order to ensure there are a range of skills and backgrounds. St Giles is overseeing the team on behalf of primary care. St Giles with partners have had the freedom to create an evaluation model that while consistent with what the NHS needs to know, also values the stories of individuals and their achievements and of the local community. The project overview and contracting of social prescribing has been within a framework that enables emergent change.

The team went live in April 2020 and therefore were immediately challenged by the impact of COVID-19. St Giles works closely with Support Staffordshire who lead on social prescribing in other parts of the county and there is a real sense of shared learning and understanding of navigating the balance between the NHS framework and a public health approach.

Over the first 6 months, 247 referrals have been received from GPs to the team. It is too early to determine whether this model will, like bereavement, over time enhance the legitimacy of a public health approach (Fig. 18.2).

What appears to be emerging from the data, however, is consistent with Julian Abel and Cormac Russell's view—that social connectedness is what people are craving.

Part of the role of the social prescribers will be supporting people to reconnect to their communities as we emerge from COVID-19, providing confidence and reassurance.

From a service redesign or realignment perspective, the value in understanding institutional change means that the conversations with partners explore the needs of a statutory system alongside the societal impact that is hoped for. The language used in the discussions can challenge beliefs and norms and design processes that are enabling and exploratory, rather than implementing social prescribing in the way that it is perhaps written at the time. Aligning St Giles' involvement in social prescribing with examples from Frome and via established networks and often new partners is part of what provides a real opportunity of deinstitutionalizing social support and truly aiming to grow associational life.

Conclusion

The aim of this chapter is to provide a different perspective on service development. It describes how new models of care, embedded in a public health approach, can grow alongside traditional, institutionalized services, and that this creates a possibility of generating legitimacy in a new way of working and growing confidence in healthcare leaders and communities in embracing them. Where an institution, whether that be an organization, a health system, or a profession, is working within a long-standing and dominant narrative, service change, particularly one that challenges embedded views, requires a more complex model of transformation.

Case study 1 on bereavement shows how a public health approach emerged alongside a more traditional model of 'counselling' and how this influenced the team, their ethos of care, and their response to people needing bereavement support. However, this is still challenging as the way we evaluate specialist palliative care services doesn't work for community development activity.

Case study 2 on social prescribing, while a contentious term, demonstrates how a new public policy provided a way of transitioning, or attempting to, from a new strategy written and developed in an institutional context to delivery within the ethos of a public health/community development approach. This example shows how institutional entrepreneurs are key in reshaping the status quo. In Balance Street Health Centre in Uttoxeter, the public health approach to palliative and end of life care was understood and therefore there was the ability to spot the opportunity to move this agenda forward with like-minded partners on a position of trust and shared values.

Organizational institutionalism as a theory and with the models that make it accessible as a model of change (Greenwood et al., 2002; Hodges and Read, 2018) challenge us to think more deeply about social value, professional identity, norms both behavioural and procedural. The concept of legitimacy provides a language in order to address these sorts of questions.

There is much work still to do in interfacing a public health approach alongside specialist palliative care services.

The challenge of evaluation is the next stage of our thinking and work in the public health approach to palliative care. For example, is the evaluation of bereavement help points based on the well-being of the local community, rather than how many referrals have been received and short-term satisfaction results? Designing a model of service evaluation that satisfies health system leaders and demonstrates the value and legitimacy of community development as part of an integrated care model is part of demonstrating technical viability, a critical part of deinstitutionalizing and realigning care.

Organizational history tells us that social movements become organized and can then become institutionalized; hospices are an example of this. That doesn't mean that new concepts and philosophies can't emerge but they do so in an institutionalized context. St Giles is under no illusion that the progress that has been made regarding the public health approach is not also at risk of becoming organized and possibly institutionalized, but hopes that it is the communities who own the organizing with support as and when required to grow resilience and well-being in the community alongside specialist care provision for those who need it.

REFERENCES

Abel, J. 2017. A public health approach to palliative and end of life care. Presentation at conference, St Giles Hospice, Lichfield.

Abel, J., Sallnow, L., Murray, S., and Kerin, M. 2016. *Each Community is Prepared to Help: Community Development in End of Life Care—Guidance on Ambition Six.* London: National Council for Palliative Care.

Barker, I. 2017. Chart: characteristics of frequent attenders at general practice. The Health Foundation. [Online] Available at: https://www.health.org.uk/chart/chart-characteristics-of-frequent-attenders-at-general-practice

Clark, D. 2002. Between hope and acceptance: the medicalisation of dying. *BMJ*, 324, 905–907.

Clark, D. 2016a. *To Comfort Always: A History of Palliative Medicine Since the Nineteenth Century.* Oxford: Oxford University Press.

Clark, D. 2016b. *To Comfort Always': Lessons From the Past to Inform the Future.* Liverpool: Hospice UK.

Clark, D., Small, N., Wright, M., Winslow, M., and Hughes, N. 2005. *A Bit of Heaven for the Few: An Oral History of the Modern Hospice Movement.* Lancaster: Observatory Publications.

Clemente, M. and Roulet, T. J. 2015. Public opinion as a source of deinstitutionalisation: a 'sprial of silence' approach. *Academy of Management Review*, 40, 96–114.

Conway, S. 2012. Public health developments in palliative care services in the UK. In: Sallnow, L., Kumar, S., and Kellehear, A. (eds.) *International Perspectives on Public Health and Palliative Care*, pp. 85–97. London: Routledge.

Cottam, H. 2018. *Radical Help: How We Can Remake the Relationships Between Us and Revolutionise the Welfare State.* London: Virago Press.

Department of Health. 2008. End of life care strategy. [Online] Available at: https://www.gov.uk/government/uploads/system/uploads/attachment_data/file/136431/End_of_life_strategy.pdf

Fordham, S., Dowrick, C., and May, C. 1998. Palliative medicine: is it really specialist territory? *Journal of the Royal Society of Medicine*, 91, 569–572.

Garud, R., Hardy, C., and Maguire, S. 2007. Institutional entrepreneurship as embedded agency: an introduction to the special issue. *Organisation Studies*, 28, 957–969.

Greenwood, R., Suddaby, R., and Hinings, C. 2002. Theorizing change: the role of professional associations in the transformation of institutionalised fields. *Academy of Management Journal*, 45, 58–80.

Commission into the Future of Hospice Care. 2013. *Future Ambitions for Hospice Care: Our Mission and Our Opportunity.* London: Help the Hospices.

Hodges, E. 2019. A mixed methods study exploring organisational factors influencing the development of services for people with dementia in English hospices. Doctoral thesis, Keele University. [Online] Available at: https://eprints.keele.ac.uk/7137/

Hodges, E. and Read, S. 2018. How might organisational institutionalism support the challenges of the modern hospice? *International Journal of Health Planning and Management*, 33, 768–774.

Hospice UK. 2015. *Hospice Enabled Dementia Care.* London: Hospice UK.

Hospice UK. 2016. *Hospice Care in the UK.* London: Hospice UK.

Hospice UK. 2017a. *Heart Failure and Hospice Care: The First Steps.* London: Hospice UK.

Hospice UK. 2017b. *Open Up Hospice Care.* London: Hospice UK.

Hospice UK. 2020. Parliamentary briefing—ensuring charitably funded hospices have sufficient funding. [Online] Available at: file:///C:/Users/emma.hodges/Downloads/hospice-uk-briefing--debate-on-hospice-funding-oct-2020.pdf

Kellehear, A. 1999. *Health Promoting Palliative Care.* Melbourne: Oxford University Press.

Parkes, C.M. (1986). Bereavement: Studies of Grief In Adult Life. London: Tavistock Publications.

Muzio, D., Brock, D. M., and Suddaby, R. 2013. Professions and institutional change: towards and institutionalist sociology of the professions. *Journal of Management Studies*, 50, 699–721.

National Institute for Health and Care Excellence. 2004. Supportive and palliative care for adults with cancer. [Online] Available at: https://www.nice.org.uk/guidance/csg4

NHS England. n.d. Primary care networks. [Online] Available at: https://www.england.nhs.uk/primary-care/primary-care-networks/

NHS England. 2019. The NHS long term plan. [Online] Available at https://www.longtermplan.nhs.uk/wp-content/uploads/2019/08 NHS Long Term Plan v1.2

Powell, W. and DiMaggio, P. J. 1991. *The New Institutionalism Organisational Analysis.* Chicago, IL: The University of Chicago Press.

Russell, C. 2017. The tale of Con Carey. Presentation at conference, St Giles Hospice, Lichfield.

Russell, C. 2020a. *Rekindling Democracy*. Bend, OR: Cascade Publishing.

Russell, C. 2020b. We don't have a health problem we have a village problem. *Community Medicine,* 1, 1–12. Available at: https://www.nurturedevelopment.org/wp-content/uploads/2018/09/we-dont-have-a-health-problem-we-have-a-village-problem8259.pdf

Sallnow, L., Kumar, S., and Kellehear, A. (eds.) 2012. *International Perspectives on Public Health and Palliative Care.* Abingdon: Routledge.

Selznick, P. 1957. *Leadership in Administration: A Sociological Interpretation*. Berkeley, CA: University of California Press.

Sleeman, K. 2016. Hospices: too good to be true and too small to be useful? [Online] Available at: https://katherinesleeman.wordpress.com/2016/03/01/hospices-too-good-to-be-true-and-too-small-to-be-useful/

Stroebe, M.S., Stroebe, W. and Habsson, R.O. (1993). Handbook of Bereavement: Theory, Research and Intervention. Cambridge: Cambridge University Press.

Suchman, M. C. 1995. Managing legitimacy: strategic and institutional approaches. *Academy of Management Review*, 20, 571–610.

The King's Fund. 2020. What is social prescribing? [Online] Available at: https://www.kingsfund.org.uk/publications/social-prescribing?

Walter, T. 1999. *On Bereavement: The Culture of Grief*. Buckingham: Open University Press.

Worden, J. W. 1991. *Grief Counselling and Grief Therapy* (2nd Edn). London: Routledge.

19

Public health approaches to bereavement support

Samar Aoun and Bruce Rumbold

Introduction

Until recently, surprisingly little was known about bereavement as it is lived out in everyday life. We were well informed about the minority who sought support from professional services, but not about the majority who do not seek these services. Bereavement was understood more as a problem to be solved rather than an experience to be engaged. Our perceptions and strategies for all were largely shaped by the complications that can arise for some, and we paid correspondingly less attention to the experience and resources used by the majority, those who learn to live, for the most part constructively, with their loss.

Over the past 7 years, our research team has explored population responses to bereavement using a public health approach. That is, we have adopted a whole population perspective, enquiring into the varied responses and sources of support—not merely health services—available to and used by people experiencing bereavement. This approach stands in contrast with a majority of previous studies that have focused on people presenting for help at counselling services. Our interest in bereavement care first emerged around the place of bereavement in palliative care models, and the apparently uniform strategies being adopted by palliative care services in their bereavement follow-up. We soon identified studies that raised questions about the effectiveness of 'best practice' strategies for bereavement care in general and observed that the evidence undergirding these strategies was selective. Most contemporary knowledge about bereavement came from people who had sought psychological support, and the treatments devised for their grief were being offered to the general community through the emerging specialty of grief counselling. Mourning, which traditionally had been managed by shared social rituals, was now being regulated through interventions with individuals. There was some evidence that people who did not seek counselling support found other means to express their grief, through practical action often linked with memorialization.

There were, however, virtually no studies investigating the bereavement responses of a cross-section of the population. We conducted a systematic review on complicated grief (Lobb et al., 2010) which showed that 10–20% of bereaved people who were service users experience complicated grief. The systematic review confirmed the need for targeted research to address the gaps in knowledge that exist in the area of complicated grief. Without it, health professionals and service providers endeavour to provide interventions and services based on anecdotal experiences and trial-and-error approaches. Furthermore, when we looked at the practice of bereavement support in several countries including Australia, the US, Canada, the UK, and Japan, we found questions about providing universal versus targeted support; a lack of clear evidence driving service delivery; informal or no risk assessment; and limited or no evaluation of services (Breen et al., 2014).

The public health model for bereavement support

The first step was to think about bereavement in a public health or population health framework. Typically, a public health approach identifies three levels of intervention for any given health issue: strategies addressed to the whole population, strategies for groups at significant risk, and strategies for people already experiencing disorder. Interventions appropriate to each category are then identified (Schut et al., 2001).

We also found that the National Institute for Health and Care Excellence in the UK had proposed a three-tiered approach to supporting bereaved people (National Institute for Health and Care Excellence, 2004). Family and friends can offer support such as information to those with normal grief, and volunteers and self-help groups if trained can give non-professional support for bereaved people with more need for reflection on loss. The third group with more complex needs which might lead to complicated grief would need the professional support and specialist interventions. In a more defined hospice setting, a retrospective audit reported that 54% of their bereaved clients were deemed to be low risk, 33% were seen by volunteers, and 9% were seen by bereavement staff or other professionals (Relf and Lines, 2005).

The conceptual public health model for bereavement support combines these sources of information (Aoun et al., 2012) in its three-tiered approach to bereavement risk and need for support, wherein the low-risk group (first tier) would need support principally from family and friends, the moderate-risk group (second tier) would need support from the wider community including some general support from various professionals, and the high-risk group (third tier) would need support from mental health services. The operationalization of this model would provide evidence to guide the development and allocation of cost-effective bereavement support services, which is identified as an important gap in the literature (Mather et al., 2008; Breen et al., 2014).

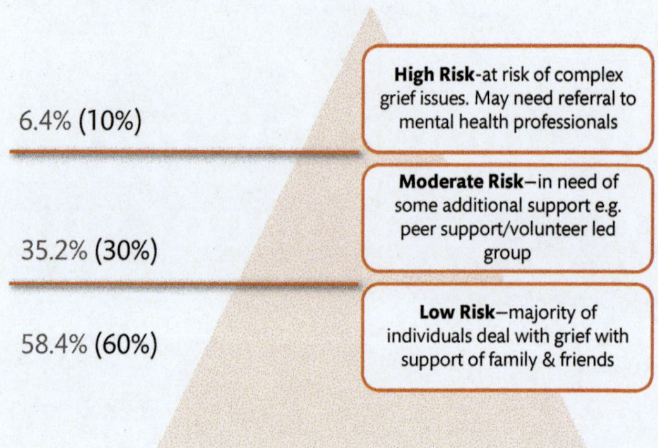

Fig. 19.1 The public health model for bereavement support—predicted proportions (in brackets) and actual proportions for the three risk groups.
Reproduced from Aoun, S. M., Breen, L. J., Howting, D. A., Rumbold, B., McNamara, B. & Hegney, D. 2015. Who needs bereavement support? A population based survey of bereavement risk and support need. *PLoS One*, 10, e0121101.

Testing the model

The next step was to test the model using population-based data. As these data were not available from death registries in Australia because of privacy issues, a partnership was formed with a group of family-owned funeral service providers who were willing to give access to their non-identified databases. An anonymous postal survey collected information from clients of six funeral providers in four Australian states (2014–2015), 6–24 months after the death of their family member or friend. The survey was posted by the funeral providers. A total of 1139 bereaved family members responded. However, some of the findings described here are based on data analyses from four funeral providers, who were willing to participate first, comprising 678 bereaved respondents.

A questionnaire was developed to obtain demographic information on the bereaved and deceased; the experience of caring for a person with a terminal illness; the supports people accessed; supports they would have liked to have been able to access; their perceived needs and whether these were met; and their current feelings about the loss. The questionnaire included a validated risk assessment screening measure (PG-13) for prolonged grief disorder (PGD) (Prigerson et al., 2009).

Who needs and who provides bereavement support?

The study identified and described the profiles of bereavement risk and support needs of a community sample in Australia and tested the fit of the data with the three-tiered public health model for bereavement support. Based on the literature, the model predicted that 60% of the sample would be low risk, 30% moderate risk, and 10% high risk. Actual figures were very close at 58.4%, 35.2%, and 6.4% respectively. The analysis of the demographic characteristics, experience, and impact of caring and bereavement, and satisfaction with support received from a variety of sources, revealed differential experiences and needs that align with the expectation of low, moderate, and high bereavement support need, as articulated in the public health model (Aoun et al., 2015) (Fig. 19.1).

The validated PG-13 meant that we were able to determine a population rate of complicated grief (high risk) in this survey of 6.4%. This rate is similar to those reported in other countries' population-based surveys, 7.6% in Denmark (Nielsen et al., 2017) and 6.7% in Germany (Kersting et al., 2011), though the differences may be due to different follow-up periods in each study. In addition, the low- and moderate-risk groups can be distinguished clearly on the basis of PG-13 scores as well as the sources of support (mental health professional sources for high risk, community support for moderate risk, and family and friends for low risk). Additionally, the profiles provided a context for the scores: low scores typically arose from losses that were expected and less disruptive to daily routines (e.g. the death of an aged parent); moderate scores typically arose from deaths that were both expected and everyday-disruptive (e.g. the death of an ageing and ill partner); and deaths that are both unexpected or resisted and disruptive (such as a child or a younger spouse) led to high scores on the PG-13 (Aoun et al., 2015).

A public health approach to bereavement support advocates for partnerships between formal services and informal networks and therefore the sources of bereavement support were classified as informal support, community support, and professional support. Informal support included support offered by family, friends, funeral directors, financial or legal advisors, religious or spiritual advisors, the internet, or literature. (Funeral, financial, and legal professionals were classified as informal support because their services did not assume a health-style duty of care.) Community support included support offered by general practitioners (GPs), nursing homes, hospitals, pharmacists, community groups, palliative care providers, or school-based advisors. Professional support included support offered by trained counsellors, bereavement support groups, social workers, case coordinators, psychologists, and psychiatrists. The majority of the bereaved respondents in each of the three risk groups accessed support from family and friends (88–94%), followed by funeral directors (82%) and GPs (56%) (Fig. 19.2). Access to mental health professional sources of support (counsellor, social worker, psychologist, and psychiatrist) was more frequently reported by the high-risk group. The moderate-risk group was particularly visible in the support accessed from community groups and palliative care services (Aoun et al., 2015).

Helpfulness of support obtained from different sources

As mentioned, the most frequently used sources of support were in the informal category such as family, friends, and funeral providers. While the professional category sources were the least used, they had the highest proportions of perceived unhelpfulness. Nearly half of those who used psychiatrists found them unhelpful (46%), and over a third of respondents who used the following services rated them unhelpful: bereavement support group (41%), case coordinator (39%), social worker (38%), and school-based advisor (36%). Similar high rates of unhelpfulness were reported in the community

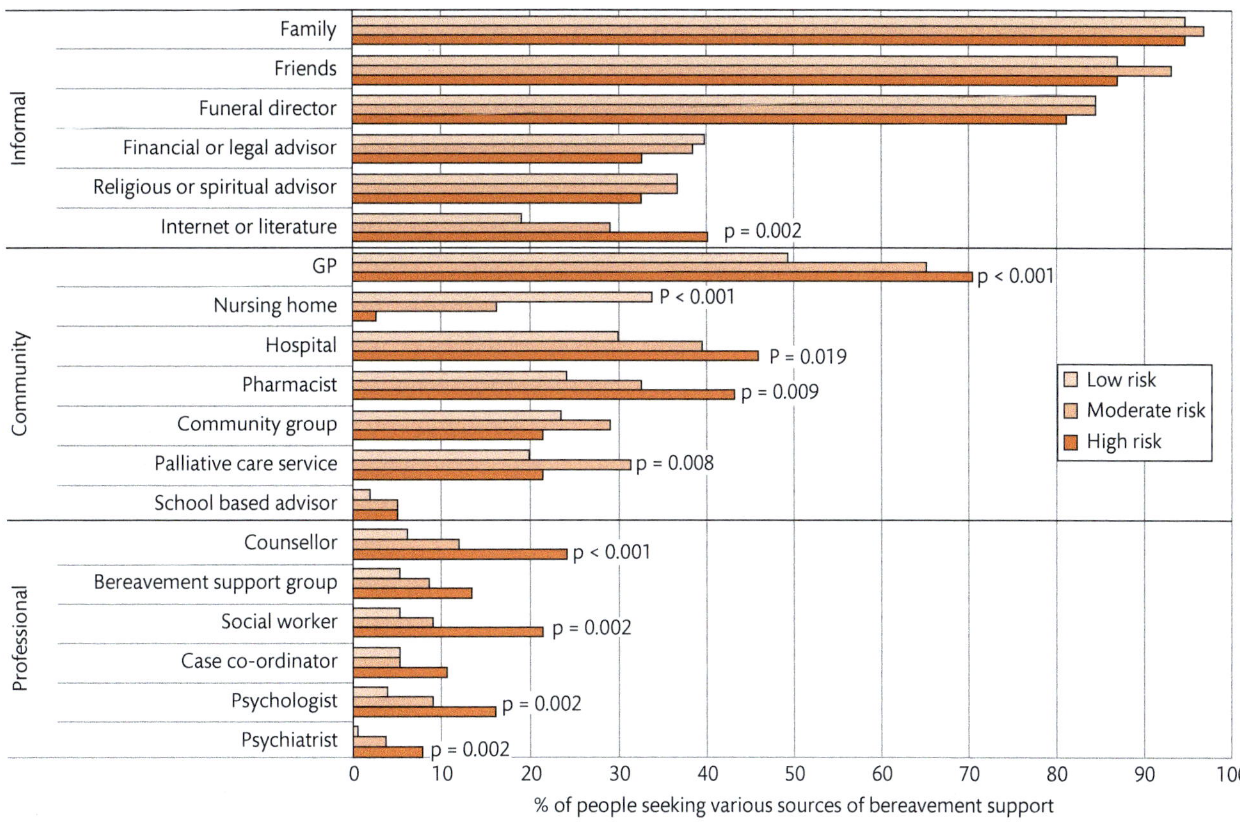

Fig. 19.2 Sources of bereavement support accessed by the three risk groups.

Reproduced from Aoun, S. M., Breen, L. J., Howting, D. A., Rumbold, B., McNamara, B. & Hegney, D. 2015. Who needs bereavement support? A population based survey of bereavement risk and support need. *PLoS One*, 10, e0121101.

category and in particular, a community group (40%), community pharmacist (39%), and palliative care service (33%). By contrast, the lowest proportions of unhelpfulness were in the informal category where only 8% found family unhelpful, followed by the funeral provider (8.7%) and friends (11.7%) (Fig. 19.3) (Aoun et al., 2018).

In the informal sources of support, the findings revealed that attachment (emotional or affectionate bond, often provided by spouse/partner or close family) was the form of social support most frequently endorsed as helpful by respondents, suggesting that the majority of bereaved individuals value emotional support from those closest to them. This was followed in terms of frequency by reliable alliance (tangible assistance such as providing meals and transport often offered by family members) and social integration (perceived sense of belonging often provided by friends). In examining the unhelpful support, it seems that feeling unsupported was more than just the absence of support. While people did mention absence of support, they also mentioned receiving insensitive comments, unwanted advice, and felt lack of empathy. However, fewer bereaved people had experienced unhelpful support (compared to helpful support) and that was mainly from government, financial, and legal institutions (Aoun et al., 2018).

What makes social networks fit for providing bereavement support? Not everyone who receives bereavement support needs it and not everyone who needs bereavement support receives it. It was important to know not only who best provided bereavement support, but more so who was perceived by bereaved people to have offered them the type and amount of support they needed, at the time they needed it. In other words, assessment of the goodness of fit between need and response was important (Aoun et al., 2019a). Improving the fit between the bereaved person's needs and the support offered will thus involve identifying and enhancing the caring capacity of existing networks. An important strategy for achieving this is to train community members in mapping and developing these naturally occurring networks or circles of care (Abel et al., 2013; Abel, 2018). Some such networks will include relationships of long standing, others may be networks formed during a period of caring (Aoun et al., 2019a).

The most systematic development of social network enhancement has been the connectors project in general practice in Frome, Somerset, UK (Abel et al., 2018). The intervention involved rigorous identification of all those in need, not limited by age or diagnosis, followed by care planning and referral to a community development service for goal setting and social network enhancement. Health connectors were the bridge between clinic and community; community connectors are conversation partners/promoters of the programme. The research team was able to demonstrate over a 3-year period a 14% reduction of unplanned admissions to emergency departments, compared with a 28.5% increase in the remainder of Somerset.

One Australian initiative involving training community members is the compassionate communities connectors model for end of life care which is a community and health service partnership in the South West of Western Australia (Aoun et al., 2020a). This initiative aims to develop, implement, and evaluate a model of community

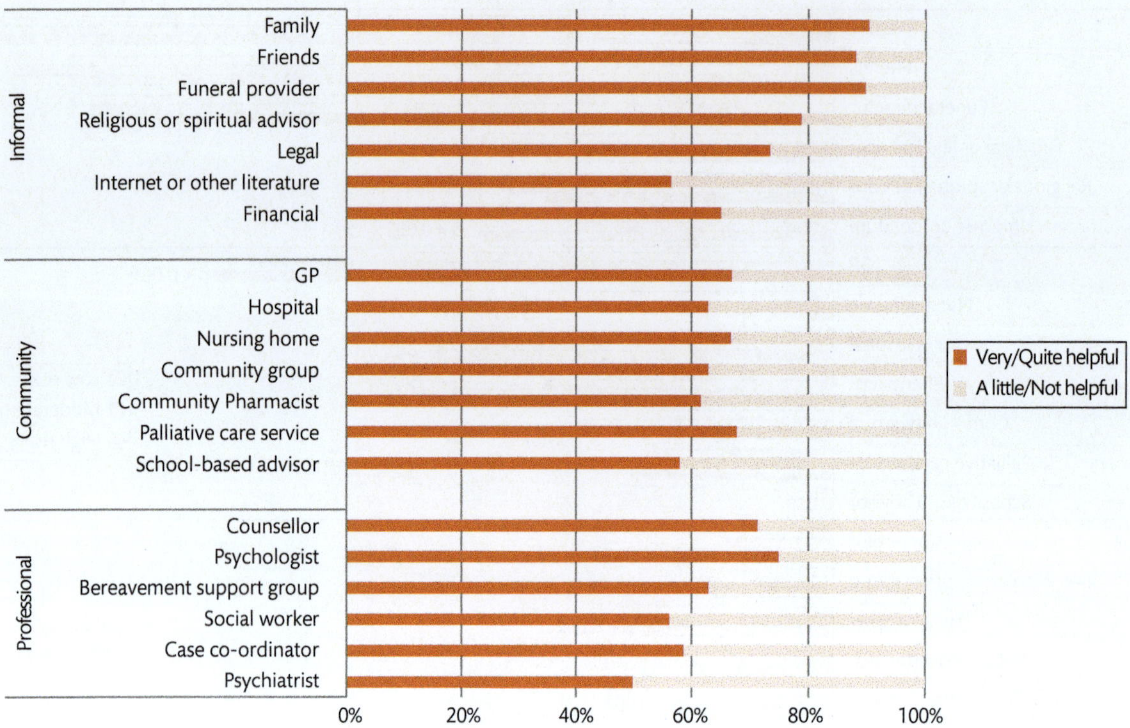

Fig. 19.3 Sources of support accessed and perceived as helpful or unhelpful.

Reproduced with permission from Aoun SM, Keegan O, Roberts A, Breen L (2020). The impact of bereavement support on wellbeing: a comparative study between Australia and Ireland. *Palliative Care and Social Practice*. Vol. 14: 1–14 DOI: 10.1177/2632352420935132.

volunteers, identified as compassionate communities connectors, to support people living with advanced life-limiting illnesses/palliative care needs. The approach seeks to map and mobilize people's personal networks of care through the connectors enlisting caring helpers (community volunteers). The primary outcome is the effect of the intervention on social connectedness. Secondary outcomes are the intervention's effect on unplanned hospital utilization, caregiver support needs, advance care plans, and satisfaction with intervention for patients/carers, volunteers, and service providers. It is expected that this intervention will enhance patient, carer, and family social, psychological, and practical support and reduce the need for dying people to be admitted to a hospital. As exemplified by compassionate communities policies and practices (Kellehear, 2005, 2013), establishing collaboration between community networks and professional services is vital for effective and sustainable bereavement care.

Bereavement care in palliative care

In many countries, the most coherent approach to bereavement support is given by palliative care services, which emphasize the care of patients with terminal illnesses and their family caregivers before and after the patient's death (Palliative Care Australia, 2005; World Health Organization, 2007; National Hospice and Palliative Care Organization, 2008). Standards for bereavement care propose that support should be matched to risk and need. However, as noted previously, studies demonstrate that many palliative care services continue to adopt a generic approach in offering support to bereaved families.

In the Australian survey (Aoun et al., 2017), the support for family caregivers before and after their relative's death was not considered optimal. Incorporating questions on a number of guidelines for the psychosocial and bereavement support of family caregivers (Hudson et al., 2010), only 39.4% of the bereaved reported being specifically asked about their emotional/psychological distress prior to bereavement, and just half of the bereaved perceived they had enough support from palliative care services. Half of the bereaved had a follow up contact from the service at 3–6 weeks, and a quarter had a follow-up at 6 months. Overall, only a third of respondents rated the support from palliative care services as helpful. Their qualitative feedback underlined the limited helpfulness of the generic approach to bereavement support, which was often described as impersonal or just standard practice. Respondents drew equally on their informal and community networks whether they used or did not use palliative care services (Aoun et al., 2017).

Findings further showed that timeliness and consistency of relationship were crucial to building rapport and trust in the service's ability to help post bereavement, as was a focus on the specific rather than the generic needs of the bereaved. In light of these limitations, palliative care services might do better investing their efforts principally in assessing and supporting family caregivers during the pre-bereavement period and developing community capacity and referral pathways for bereavement care.

Application to special population groups: motor neurone disease

The survey was adapted for use with those bereaved by motor neurone disease (MND). An anonymous national population-based cross-sectional postal and online survey of bereavement

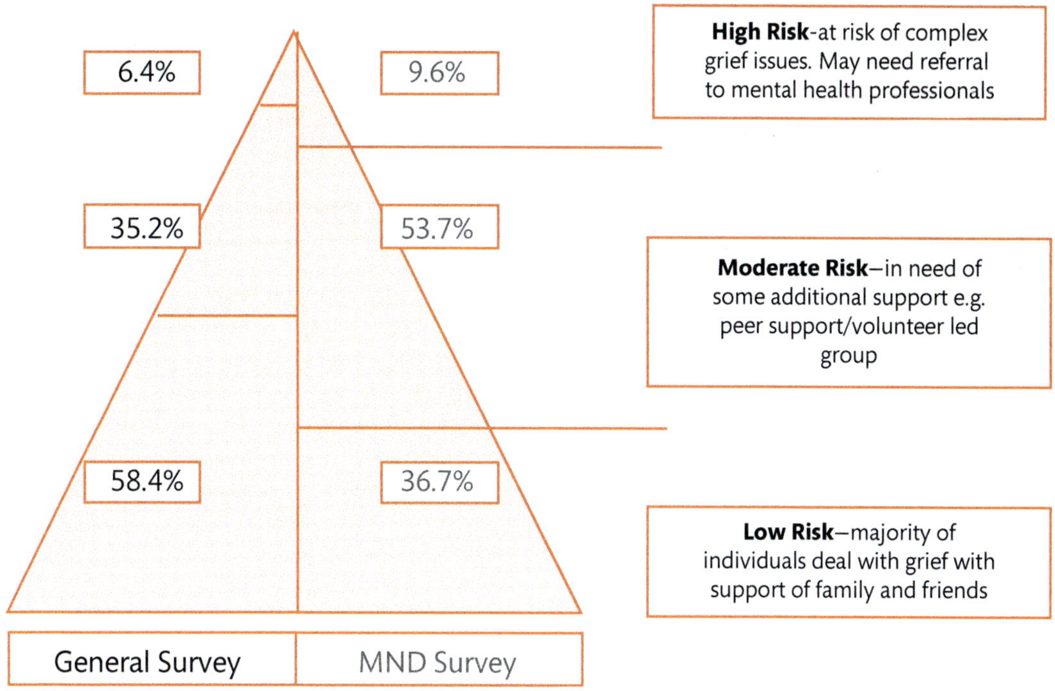

Fig. 19.4 Comparison of proportions in the three grief risk groups of the MND bereaved population and the general bereaved population.
Reproduced with permission from Aoun, S. M., et al. 2020. Grief, depression, and anxiety in bereaved caregivers of people with motor neurone disease: a population-based national study. *Amyotrophic Lateral Sclerosis and Frontotemporal Degeneration*, 21: 593–605

experiences of family caregivers who lost a relative/friend to MND was conducted in 2019. Recruitment was through all MND associations in Australia. The most frequently used sources of support by the 393 respondents were those in the informal category such as friends (98%), family (96%), and funeral providers (72%). In the community category, the most used services were those of the MND associations (78%) and GPs (74%) followed by palliative care services (45%). Professional resources were the least frequently used, with case coordinators (23%), counsellors (22%), and social workers (19%) the most consulted. Professional sources were perceived to be the least helpful while informal sources were perceived as more helpful (Aoun et al., 2020b).

MND caregivers were found to have higher bereavement risk than the general bereaved population, with 9.6% in the high-risk group or having PGD (vs 6.4%) and 54% at moderate risk (vs 35%) (Fig. 19.4). Over one-half of those who reported not receiving enough support experienced significant worsening of their mental health ($p = 0.008$), and just under 40% reported worsening physical health ($p = 0.049$) (Aoun et al., 2020c). Perceived insufficiency of support was higher for those at high bereavement risk. Being in the PGD group was 8 or 18 times more likely when the respondent had anxiety or depression, respectively. Poor family functioning significantly increased the likelihood of PGD by a factor of four. Other significant predictors of PGD were a recent bereavement (<12 months), being a spouse/partner of the deceased, insufficient support during the disease journey, the deceased being under 60 years of age, and a shorter period of caring (<1.5 years).

It is worth mentioning here the role of the not-for-profit or third-sector organizations that represent the concerns of specific groups, such as those of MND caregivers in this study. MND associations provide support during the illness experience for people with MND and their families and are ideally placed to do so in bereavement. Additionally, these types of organizations can connect both professional and community resources in a way that clinicians alone, or community actors, cannot. They are sufficiently structured and accountable to be acceptable partners for clinical services, but they are also responsive to their membership base and flexible enough to make an immediate response to expressed needs—something that is particularly important given the rapidly shifting nature of MND. However, this requires MND associations to include bereavement care as an integral part of their role, expanding the period of support and accessing additional training and necessary resources (Aoun et al., 2020b).

Application in other countries: comparison with Ireland

Until recently, there was a dearth of national and international data on the impact of social support on physical, mental, and financial outcomes. The utility of this population-based public health approach has been demonstrated in societies other than Australia. For example, a recent study in Ireland was based on the Australian population-based cross-sectional study of bereavement experiences. It entailed a telephone survey of a stratified sample of 908 adults (18+ years) living in the Republic of Ireland.

Despite the different recruitment methodologies and the different age distribution of the bereaved and their relationship to the deceased between the Irish and Australian studies, the vast majority of bereaved people in Ireland also relied on informal supporters, particularly family and friends (Aoun et al., 2020d). This is in line with a public health approach to bereavement support. Irish respondents

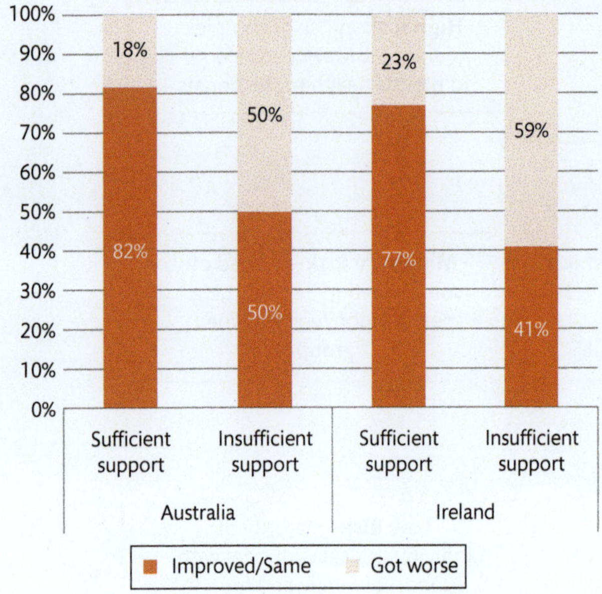

Fig. 19.5 Sufficiency of support and self-reported mental well-being: Australia and Ireland.

Reproduced with permission from Aoun SM, Keegan O, Roberts A, Breen L (2020). The impact of bereavement support on wellbeing: a comparative study between Australia and Ireland. *Palliative Care and Social Practice*. Vol. 14: 1–14 DOI: 10.1177/2632352420935132.

also rated professional supports, such as counsellors, psychiatrists, psychologists, and social workers poorly. The impact of the perceived insufficiency of support on health deterioration was also very similar in the two studies (Fig. 19.5). A relationship between self-reported post-bereavement mental and physical health and perceived support during bereavement was observed. Those who rated their health as deteriorated also attested a lack of support in bereavement.

Reception of the model and impact on policy and practice

Service providers, at the national and international levels, received the model with a sense of relief as it gave them more focus on the bereavement needs they are able to service within their capacity. The public health approach emphasizes the capacity of social networks and communities to respond to bereaved people and positions bereavement care as a shared responsibility between communities and health services (Rumbold and Aoun, 2014). This reduces unnecessary over-professionalization of bereavement care and improves services' capacity to respond to those who actually do need them. Comments from service providers reflect this feeling of relief: 'Thanks so much, I am enjoying your research so much! We've been using it at the service too—that triangle says so much.' This means less reliance on anecdotal experiences and trial-and-error approaches (Lobb et al., 2010) and improved services' capacity to respond to those who actually do need them (Aoun et al., 2015).

The UK National Bereavement Alliance were the first to reach out with their work based on this model: 'We are currently developing a guide for commissioners of area-based bereavement services, and I am drawing heavily on your population-based survey of bereavement risk and support need. Your work is proving very helpful to us here in the UK.' Furthermore, in their published policy guide to commissioning services (National Bereavement Alliance, 2017) and 'Care After Caring' document (National Bereavement Alliance, 2019), they report that 'the public health approach emphasizes mechanisms that help get the right support for the right people at the right time'. In addition, they drew on the public health model when revising/expanding the National Institute for Health and Care Excellence model of care (National Bereavement Alliance, email personal communication).

At the Australian policy level, the research has informed the development of Standard 6 on 'Grief support' in the revised National Palliative Care Standards in Australia (Palliative Care Australia, 2018). In particular 'the service develops strategies and referral pathways in partnership with other providers in the community' and 'referrals to mental health specialists and counselling professionals are made when clinically indicated'. More recently, Palliative Care Australia produced a position statement on palliative and coronavirus disease 2019 (COVID-19) with emphasis on grief, bereavement, and mental health encompassing the public health model for bereavement support (Palliative Care Australia, 2020).

At the international level, the research has informed the work of the bereavement care Taskforce of the European Association of Palliative Care to develop best practice guidelines (Guldin et al., 2015). The taskforce reported that the public health framework offers a structure within which bereavement support should be considered, designed, and operationalized (in palliative care and elsewhere).

For Ireland, the findings from their survey triggered the development of standards for bereavement care which provided a framework for services, a guidance on level of service provision, and associated staff competencies and training needs. Their report 'Enhancing Adult Bereavement Care across Ireland' endorsed the 'pyramid model' (as in Fig. 19.1) as a way forward for a national framework to shape bereavement care policy, planning, and service delivery (McLoughlin, 2018). This framework was developed through a national collaborative process, involving both state and voluntary organizations, at all levels of service provision. It is the first step in a process to enhance bereavement care provision across Ireland and will be used as a guide in further developments, such as national standards and mapping of service provision across Ireland (The Irish Hospice Foundation, 2020).

Funerals and memorials

The funeral industry has been particularly interested in making a contribution to communities and becoming more intentional about bereavement support. This is not surprising when the funeral providers were reported as the third most frequently used source of support after family and friends and also described as mostly helpful in their support (Aoun et al., 2019b). This appreciation by the bereaved is seemingly related to funeral providers' shaping of the chaos of the early days of bereavement and related to helpful aspects of instrumental support, professionalism, informational support, communication, and emotional support. Furthermore, 30% of respondents suggested funeral service providers should adopt a proactive approach to clients' bereavement needs and foster an ongoing relationship in support of the bereaved. In Western Australia, suicide postvention training is currently underway for funeral providers' staff to respond appropriately to bereavement caused by suicide. This new relationship between the Australian funeral service industry and suicide postvention agencies is an example of community-based groups and more formal support services coming together to form partnerships as advocated by the public health model. Funeral service providers are one of those assets that have a key role to play in building community—capacity around death, dying and bereavement (Aoun et al., 2019b).

The Australasian Crematoria and Cemeteries Association commissioned our team to carry out a study to better understand the influence of memorialization on grief and bereavement. Findings revealed that the community is 'reclaiming' death, dying, and bereavement and hence memorialization practices. Therefore, reframing the role of the industry within such community-based approaches may help it respond more adequately to the cultural and market changes currently affecting the industry and the changing role of service providers in sharing this space with other players (Lowe et al., 2019). In using the public health model to include memorialization needs based on bereavement risk, the following trends were identified from the synthesized findings of this study: bereaved people with high memorialization needs may require a private memorial in a public space, highly personalized memorial rituals, close proximity to the remains, and rituals enacted daily. Those with moderate memorialization needs may benefit from a public memorial in a private space, personalized memorial rituals, access to remains, and rituals that decline in frequency over time. Those with low memorialization needs may prefer a public memorial in a public space and standardized rituals that are enacted on occasion. This model may guide service providers in understanding the potential benefits of matching specific memorialization practices to clients' bereavement risks and support needs. Cemeteries, crematoria, and the funeral industry have resolved to shape a more contemporary industry and to become more intentional about their social contributions as educators, facilitators, and consultants on meaningful, effective, and therapeutic rituals for bereaved Australians (Rumbold et al., 2019).

Through the lens of the pandemic

Recent publications on the effect of COVID-19 on grief and bereavement have projected an increase in the risk of PGD (Eisma et al., 2020; Wallace et al., 2020) because of the difficult and unexpected circumstances of the deaths, reduction of physical social support, and diminished mourning rituals to name a few factors. Such projections certainly cannot be discounted, but they also fail to take account of the resilience indicated by the population survey findings, the diversity of support upon which people draw in learning to live with loss. Whatever the circumstance, people still manage to connect in different ways. For example, memorial rituals previously peripheral have become central to funeral participation during COVID-19: streaming the funeral service online, conducting a personal memorial at home, sending flowers or a sympathy card, signing an online guest book, making a donation in the name of the deceased, writing or recording a message to be read out or played at the funeral, and using social media to connect with funeral attendees afterward as a means of social support (Australian Centre for Grief and Bereavement, 2020; Lowe et al., 2020). Somewhat paradoxically, the loss of opportunities to say farewells itself becomes a source of social connection as people post their accounts on social media and support each other in sharing their wishes about what might have been.

Whether these different ways of remembering and supporting each other will prove to be effective in the longer term depends in part on how capable and comfortable mourners are in exposing their inner reflections to the shared digital world. Even before the pandemic, there was evidence that many people were embedding memorialization in their everyday lives more than in shared public events and static memorials. It appears that the restrictions placed upon many familiar memorialization practices have made room for creative new expressions of innovative memorialization, making these new expressions more widely available and more likely to continue to serve individuals, families, and communities in a post-pandemic future (Lowe et al., 2020).

Some of the opportunities created with COVID-19's sharp focus on death, dying, loss, and grief are potential improvements in death literacy within the community enabling more preparedness and ability to die at home if it is in line with a person's wishes, and improvements in grief literacy (Aoun, 2020; Breen et al., 2020), community understanding in supporting the bereaved, recognition of grief-related issues and appropriate help-seeking.

If we were to make an informed guess or extrapolation on changes to the three risk levels under the pandemic, based on the studies outlined previously, especially similarities with a progressive and fatal disease like MND—when caregivers experience insufficient support during the disease journey, and a short period of caregiving—the largest increase would be in the moderate-risk group, unless there are predisposing factors to be in the high-risk group such as having anxiety, depression, or poor family functioning (Fig. 19.6). However, many of the projections of increased PGD may overestimate the importance of professional support, and correspondingly underestimate what family, friends, and neighbours can provide.

Responses to the pandemic have been in most places—albeit with some notable exceptions—shaped by public health guidance concerning pandemic control. Public health strategies to address the well-being of shutdown communities have been less evident, although the importance of social connection, a recurring theme in popular media, is arguably a public health message.

Public health strategies like compassionate communities retain their value but need to develop new approaches when face-to-face encounters are minimal and physical strategies for support are limited. Compassionate communities approaches have driven increased community engagement in tasks that were in the modern era limited to close family members or consigned to professional services. But now sitting with the dying, offering respite care in the home, cleaning the home of a caregiver, laying out a body, keeping a body at home, and offering companionship in grief, are all suspended, or modified. Of course, there have been more radical expressions of compassion that reshape community life, among them staff members of care homes moving in to share lockdown with their residents.

A public health approach to bereavement care should shape policy and action as we emerge from the pandemic. The focus of this approach is upon the assets that remain available or can be mobilized as support, upon what is possible more than what has been lost. The support of family and friends continues to be central, so

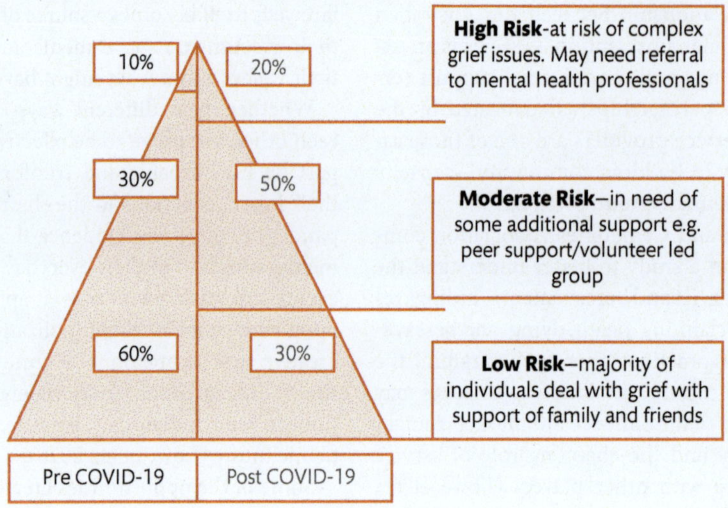

Fig. 19.6 Pre-pandemic and estimated post-pandemic proportions of risk groups.

Reproduced from Professor Samar Aoun, Keynote presentation entitled: Public Health Approaches to Bereavement Care—through the lens of the pandemic, at the second international research seminar on public health research in palliative care: Towards Solutions for Global challenges, 17–18 November 2020.

opening up and maintaining communication is vital. At present, with much contact being digitally mediated, communication has to be much more intentional—we can no longer rely on bumping into people in shops or on the street. Spontaneity may be reduced, but creativity increased. Public health approaches that aim to increase social support and community engagement are being re-set. COVID-19 has returned virus-related deaths to medical control, and significant levels of complicated grief could also increase clinically managed grieving. However, at the time PGD emerges (from 6 months after death), there should also be more options for face-to-face support. Strategies for moving out of lockdown need also to attend to strategies to restore the interpersonal dimensions of care.

Conclusion

The findings from this programme of work provide empirical evidence for building a community's capacity to provide the type of social and practical support advocated by the compassionate communities approach, which relies on identifying and developing local caring networks around the dying person and their family. This body of work, innovative in content, conceptual model, and recruitment approach, has challenged the existing bereavement support structure and provision and has already influenced practice and policy in Australia, the UK, and Ireland.

This public health model also shifts providers' perspective of bereavement care. Rather than organize strategies around the potential for complications, it takes into account the fact that most people manage to live with and through bereavement without developing mental health problems and often enhancing their social connectedness. The resources or assets available to them in their everyday lives are sufficient to meet their needs. The community needs to own its central role in end of life and bereavement care, with healthcare professionals advising, supporting, and contributing as required. A public health perspective means that healthcare contributions alone are not a sufficient basis for creating healthy communities and formulating health strategies. Informal care is the bedrock, with formal services supplementing this support. If palliative care services wish to serve the majority of their bereaved clients, they should attend to developing community capacity rather than providing specialized bereavement services of their own. A bereavement care policy informed by this public health perspective should have its foundation in the strengthening and support of the principal resource for bereavement care, the community social networks.

The findings have shown a mixed reception for formal support around different expectations, most likely because some formal providers fail to notice, or enquire about, the support that already exists. Thus, counsellors may focus on emotional support, not understanding that emotional support is largely in place, and that what clients need is strategic support to help them negotiate their changed world, not merely to adjust their emotions. In this respect, grief counselling continues to display its origins in psychiatric studies of bereavement: interest in painful emotions, in inner conflicts, and individual coping. Certainly, grief therapies have moved from their psychodynamic roots to take account of continuing bonds and dual process, but they still seem biased towards emotional enquiry rather than attending to strategies for everyday living with loss. Counsellors, or other professionals, need to remember that they are being consulted not to deal with grief as a separable event, but as one aspect of a tangible, multidimensional loss with which that bereaved person has to live (Breen et al., 2018).

The wider intention of this chapter is to illustrate the importance of a population health perspective as a key component of a public health approach. If policy and practice are to be inclusive, our approach to any issue needs to consider how and where that issue arises within our society, who is affected by it, and how resources are used to address it. A population health approach, as we have seen here, raises questions about access to care and the appropriate use of resources. These in turn are questions about equity, which we have not addressed explicitly in the studies described here, but which are an integral part of a public health approach to bereavement, as Paul and Vaswani (2020) show. A public health approach also exposes the inadequacy of policy that focuses exclusively upon services a government can fund and deliver, which by implication marginalizes or ignores the contribution of the community. The concern of public health is health for all, which involves attending to the complex systems of care that form within communities. Effective and sustainable care requires collaboration between formal services and informal approaches to care, often mediated by third-sector organizations that represent the concerns of specific groups of caregivers. It also requires a sense of connection and mutual responsibility within communities—a stance inherent to compassionate communities—preferably fostered by leadership that strives to unite rather than divide. Population health and a nation's political climate are intrinsically connected, as the pandemic has shown.

REFERENCES

Abel, J. 2018. Compassionate communities and end-of-life care. *Clinical Medicine,* 18, 6.

Abel, J., Kingston, H., Scally, A., Hartnoll, J., Hannam, G., Thomson-Moore, A., et al. 2018. Reducing emergency hospital admissions: a population health complex intervention of an enhanced model of primary care and compassionate communities. *British Journal of General Practice,* 68, e803–e810.

Abel, J., Walter, T., Carey, L. B., Rosenberg, J., Noonan, K., Horsfall, D., et al. 2013. Circles of care: should community development redefine the practice of palliative care? *BMJ Supportive & Palliative Care,* 3, 383–388.

Aoun, S., Breen, L., O'Connor, M., Rumbold, B., and Nordstrom, C. 2012. A public health approach to bereavement support services in palliative care. *Australian and New Zealand Journal of Public Health,* 36, 14–16.

Aoun, S. M. 2020. Bereavement support: from the poor cousin of palliative care to a core asset of compassionate communities. *Progress in Palliative Care,* 28, 107–114.

Aoun, S. M., Abel, J., Rumbold, B., Cross, K., Moore, J., Skeers, P., et al. 2020a. The compassionate communities connectors model for end-of-life care: a community and health service partnership in Western Australia. *Palliative Care and Social Practice,* 14, 2632352420935130.

Aoun, S. M., Breen, L. J., Howting, D. A., Rumbold, B., Mcnamara, B., and Hegney, D. 2015. Who needs bereavement support? A population based survey of bereavement risk and support need. *PLoS One,* 10, e0121101.

Aoun, S. M., Breen, L. J., Rumbold, B., Christian, K. M., Same, A., and Abel, J. 2019a. Matching response to need: what makes social networks fit for providing bereavement support? *PLoS One,* 14, e0213367.

Aoun, S. M., Breen, L. J., White, I., Rumbold, B., and Kellehear, A. 2018. What sources of bereavement support are perceived helpful by bereaved people and why? Empirical evidence for the compassionate communities approach. *Palliative Medicine,* 32, 1378–1388.

Aoun, S. M., Cafarella, P. A., Rumbold, B., Thomas, G., Hogden, A., Jiang, L., et al. 2020b. Who cares for the bereaved? A national survey of family caregivers of people with motor neurone disease. *Amyotrophic Lateral Sclerosis and Frontotemporal Degeneration,* 22, 12–22.

Aoun, S. M., Keegan, O., Roberts, A., and Breen, L. J. 2020d. The impact of bereavement support on wellbeing: a comparative study between Australia and Ireland. *Palliative Care and Social Practice,* 14, 2632352420935132.

Aoun, S. M., Kissane, D. W., Cafarella, P. A., Rumbold, B., Hogden, A., Jiang, L., et al. 2020c. Grief, depression, and anxiety in bereaved caregivers of people with motor neurone disease: a population-based national study. *Amyotrophic Lateral Sclerosis and Frontotemporal Degeneration,* 21, 593–605.

Aoun, S. M., Lowe, J., Christian, K. M., and Rumbold, B. 2019b. Is there a role for the funeral service provider in bereavement support within the context of compassionate communities? *Death Studies,* 43, 619–628.

Aoun, S. M., Rumbold, B., Howting, D., Bolleter, A., and Breen, L. J. 2017. Bereavement support for family caregivers: The gap between guidelines and practice in palliative care. *PLoS One,* 12, e0184750.

Australian Centre for Grief and Bereavement. 2020. Grief and bereavement and COVID-19. [Online]. Available at: https://aged.grief.org.au/

Breen, L. J., Aoun, S. M., O'Connor, M., and Rumbold, B. 2014. Bridging the gaps in palliative care bereavement support: an international perspective. *Death Studies,* 38, 54–61.

Breen, L. J., Croucamp, C. J., and Rees, C. S. 2018. What do people really think about grief counseling? Examining community attitudes. *Death Studies,* 43, 611–618.

Breen, L. J., Kawashima, D., Joy, K., Cadell, S., Roth, D., Chow, A., and MacDonald, M. E. 2020. Grief literacy: a call to action for compassionate communities. *Death Studies,* 19 March, 1–9. doi: 10.1080/07481187.2020.1739780. Epub ahead of print.

Eisma, M. C., Boelen, P. A., and Lenferink, L. I. 2020. Prolonged grief disorder following the coronavirus (COVID-19) pandemic. *Psychiatry Research,* 288, 113031.

Guldin, M., Murphy, I., Keegan, O., Monroe, B., Lacasta-Reverte, M., and Benkel, I. 2015. Bereavement services in palliative care in Europe: a survey study by the European Association for Palliative Care bereavement taskforce. *European Journal of Palliative Care,* 22, 185–189.

Hudson, P., Remedios, C., Zordan, R., Thomas, K., Clifton, D., Crewdson, M., et al. 2010. *Clinical Practice Guidelines for the Psychosocial and Bereavement Support of Family Caregivers of Palliative Care Patients.* Melbourne: Centre for Palliative Care.

Kellehear, A. 2005. *Compassionate Cities: Public Health and End-of-Life Care.* Abingdon: Routledge.

Kellehear, A. 2013. Compassionate communities: end-of-life care as everyone's responsibility. *QJM: An International Journal of Medicine,* 106, 1071–1075.

Kersting, A., Brähler, E., Glaesmer, H., and Wagner, B. 2011. Prevalence of complicated grief in a representative population-based sample. *Journal of Affective Disorders,* 131, 339–343.

Lobb, E. A., Kristjanson, L. J., Aoun, S. M., Monterosso, L., Halkett, G. K., and Davies, A. 2010. Predictors of complicated grief: a systematic review of empirical studies. *Death Studies,* 34, 673–698.

Lowe, J., Rumbold, B., and Aoun, S. M. 2019. Memorialization practices are changing: an industry perspective on improving service outcomes for the bereaved. *OMEGA,* 38, 62–67.

Lowe, J., Rumbold, B., and Aoun, S. M. 2020. Memorialisation during COVID-19: implications for the bereaved, service providers and policy makers. *Palliative Care and Social Practice,* 14, 1–9.

Mather, M. A., Good, P. D., Cavenagh, J. D., and Ravenscroft, P. J. 2008. Survey of bereavement support provided by Australian palliative care services. *Medical Journal of Australia,* 188, 228–230.

McLoughlin, K. 2018. *Enhancing Adult Bereavement Care Across Ireland: A Study.* Dublin: The Irish Hospice Foundation.

National Bereavement Alliance. 2017. A guide to commissioning bereavement services in England. [Online] Available at: https://nationalbereavementalliance.org.uk/wp-content/uploads/2017/07/A-Guide-to-Commissioning-Bereavement-Services-in-England-WEB.pdf

National Bereavement Alliance. 2019. Care after caring: supporting family carers facing and following bereavement. [Online] Available at: https://nationalbereavementalliance.org.uk/wp-content/uploads/2019/06/Care-after-Caring-for-carers-organisations-v2-1.pdf

National Hospice and Palliative Care Organization. 2008. *Guidelines for Bereavement Care in Hospice*, 2nd ed. Alexandria, VA: National Hospice and Palliative Care Organization.

National Institute for Health and Care Excellence. 2004. Guidance on cancer services: improving supportive and palliative care for adults with cancer. The manual. [Online] Available at: https://www.nice.org.uk/guidance/csg4/resources/improving-supportive-and-palliative-care-for-adults-withcancer-773375005

Nielsen, M. K., Neergaard, M. A., Jensen, A. B., Vedsted, P., Bro, F., and Guldin, M.-B. 2017. Predictors of complicated grief and depression in bereaved caregivers: a nationwide prospective cohort study. *Journal of Pain and Symptom Management*, 53, 540–550.

Palliative Care Australia. 2005. *Standards for Providing Quality Palliative Care for All Australians*. Canberra: Palliative Care Australia. Available at: https://palliativecare.org.au/wp-content/uploads/2015/07/Standards-for-providing-quality-palliative-care-for-all-Australians.pdf

Palliative Care Australia. 2018. *National Palliative Care Standards*, 5th ed. Canberra: Palliative Care Australia.

Palliative Care Australia. 2020. *Palliative Care and COVID-19. Grief, Bereavement and Mental Health*. Canberra: Palliative Care Australia.

Paul, S. and Vaswani, N. 2020. The prevalence of childhood bereavement in Scotland and its relationship with disadvantage: the significance of a public health approach to death, dying and bereavement. *Palliative Care and Social Practice*, 14, 2632352420975043.

Prigerson, H. G., Horowitz, M. J., Jacobs, S. C., Parkes, C. M., Aslan, M., Goodkin, K., et al. 2009. Prolonged grief disorder: psychometric validation of criteria proposed for DSM-V and ICD-11. *PLoS Med*, 6, e1000121.

Relf, M. and Lines, C. 2005. Who uses bereavement care. Presentation at the 7th International Conference on Grief and Bereavement in Contemporary Society, London, UK.

Rumbold, B. and Aoun, S. 2014. Bereavement and palliative care: a public health perspective. *Progress in Palliative Care*, 22, 131–135.

Rumbold, B., Lowe, J., and Aoun, S. M. 2019. Funerals, memorials and bereavement care. *Bereavement Care*, 38, 62–67.

Schut, H., Stroebe, M. S., Van Den Bout, J., and Terheggen, M. 2001. The efficacy of bereavement interventions: determining who benefits. In: Stroebe, M. S., Hansson, R. O., Stroebe, W., and Schut, H. (eds.) *Handbook of Bereavement Research: Consequences, Coping, and Care*, pp. 705–737. Washington, DC: American Psychological Association.

The Irish Hospice Foundation. 2020. *Adult Bereavement Care Pyramid: A National Framework*. Dublin: The Irish Hospice Foundation.

Wallace, C. L., Wladkowski, S. P., Gibson, A., and White, P. 2020. Grief during the COVID-19 pandemic: considerations for palliative care providers. *Journal of Pain and Symptom Management*, 60, e70–e76.

World Health Organization. 2007. *WHO Guide for Effective Programmes: Palliative Care*. Geneva: World Health Organization.

20

Public health palliative care, equity-oriented care, and structural vulnerability

Holly Prince, Kathy Kortes-Miller, Kelli I. Stajduhar, and Denise Marshall

Introduction

Hospice care, palliative care, and end of life (EOL) care are increasingly understood to be basic human rights (Stajduhar et al., 2019). Yet despite emphasis globally on improving 'access', we still have a profound lack of equity across the world. Many people and communities face significant, enduring structural and systemic barriers that severely affect access to health and social care, create health disparities, and impinge on people's quality of life. Consequently, framing hospice care, palliative care, and EOL care around equity and social justice issues are fundamental to the public health palliative care (PHPC) approach (Abel and Kellehear, 2018).

The PHPC approach is, at its core, a focus on equity, inclusivity, and diversity. The PHPC movement seeks to reclaim the natural course of dying and in the process, re-engage 'communities' to take on a larger role in caring for their own. For some communities, this means revisiting what has been lost or was never included in the evolution of modern mainstream palliative care. There are several promising initiatives being developed globally to enact a PHPC approach, but there is less attention on groups that could greatly benefit from participatory and community-based approaches embedded within PHPC and that are currently poorly served by palliative care in general. This reclaiming requires an understanding of basic precepts that affect equity and health. Many populations worldwide experience health inequities related to their palliative care and EOL needs; those with mental health issues, substance use disorders, those incarcerated, Indigenous peoples, lesbian, gay, bisexual, transgender, queer and Two-Spirited (LGBTQTS+) communities, and people facing homelessness, among others. In this chapter, we describe key contemporary concepts related to equity and health. We then situate these concepts within palliative and EOL care and PHPC. Next, we highlight examples of three groups of people who experience inequities in palliative and EOL care whose realities and experiences underscore the need for collective focus. A final discussion consolidates overarching themes to provide direction for broad, enduring, and global application.

Contemporary concepts related to equity and health

In 1992, Margaret Whitehead published an influential paper on equity and health that defined health inequities as differences in health that are unnecessary, unfair, and unjust. Whitehead offered three definitions of equity in healthcare: equal access to available care for equal need, equal utilization for equal need, and equal quality care for all (Whitehead, 1992). More recently, the World Health Organization has articulated a mandate of 'strengthening health equity' to focus collective attention on the fundamental global and national structures of social hierarchy and the socially determined conditions in which people grow, live, work, and age (Stajduhar, 2019). Stadjuhar and others remind us that societies comprise a diverse array of individuals whose social (e.g. gendered, racialized), economic, political, and cultural (e.g. classism, colonialism) power hierarchies result in differing degrees of privilege and oppression. It can be seen then that health equity carries moral, legal, and social connotations and calls upon society's obligation to improve unequal health outcomes (Stajduhar, 2019).

An individual's position of power, their experience of privilege or marginalization within a society, is informed by their social location. When these experiences intersect, as they often do, this can add to the impact of (dis)advantage and be reflected in individuals' health status (Hankivsky and Christoffersen, 2008). Such forces of oppression result in various negative health outcomes resulting from ongoing violence, trauma, and harm (Stajduhar et al., 2019). Trauma, defined broadly as 'experiences that overwhelm an individual's capacity to cope' (BC Provincial Mental Health and Substance Use Planning Council, 2013, p. 6), is an important construct to understand when considering oppression and negative health outcomes. Trauma is often a precursor to people's experiences of marginalizing conditions such as homelessness, substance use, and mental health issues (Farag and Buchanan, 2020). Privilege—the special advantages that some people have that are not enjoyed by everyone (Stajduhar et al., 2019)—is often unconscious and unrecognized due to socialization and having not experienced the oppressive side. Privilege is deeply rooted in our societies, is widely institutionalized, and imbues people's everyday experiences, including those in the health and social care systems.

More recently, the term '*structural vulnerability*' has been articulated to describe a person's or group's lower position within social hierarchies, which may amplify vulnerability, risk, and harm (Quesada et al., 2011; McNeil et al., 2015). People who experience structural vulnerability are disproportionately impacted by trauma through individual experiences and systems of power in society (Farag and Buchanan, 2020). Equity-oriented research shows that structurally vulnerable groups face significant barriers in having their palliative care and EOL needs met (Reimer-Kirkham et al., 2016; Stajduhar et al., 2019). Most palliative care services are currently designed to serve the dominant culture within a population, which often excludes those with differing structural, social, and individual conditions and fails to recognize diversity. In this manner, a cohort of people and communities is seen as 'doubly vulnerable', needing palliative care services and experiencing deficits in the social determinants of health that result in multiple health disparities when facing EOL. These disparities may include lack of access to palliative care until very late in the illness trajectory (Ahmed et al., 2004; Reimer-Kirkham et al., 2016). Current research underscores that without recognizing structural vulnerability, the advancement of equitable access to quality hospice care, palliative care, and EOL care will not be achievable (Stajduhar et al., 2019). Thus, an *equity-oriented* approach to PHPC demands that we attend to *who* current palliative care, hospice care, and EOL care programmes and services are working for and *whom they are failing* (Reimer-Kirkham et al., 2016). The very success of the PHPC approach depends on this.

Equity-oriented healthcare is comprised of at least three key dimensions: (1) *trauma- and violence-informed care*, (2) *cultural safety* and *cultural humility*, and (3) *harm reduction* (Browne et al., 2018). *Trauma-informed care* occurs when programmes, organizations, and systems realize the widespread impact of trauma; understand paths for recovery; recognize the signs and symptoms of trauma in patients, families, and staff; and respond by fully integrating knowledge about trauma into policies, procedures, and practices. By doing so, the focus is to actively resist re-traumatization. Recent work has seen the development of *violence-informed care*, an awareness that grew out of trauma-informed care. Violence-informed care draws attention to the traumatic effects of living with violence of any kind, including structural violence. This harm can result from the ways that societies are organized. A core focus of *trauma- and violence-informed care* is creating safety for people who have faced or are facing personal or structural violence (Levine et al., 2021). Patients receiving hospice care, palliative care, or EOL care may have experienced trauma as a direct result of diagnosis and medical intervention, for example, or by being stigmatized by healthcare providers. Previous personal or structural traumas can be reactivated, especially in the face of anxiety, pain, delirium, or even by hospitalization. Palliative care providers, volunteers, and communities, whose focus is already to alleviate pain, distress, and suffering, are uniquely positioned to integrate trauma-and violence-informed care, recognizing that many people may be survivors of a traumatic healthcare experience, for example, and acknowledging that it is not necessary to know the details of a person's trauma and violence history to provide them with trauma- and violence-informed care.

Cultural safety emerged as a construct in New Zealand in the 1980s in response to recognizing poor health outcomes of Māori people and their dissatisfaction with health care. Cultural safety provides quality care by addressing power dynamics in relationships while centring on patients' rights (Papps and Ramsden, 1996). It is an outcome that 'results in an environment free of racism and discrimination, where people feel safe when receiving health care' (First Nations Health Authority, 2016, p. 5). *Cultural humility* has been defined as a 'lifetime commitment to self-evaluation and critique, to redressing the power imbalances' (Trevalon and Murray-García, 1998, p. 123) that may be inherent in a provider–patient dynamic. Such a commitment seeks to 'develop mutually beneficial and non-paternalistic partnerships with communities on behalf of individuals and defined populations' (p. 123). As the focus is on the provider–patient relationship and not on the provider's knowledge or attitude, cultural humility seeks to challenge and address power imbalances by engaging in teaching and learning strategies for mutual respect. It has been aptly described as 'humbly acknowledging oneself as a learner when it comes to understanding another's experience' (First Nations Health Authority, 2016, p. 7). Cultural humility seeks to make conscious and known the personal and systemic biases that create environments that may be unconsciously perpetuated (Diangelo, 2018). As a result, cultural humility holds institutions accountable.

The World Health Organization (2021) defines *harm reduction* as a set of policies, programmes, services, and actions that aim to reduce the harm to individuals, communities, and society related to drugs, including the prevention of infectious diseases such as HIV and hepatitis C. More contemporary definitions of harm reduction suggest that it is an approach to care that promotes non-judgement, dignity, self-determination, and autonomy. Rooted in social justice movements aimed at respecting the rights of people who use drugs, harm reduction incorporates a spectrum of strategies that include safer drug use, managed use, abstinence, and meeting people who use drugs where they are at (McNeil et al., 2012b). A key principle of harm reduction is acknowledging and affirming that people who use drugs are themselves the primary agents of reducing the harms of their drug use. It includes recognizing that poverty, class, racism, past trauma, sex-based discrimination, and other social inequalities affect both people's vulnerability to, and capacity for, effectively dealing with drug-related harms (Pauly, 2008). Harm reduction is considered a central component of public health strategies in most countries in the Global North. Therefore, PHPC, by definition, must consider harm reduction as a centralizing concept in the care of people who are structurally vulnerable.

To summarize, health inequities result from systemic and structural issues that position certain groups of people at a disadvantage. This disadvantage is exacerbated when people are diagnosed with a life-limiting condition. People working within hospice, palliative, and EOL care, with a commitment to PHPC approaches, need to consider how to develop, adapt, and translate equity-oriented approaches within PHPC to address the needs of people experiencing structural vulnerability, and fully embrace what it means to provide inclusive care to diverse populations. Three such populations are the focus of the remainder of the chapter. They provide practical examples and ways in which the key dimensions of equity-oriented care (i.e. trauma- and violence-informed care, cultural safety and cultural humility, and harm reduction) can be used as an orienting frame for PHPC for people who are structurally vulnerable. A focus on emerging models, practice, exemplars, and evidence of such initiatives is discussed.

Communities of people facing structural vulnerability

There are many individuals and communities of people facing health inequities. These inequities are evident in mortality and morbidity outcomes at individual and population levels (Krieger, 2014; Arcaya et al., 2015) and create conditions that can be challenging to the provision of palliative care. Here, we describe three communities/groups of people who experience structural vulnerability as a focus, highlighting the inherent strengths and capacities within these groups and outlining emerging developments and evolving practices and/or new evidence that may foster equity-oriented PHPC for the future. While having global application, our discussion is embedded within our experiences in the Canadian context and our own social locations as scholars in palliative care who are working with communities of people experiencing structural vulnerability. Collectively, we represent gay and cisgender identities, are of European settler and Indigenous heritage, and have a strong PHPC and social justice orientation to our work. Each of the authors of this chapter contributes work rooted in long-standing health disparities.

Indigenous peoples

See Box 20.1 for an illustrative case study.

Setting the context

There are more than 370 million Indigenous peoples worldwide living in over 90 countries (United Nations, 2009). Indigenous peoples consist of diverse nations with unique cultural, political, spiritual, and social worldviews, speaking over 4000 languages.

Box 20.1 Case study: Margaret

Margaret, 72, is from a small Indigenous community in northern Canada, accessible only by air. Her primary language is Cree, but she is also fluent in English due to her early educational experiences in the Canadian Indian Residential School System. Margaret comes from a large extended family who all live in the community. She is the primary caregiver to three of her granddaughters, who have lived with her since they were young. Margaret follows a traditional way of life and can be normally found on the land, picking medicines, harvesting berries, and fishing and hunting. She is a well-respected Elder and Knowledge Carrier who shares her knowledge of ceremonies and medicines with her community. Margaret was diagnosed with diabetes at age 37. She uses both insulin and traditional medicine in the treatment of her disease. A physician who comes to Margaret's community once a month recently met with her to review her prognosis. He explained to Margaret that her kidneys are failing and that her life will be shortened without dialysis. As dialysis is not available in her community, she would need to move to the nearest urban centre for treatment. Her community has agreed to organize a place for Margaret to stay in the city, but she would be living on her own. As community funding is scarce, returning home for periods of time will not be an option.

Indigenous peoples worldwide are among the most marginalized populations and suffer from higher rates of infant and child mortality, maternal morbidity and mortality, chronic illness and infectious disease, and lower life expectancy than their non-Indigenous counterparts (Gracey and King, 2009; United Nations, 2016). Indigenous peoples face similar experiences with colonization, loss of ancestral land, and structural violence, which are prominent factors contributing to poor health (Valeggia and Snodgrass, 2015; Browne et al., 2016). Overall, Indigenous peoples' access to equitable healthcare continues to be one of the most challenging and complex areas to address globally (United Nations, 2016). By design, Westernized health systems and services often fail to address these structural and social inequities as part of healthcare delivery (Browne et al., 2016). These factors may increase the overall burden of disease that needs to be addressed as EOL approaches.

In Canada where Margaret lives, over 150 years of settler-colonialism, national policies, and legislation including the Indian Act, the reserve (land) system, the Indian Residential School system, and the child welfare system were designed to assimilate Indigenous peoples into Euro-Canadian culture, resulting in inter-generational trauma, struggles with poverty, violence, addictions, suicide, and poor health outcomes. The planning, design, and imposition of Western medicine on Indigenous peoples in Canada further reinforced colonialism by invalidating effective Indigenous knowledges, practices, and caregiving models and fostering deeply internalized feelings of oppression. Purposeful disregard of Indigenous healers, and the dependence on professional hierarchy, has exerted control over Indigenous people (Hudson-Rodd, 1998). Furthermore, racial segregation has resulted in Western health systems, effectively devaluing Indigenous health. Currently, Indigenous people receive less care than other citizens and at a lower cost, as evidenced in current funding allocations (Gunn, 2016).

With respect to Indigenous peoples' needs at EOL, national groups in Canada state that current healthcare delivery models are not meeting Indigenous people's healthcare needs (Assembly of First Nations, 2016). In addition, current barriers and challenges to EOL care for Indigenous peoples include a lack of healthcare providers and culturally safe education and programmes (Hampton et al., 2010; Fruch et al., 2016; Cajax et al., 2018; Kelley et al., 2018; Prince et al., 2019). Existing palliative care services are often not culturally reflective of Indigenous communities' values and beliefs related to dying, death, grief, and bereavement and do not reflect the social and cultural aspects of caregiving within Indigenous communities.

Indigenous communities need to reclaim and revitalize Indigenous knowledges and healthy caregiving networks and mobilize local capacities through community-based and community-led processes and initiatives to improve care and health outcomes. As the critical issue for Indigenous peoples' poor health is a direct result of settler-colonialism, it is imperative to address and challenge these structural systems (Reading and Wein, 2009; Reading, 2018). Racist ideologies and discourse are often entrenched within current healthcare systems with little understanding of colonization's continued harmful role on Indigenous peoples' health (Browne et al., 2016). The ongoing impacts of colonization continue to have a deeply internalized, disempowering effect on Indigenous community members' confidence to provide care and healing to one another, as well as in their ability to engage with their traditional knowledge and ways of healing (Decourtney et al., 2003; Macdonald and Steenbeek, 2015).

As a result, Indigenous scholars state that decolonization is needed to contend with these issues and re-empower Indigenous communities (Simpson, 2008; Tuck and Yang, 2012; Coulthard, 2014).

Towards equity-oriented approaches to palliative care

Indigenous peoples must lead the way forward in developing approaches to caring for people at the EOL to achieve equitable and culturally safer care (DeCourtney et al., 2003; McGrath, 2007; Fruch et al., 2016; Kelley et al., 2018; Nadin et al., 2018). Indigenous communities are now starting to reclaim their cultural and community-based knowledge about EOL (Hampton et al., 2010; Duggleby et al., 2015; Fruch et al., 2016; Anderson and Woticky, 2018; Kelley et al., 2018). This also helps deconstruct colonial ideologies. Simpson stresses that 'Indigenous Knowledge is critical for resurgence', and that through Indigenous knowledge we can begin to 'combat colonialism, decolonize, and re-Indigenize' (Simpson, 2008, p. 75).

Through community-based initiatives, Indigenous communities are developing caregiving models and practices based on individual, family, and community worldviews (DeCourtney et al., 2003; Fruch et al., 2016; Hordyk et al., 2017; Kelley et al., 2018; Nadin et al., 2018). In Canada, a PHPC approach was used by the 'Improving EOL Care in First Nations Communities' project (Kelley et al., 2018). This project was successful in developing local community-based programmes and teams to care for people at the EOL in four First Nations communities, as well as creating a practical workbook of research-informed strategies for developing similar programmes in other First Nations communities. The project was based on community engagement and development, mobilized existing capacities within Indigenous communities, and focused on integrating care into existing social frameworks to overcomes cultural differences.

These models recognize that dying is a social event with caregiving provided by family and community. This concept of kinship is woven throughout the fabric of the culture. It is powerful to note that as Indigenous peoples face dying and EOL, family and community connections may be valued more than access to specialty services (Cajax et al., 2018). The involvement of family and community may also reflect respect for traditional protocols and values at the EOL (DeCourtney et al., 2003; McGrath, 2007).

Such initiatives must be strengthened by accepting Indigenous concepts of health and well-being and support given to Indigenous health systems as strategies to increase access and coverage of healthcare (United Nations, 2016). Over a decade ago, the United Nations declared that the structural systems and policies imposed through colonization need to be challenged through what it called a 'full recognition and exercise of Indigenous peoples' collective rights to communal assets and self-determination' (United Nations, 2009, p. 159). This includes Indigenous peoples 'right to be actively involved in developing and determining their health programmes; their right to traditional medicines, maintain their health practices, and the equal right to the enjoyment of the highest attainable standard of physical and mental health' (United Nations, 2016, p. v). It is understood that this includes EOL care. At this juncture, healthcare systems, organizations, and providers must now be willing to challenge their own power structures and their cultural identities to address culturally safer care for Indigenous peoples at EOL.

Box 20.2 Case study: Margaret, continued

Margaret remembers when she was forced to leave her community to attend the Indian Residential School. Now at this vulnerable time in her life, she feels as though she is being forced to leave her community once again, this time for healthcare. Margaret has decided not to pursue dialysis. She has decided to stay at home, surrounded by her family, community, culture, and language. Her relationship and connection to the land are extremely important to her. It is what she values most in her life. Her family and community support her decision and have begun to rally local services to support Margaret.

Programmes and services designed to support Indigenous peoples at the EOL, grounded in Westernized knowledge, will never be truly 'safe' for Indigenous peoples. Unless healthcare systems are completely dismantled and rebuilt by Indigenous peoples, the term culturally *safer* care may be more appropriate as it shows that there has been some effort by the system to recognize and challenge the structural processes that maintain the colonial state of inequities (Elder A. McLeod, personal communication, 20 November 2019). Through the lens of trauma-informed care, systems and organizations can begin to recognize and challenge the widespread impact of colonization and the consequent harm and trauma that ensued, impacting EOL care and creating culturally safer care for people impacted by this type of structural violence. Margaret's case study continues in Box 20.2.

LGBTQTS+ communities

See Box 20.3 for an illustrative case study.

Setting the context

Over the past few decades, the social climate regarding LGBTQTS+ people has become increasingly positive and accepting, especially

Box 20.3 Case study: Colin and Michael

Colin and Michael were married 10 years ago, a day Colin remembers with much fondness. He describes it as a celebration most people will not forget. Unlike his husband Michael, who was 'out and proud' for most of his life and a vocal advocate during the HIV/AIDS epidemic, Colin, now 75, has only openly acknowledged being gay for the last 20 years. Before that, Colin was married to a woman for many years and had two children, now adults. It was a health scare with cancer that changed Colin's perspective, propelling him to come out and live openly as a gay man. Through Michael, Colin has been welcomed into a new community where he feels connected and active. He has even joined a gay men's choir! It has helped ease the hurt and isolation that resulted when he first came out, as he lost many friends and family relationships as a result of doing so. Unfortunately, Colin learned recently that his cancer has recurred and is now advanced. There will be no further treatment. Michael's own health challenges make it unlikely that Colin can be cared for at home through to the time of his death. He is frightened about dying but even more worried about how the local hospice will accept him at the EOL. He has had negative healthcare experiences in his own town since coming out. Michael is angry, having worked hard to advocate for LGBTQTS+ rights, that the man he loves faces these very real worries at the EOL.

in Western societies. There are various terms used to refer to this community around the world and within countries. The term LGBTQTS+ has been chosen for this chapter. Despite positive movement, health and social inequalities between LGBTQTS+ and non-LGBTQTS+ individuals are still present (Fredriksen-Goldsen et al., 2013, 2014). These inequities are particularly relevant for older LGBTQTS+ adults, many of whom have lived most of their lives in a climate where there was much less acceptance of LGBTQTS+ persons. Ramifications of these negative experiences are very much present around the world and still visible decades later. One example relates to Canada's Criminal Code prior to 1969. At that time, homosexual acts were criminalized, which resulted in many older LGBTQTS+ people encountering social and legal ramifications that threatened their personal safety (Brotman et al., 2003). Internationally, homosexuality was categorized as a sociopathic personality disorder in the *Diagnostic and Statistical Manual of Mental Disorders* (Silverstein, 2009) until 1973. Many older LGBTQTS+ adults have been in work situations where the goal was to purge LGBTQTS+ people from employment (Knegt, 2018) or community situations such as conversion therapy where the attempt was to force them into heterosexual identities (Drescher et al., 2016).

The LGBTQTS+ communities have specific health issues as compared to cisgender heteronormative populations. Some of these issues are linked to negative societal attitudes to the LGBTQTS+ communities, which has meant that they are less likely to access healthcare (Fredriksen-Goldsen et al., 2010, 2014). Several countries, including Canada and the US, have data revealing that the LGBTQTS+ populations are underserved with regard to healthcare needs, including at the EOL. One of the main barriers to healthcare access results from these traumatic experiences and/or the expectation of discriminatory and harmful treatment from a healthcare system that has not served them well in the past (Sabin et al., 2015). These barriers can prevent people from disclosing their sexual orientation and/or gender identity to their healthcare providers, despite the fact that this information can help their providers identify health risks (Gardner et al., 2014; Putney et al., 2018). Minority stress theorists describe that the added stressors of discrimination, internalized heterosexism, and concealment of identity that LGBTQTS+ individuals experience during health encounters negatively impact their overall psychological well-being (Boulé et al., 2020). There appears to be a correlation between concealment and internalized heterosexism that results in this psychological distress (Hoy-Ellis and Fredriksen-Goldsen, 2016). A sense of not 'fitting in' and feeling unable to be oneself based on past stigmatization creates a heightened fearful awareness of the possibility of being rejected by others (Meyer, 2003; Fabbre and Gaveras, 2020). Consequently, LGBTQTS+ communities experience social exclusion and health disparities directly related to their sexual orientation and gender identity, which, when intersected with other social locations, exposes multiple forms of oppression (Fredriksen-Goldsen et al., 2014; Boulé et al., 2020).

In addition to the array of worries and fears that people may have towards EOL, the lived experience of LGBTQTS+ people, as described previously, creates additional burdens that affect their palliative care needs and contributes to their structural vulnerability. Contemporary research has highlighted that a host of negative emotions that older LGBTQTS+ adults may experience as they near EOL include disenfranchisement, isolation, and anxieties of being discriminated against due to sexuality (Brotman et al., 2007; Kimmel, 2014; Arthur, 2015). Many LGBTQTS+ older persons enter their later years of life without a traditional biological family system who might be accessed to assist with care or support with preparing for EOL (de Vries and Gutman, 2016). One outcome of this is that many LGBTQTS+ individuals will prefer or request the presence and inclusion of non-biological social support as they near EOL, compared to heterosexuals (MetLife Mature Market Institute and Lesbian and Gay Aging Issues Network of the American Society on Aging, 2010). Furthermore, members of LGBTQTS+ communities may have less access to traditional forms of informal caregiving and have higher needs for institutional care than heterosexual and gender-conforming older persons (de Vries and Gutman, 2016). LGBTQTS+ individuals are also more likely to identify or choose a close friend as their legal EOL decision maker versus a biological family member (Arthur, 2015).

Place of death has also been identified as a major concern and fear for older LGBTQTS+ adults, especially when discussing the care they might receive in institutionalized settings such as long-term care (Witten, 2014). Given reports about harassment and discrimination from healthcare providers or residents of long-term care homes that can be connected to sexual orientation or gender identity, place of death is a major concern and fear of older LGBTQTS+ adults and results in fewer LGBTQTS+ individuals accessing long-term care facilities due to this fear of mistreatment and harm (Arthur, 2015; Brotman et al., 2007). These experiences and fears may result in inequitable access to palliative and EOL care services, as the existing services are not aligned with LGBTQTS+ individuals' desire to have a safe, meaningful, and autonomous experience at the end of their lives. A research-based report from Alzheimer's Australia (2014) reveals that some transgendered older adults would rather take their own lives than risk entering long-term care (Barret et al., 2015). As a result, researchers such as de Vries and Gutman (2016) have argued that the need for preparation for the EOL is greater in the LGBTQTS+ communities. The structural vulnerabilities that impact LGBTQTS+ peoples at EOL include past and current traumas, as well as personal and institutional violence.

Towards equity-oriented approaches to palliative care

A PHPC approach requires cultivating spaces that promote cultural humility and safety in LGBTQTS+ ageing care. The current literature on ageing well and wellness at EOL for LGBTQTS+ people highlights the need for increased education for service providers related to LGBTQTS+ cultural competency, with the goal of reducing heteronormativity within health and social care systems (Aldredge and Conlon, 2012; Arthur, 2015; Griebling, 2016; Wilson et al., 2018). Increased education opportunities concentrating on increasing culturally safe care in this area have resulted in more positive care experiences for both the care provider and patient. Research by Porter and Krinsky (2014) indicates that such education can increase the levels of comfort a service provider feels when treating or providing care to an individual who is LGBTQTS+ , which is a step towards creating a safer environment in which to meet their health and social care needs. Additionally, Wilson and colleagues (2018) support the need for these educational initiatives to be widely promoted so that LGBTQTS+ individuals know that this education is occurring and ideally may witness some of the improvements within systems that have historically been oppressive towards them.

It is important to utilize a lens of trauma- and violence-informed care when seeking to understand the past healthcare-related experiences of LGBTQTS+ people, and to give expression to their hopes and fears when constructing or offering approaches to EOL care for these citizens. Given our current literature, which speaks to these citizens' true fear of lack of autonomy, fears of dying alone, in pain, in a location that does not recognize LGBTQTS+ rights and only focuses on heteronormative health and social support, it is essential that healthcare providers recognize that sexual orientation and gender identity are key determinants of health (de Vries and Gutman, 2016). This recognition is particularly significant in relationship to discrimination and social inclusion. To achieve this, Wilson and colleagues strongly recommend that the lived experiences of people who identify as LGBTQTS+ are included in educational offerings. This inclusion of lived experiences can be accomplished through in-person participation but also through the use of knowledge mobilization tools such as digital stories. The inclusion of real stories will work towards reducing stigma and discrimination (Wilson et al., 2018).

Older LGBTQTS+ adults possess unique needs and expectations as they age and move towards the EOL. To ensure equitable care and positive experiences throughout the ageing continuum, there needs to be acknowledgement of intersectionality and varying social locations (Wilson et al., 2018). Research conducted by Wilson and colleagues (2018) found that fears around staying out of the closet and around institutionalization, coupled with the need for different social support networks, play a salient role in some of the challenges older LGBTQTS+ adults face in accessing care that meets their needs. Recent work by Fredriksen-Goldsen and colleagues (2018) reveals that confirmation of identity positively impacts mental health status and experiences of victimization impact the openness of individuals. From a practical perspective, a study by Wilson and colleagues (2018) demonstrated the seemingly simple act of including symbols, such as a rainbow flag, can be a powerful move towards identifying an LGBTQTS+ friendly organization and creating the much needed inclusive, safer space.

Palliative care programmes, services, and initiatives need to recognize and promote inclusion at EOL to begin to attend to the specific needs of LGBTQTS+ individuals. These groups need to know that there will be an inclusive health and social care system accessible to them that will respond to their unique needs and fears and facilitate good EOL care in a safe and equitable manner. Thus, a PHPC approach for LGBTQTS+ people at the EOL actively facilitates an increase in cultural safety and provision of trauma-informed care. There is a need for PHPC to facilitate an increase in structural competency by creating safe spaces for and building rapport with LGBTQTS+ individuals, based on understanding their structural vulnerability. It is clear, many LGBTQTS+ people do not want to have to return to the closet at the end of their lives. PHPC must have a key role in promoting opportunities for social connectedness, inclusive, safe spaces, and a true sense of community at the EOL. Colin and Michael's case study continues in Box 20.4.

Box 20.4 Case study: Colin and Michael, continued

Colin and Michael went to visit their local hospice during an open day. They found a rainbow flag posted on many windows of the hospice. A hospice volunteer greeted them, and Michael directly asked if they had any LGBTQTS+ people in their care. The volunteer shared that members of the LGBTQTS+ community were hosting an upcoming death cafe at the hospice. She also provided them with some information about advance care planning and some educational materials specifically designed to address some of the unique needs of LGBTQTS+ people at the EOL. While not alleviating all of their fears by any means, both Colin and Michael felt this interaction was surprisingly pleasant and a good starting point for them. They decided to add this local hospice to their list of options to consider when Colin's health deteriorated.

People experiencing homelessness

See Box 20.5 for an illustrative case study.

Setting the context

Homelessness is described as a 'situation of an individual, family or community without stable, safe, permanent, appropriate housing, or the immediate prospect, means and ability of acquiring it' (Gaetz et al., 2012). Whereas 'the homeless' are often pictured as those relatively few, visibly homeless people (usually men) asleep on flattened cardboard in alleyways or hidden from view in emergency shelters, homelessness is defined along a continuum from those sleeping rough and completely unsheltered to those who are emergency sheltered (i.e. people staying in overnight shelters, and shelters for those experiencing family violence), provisionally sheltered (i.e. people whose accommodation is temporary), and at risk of homelessness (i.e. those who are not homeless but whose current economic situation or housing instability would put them at risk) (Gaetz et al., 2012).

Box 20.5 Case study: Charlie

Charlie, 46, wound up in hospital after his medical issues, including liver cancer and chronic obstructive pulmonary disease, became too much for his housing provider to handle. He was transferred to a transitional care unit for months and then was discharged due to drinking and aggressive verbal behaviour. A case management team arranged for Charlie to live in a motel, but after the owners raised the rent, he moved into a homeless shelter, considered a temporary arrangement. When his health declined further, Charlie was finally moved into supported housing but was unable to access community healthcare services 'at home' because of providers' fears of the housing complex being unsafe. When he became more short of breath and in pain, his housing provider called the ambulance and Charlie was admitted to hospital. He continued to drink heavily while in the hospital, which made hospital staff uncomfortable. Security guards were frequently called to remove his visitors, his 'chosen family', from the hospital because of concerns for safety. Most were banned from re-entry. In the last 2 years of his life, Charlie had moved five times and spent more than half a year in hospital. Charlie died alone in hospital without having the opportunity to say goodbye to his chosen family. For unclear reasons, his belongings were thrown in the garbage and his body was cremated, despite his expressed wish to his chosen family that he wanted to be buried and have a celebration of life.

People who experience homelessness have higher rates of disease and poorer health status compared to a more privileged, higher-income, and securely housed population (Guirguis-Younger, 2014; Hwang and Burns, 2014). They have more ageing-related conditions than those who are decades older (Brown et al., 2016). They also have disproportionately high rates of advancing chronic illness across the spectrum of causes including cardiovascular, kidney, and lung disease, many cancers, HIV/AIDS, and hepatitis C (Guirguis-Younger et al., 2014). These disparities are often coupled with high rates of serious and debilitating mental illness and/or substance use disorders, placing people at even greater risk of poor health outcomes and death (Hwang and Burns, 2014).

People who experience homelessness are a population that should be given consideration within the context of palliative care. They still face significant challenges in accessing care, including at the EOL. While some receive care and die in hospice and palliative care settings, homeless people are much more likely to die in hospital or alone, on the street and in vehicles, or in shelters or transitional housing (McNeil et al., 2012a; Stajduhar et al., 2019). Moreover, stigmatization and discrimination often dissuade homeless people from accessing health services, including palliative care (McNeil, Guirguis-Younger, et al., 2012; Shulman et al., 2018; Stajduhar et al., 2020b). Policies and regulations that are customary in most institutions (e.g. substance use policies, visitor policies that do not support the involvement of 'street family') worsen the effect of the myriad barriers that people who are homeless face (Giesbrecht et al., 2018; Stajduhar et al., 2020a). These issues are compounded by discrimination from healthcare professionals on the grounds of HIV or hepatitis C status, racial background, substance use, and mental illness (Song et al., 2008; Donald and Stajduhar, 2019). Research with marginalized and vulnerable populations shows that they distrust health professionals, are fearful that abstinence from drugs and alcohol will be a condition of accessing care, and fear that requests for pain relief will be viewed as drug-seeking (Hudson et al., 2016); access barriers also occur because their situations necessitate prioritizing other basic needs over their health such as finding food or shelter (Stajduhar et al., 2019). The assumptions that palliative care is based on the presence of safe and secure housing, family supports, and income for ancillary costs associated with dying do not apply to this population (Stajduhar, 2019).

Homelessness affects diverse populations. While highly heterogeneous in terms of age, gender, sexuality, and ethno-racial background, across the Global North, homelessness is on the rise (Cohen et al., 1989; Crane et al., 2005; Culhane et al., 2013). Homelessness is caused by a complex and interrelated set of structural factors, systems failures, and personal and relational circumstances. A lack of adequate income, access to affordable housing, and the unavailability of subsidized housing have all contributed to homelessness, as have neoliberal policies that emphasize a reduced role of the state in providing services and protection for citizens, and that have failed to address the needs of people living in poverty (Johnstone et al., 2017). Systems failures such as difficult transitions from child welfare, inadequate discharge planning for people leaving hospitals, and lack of supports for people with mental health and addictions or immigrants and refugees, contribute to people 'falling through the cracks', sometimes creating pathways into homelessness (Gaetz, 2014). Individual and relational factors such as traumatic events (e.g. house fire, job loss), early childhood adverse experiences, association with the criminal justice system, family violence and abuse, non-heterosexual sexual identity, and mental health and addictions challenges are all factors that are associated with homelessness (Shinn, 2007; Fazel et al., 2014). Understanding the range of ways in which homelessness can occur is critically important for palliative care providers and the larger community to avoid falling into the trap of assuming that a single individual is at fault or to blame for their circumstances.

Towards equity-oriented approaches to palliative care

As outlined at the beginning of this chapter, the concept of structural vulnerability directs attention to understanding how external forces (e.g. poverty, homelessness, criminalization, racialization, colonization, etc.) can alter a person's life and can also change itself as a response to a new environment (e.g. policy or healthcare reforms, economic restructuring). Although palliative care providers and organizations may not have the power to affect the multiple determinants of health and may not be able to erase the harm of inequities on people's health and quality of life, they can address health inequities directly during clinical encounters or programme design. People experiencing inequities such as homelessness need approaches to care that recognize structural and system barriers—what Metzl and Hansen (2013) term 'structural competency'—or an awareness of how social, political, and economic structures may influence interactions between clinicians and patients. This means envisioning and implementing structural interventions. An equity-oriented palliative approach to care is one way to consider how this might be accomplished.

Take, for example, the case of Charlie, the 46-year-old who moved multiple times before his life ended (Box 20.5). What supports and approaches could enable Charlie to stay at 'home' surrounded by the housing workers he had known and trusted as he came to the end of his life? In what ways might PHPC, or even conventional palliative care, work to support Charlie and his housing providers at EOL, so that he could remain connected to his chosen family? How might harm reduction approaches have been implemented to allow Charlie to live his final days of life in ways he desired? How might Charlie's community of care have been engaged to ensure his EOL wishes were respected? How might the trauma experienced by his chosen family have been avoided when they found out that his worldly belongings were discarded and his wish for a funeral unknown because nobody asked what was important to him? An equity-oriented approach could begin with addressing perceptions of risk and fears that healthcare providers had that would enable Charlie to be cared for in surroundings that were supportive of him. An equity-oriented approach could enable creative strategies to address access to care barriers, such as joint visits between housing providers in the community and home and palliative care providers, to facilitate relationship building in new settings. An equity-oriented approach could enable a chosen family to be consulted and be a part of Charlie's EOL experience. Equity-oriented advance care planning could ensure that Charlie's wishes were known and respected.

Additionally, palliative care organizations committed to PHPC approaches and development of compassionate communities could enlist the collectivist spirit embedded in those interventions to work alongside community groups supporting people who are homeless to mobilize strategies to better support their EOL experiences. Promising mobile palliative care services are emerging across many countries, including Canada, such as the Palliative Outreach Resource Team (PORT) in Victoria, British Columbia, the Allied Mobile Palliative Care Program (CAMMP) in Calgary, Alberta, and the Palliative Education and Care for the Homeless (PEACH) in Toronto, Ontario. Each has teams working together with academics (see https://www.equityinpalliativecare.com/) and alongside inner-city community-based organizations to support social care workers (i.e. housing, shelter, and support workers, including mental health, addictions, and harm reduction workers) and chosen family (e.g. street family). In other words, the palliative care community could work with those people who have the most contact with people who experience structural vulnerability. St Mungo's, a UK charity that provides accommodation and support to people experiencing homelessness, has worked to foster approaches to care that involve health, housing, social care, and drug and alcohol services to integrate palliative approaches into their care work, working alongside people who experience homelessness to ensure that people's wishes are respected and attended to at the EOL (https://www.mungos.org/). The goal is to integrate palliative approaches to care across health and social service sectors to reduce the silos in which many homeless people fall.

The approaches embedded within such innovations are consistent with the PHPC approach, engaging the strengths of the community to create broader awareness of death and dying and compassion for those who are vulnerable and at the EOL. Using strengths- and community-based, equity-oriented and harm reduction approaches, these initiatives strive to address the problems created and sustained through political, economic, and social systems of disadvantage. These initiatives concentrate on those issues that can be addressed to promote quality of life for those who are homeless, dying, and rendered vulnerable on the basis of the intersection of structural inequities (e.g. poverty, homelessness) and marginalizing experiences such as mental illness and substance use disorders.

Moving towards equity-oriented palliative care: a core feature of public health palliative care

One of the core tenets of a public health approach to palliative care is identity politics. That is, the focus on barriers that specific groups face in their struggle for equality. We began our chapter outlining contemporary concepts related to the care of people who experience structural vulnerability and focused our attention on three groups and the contexts which influence access to high-quality palliative care. While we have been encouraged by recent developments worldwide to better understand and work alongside communities of people experiencing structural vulnerability, the historical, good-willed, and well-intentioned tendency within palliative care to rescue people in the name of 'quality palliative care for all' needs to be tempered if we are to avoid retraumatization of communities of people who experience structural vulnerability. For those aiming for a public health approach to care across their societies and jurisdictions generally, and in working with structurally vulnerable people specifically, we would be wise to ask: Why do I want to work with this population and where is my motivation to do this coming from? Have I sought to understand, deeply, the contexts in which structurally vulnerable people live? If I am to engage in this work, how can I create the space for structurally vulnerable people to live—and die—in ways that they value? How can our palliative care services and programmes work alongside people who are structurally vulnerable and those who work with them closely to support care provision?

Diangelo (2018) reminds us that human bias is always at play because all humans have bias. Our thoughts and feelings, stereotypes, and generalizations based on little experience can be projected onto everyone in a group. This is a kind of prejudice and prejudgement of a person based on the social groups to which they belong (Diangelo, 2018). Discrimination is an action based on that prejudice. To that end, when providing palliative care to a person experiencing structural vulnerability, our best way forward may well be to first question our own unconscious bias, our own socialization, and how it has affected our own views of people—for example, those who are Indigenous, LGBTQTS+, or homeless. Palliative care providers would best be advised to explore what Diangelo coined the 'ubiquitous socializing power' of the dominant culture (Diangelo, 2018, p. 129). While none of us working in healthcare or palliative care might have chosen this socialization, we are, nonetheless, responsible for our role in it. To say we treat everyone the same in our palliative care services, programmes, and EOL initiatives reveals a lack of understanding of this socialization. Social systems and socialization are embedded in our cultures and our institutions. Oppression from our very well-intended services, programmes, and initiatives can result because a person or a group lacks social or institutional power to transform the prejudice and discrimination they experience, such as the heterosexism issues outlined in the section around LGBTQTS+ communities. Fortunately, all systems of oppression are adaptive and able to adjust. The challenge for PHPC is to not fall into the trap of what Diangelo calls 'small adaptations', which may serve only to reassure a dominant culture that their intent and overt acknowledgements are sufficient, whereas the roots of oppression remain deep (Diangelo, 2018). In addition, while we may have been socialized to believe that people who experience structural vulnerability 'matter', our actions often reveal much more of a charity focus than a focus on addressing the underlying structural and systemic issues involved that could create the conditions in which those who are marginalized and vulnerable could be fully engaged in developing models of care that work for them. Ultimately, without insight into our motivations and drivers and our own unconscious biases and socializations, we risk developing charitable models that are self-serving and can be retraumatizing instead of working *alongside* people to foster the best palliative care possible for people and their chosen family.

The very genesis of palliative care was founded on what we contemporarily describe as the 'structural and social determinants of health', and PHPC is an intentional focus back on that social side. To meet those intentions, however, PHPC approaches must tend to the systemic and structural issues that lead to structural vulnerability in the first place. Are our programmes, initiatives, and services really investing time and talent into addressing these inequities? If we believe that people have their own inherent personal and community agency and wisdom, are we truly fostering ally-ship with them for their palliative care and EOL needs? Are we really prepared to challenge power structures and our own biases, assumptions, and prejudices that may contribute to a lower quality of healthcare for some people? How can we engage in mutual empowerment and respectful partnership building with the people that we serve? When considering a public health approach, mobilizing the specific communities' experiences, wisdom, and care models is essential to serving these populations at the EOL. Kreztmann and McKnight (1996) described such mobilization in their articulation of asset-based community development, a process that first and foremost views people (including those who experience structural vulnerability) as fully capable of informing and engaging in solutions to resolve some of the key struggles experienced by marginalized people at the EOL (Russell, 2011; Klee et al., 2014).

If PHPC is to be the 'way forward' or perhaps more aptly, our 'great remembering', this will need to include a commitment to equity-oriented approaches to care. In this chapter, we provided three examples of populations or communities of people who benefit greatly when key dimensions of equity-oriented approaches to care are considered. These three groups are by no means the only ones that face inequities and disparities; they are examples of the central struggles that people who are structurally vulnerable face on a daily basis in their efforts to obtain quality care at the EOL. If PHPC is to embrace what it means to care for our own, it is essential that consideration of people who experience structural vulnerability is included in all of their diversity.

Resources

Indigenous resources

https://eolfn.lakeheadu.ca/
https://livingmyculture.ca/culture/
http://www.aboriginalendoflifecare.com/index.html

LGBTQTS+ resources

http://www.sfu.ca/lgbteol.html
https://hospicefoundation.org/End-of-Life-Support-and-Resources/Coping-with-Terminal-Illness/How-to-Choose/LGBT-Resources
https://www.mariecurie.org.uk/professionals/palliative-care-knowledge-zone/equality-diversity/lgbt-end-life
https://clri-ltc.ca/lgbtq/
https://clri-ltc.ca/resource/crossing-the-rainbow-bridge/
https://jmla.pitt.edu/ojs/jmla/article/view/766

People experiencing homelessness resources

http://www.homelesspalliativecare.com/overview-and-faqs/
https://www.equityinpalliativecare.com
https://www.homelesshub.ca/

REFERENCES

Abel, J. and Kellehear, A. 2018. Palliative care: the new essentials. *Annals of Palliative Medicine*, 7, S3–S14.

Ahmed, N., Bestall, J., Ahmedzai, S., Payne, S., Clark, D., and Noble, B. 2004. Systematic review of the problems and issues accessing specialist palliative care by patients, carers and health and social professionals. *Palliative Medicine*, 18, 525–542.

Aldredge, P. A. and Conlon, A. 2012. Reflections: gay men and lesbians at end-of-life. *Journal of Social Work in End-of-Life & Palliative Care*, 8, 113–118.

Anderson, M. and Woticky, G. 2018. The end of life is an auspicious opportunity for healing: decolonizing death and dying for urban Indigenous people. *International Journal of International Journal of Indigenous Health*, 13, 48–60.

Arcaya, M. C., Arcaya, A. L., and Subramanian, S. V. 2015. Inequalities in health: definitions, concepts and theories. *Global Health Action*, 8, 27106.

Arthur, D. P. 2015. Social work practice with LGBT elders at end of life: developing practice evaluation and clinical skills through a cultural perspective. *Journal of Social Work in End-of-Life & Palliative Care*, 11, 178–201.

Assembly of First Nations. 2016. Study on the right to health and Indigenous peoples with a focus on children and youth. Submission of the Assembly of First Nations to the UN Expert Mechanism on the Rights of Indigenous Peoples. [Online] Available at: https://digitallibrary.un.org/record/848142?ln=en

Barrett, C., Crameri, P., Lambourne, S., Latham, J. R., and Whyte, C. 2015. Understanding the experiences and needs of lesbian, gay, bisexual and trans Australians living with dementia, and their partners. *Australasian Journal on Ageing*, 34, 34–38.

BC Provincial Mental Health and Substance Use Planning Council. 2013. Trauma-informed practice guide. [Online] Available at: https://bccewh.bc.ca/wp-content/uploads/2012/05/2013_TIP-Guide.pdf

Boulé, J., Wilson, K., Kortes-Miller, K., and Stinchcombe, A. 2020. 'We live in a wonderful country, Canada, but … ': perspectives from older LGBTQ Ontarians on visibility, connection, and power in care and community. *International Journal of Aging and Human Development*, 91, 235–252.

Brotman, S., Ryan, B., Collins, S., Chamberland, L., Cormier, R., Julien, D., et al. 2007. Coming out to care: caregivers of gay and lesbian seniors in Canada. *Gerontologist*, 47, 490–503.

Brotman, S., Ryan, B., and Cormier, R. 2003. The health and social service needs of gay and lesbian elders and their families in Canada. *Gerontologist*, 43, 192–202.

Browne, A., Varcoe, C., Lavoie, J., Smye, V., Wong, S. T., Krause, M., et al. 2016. Enhancing health care equity with Indigenous populations: evidence-based strategies from an ethnographic study. *BMC Health Services Research*, 16, 544.

Brown, R. T., Hemati, K., Riley, E. D., Lee, C. T., Ponath, C., Tieu, L., et al. 2016. Geriatric conditions in a population-based sample of older homeless adults. *Gerontologist*, 57, 757–766.

Cajax, C. S., Schill, K., and Janke, R. 2018. Priorities and challenges for a palliative approach to care for rural Indigenous populations: a scoping review. *Health and Social Care in the Community*, 26, e329–e336.

Cohen, C. I., Sokolovsky, J., Roth, E., Teresi, J., and Holmes, D. 1989. *Old Men of the Bowery: Strategies for Survival Among the Homeless*. New York: Guilford Press.

Coulthard, G. 2014. *Red Skin White Masks: Rejecting the Colonial Politics of Recognition*. Minneapolis, MN: University of Minnesota Press.

Crane, M. 1999. *Understanding Older Homeless People: Their Circumstances, Problems and Needs*. Buckingham: Open University Press.

Culhane, D. P., Metraux, S., Byrne, T., Stino, M., and Bainbridge, J. 2013. Aging trends in homeless populations. *Contexts*, 12, 66–68.

DeCourtney, C. A., Jones, K., Merriman, M. P., Heavener, N., and Branch, P. K. 2003. Establishing a culturally sensitive palliative care program in rural Alaska native American communities. *Journal of Palliative Medicine*, 6, 501–510.

de Vries, B. and Gutman, G. 2016. End-of-life preparations among LGBT older adults. *Generations*, 40, 46–48.

Diangelo, R. 2018. *White Fragility*. Boston, MA: Beacon Press.

Donald, E. and Stajduhar, K. 2019. A scoping review of palliative care for persons with severe persistent mental illness. *Palliative Supportive Care*, 19, 1–9.

Drescher, J., Schwartz, A., Casoy, F., McIntosh, C. A., Hurley, B., Ashley, K., et al. 2016. The growing regulation of conversion therapy. *Journal of Medical Regulation*, 102, 7–12.

Duggleby, W., Kuchera, S., MacLeod, R, Holyoke, P., Scott, T., Holtslander, L., et al. 2015. Indigenous people's experiences at the end of life. *Palliative Supportive Care*, 13, 1721–1733.

Fabbre, V. D. and Gaveras, E. 2020. The manifestation of multilevel stigma in the lived experiences of transgender and gender nonconforming older adults. *American Journal of Orthopsychiatry*, 90, 350–360.

Farag, A. and Buchanan, N. 2020. Trauma informed palliative care. Academic journal club, Division of Palliative Care, McMaster University, Canada.

Fazel, S., Geddes, J. R., and Kushel, M. 2014. The health of homeless people in high-income countries: descriptive epidemiology, health consequences, and clinical and policy recommendations. *Lancet*, 384, 1529–1540.

First Nations Health Authority. 2016. Creating a climate for change: cultural safety and humility in health services delivery for First Nations and Aboriginal peoples in British Columbia. [Online] Available at: https://www.fnha.ca/wellness/cultural-humility

Fredriksen-Goldsen, K. I., Jen, S., Bryan, A. E., and Goldsen, J. 2018. Cognitive impairment, Alzheimer's disease, and other dementias in the lives of lesbian, gay, bisexual and transgender (LGBT) older adults and their caregivers: needs and competencies. *Journal of Applied Gerontology*, 37, 545–569.

Fredriksen-Goldsen, K. I., Kim, H. J., Barkan, S. E., Muraco, A., and Hoy-Ellis, C. P. 2013. Health disparities among lesbian, gay, and bisexual older adults: results from a population-based study. *American Journal of Public Health*, 103, 1802–1809.

Fredriksen-Goldsen, K. I. and Muraco, A. 2010. Aging and sexual orientation: a 25-year review of the literature. *Research on Aging*, 32, 372–413.

Fredriksen-Goldsen, K. I., Simoni, J. M., Kim, H. J., Lehavot, K., Walters, K. L., Yang, J., et al. 2014. The health equity promotion model: reconceptualization of lesbian, gay, bisexual, and transgender (LGBT) health disparities. *American Journal of Orthopsychiatry*, 84, 653–663.

Fruch, V., Monture, L., Prince, H., and Kelley, M. L. 2016. Coming home to die: Six Nations of the Grand River Territory develops community-based palliative care. *International Journal of Indigenous Health Research*, 11, 50–74.

Gaetz, S. 2014. *Coming of Age: Reimagining the Response to Youth Homelessness in Canada*. Toronto: The Canadian Observatory on Homelessness Press. Available at: https://www.homelesshub.ca/comingofage

Gaetz, S., Barr, C., Friesen, A., Harris, B., Hill, C., Kovacs-Burns, K., et al. 2012. *Canadian Definition of Homelessness*. Toronto: Canadian Observatory on Homelessness Press. Available at: https://www.homelesshub.ca/sites/default/files/COHhomelessdefinition.pdf

Gardner, A. T., de Vries, B., and Mockus, D. S. 2014. Aging out in the desert: disclosure, acceptance, and service use among midlife and older lesbians and gay men. *Journal of Homosexuality*, 61, 129–144.

Giesbrecht, M., Stajduhar, K., Mollison, A., Pauly, B., Reimer-Kirkham, S., McNeil, R., et al. 2018. Hospitals, clinics, and palliative care units: place-based experiences of formal healthcare settings by people experiencing structural vulnerability at the end-of-life. *Health and Place*, 53, 43–51.

Gracey, M. and King, M. 2009. Indigenous health. Part 1. Determinants and disease patterns. *Lancet*, 374, 65–75.

Griebling, T. L. 2016. Sexuality and aging: a focus on lesbian, gay, bisexual, and transgender (LGBT) needs in palliative and end of life care. *Current Opinion in Supportive and Palliative Care*, 10, 95–101.

Guirguis-Younger, M., Hwang, S. W., and McNeil, R. 2014. *Homelessness & Health in Canada*. Ottawa: University of Ottawa Press.

Gunn, B. 2016. Ignored to death: systemic racism in the Canadian healthcare system. Submission to EMRIP the Study on Health. [Online] Available at: https://www.ohchr.org/Documents/Issues/IPeoples/EMRIP/Health/UniversityManitoba.pdf

Hampton, M., Baydala, A., Bourassa, C., McKay-McNabb, K., Placsko, C., Goodwill, K., et al. 2010. Completing the circle: elders speak about end-of-life care with Aboriginal families in Canada. *Journal of Palliative Care*, 26, 6–14.

Hankivsky, O. and Christoffersen, A. 2008. Intersectionality and the determinants of health: a Canadian perspective. *Critical Public Health*, 18, 271–283.

Hordyk, S. R., Macdonald, M. E., and Brassard, P. 2017. End-of-life care in Nunavik, Quebec: Inuit experiences, current realities, and ways forward. *Journal of Palliative Medicine*, 20, 647–655.

Hoy-Ellis, C. P. and Fredriksen-Goldsen, K. I. 2016. Lesbian, gay, & bisexual older adults: Linking internal minority stressors, chronic health conditions, and depression. *Aging & Mental Health*, 20, 1119–1130.

Hudson, B. F., Flemming, K., Shulman, C., and Candy, B. 2016. Challenges to access and provision of palliative care for people who are homeless: a systematic review of qualitative research. *BMC Palliative Care*, 15, 18.

Hudson-Rodd, N. 1998. Nineteenth century Canada: indigenous place of dis-ease. *Health & Place*, 4, 55–66.

Hwang, S. and Burns, T. 2014. Health interventions for people who are homeless. *Lancet*, 384, 1541–1547.

Johnstone, M., Lee., E., and Connelly, J. 2017. Understanding the meta-discourse driving homeless policies and programs in Toronto, Canada: the neoliberal management of social service delivery. *International Social Work*, 60, 1443–1456.

Kelley, M. L., Prince, H., Nadin, S., Brazil, K., Crow, M., Hanson, G., et al. 2018. Developing palliative care programs in Indigenous communities using participatory action research: a Canadian application of the public health approach to palliative care. *Annals of Palliative Medicine*, 7, S52–S72.

Kimmel, D. 2014. Lesbian, gay, bisexual, and transgender aging concerns. *Clinical Gerontologist*, 37, 49–63.

Klee, D., Mordey, M., Phuare, S., and Russell, C. 2014. Asset based community development-enriching the lives of older citizens. *Working with Older People*, 18, 111–119.

Knegt, P. 2018. The fruit machine: why every Canadian should learn about this country's 'gay purge.' *CBC News*. 30 May. [Online] Available at: https://www.cbc.ca/arts/the- fruit-machine-why-every-canadian-should-learn-about-this-country-s-gay-purge-1.4678718

Kreztmann, J. and McKnight, J.P. 1996. Asset-based community development. *National Civic Review*, 85, 23–29.

Krieger, N. 2014. Discrimination and health. *International Journal of Health Services*, 44, 643–710.

Levine, S., Varcoe, C., and Browne, A. J. 2021. "We went as a team closer to the truth": impacts of interprofessional education on trauma- and violence-informed care for staff in primary care settings. *Journal of Interprofessional Care*, 35, 46–54.

MacDonald, C. and Steenbeek, A. 2015. The impact of colonization and western assimilation on health and wellbeing of Canadian Aboriginal people. *International Journal of Regional and Local History*, 10, 32–46.

McGrath, P. 2007. Aboriginal cultural practices on caring for the deceased person: findings and recommendations. *International Journal of Palliative Nursing*, 13, 418–425.

McNamara, T., Wadell, C., and Colvin, M. 1994. The institutionalisation of the good death. *Social Science & Medicine*, 39, 1501–1508.

McNeil, R. and Guirguis-Younger, M. 2012. Illicit drug use as a challenge to the delivery of end-of-life care services to homeless persons: perceptions of and social services professionals. *Palliative Medicine*, 26, 350–359.

McNeil, R., Guirguis-Younger, M., and Dilley, L. B. 2012a. Recommendations for improving the end-of-life care system for homeless populations: a qualitative study of the views of Canadian health and social services professionals. *BMC Palliative Care*, 11, 14.

McNeil, R., Guirguis-Younger, M., Dilley, L. B., Aubry, T. D., Turnbull, J., and Hwang, S. W. 2012b. Harm reduction services as a point-of-entry to and source of end-of-life care and support for homeless and marginally housed persons who use alcohol and/or illicit drugs: a qualitative analysis. *BMC Public Health*, 12, 312.

McNeil, R., Kerr, T., Anderson, S., Maher, L., Keewatin, C., Milloy, M. J., et al. 2015. Negotiating structural vulnerability following regulatory changes to a provincial methadone program in Vancouver, Canada: a qualitative study. *Social Science & Medicine*, 133, 168–176.

MetLife Mature Market Institute and Lesbian and Gay Aging Issues Network of the American Society on Aging. 2006. *Out and Aging: The MetLife Study of Lesbian and Gay Baby Boomers*. Westport, CT: MetLife Mature Market Institute.

Metzl, J. M. and Hansen, H. 2013. Structural competency: theorizing a new medical engagement with stigma and inequality. *Social Science & Medicine*, 103, 126–133.

Meyer, L. H. 2003. Prejudice, social stress, and mental health in lesbian, gay and bisexual populations: conceptual issues and research evidence. *Psychological Bulletin*, 129, 674–697.

Nadin, S., Crow, M., Prince, H., and Kelley, M. L. 2018. Wiisokotaatiwin: development and evaluation of a community-based palliative care program in Naotkamegwanning First Nation. *Rural and Remote Health*, 18, 4317.

Papps, E. and Ramsden, I. 1996. Cultural safety in nursing: the New Zealand experience. *International Journal in Quality Health Care*, 8, 491–497.

Pauly, B. 2008. Harm reduction through a social justice lens. *International Journal of Drug Policy*, 19, 4–10.

Porter, K. E. and Krinsky, L. 2014. Do LGBT aging trainings effectuate positive change in mainstream elder service providers? *Journal of Homosexuality*, 61, 197–216.

Prince, H., Nadin, S., Crow, M., Maki, L., Monture, L., Smith, J., et al. 2019. "If you understand you cope better with it": the role of education in building palliative care capacity in four First Nations communities in Canada. *BMC Public Health*, 19, 768.

Putney, J. M., Keary, S., Hebert, N., Krinsky, L., and Halmo, R. 2018. "Fear runs deep:" the anticipated needs of LGBT older adults in long-term care. *Journal of Gerontological Social Work*, 61, 887–907.

Quesada, J., Hart, L. K., and Bourgois, P. 2011. Structural vulnerability and health: Latino migrant laborers in the United States. *Medical Anthropology*, 30, 339–362.

Reading, C. 2018. Structural determinants of Aboriginal peoples' health. In: Greenwood, M., de Leeux, S., and Lindsay, N. M. (eds.) *Determinants of Indigenous Peoples' Health in Canada: Beyond the Social*, pp. 3–18. Toronto: Canadian Scholars' Press.

Reading, C. L. and Wien, F. 2009. *Health Inequalities and Social Determinants of Aboriginal Peoples' Health*. Prince George: National Collaborating Centre for Aboriginal Health.

Reimer-Kirkham, S., Stajduhar, K., Pauly, B., Giesbrecht, M., Mollison, A., McNeil, R., et al. 2016. Death as a social justice issue: perspectives on equity informed palliative care. *Advances in Nursing Science*, 39, 293–307.

Russell, C. 2011. Pulling back from the edge: an asset-based approach to ageing well. *Working with Older People*, 15, 96–106.

Sabin, J. A., Riskind, R. G., and Nosek, B. A. 2015. Health care providers' implicit and explicit attitudes toward lesbian women and gay men. *American Journal of Public Health*, 105, 1831–1841.

Shinn, M. 2007. International homelessness: policy, socio-cultural, and individual perspectives. *Journal of Social Issues*, 63, 657–677.

Shulman, C., Hudson, B. F., Low, J., Hewett, N., Daley, J., Kennedy, P., et al. 2018. End-of-life care for homeless people: a qualitative analysis exploring the challenges to access and provision of palliative care. *Palliative Medicine*, 32, 36–45.

Silverstein, C. 2009. The implications of removing homosexuality from the DSM as a mental disorder. *Archives of Sexual Behaviour*, 38, 161–163.

Simpson, L. 2008. Our elder brothers: the lifeblood of resurgence. In: Simpson, L. (ed.) *Lighting the Eighth Fire*, pp. 73–88. Winnipeg: Arbeiter Ring Publishing.

Song, J., Wall, M. M., Ratner, E. R., Bartels, D., Ulystad, N., and Gelberg, L. 2008. Engaging homeless persons in end of life preparations. *Journal of General Internal Medicine*, 23, 2031–2045.

Stajduhar, K. I. 2019. Provocations on privilege in palliative are: are we meeting our core mandate? *Progress in Palliative Care*, 28, 89–93.

Stajduhar, K. I., Giesbrecht, M., Mollison, A., and d'Archangelo, M. 2020b. "Everybody in this community is at risk of dying": an ethnographic exploration on the potential of integrating a palliative approach to care among workers in inner city settings. *Palliative and Supportive Care*, 18, 670–675.

Stajduhar, K. I., Giesbrecht, M., Mollison, A., Dosani, N., and McNeil, R. 2020a. Caregiving at the margins: an ethnographic exploration of 'family' caregivers' experiences providing care for structurally vulnerable populations at the end-of-life. *Palliative Medicine*, 34, 946–953.

Stajduhar, K. I., Mollison, A., Giesbrecht, M., McNeil, R., Pauly, B., Reimer-Kirkham, S., et al. 2019. "Just too busy living in the moment and surviving": barriers to accessing health care for structurally vulnerable populations at end-of-life. *BMC Palliative Care*, 18, 11.

Trevalon, M. and Murray-García, J. 1998. Cultural humility versus cultural competence: a critical distinction in defining physician training outcomes in multicultural education. *Journal of Health Care for the Poor and Underserviced*, 9, 117–125.

Tuck, E. and Yang, K. W. 2012. Decolonization is not a metaphor. *Decolonization: Indigeneity, Education & Society*, 1, 1–40.

United Nations. 2009. State of the world's Indigenous peoples. Department of Economic and Social Affairs, United Nations. [Online] Available at: https://www.un-ilibrary.org/content/books/9789210548434

United Nations. 2016. State of the world's Indigenous peoples: Indigenous peoples' access to health services. Department of

Economic and Social Affairs, United Nations. [Online] Available at: https://doi.org/10.18356/7914b045-en
Valeggia, C. R. and Snodgrass, J. J. 2015. Health of Indigenous peoples. *Annual Review of Anthropology*, 44, 117–135.
Whitehead, M. 1992. The concepts and principles of equity and health. *International Journal of Health Services*, 22, 429–445.
Witten, T. M. 2014. It's not all darkness: robustness, resilience, and successful transgender aging. *LGBT Health*, 1, 24–33.
Wilson, K., Kortes-Miller, K., and Stinchcombe, A. 2018. Staying out of the closet: LGBT older adults' hopes and fears in considering end-of-life. *Canadian Journal on Aging/La Revue Canadienne Du Vieillissement*, 37, 22–31.
World Health Organization. 2021. Harm reduction. [Online] Available at: https://www.euro.who.int/en/health-topics/communicable-diseases/hivaids/policy/policy-guidance-for-areas-of-intervention/harm-reduction

21

Public health palliative care design and practice in low- and middle-income countries

Suresh Kumar and Jairam Kamala Ramakrishnan

Introduction

Palliative care is a recognized component of the right to the highest attainable standard of health, which is protected in article 12 of the United Nations International Covenant on Economic, Social and Cultural Rights, and in article 24 of the United Nations Convention on the Rights of the Child. Public health is often defined as a discipline focused on promoting and protecting health of people and communities spanning science and art. It is argued that public health is not only a professional practice or discipline but everybody's business as an act of a social being living in communities.

This chapter considers how palliative care is embedded within public health of the latter kind in contexts where material resources are limited, whether considered in terms of income poverty or deprivation indices. Palliative care is built on compassionate professional care and requires networks and relations of community supports (Lewis et al., 2014). At the outset, we make the argument that income poverty does not mean, and should not mean, poverty of community supports and relationships. However, income poverty may pose challenges to utilization of existing supports and relationships.

In addressing public health palliative care in resource-constrained settings, our approach is to first set out the context of action. This implies a sphere of action of a government or governing authority who is responsible for population health and has the means at its disposal for public health actions. These are typically geographically boundaried areas such as cities, regions, provinces, or countries. Addressing social determinants of health in such contexts is an essential public health approach and which requires monetary resources. However, there may be other non-monetary resources that may be available such as social capital which have a role in developing 'community-partnered' palliative care. Social capital is defined by the Organisation for Economic Co-operation and Development as 'networks together with shared norms, values and understandings that facilitate co-operation within or among groups' (2001, p 41). Social capital is a useful concept that helps in understanding how a community utilizes the inherent networks to achieve collective results. Although research into the relation between social capital and health has built up in the past decade (Choi et al., 2014), early indications are that social capital predicts better physical and mental health and probably has a protective role against mortality (Ehsan et al., 2019). There are indications that, specifically, community level trust and reciprocity may have a health impact (Choi et al., 2020). We will consider under the following two main sections an approach to designing and practising community-partnered palliative care in contexts facing material poverty.

- Palliative care as part of formal systems of care.
- Palliative care as essential compassionate care within communities.

Palliative care within formal systems of care

Within low- and middle-income countries (LMICs), the main barriers to providing palliative care within existing health and care systems include:

- *Structural and functional weaknesses of the health system*: problems with universal health coverage contribute to the burden of avoidable suffering due to delays in treatable or preventable health conditions. Thus, people who might have otherwise received curative care may end up with suffering in need of palliative care. Inadequate human resources capacity or skills as well as limited availability of medicines can also compound this avoidable suffering. Finally, quality monitoring and improvement systems are generally less developed in many LMICs and may limit adaptation of practice according to developing evidence.
- *Poor living conditions* which are more causally related to material poverty can contribute to increased health-related suffering through higher morbidity and poorer access to healthcare. These span domains of housing, education, employment, and

nutrition-related factors. In terms of social needs, LMICs have less robust social protection measures which can easily throw individuals and families into abject suffering. Many families who maintain basic sustenance often have a precarious existence, one illness away from abject poverty.

Palliative care as compassionate caring communities

Informal caring is the fundamental building block for health and social care in the community. This involves family, friends, or neighbours. Proximity of geography or proximity of kinship may be the spokes in the network. This informal care system is strengthened in numbers and capacity by connectedness and support of the individual or family in the community.

Existing systems of care: formal and informal

Worldwide, there are many patients going through illness and suffering who are cared for in their respective households without support or intervention from health or social care systems. In low-income settings, such patients and families often remain suffering at home except for occasional visits to a health facility when the need becomes extreme or unmanageable and/or the income makes access to care temporarily affordable. In individualistic communities in high-income settings this care function is devolved through statutory systems of social welfare. In collectivistic cultures such as the global South, informal social protection systems function to meet the need unmet by scarce formal welfare systems (Oware, 2020).

Informal care generally occurs in isolation rather than collectively whether in high-income or low-income settings. However collective action through patient (service user) and family support organizations has developed gradually in high-income settings in recent decades. Although by no means widespread in affluent settings, such movements are rare in low-income settings. Such organization of patient and families can be seen as joining hands to strengthen informal care and also hold health system and professionals as partners in care, even to challenge and hold them accountable in some instances.

Design and development of community participatory palliative care

More than four decades on from the Alma Ata declaration, the lofty ideals of 'requiring and promoting maximum community and individual self-reliance and participation in the planning, organization, operation and control of primary health care' remain a dream. Community engagement is highlighted as an essential component to achieve universal health coverage and seen as both a process and outcome. There are four approaches to community engagement:

> Level 1. *Community-oriented*: the community is *informed* and mobilized to participate in addressing immediate short-term concerns with strong external support.
>
> Level 2. *Community-based*: the community is *consulted and involved* to improve access to health services and programmes by locating interventions inside the community with some external support.
>
> Level 3. *Community-managed*: there is *collaboration* with leaders of the community to enable priority settings and decisions from the people themselves with or without external support of partners.
>
> Level 4. *Community-owned*: community assets are fully mobilized and the community is *empowered* to develop systems for self-governance, establish and set priorities, implement interventions and develop sustainable mechanisms for health promotion with partners and external support groups as part of a network. (World Health Organization, 2020, p. viii)

In this context, we use the term '*community-partnered palliative care*' to denote an important feature—participation in planning, organization, operation, and control of palliative care services—which places such care across levels 3 and 4 previously described above. We do not include services that fall into levels 1 and 2. Our focus is on the ownership of services by members in the community who are not purely healthcare staff. While representation of community members in organizational boards or decision-making bodies is a good start, until community members have a key role in decision-making rather than as token gesture, it is not truly community-partnered palliative care.

Unlike in high-income settings where the focus is on developing palliative care within the health system, there is a dual challenge facing LMICs. Firstly, a health system that is suboptimal in function and secondly, palliative care need which is largely unmet. While improving the health system remains an ongoing challenge that most LMICs grapple with, we argue that developing palliative care cannot and must not wait for health system to develop to the best standard feasible. Such an approach will consign millions of patients and families to unnecessary suffering, for whom such a development will come too late. We instead propose that care be built around what exists in different capacities in such communities; while development of the health system will be welcome and essential, at least those suffering now are able to experience some relief and improvement in their quality of life. Building upon and developing existing informal care systems in the community should be mindful of the existing formal systems of health and care such that compatibility with the evolving health system is assured.

Even in high-income countries, developing palliative care based primarily around existing health systems overlooks the essence of health-promoting palliative care (Kellehear, 1999). The voice of the person suffering gets diminished, their agency and their family's perspective get undermined by care seen through the prism of professional care. In addition, there are concerns over access to good palliative care being determined by systemic inequities in high-income countries. Thus, caution is needed in adopting developments in palliative care in high-income contexts without adequate contextual adaptation to LMICs settings. In addition, such adaptation also risks losing out on the inherent strengths and capacities that may be dormant in the LMICs settings and remaining paralysed in the process of trying to establish a hitherto alien model.

In order to develop community-partnered palliative care, there are two elements of care that needs to come together around the patient and family. These are the formal healthcare sector and the informal care system (Fig. 21.1).

System overview

Palliative care should be situated within the reality of complex living systems. Such a system will have many inter-related domains (e.g.

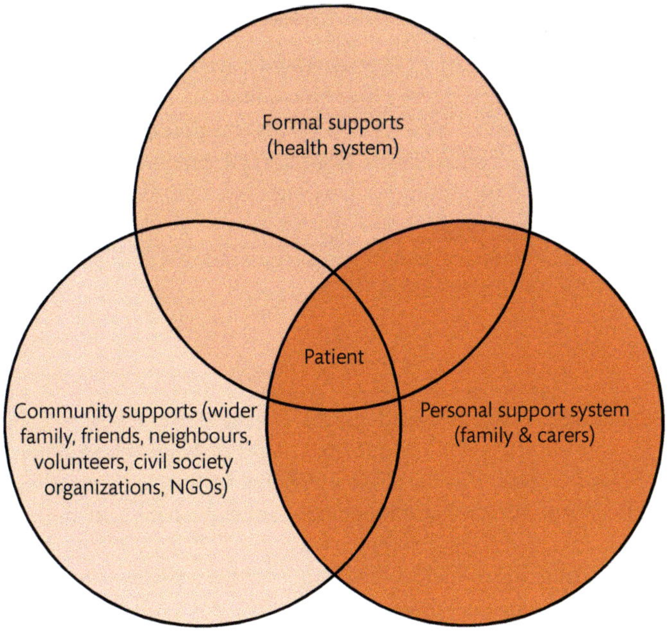

Fig. 21.1 Community-partnered palliative care.

across health, social services, education and employment, transport, finance, and business) spanning different ways of structuring activity (e.g. public, private, and third sectors).

Inputs into the system include the following actors:

- Patients and carers/family.
- Community members.
- Professionals.
- Volunteers.
- Governmental institutions and private businesses.
- Civil society organizations.

The following are some of the activities carried out by these actors:

- Seeking relief of symptoms, engaging with providers of care and support.
- Providing (physical, psychological, social, and spiritual) support and care for the patient.
- Providing information and guidance to patient and family.
- Psychological and social support for the carers.
- Organizing and managing activities.
- Funding.
- Developing policy.

The outputs of the system relevant to developing community-partnered palliative care are:

- Quality of life of patient in need of palliative care.
- Palliative care service delivery (amelioration of distress from symptoms and mitigation of negative impact on life).
- Defining care beyond the biomedical paradigm.
- Wider well-being of community (e.g. the New Economics Foundation's recommended measures).
- Community capability to address/managing care and support needs locally.

Details of system/environmental consideration

Geographical and infrastructure

- How does the terrain and natural environment impact on needs and challenges in meeting those needs?
- Transport and mobility (network of public transport etc.) in connecting people in need with the supports (care and support facilities as well as people providing care).
- Energy, water and sanitation, communication.

Sociodemographic factors

- Population distribution: age, urbanization, family systems (collectivist vs individualist structure).
- Education, literacy, unemployment, poverty levels.
- Disabilities, disadvantaged groups.
- Safety and security, legal protection.

Sociopolitical environment

- Healthcare as a political priority.
- Is there enough political leadership or consensus in identifying palliative care as a need?
- Social and cultural practices impact caring roles in society—individualistic and collectivist communities.
- Civil society organizations and participatory democracy.
- Advocacy organizations.

Health service provision

- Define the following aspects of the healthcare system (especially primary healthcare system):
  - Clinical service provision: coverage, access to preventive and curative treatments.
  - Public health measures (health of the population, preventive measures, sensitization, and education of public).
  - Healthcare administration and service management: including funding, insurance, and out-of-pocket expenditure.
  - Training and development of healthcare workers.
  - Regulation of healthcare practice and products (including medicines).
- Inter-relationship of private, public, and non-governmental organization (NGO) healthcare providers.
- Does the funding/financing of healthcare provide any leverage for cooperation?
- Which are the key players in healthcare?

For an individual in need of palliative care, what systems currently get involved to meet her needs and those of her family?

- Food and shelter/accommodation, caring for dependents.
- Medical or healthcare needs: including participation in decision-making.
- Well-being needs: social participation, recreation/stimulation, spiritual needs.
- Developmental needs: education, employment, etc.
- Religious systems.

There may be a range of different components which are involved (or not) in meeting these needs:

- Primary healthcare, hospitals, pharmacies, and complementary and allied health services including 'healers'.
- Social welfare system and other governmental agencies.
- NGOs and corporate social responsibilities.
- Workplaces, businesses.
- Educational institutions.

Geographical and infrastructure:

- Globalization affects health through changes in social stratification, differential exposure or vulnerability, health system characteristics, and differential consequences.

Sociodemographic factors:

- The key to improved health equity lies in optimizing urban settings for health. Urbanization can be a positive determinant of health in the appropriate circumstances.
- Employment: strengthening fair access to employment and the other dimensions of decent work can improve health inequities of workers and their families.
- Social exclusion leads to unequal access to resources, capabilities, and rights which leads to health inequalities.

Sociopolitical environment:

- Building governance, whereby all sectors take responsibility for reducing health inequities, is essential to achieve this goal. Intersectoral action—that is, effectively implementing integrated work between different sectors—is a key component of this process.
- The participation of communities and civil society groups in the *design* of public policies, in the *monitoring* of their implementation, and in their *evaluation* is essential to action on social determinants of health (Fig. 21.2).

Health service provision:

- Making health services more accessible, available, affordable, and higher quality can reduce health inequities.
- Improving health system performance requires continuous support and concerted efforts from several actors—including the international organizations, governments, civil society organizations, and academia.
- Participation of communities in service delivery is important for reducing health inequities.

Approach to interventions for strengthening community-partnered palliative care

An initial assessment should inform how the above-described components interface with the informal (families, neighbours) systems of care to meet the needs of the individual and family. The individuals or group initiating development activity need to be aware of their value systems and potential bias.

The strengths of each component and the challenges in participation (or potential obstruction) of each component should be evaluated. This will help in formulating proposals for change in the current system to incorporate palliative care. For example, an initiative could be started through an NGO or through a wider health system-based approach, but the impact and relationship to the wider system should be monitored through easily measurable and meaningful parameters.

Our approach to developing community-partnered palliative care aims to bring the professional aspects of care (healthcare workers) together with informal support systems in the community to enhance efficiency and effectiveness of the system. A community-based approach recognizes an individual in need of palliative care at the functional centre of the care process.

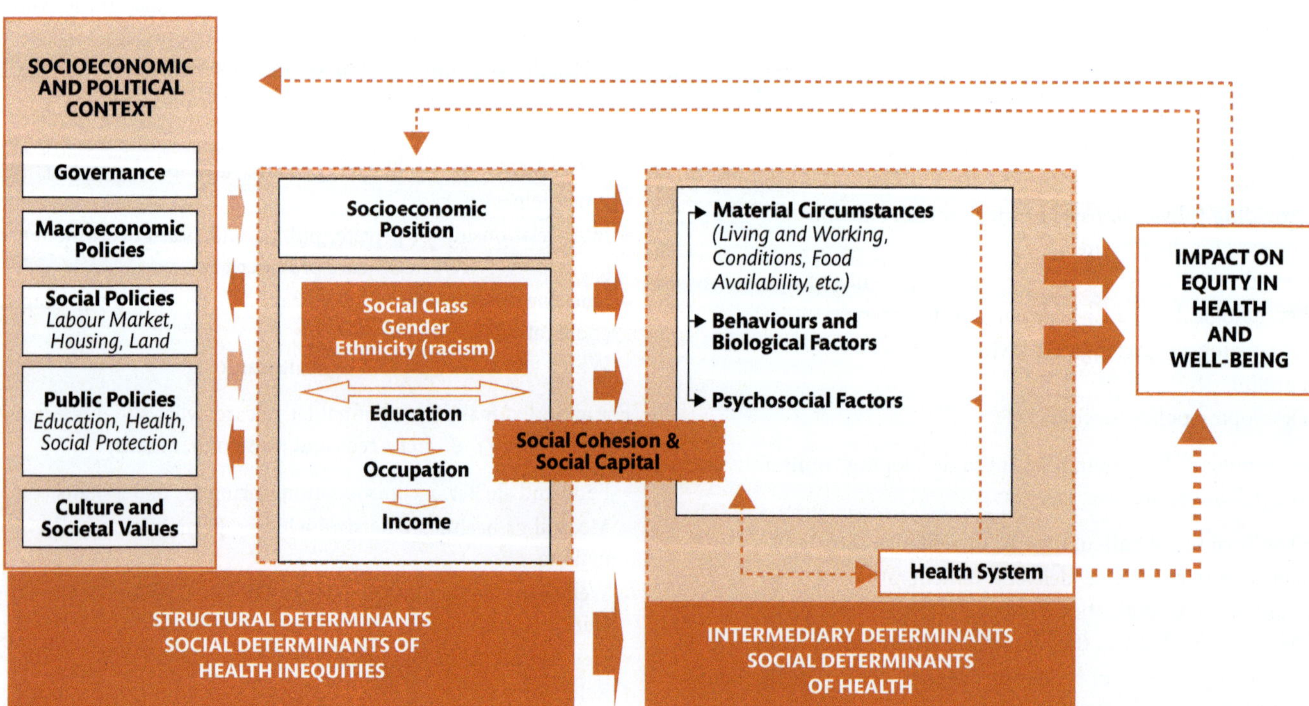

Fig. 21.2 Conceptual framework developed by Commission on Social Determinants of Health.

Reproduced with permission from Concern: A Conceptual Framework for Action on the Social Determinants of Health. Social Determinants of Health Discussion Paper 2. World Health Organization. Available at https://www.who.int/publications/i/item/9789241500852

A patient is naturally based at home or living place, supported by family, friends, and neighbours. Health systems and professionals should play a role in supporting this primary support system to reduce the patient's distress and suffering. The wider community has a role in supporting the patient's needs through social solidarity. In addition, the community should define and establish norms of suffering, death, and dying, not primarily by the healthcare or medical system.

A step-by-step approach to consider building palliative care in the community is elaborated here. It may be valuable to have mentoring support from existing projects.

1. *Making the case that coordinating responsibilities between medical facilities and the community leads to better health outcomes.* The partnership approach of community and healthcare professionals collaborating to provide care is an essential first step. This step can be broken down into the following components:
   1.1 *Establish a local core group*: there must be at least one person with dedicated time and commitment to take up the initiative. A local core group must have legitimacy in the community, and have organizational and technical competence. The local core group must assess the potential within the community for palliative care. Careful consideration must be given to evaluate the pros and cons of outsourcing the activities to any existing groups as against developing community-based palliative care. Pros and cons of allying with or potential partnerships with other organizations can be considered. Once the core group is well established, goals must be identified and a core committee formed to drive this. The core committee should have defined roles and job descriptions. A seed vision statement may be formulated to capture the commonalities.
   1.2 *Initiate a demonstration project*: once the core committee is in place, a demonstration project should be initiated. This early phase will benefit from mentorship from external experts with experience in setting up community-partnered palliative care. A demonstration project should coordinate medical palliative care and community care and show an impact on at least 25–30 patients if implemented, based on the guideline provided for setting up a demonstration (Box 21.1). If an external expert is involved, they need to engage at high intensity with the core committee at the beginning. This mentoring role is best continued 'on tap' typically for a duration for up to 2 years until the demonstration project is established. Proposed key performance indicators/success criteria may include number of patients seen,

Box 21.1 Guidelines to set up a demonstration project in community-partnered palliative care

Step 1

Identify the core components of palliative care project:

A. Management/coordination (useful to have representation from B and C).
B. Clinical professionals (includes a doctor and nurse who provide clinical service, but also involvement of sensitized professionals who will serve as sources of referrals from within health system).
C. Community leaders and volunteers.

While role A may be carried out by professionals or community leaders, it is key to recognize A, B, and C each as a core function in its own right.

Step 2

Identify tasks for each group including:

- Fundraising (source, locally relevant methods, and sustainability), liaising with existing health system (public/private/NGO service providers), scoping of type of clinical service to be provided (outpatient service, home care, or a mix of the two) and frequency (once a week, twice a week), and budget. Media and publicity engagement (A).
- Identify doctor and nurse (even if both not available, can start with one); organizing their training (A).
- Connect with support and supervision in palliative care practice especially in the early phase (B).
- Sensitize health system to the availability of services (B + A).
- Community engagement, developing a wider pool of volunteers, training of volunteers from different groups in the community (C + A).

Step 3

Set-up of clinical service:

- Referral pathway (how can people in need be referred to the new project?)—from within health system or directly from community.
- Space for clinical service (outpatient), office, and pharmacy.
- Medicines and equipment supply and storage.
- Transport, communication, and logistics for home care (home care may be a quick and easy win while awaiting or even in the absence of outpatient care).
- Licensing, regulations, stock keeping, and clinical records.
- Links with specialists (oncology/physician/surgeon/mental health) for specialist opinion/consultation if needed.

Set-up of social support network:

- To meet basic needs: food, clothes, and education material for children.
- Access to social support through volunteers and linking to available state welfare systems.
- Equip community volunteers for providing basic psychosocial care (this can start even in the absence of a core clinical service).

Sustainability:

- Fundraising: large-scale donations from key individuals/organizations versus small-scale donations from a wide base in the community (materials, functional support, or money).
- Clinical-community links: regular community meetings involving community leaders/volunteers and clinical team.

Step 4

- Further service development or adapting the model based on resources and needs.
- Ethical framework and transparency of decision-making.
- Evaluation and monitoring indicators of impact:
  - A system in place for feedback from patients and families to inform continuing quality improvement.
  - Number of patients and families supported; measures on quality of life in individual cases (easy to use and valid to setting outcome measures?).
  - Engagement with community and professionals (e.g. awareness, participation, and access to service rated by them).
  - Volunteer activity: number of community members participating in regular meetings, increase in number of volunteers, number of volunteers actively engaged in patient support, from community members/referring.
  - Social well-being measures (e.g. assessed at baseline and periodically among staff, volunteers, patients, and families).

numbers trained, volunteers active, community organizations involved, funding/financial sustainability, and/or participation from medical groups.

1.3 *Collaboration with stakeholder/policy makers/decision makers established*: at this stage, potential collaborators among policy makers, stakeholders, and decision makers must be identified. Communication is established with them to share available evidence from the demonstration project. A regular feedback loop between the core committee and policy makers should be established. This will serve as ground work for the main outcome in this step: a charter on the inclusion of palliative care in policy document or vision statement of the decision makers.

2. *Enabling the medical service provision as part of shared palliative care*: this step envisions equipping the healthcare professionals to provide palliative care through necessary training and accountability. The components may include:

2.1 *On-the-job training in palliative care is implemented for healthcare workers*: the core committee should identify healthcare workers for sensitization to palliative care. These healthcare workers are provided with a basic 3-day training course in palliative care. Manual or training modules used for training must be fit for context. If it is not developed in the local context, it must be adapted for the context in consultation with some of the identified healthcare workers who could be future trainers. A feedback system must be put in place to gather healthcare worker feedback and any patient-reported outcome measures from implementation. Healthcare workers are encouraged to collaborate as a peer group through social media or another platform.

2.2 *Funding identified and allocated for regular palliative care training programme*: training of professionals in palliative care is agreed as a priority by the core committee. The core committee determines funding required based on cost estimation of training of healthcare workers in palliative care. Funding commitment is made by the core committee for 2 years with a calendar of training.

2.3 *Mechanism for accountability set out in formal document between local group and government including coordination of palliative care between community and medical staff*: the core committee establishes links with government, academics, and professional stakeholders and shares good practice on development of palliative care, highlighting working in partnership. The expected outcome is a memorandum of understanding between the core group and government and a standard operating protocol that describes the governance structure, explaining the process and ways of working between healthcare system and the community volunteers. Roles and responsibilities of various stakeholders and medical professionals are defined and agreed. Clear roles and boundaries for volunteers are set out in the document. Relationships between various organizations must be documented and agreed. The process followed while delivering palliative care services in the region should be clearly articulated. Guidelines must be set for monitoring projects, evaluation of outcome, financial responsibility, administrative and legal issues, etc.

2.4 *Thirty per cent of medical and nursing schools integrate palliative care curriculum into their core syllabus*: a request is submitted to various stakeholders to include palliative care in the professional syllabus. Typically based on the request and a range of health education system factors, a body will be formed to evaluate the course content and syllabus. Course content will be then submitted for formal evaluation and upon approval will become part of the syllabus.

3. *Laying the foundation for community care provision as part of shared palliative care*: this is the most critical component in building community-partnered palliative care as it determines how much the community will partner with the healthcare system.

3.1 *Recruitment of priming group of community volunteers/caregivers*: the priming group of volunteers is identified by the core committee. Members of the core committee engage with identified groups in the community—from universities, religious or political groups, civil society organizations, etc. Palliative care sensitization is provided within such groups. The aim is to seek support through formation of a group constituted by members from these varied groups. At least 10–20 volunteers recruited from two or more social groups (age, gender, civil society organization, etc.) would be a reasonable number to aim for in the first instance. This component should not require fundraising and is a low-cost activity.

3.2 *Train the priming group of volunteers using a structured training manual*: the first group of community volunteers are trained (by an external trainer or a core committee member who is already trained). The training uses a structured volunteer training manual created in or adapted to the context. The training can be run in batches to allow those who miss sessions to catch up and complete training in follow-up batches. The desired outcome is that at least half the recruited priming group complete volunteer training. In this process, the core committee maintains a register with a list of volunteers who have completed training. Among the volunteers, those with potential to be trainers should be identified early on and nurtured. In addition, volunteers should also be identified with designated roles (focal person) in expanding the community component (e.g. fundraising, networking, linking with policy makers, other civil society organizations, and media).

3.3 *Develop a pool of trainers from the primed group*: training of trainers with structured protocol to continuously train batches of volunteers. Expert training facilitator trains identified volunteers to become the local trainers. This starts with discussion about the training manual, material and content for activities used in training, and participating as co-facilitator with the expert trainer in training. Following this, the trainer carries out training with supervision or support from the expert facilitator. The expected outcome is at least five local trainers who have conducted at least two training sessions independently for volunteers.

3.4 *Training for trainers and volunteers is funded and coordinated by the local core groups*: regular training of volunteers is a core activity of the group. The core committee will identify specific funding to continue training volunteers and refresher trainings for existing volunteers. A training programme with a defined number of courses, new/refresher, and number of participants is generated. Availability of funding for the training must be ensured, and a system is put in place to collect training feedback on a regular basis. The expected outcome is a training calendar for 1 year available with funding for training earmarked. A training coordinator must be identified in the volunteer cohort who is able to liaise with other training centres locally or externally.

3.5 *Role of community volunteer in the project is clearly outlined*: when at least a few volunteers have finished training and are available to join the palliative care programme, the roles must be clearly documented. Core committee and volunteers jointly set the ground rules and document the roles and responsibility. If a memorandum of understanding and standard operating protocol are available, the defined roles and responsibility are updated in the memorandum of understanding and standard operating protocol. This step is realized when volunteers are working with professionals in providing patient care and have a copy of the document setting out their roles and responsibilities.

3.6 *Establish sustainable mechanism for caregivers' self-organization that incorporates continuous feedback to improve quality of training and care, social auditing, and sharing good practice to wider areas*: the core committee determines that quality improvement is an integral part of the service. The different components of quality improvement are identified including audit, training, and user feedback from patients and families. Patients and families are provided with a platform to come together to provide feedback and share experiences. Feedback from the patient and family platform are reviewed on a monthly basis by the core committee. The core committee identifies an external agency or institution to carry out a social audit and generates a report of good practice and areas to improve. The expected outcome of this step is that a regular review system is in place (either a committee/regular meetings) to consider feedback from patients, families, and volunteers to check the quality of care provided and quality of training given.

4. *Ensuring smooth and coordinated implementation of shared palliative care at a larger scale* (optional for programmes wishing to expand and scale up). This step is aimed at scaling up of community-partnered palliative care at region or provincial or country level.

4.1 *Identify and sensitize key allies among policy and decision makers and medical and community leadership on the approach of community-partnered palliative care and potential demonstration project*: this is initiated when the core committee determines that scale-up of palliative care is a target. Key allies are identified across sectors: health professional groups, community leaders informal, policy makers (elected representatives and administrative/managerial), civil society organizations, businesses, and educational establishments. A few key allies are sensitized to start with, aiming to develop a critical mass who accept scale-up of palliative care as a goal. The outcome desired is a prepared action plan based on assessment of allies/opportunities to advance the community palliative care agenda. Following on from this, a key stakeholder (usually governmental or other institutional actor with capacity) with a leadership role can plan a scale-up of palliative care.

4.2 *Set up a coordination committee with membership from this group (of higher-level stakeholders) to oversee the scale-up (geographical or domains of care)*: when a larger actor (e.g. government/institution) declares intention to scale-up palliative care, core committee offers to provide guidance/expertise in the process. They recommend formation of a coordination committee of higher-level stakeholders. This coordination committee is likely to include membership from the core committee. The coordination committee agrees on indicators of successful scale-up. A suite of suggested indicators of successful scale-up is prepared (Table 21.1).

4.3 *A mechanism for continuous evaluation and learning from scale-up process is established within the committee*: evaluation and learning are identified as a key part of scale-up within the coordination committee (the core committee member has an advocacy role in this). A mechanism is established for scale-up evaluation and learning by the coordination committee; this must include:

- An annual service audit (internal professional practice audit to improve quality).
- A social audit (external audit by independent agency/organization).

4.4 *Sustainability of the scale-up through community, institutional, or governmental mechanism*: sustainability of scale-up (with regard to funding, human resources/professional, and community involvement) is explicitly identified within the scale-up process by the coordination committee (the core committee member has an advocacy role in this).

Examples of community palliative care in low- and middle-income countries

Uganda

Though Uganda still faces challenges with only about 10% of patients in need of palliative care accessing it, the evolving model is different from conventional Western palliative care system (Palliative Care Association of Uganda, 2017).

In Uganda, community volunteers supplement the work of palliative care teams and identify patients in need of palliative care, particularly in rural settings where the hospice teams may not easily be reached. In addition, they help to provide physical, emotional, and spiritual care for patients while in their own homes (Jack et al., 2012). Being part of the community and aware of the inherent values and norms, these volunteers give culturally acceptable care and, therefore, patients and their families are willing to participate in the palliative care activities. Volunteers also provide information to the communities regarding cancers and HIV and advise on family planning, health promotion, preparing wills, and using herbal medicines. Volunteers are often recruited through churches, and they call on their church networks for support (Grant et al., 2011).

Table 21.1 Tentative list of indicators of success in community palliative care

Domain	Measurable criteria
Sustainability/community engagement	• Financial *sustainability*—no funding shortfall in running the project • Are there links with other community-based organizations and public health system? Are there shared activities/memorandums of understanding? • Staff satisfaction and turnover of staff • Volunteerism: • How many volunteers in proportion to patients? • How much time/how many patients per volunteer? • How long do volunteers stay in the project? • Is the project *inclusive* (participation from a range of interest groups—political/religious/social)? • Does the project reflect the community with respect to *diversity* (ethnic/language/disadvantaged groups)?
Quality, outcomes for individuals, families, communities	• Increase in number of patients and families supported • Quality of life measures (WHO-QOL, EQ-5D, Distress Thermometer); measures of symptom relief and number of hospitalizations needed • Survey of patients/families on impact of the project (physical/psychological/social/spiritual needs being met) • Proxy measures of community cohesion (social capital—Integrated Questionnaire) • Staff satisfaction and turnover of staff (also in team characteristics) • Existence of a quality improvement component within the project
Accessibility	• Is home care available for patients? • Out-of-hours access—direct or remote (telephone or other) • Disability-friendly access to professional and community support available for *patients and families* • Is the project disability friendly in engaging with *staff and volunteers*?
Team characteristics	• Staff turnover • Staff satisfaction • Team effectiveness questionnaires (e.g. https://www.londonleadershipacademy.nhs.uk/sites/default/files/Team_effectiveness_diagnostic-LAL1.pdf)
Project management characteristics	• Does the project have a core/executive committee? • Is there a clear project plan document available? • Are the visions/objectives/milestones of the project specified? • Is there a structure/function for management of the project? • Is there an identified group for technical expertise?

Kerala, India

The community-based palliative care programme in Kerala, owned and run by multiple civil society groups, political parties, religious groups, and local governments, is an example of the full extent of community ownership. Kerala now has more than 1000 palliative care units linked to local government institutions and more than 400 units run by local community groups. Local community groups own programmes in a non-hierarchical system. New players continue to enter the scene (Kumar, 2020).

A key player in delivery of palliative home care services along with volunteers from the community is the community palliative nurse. This is usually a woman, from the local community, employed in the palliative care programme after 3 months' structured training in palliative care. The homecare service is run either by the basic unit of public health system (primary healthcare centre) or by a community organization. In addition to trained volunteers and trained nurses, the home care service also incorporates local accredited social health activists and junior public health nurses. The team assesses the medical, emotional, and financial situation of the patient. The medical officer in charge of the primary health centre provides consultation to the team in developing the plan as needed. Accordingly, medicines are given and visits, including for emotional counselling, are scheduled. Family members are also given advice on the basic care of bedridden patients (NITI Aayog and UNDP-India, 2015).

The palliative care service delivery within this model combines the medical and nursing components with the following:

1. Regular supply of food for the starving families.
2. Support for children from families of poor patients to continue their education.
3. Transport facilities to referral hospitals.
4. Rehabilitation services supporting patients/family members in income-generating activities.
5. Financial support in emergency situations.
6. Companionship to the patient and family.
7. Link up with other social or religious organizations which can offer support.
8. Link the patient with local government to secure benefits from government schemes (Kumar and Numpeli, 2005).

Conclusion

Public health palliative care in low- and middle-income settings has a unique opportunity to root itself in the theory and practice of community participation. This plays to existing strengths available in such settings while refraining from replicating institutionalized and medically based models of palliative care in high-income settings. The community is where the suffering sits and where the solutions lie—health systems can only play a stewardship role in mobilizing the capacity for compassion and care that lies in the community.

REFERENCES

Choi, M., Mesa-Frias, M., Nuesch, E., Hargreaves, J., Prieto-Merino, D., Bowling, A., et al. 2014. Social capital, mortality, cardiovascular events and cancer: a systematic review of prospective studies. *International Journal of Epidemiology,* 43, 1895–1920.

Choi, S., Oh, J., Park, S. M., Hwang, S. E., Lee, H. Y., Kim, K., et al. 2020. Association of community level social trust and reciprocity with mortality: a retrospective cohort study. *BMC Public Health,* 20, 1793.

Ehsan, A., Klaas, H. S., Bastianen, A., and Spini, D. 2019. Social capital and health: a systematic review of systematic reviews. *SSM—Population Health,* 8, 100425.

Grant, L., Brown, J., Leng, M., Bettega, N., and Murray, S. A. 2011. Palliative care making a difference in rural Uganda, Kenya and Malawi: three rapid evaluation field studies. *BMC Palliative Care,* 10, 8.

Jack, B. A., Kirton, J. A., Birakurataki, J., and Merriman, A. 2012. The personal value of being a palliative care community volunteer worker in Uganda: a qualitative study. *Palliative Medicine,* 26, 753–759.

Kellehear, A. 1999. Health-promoting palliative care: developing a social model for practice. *Mortality,* 4, 75–82.

Kumar, S. 2020. Community participation in palliative care: reflections from the ground. *Progress in Palliative Care,* 28, 83–88.

Kumar, S. and Numpeli, M. 2005. Neighborhood network in palliative care. *Indian Journal of Palliative Care,* 11, 6–9.

Lewis, J. M., DiGiacomo, M., Currow, D. C., and Davidson, P. M. 2014. Social capital in a lower socioeconomic palliative care population: a qualitative investigation of individual, community and civic networks and relations. *BMC Palliative Care,* 13, 30.

NITI Aayog and UNDP-India. 2015. *Arogyakeralam Palliative Care Project: Ensuring Care and Support for the Chronically Ill & Infirm in Kerala.* New Delhi: NITI Aayog.

Organisation for Economic Co-operation and Development. 2001. *The Well-Being of Nations: The Role of Human and Social Capital.* Paris: Organisation for Economic Co-operation and Development.

Oware, P. M. 2020. Informal social protection actors: a focus on women self-help groups in Kenya. *International Social Work,* 63, 612–625.

World Health Organization. 2020. *Community Engagement: A Health Promotion Guide for Universal Health Coverage in the Hands of the People.* Geneva: World Health Organization.

SECTION 5

Evidence base

22

The evidence for the effectiveness of a public health palliative care approach

Joseph Sawyer and Libby Sallnow

Introduction: defining the parameters of a public health approach to palliative care

Within this chapter we seek to trace the origins of public health and palliative care in order to define the current working parameters of the relationship. We go on to examine the practice and evidence base that informs such a relationship and its impact, acknowledging some of the inherent tensions and scope for future work.

The emergence of palliative care as a specialty can be traced back to studies describing the experience of dying patients (Marie Curie Memorial Foundation, 1952; Townsend, 1962; Hinton, 1964; Glaser and Strauss, 1966) and the impact of death on the family unit (Kübler-Ross et al., 1972). Following these early descriptions, Dame Cicely Saunders developed her seminal ideas on total care (Saunders, 2006). In what was a break from traditional biomedical models of care, she focused on holistic care, a concept that incorporated the domains of physical, psychological, social, and spiritual support. This helped form the founding philosophy of hospice and palliative care and since then the speciality has grown in strength. In 1987, palliative medicine was recognized in the UK as a subspecialty of medicine by the Royal College of Physicians and in 2014 the World Health Organization (WHO) recommended that all countries include palliative care in their undergraduate curricula and national health policies (WHO, 2014). Palliative care is now an established international specialty service designed to recognize and support the needs of the dying.

Despite this, the movement continues to face challenges and criticisms. Many feel that palliative care is poorly understood and, while it is established in many high-income settings, many people from across the world struggle to access its services (The Economist Intelligence Unit, 2015). In the UK, the hospice movement has been described as 'too good to be true and too small to be useful' (Douglas, 1992) while inequity in provision relating to age (Burt and Raine, 2006), diagnosis (Mitchell et al., 2004; Abel and Kellehear, 2016), gender (Gott et al., 2020), ethnicity (Koffman et al., 2007), and sexuality (Bristowe et al., 2016) have been demonstrated.

Such problems are compounded by changing demographics. With the global population set to age further over the next 20 years, there is likely to be an increased demand for palliative care services to support the comorbidities associated with old age (Etkind et al., 2017). In many settings, excluding the US, the hospice movement remains focused on inpatient activity with high-intensity care over a short period. This is well suited to the needs of those with cancer; however, conditions such as dementia, frailty, and chronic organ failure follow a more undulating course based more in the community (Murray et al., 2005).

At the same time, the capacity of professional services to care for people in their own homes is diminishing (Abel and Kellehear, 2016). Indeed, it has been argued that the community component of care originally alluded to by Dame Cicely Saunders (1998) has become restricted in its interpretation. Hospice volunteers, for whom palliative care services remain reliant upon (Vanderstichelen et al., 2020), have come to represent community input (Burbeck et al., 2014) yet their role is largely governed by management in order to augment the functioning of the organization as opposed to facilitating an ongoing partnership of activity with the community.

The specialty of palliative care has also faced questions relating to a perceived professionalization of death (Kearney, 1992; Sawyer and Taylor, 2018). A reliance on evidence-based medicine and multiprofessional teams as a vehicle to achieve a 'good death' has perhaps come at the expense of engaging at the deeper level of what it means to provide human care (Kearney, 1992). At the same time, traditional, long-standing social structures of care have been undermined and neglected. This has led to a narrative that highlights the objective lack of compassion in current healthcare services (Francis, 2013).

A closer evaluation of the parameters by which palliative care services have come to be judged therefore show the service has struggled to develop beyond its early successes. Successive reports commissioned to address such issues continue to focus on the problems relating to access without addressing measures that may overcome them. The response, however, has been invigorated by a 'new public health approach' to palliative care that re-imagines the question of access by asking what can be done by people within their own communities in order to find social solutions for socially mediated problems (Kellehear, 1999; Leadbeater and Garber,

2010; Commission into the Future of Hospice Care, 2013; Abel and Kellehear, 2016). Such ideas are the product of an evolution of thinking in public health. Following the period of industrialization, there was a move beyond traditional public health measures of disease prevention and control to an appreciation of the wider social determinants of health in preventative terms (Ashton and Seymour, 1988). This culminated in the Ottawa Charter (WHO, 1986) where health education and more radical ideas relating to community development found themselves at the fore. Current practice in public health now involves a diverse field that draws on community development and capacity building, social capital, and social ecology alongside ideas on health promotion.

The close articulation between broad-ranging specialties such as palliative care and public health has posed challenges in providing theoretical clarity (Dempers and Gott, 2017b). This has been compounded by seemingly different interpretations of such an articulation that have evolved over time and remain in a consistent state of flux. The points of difference would seemingly revolve around which 'foundation' of public health is best suited to palliative care (Dempers and Gott, 2017b). Some commentators continue to express concern that palliative care is poorly understood and requires greater integration into healthcare systems with more clearly defined and measurable outcomes (Payne, 2007; Stjernsward, 2007; Whitelaw and Clark, 2019); this has been termed the 'WHO approach' (Dempers and Gott, 2017b) and is focused on more traditional models of public health. Others suggest that palliative care must move beyond the bedside and work to reclaim illness, loss, and mortality as social experiences shaped by culture, geography, beliefs, and relationships (Kellehear, 1999; Abel et al., 2013). This is more widely known as a 'health-promoting approach' or a 'new public health approach' (Dempers and Gott, 2017b). Central themes to the latter focus on a widened understanding of death as a shared social process that is negotiated through new partnerships between communities and services. Such partnerships draw on the participatory principles of a new public health and translate into greater capacity for communities to provide the care and support necessary at the end of life. By way of example, some of the major approaches of this relationship will now be outlined with an accompanying critique of the corresponding evidence base in its current form. Developing an evidence base poses a unique set of challenges for those looking to assess and evaluate this idea. Beyond the challenges faced by health service research methods to showcase effectiveness in what is a complex and multifaceted domain, there lie further issues to address including how we conceptualize, define, and measure concepts such as social capital, community, and death literacy. We will endeavour to highlight these problems and where possible discuss solutions or potential alternatives.

Communities as independent agents of care

A new public health approach has led to the emergence of 'community' as a recurrent theme (Kellehear, 2005; Abel et al., 2013; Abel, 2018). Many studies now refer to communities as independent agents of care provision, as opposed to passive recipients of education and other medical interventions bestowed upon them through legislative change (Leonard et al., 2015; Mills et al., 2015; Rosenberg et al., 2016; Gott et al., 2018). This represents a shift away from the development of formal services towards community engagement, where the growth of social networks can occur as a product of communities being active in end of life care (Horsfall et al., 2014). In this context 'communities' tend to refer to people or places or both; however, there are challenges in defining community within such a context (Dempers and Gott, 2017b).

The link with communities is strengthened by conceptualizing death as a process that shares an interdependence and social connection with processes of grief, caregiving, and bereavement. A new public health approach therefore rejects the subspecialization of palliative care and bereavement care into separate entities and constructs a paradigm that embraces the totality of end of life experiences, placing them together as shared social experiences embedded within community life (Kellehear, 2007; Horsfall et al., 2013; Rumbold and Aoun, 2014; Kelley et al., 2018; Aoun, 2019; Huang et al., 2019).

Evidence for such ideas lie within the work done by Gott and colleagues (2018) who have studied the role of community at the end of life for people in old age. In a study involving interviews with caregivers for people aged over 80 they conceptualized community as a 'group or network of persons who are connected (objectively) to each other by relatively durable social relations that extend beyond immediate genealogical ties and who mutually define that relationship (subjectively) as important to their social identity and social practice' (Gott et al., 2018, p. 71). Analysis sought to identify three commonly differentiated forms of community, namely communities of place, interest, and age. They were able to demonstrate a wide range of tasks carried out by people from within an inner network often relating to family. In what brings some empirical questioning to the role of community, they also demonstrate the limited involvement and response of the outer or wider community network. This was due to unique barriers and also an observed 'active withdrawal' from community towards the end of life. That people were found to actively withdraw from community life poses interesting questions for a new public health approach to palliative care. The study references the importance of reciprocity for this group of people in the cultural context in which the study was conducted. Not being able to reciprocate acts of care was perceived as a source of distress and can ultimately lead to acts of care being 'done to' rather than 'by and for', a model that has echoes of professionally based services from which new public health measures are meant to be moving away from. In order for new public health approaches to be more effective in this context, there is a need to better understand the role of community in advanced age. Social networks can then be strengthened in ways sensitive to the unique set of circumstances people of old age find themselves within.

In Australia, Grindrod and Rumbold (2018) have outlined a comprehensive community development project that identifies local end of life needs and meets them through community resource. Using in-depth interviews and focus groups, they examined carers' experience of home-based dying with particular reference to supportive networks during this time. Using a public health framework, an evidence-informed community development model was created. This body of work showed that people are often reluctant to ask for or accept help from informal networks despite an apparent need. A willingness of such networks to provide support was limited by uncertainty as to what to offer and the possibility of infringing on people's privacy. The study therefore promotes the idea that such social norms need to change if we are to build community capacity. They conclude this can be achieved through the use of established community development strategies. Generating partnerships, forums for discussion and the sharing of information while facilitating the development of social networks are vehicles to deliver the five principles of their 'Healthy End of Life Project' (HELP) guide. In a follow-up paper, Grindrod (2020) maps national, state, regional, and locally based assets with the potential to help build a community's capacity to contribute to and improve end of life care. They argue that newly developed capacity supplements and strengthens the services delivered by health and palliative care services while recognizing that both formal and informal support are required for optimal quality end of life care. Through the collective review of their various public health and palliative care projects they suggest change is achieved by using evidence-based public health principles and methods, alongside asset-based partnerships and a capacity-building approach. Uptake is enhanced through solution-focused methods that reduce or remove barriers to sector engagement and by reframing existing systems, structures, and networks to incorporate end of life policy and practice.

This work generates interesting questions when compared to the study of community-based care in advanced age by Gott and colleagues (2018) that demonstrated an active withdrawal from community at the end of life. Balancing the privacy and intimacy of death and dying alongside profoundly social processes and implications is perhaps more complex than initially assumed. Wholesale cultural changes are also difficult to achieve and have to be tailored to context and the individual needs of a community. Such unresolved complexities preclude the large-scale roll out of community-based interventions and remain a stumbling block for new public health measures in palliative care.

Central to the argument of communities being independent agents of care is the idea that the end of life is a shared social process. This is described in detail among much of the theoretical work on new public health approaches to palliative care (Kellehear, 2007, 2016, 2019; Conway, 2008; Rosenberg, 2011; Abel et al., 2013; Horsfall et al., 2013; Rumbold and Aoun, 2014; Noonan et al., 2016; Sallnow et al., 2016a, 2016b; Dempers and Gott, 2017a; Abel, 2018; Aoun et al., 2018; Bunce, 2018; Horsfall, 2018; Kelley et al., 2018). Authors draw upon the idea of the universality of death and a shared impermanence held between all living things (Kellehear, 2007; Mills et al., 2015). Death, therefore, is not seen as contingent on a medical diagnosis and is not characterized simply by the absence of life, beyond which there is social vacuum. Rather, it is argued that death can be 'full of life' through the multitude of interpersonal experiences that the process of dying, caring, and bereavement brings (Kellehear, 2007). These experiences take place in the embodied realm of the living and are predominantly social in nature.

Evidencing these phenomena in 'scientific terms' is perhaps a more abstract question and relates to the need for more innovative and creative research methodologies in this area (see Chapter 24). There are multiple qualitative studies that help to convey the social narrative of death, dying, and grief (Kellehear, 2007, 2016, 2019; Conway, 2008; Rosenberg, 2011; Abel et al., 2013; Horsfall et al., 2013; Rumbold and Aoun, 2014; Noonan et al., 2016; Sallnow et al., 2016a; Dempers and Gott, 2017a; Abel, 2018; Aoun et al., 2018; Bunce, 2018; Horsfall, 2018; Kelley et al., 2018; Sawyer et al., 2018). Authors draw upon the idea of the universality of death and a shared impermanence held between all living things (Kellehear, 2007; Mills et al., 2015). However, what is needed is a better understanding of how embracing these issues and providing social solutions can then impact outcomes. In their 2016 systematic review Sallnow and colleagues (2016a) evaluate the impact of new public health approaches. Through the careful evaluation of eight studies, they found that engaging communities can lead to improved outcomes in terms of reduced fatigue and isolation while networks can also influence place of death (a widely used proximal marker to quality of care at the end of life) and palliative care service involvement. This review had a relatively narrow focus when considering the breadth of topic and highlights the tension in what might be considered 'evidence' and indeed also what we then consider as outcomes of interest to such complex interventions. The studies included use preselected participants over quite short time frames, raising the question as to what impact is experienced beyond such parameters and the need for further work to demonstrate such effects.

Social networks and social capital

Another theme identified within the discourse of new public health approaches relates to 'assets' and the presence of social capital. The term social capital was popularized at the end of the last century by a series of authors attempting to capture what is contained with the relationships held between individuals, communities, and the state (Bourdieu, 1986; Coleman, 1988; Putnam, 2000). The focus on the social determinants of health has led to the term being adopted within the literature of healthcare where it is seen as a target for public health interventions (Johansson et al., 2012; Lewis et al., 2013; Horsfall et al., 2014; Mills et al., 2015; Rosenberg et al., 2015; Sawyer et al., 2019).

The origins and application of social capital stem from such a diverse literature that definitions have become multiple. Unifying themes focus on social capital being inherent in the structure of human relationships (Portes, 1998). To possess social capital, one must therefore be held in connection with others and an advantage is realized through these other people (Portes, 1998). Although multiple classifications continue to be debated, a three-tier system is generally described (Kawachi et al., 2004; Szreter and Woolcock, 2004). This includes bonding social capital, which describes relationships between people with characteristics in common; bridging social capital, which exists across people with different characteristics; and linking social capital, describing relationships taking place across power gradients such as between communities and institutions.

New public health approaches to palliative care seek to operationalize social capital and its varying components. In a relationship that is new and constantly evolving, a range of positive outcomes have been described from within the field of healthcare (Reeves et al., 2014; Sallnow et al., 2016a; Abel et al., 2018b; Sawyer et al., 2019). However, it has been argued that such studies have oversimplified the concept leading to a tendency for it to be seen as uniformly positive in its potential to generate outcomes of interest (Dempers and Gott, 2017b). We know from the field of sociology that is not the case, for example, high levels of bonded social capital can create close-knit communities that provide access to resources, but can also restrict individual freedoms and bar outsiders from access

(Portes, 1998). Other authors have noted that the power dynamics inherent within all relationships are often not made explicit while the influence of social class, gender, and race in such relationships is rarely accounted for (Bourdieu, 1986; Wakefield and Poland, 2005).

The evidence base for developing social networks and social capital has developed significantly over recent years with a series of large-scale quantitative studies and systematic reviews (Fletcher et al., 2011; Macdonald-Wallis et al., 2012; Sawka et al., 2013; Latkin and Knowlton, 2015; Hunter et al., 2019). Christakis and Fowler (2007, 2008) have described the spread of smoking cessation and the rise of obesity in social networks in the US, highlighting the role social relationships play in individual and community level outcomes for such issues. While Hunter and colleagues (2019) found social network interventions to be effective in both the short and the long term in improving health behaviours and outcomes, particularly in the field of sexual health. In 2010, Holt-Lunstad and colleagues undertook a large meta-analysis of the relationship between social relationships and mortality. They demonstrated a 50% increased survival for those with stronger social relationships, higher than the survival benefit conferred by many well-known public health interventions such as giving up smoking, the pneumococcal flu vaccine, or reduction in obesity (Holt-Lunstad et al., 2010).

Despite seemingly common and fertile ground for collaboration, there appears to be little crossover between such studies and the body of evidence provided from the field of sociology and social sciences. Instead, these studies speak in terms of social relationship and social networks and a practical description of their impact and associations. The underlying ideas behind social capital are not mentioned, leaving questions for social scientists as to what is actually happening within such networks to deliver observed outcomes.

In relation to palliative care, Horsfall, Noonan, and Leonard have contributed to a growing field of evidence exploring the role of carers and community networks in caring for those dying at home (Leonard et al., 2010, 2015; Horsfall et al., 2013, 2014; Noonan et al., 2016; Horsfall, 2018; Noonan, 2018). Employing mixed methods, their work has shown caregiving can be a positive experience that can contribute to the acquisition of social capital and lead to community development. Horsfall and colleagues explore the quality and effect of informal caring networks that are established or strengthened as a result of caring for a person dying at home in their 2014 paper 'Bringing our dying home' (Horsfall et al., 2014). They used network mapping in focus groups and interviews in order to create oral and visual narratives of caring and support at the end of life. The study demonstrates that carers mobilized and negotiated a complex web of relationship and that such experiences contributed to the development of social capital and a community's capacity to hold such events as the end of life. This work also gives empirical evidence to the notion that caregiving generates social capital for both a private but also a public good. The latter is of particular relevance when considering how and why communities may be able to act as independent agents in the provision of care.

This work was followed up by Leonard and colleagues in their 2015 paper that analysed how caring networks change for people with terminal illnesses being cared for at home (Leonard et al., 2015). Using third-generation social network analysis involving quantitative network mapping accompanied by recorded interview data, they were able to show an increase in the size of networks and that ties between original members of the network were strengthened. The qualitative data gave insight into the importance between members of the core and outer networks and the range of contributions made by each. Again, these data show how social capital may be strengthened through end of life caregiving which in turn may contribute to a community's capacity to provide care. The study used carers for people dying of cancer or motor neurone disease. This narrow focus does not address some of the issues faced by other people who are situated within a different social context such as those of advanced age or those with dementia. The study was also performed retrospectively and a reliance on memory of events may distort the actual unfolding of events.

In a 2019 paper, Sawyer and colleagues evaluate the role of social networks and social capital at the end of life for people affected by dementia (Sawyer et al., 2019). Employing a realist philosophy of science, they attempt to dispassionately understand how social capital may influence end of life outcomes in this context. Social capital was found to exert influence in key areas such as how the caregiving experience unfolds, transitions in the physical environment of care, and the decision-making processes underpinning such topics. Social capital was noted to be a component of a complex system that gives context specific outcomes. Such outcomes ranged from positive and rewarding care experiences to more negative and overwhelming care experiences. There was very little evidence to suggest that caregiving contributed towards a community's capacity to provide end of life care; however, this is likely secondary to an absence of available data in this area.

In a paradigmatic shift to the more commonly described burden and isolation that caregiving brings, this body of evidence suggests social capital can be developed through the build-up of trust, reciprocity, and adherence to a new set of social norms that facilitate social agency (Johansson et al., 2012). This, however, does not take into account the quality of such relationships which are not always functional and cohesive (Sawyer et al., 2019). The capacity of social capital to be operationalized by a public health approach is therefore very much dependent on a greater theoretical understanding of the tensions at hand and their sub-context. For example, how will this concept support female informal carers, marginalized groups, and those from lower socioeconomic groups? How does it accommodate dysfunctional and damaging relationships? How does it accommodate power gradients and work alongside professional services and how does this model change in relation to non-cancer-related conditions such as dementia, the effects of which fundamentally change social relationships?

The complexity associated with engaging with and operationalizing social capital is suggestive that it alone is not sufficient to guarantee community development and capacity building. Additional processes and supportive structures are necessary to develop a robust understanding and subsequent plan for integrating informal networks into caregiving.

Community engagement, development, and empowerment

Addressing the term social capital within the broader framework of community engagement, development, and empowerment goes some way in achieving this. The term community engagement is commonplace in healthcare rhetoric but can describe a variety of practices (Sallnow and Paul, 2015). Morgan (2001) has described the tensions that can exist with the use of the term community participation being used either for its cosmetic value or, simultaneously, by different actors to advance conflicting goals. Aside from tensions in terminology, there can be a discrepancy in understanding between practitioners (Sallnow and Paul, 2015).

A spectrum of shared collaborative working between communities and professional services is highlighted as a crucial component of a new public health approach to palliative care (Sallnow and Paul, 2015). Described as an 'umbrella term' (Sallnow and Paul, 2015), community engagement depicts the process by which professional services work with communities on issues relating to end of life care. Such processes exist on a spectrum of activities that extends from informing to empowering (Sallnow and Paul, 2015; Noonan et al., 2016). In the former, the community is passive with the aims limited to raising awareness. Through co-production and collaboration, it is argued that services can ultimately help empower communities. This necessitates the community taking full control of an aspect of care and using services for specialist support where it is felt to be needed (Sallnow and Paul, 2015).

Such an approach is evidenced by a community development project established in the southern Indian state of Kerala in the late 1990s. The project worked to establish an independent process of community empowerment (Kumar, 2007; Sallnow et al., 2010). Members of the community build teams that then establish themselves as independent entities capable of delivering home-based palliative care. Networks are formed between volunteers, doctors, and nurses while the human resource present within the wider community is mobilized. The model is termed the Neighbourhood Network in Palliative Care and compromises three main components: (1) community mobilization and ownership by the local community, (2) involvement of the local self-government institutions, and (3) incorporation of palliative care in the primary healthcare system (Kumar, 2013). It has been looked to as an inspiration and in 2010 it was recognized by the WHO as a collaborating centre in community participation in end of life care. Experience from such an initiative has given rise to guidance on community development (Abel et al., 2016); however, the evidence for the impact of such initiatives remains anecdotal.

The paradigm of community empowerment is, however, fraught with tensions. The institutionalization of 'empowerment' within community care and its tendency to be uncritically accepted as a universal panacea has multiple implications for both family and caregivers, especially so in the context of end of life care. For example, where people are 'empowered' to die at home, family members may be forced to relinquish traditional family-based roles in place of caregiving roles. This is an example as to how tensions can arise depending on the level at which empowerment is interpreted. Where interpretation occurs at the level of healthcare service policy and practice management, it often takes the form of healthcare interventions and service delivery approaches. Empowerment has also been shown to accentuate the highly gendered dimensions of caregiving (Williams et al., 2017). This can create cultural norms and expectations that are difficult to break free from. Empowering people to work in a more holistic and supportive manner also neglects the fact that not all people have the same thresholds to provide care and work in such a way. Those people unwilling or unable to work in this way may then be targeted or subject to discrimination (Williams et al., 2011).

In the UK, a number of hospices in the south-east of England have been working to augment social networks through the implementation of the Compassionate Neighbours project (Hospice UK, n.d.). This project recruits and trains local people to support those nearing the end of life in their own homes. Rather than creating and training people in a new role, people are supported to be 'good neighbours'. Such an intervention is thought to bring companionship, practical support, and the opportunity to help connect with others, thus building social capital. Training is significantly different to that of traditional hospice volunteering programmes and focuses on network development and self-reflection. This model is being adopted by other hospices across the UK, yet evaluative measures are still in development. Sallnow's thesis (2017) assessing the impact of this intervention provides evidence for 'collective social capital' a medium that fosters interdependence and reciprocity between communities and organizations.

The proactive building of networks, through interventions designed under the guise of the public health movement, is described as an important component to a new public health approach to palliative care (Horsfall et al., 2014; Abel and Kellehear, 2016; Abel et al., 2018a). Much in the way that the palliative care movement broke from the traditional medical structures in the 1980s, this technique employs a degree of 'disruptive innovation' that challenges the norms of public health and palliative medicine. Authors speak of using the power of 'activism' as a means of implementing a new public health philosophy; it is argued this is necessary for the movement to achieve the scale and momentum necessary to bring change (Kumar, 2013). This philosophy is projected onto a global platform where it is suggested the movement has a role in assisting poorer countries in order to meet needs for analgesia and the promotion of well-being in the face of death (Murray and Mason, 2010).

The development of such initiatives has the potential to exert significant pressure on the relationships and actions of local and national governing bodies. On the one hand, this influence is important in instigating lasting change and bringing a cultural shift through all of society. On the other, it can also create a tension between government, policy, and the wider society. The wave of social support generated by the previously mentioned Neighbourhood Network in Palliative Care has resulted in the Keralan government being forced to recognize its success and allocate funds and resources. The involvement of government, and political parties, has raised issues relating to the balance of power with people inside the movement suggesting that increased interventions can stifle the innovation and the community-owned nature of work (Kumar, 2013, 2020).

Taking this idea further, solidarity within the community could be jeopardized as publicly made resources substitute for those previously provided by the family. Empirical evidence for this phenomenon in the context of new public health approaches is lacking; however, the topic has been discussed at length in the fields of sociology and social gerontology in relation to the welfare state (Van Oorschot and Arts, 2005). Here the argument is presented in terms of 'crowding in' and 'crowding out' whereby increased services may either reduce the willingness or resources of naturally occurring networks (crowding out) or in opposition to this, work by drawing people into action in a way that positively links the growth of community support at the level of giving and receiving (crowding in) (Künemund and Rein, 1999).

Another technique described less frequently in the literature, which is perhaps in direct contradiction to the examples mentioned, is to take a deconstructive approach and target the very structures that are seen to impose a blockade on organically developed social capital. This would allow for the 'rippling out' of knowledge and experience. Such a phenomena is described in qualitative studies relating to end of life care (Horsfall et al., 2013, 2014) where it is noted that acts of care represent the 'the ordinary becoming extraordinary' (Horsfall et al., 2014). Advocates of such an approach theorize that lay networks of people perhaps want to be involved but lack the capacity due to other responsibilities or structures that impede their motivation. This notion exists beyond a romanticized level and is demonstrated in empirical studies (Horsfall et al., 2014; Noonan et al., 2016; Horsfall, 2018). There is an acceptance of the immense challenges end of life care can bring but this came with a strong sense of personal fulfilment. Instead, the source of distress and difficulty comes through the hard work that comes with trying to maintain social connections (Horsfall et al., 2014). Frequently, people are presented with obstacles from social structures that do not accommodate such desires. At best, professional services or the stream of bureaucratic interventions designed to help do actually help fill the void; at worst, they are further structures that obstruct people's desires to partake in the caregiving process (Horsfall et al., 2014).

Fundamental to this approach is the idea that, while engaging with the end of life process may invoke feelings of fear and sadness, it can also generate great courage and compassion which can help build social legacies (Kellehear, 2019). In a new public health approach to palliative care, the caring role is seen as no better catalyst to learning and education and is noted to be a key component to creating Noonan and colleagues' (2016) concept of 'death literacy'.

Compassionate communities and compassionate cities

Bringing these components of a new public health approach to palliative care together is Kellehear's theoretical framework of a compassionate community. This describes a range of approaches that focus on community development via the creation and mobilization of support networks and harnessing the influence of social capital (Kellehear, 2005). The ultimate aim of a compassionate community is to develop an active role for communities in the process of death, dying, and loss. Such an approach remains loosely defined and poorly understood yet impacts have been demonstrated in terms of making a practical difference, promoting individual learning and personal growth, as well as developing community capacity (Sallnow et al., 2016a). In the last decade, several organizations from different countries including England (Cronin, 2016; Abel et al., 2018b), Scotland (Hazelwood and Patterson, 2018), Ireland (McLoughlin et al., 2015), Austria (Wegleitner and Schuchter, 2018), India (Kumar, 2007), Canada (Pesut et al., 2017), Australia (Rosenberg et al., 2015), and Spain (Gomez-Batiste et al., 2018; Librada Flores et al., 2018) have worked to develop different implementation models for this concept.

Hospice and palliative care services have led the way in developing such an approach (Paul and Sallnow, 2013) and often provide the context to compassionate community initiatives (Barry and Patel, 2013). Usually compromising hospice-trained volunteers, there is an expectation such volunteers provide social support and are active in network building (Cronin, 2016; Sallnow et al., 2016a). Volunteers then subsequently transfer under the ownership and management of the local community. A 2020 systematic review by Librada-Flores and colleagues concluded there is currently no agreed systematic framework for the development and evaluation of a compassionate community programme (Librada-Flores et al., 2020); however, the end of life care research group affiliated to the Free University of Brussels (Vrije Universiteit Brussel) is conducting a feasibility project to develop, implement, and evaluate a model of community volunteers identified as compassionate communities connectors (Aoun et al., 2020). There have also been attempts to demonstrate an effect of compassionate community-based models on hospital admissions and other such parameters which have shown some promising results (Abel et al., 2018b; Abbey et al., 2020).

Reducing emergency hospital admissions has been a long-standing target for healthcare policy in the Western world. This takes on special precedence in the context of end of life care where people close to death may be exposed to unnecessary and exhausting interventions that can cause undue distress. From the perspective of a public health approach to palliative care, hospital admissions at the end of life elevate institutions and their respective knowledge, expertise, and resource over and above communities and their own assets thus hollowing out a community's capacity to provide security, care, and contribute to a fertile social ecology. From a health systems perspective, reducing perceived 'unnecessary' hospital admissions can also be argued as a positive from an economic perspective, with rising admissions linked to heavy financial costs.

In a cohort retrospective analysis, a single general practitioner practice in Frome, Somerset, England, targeted people at risk of unplanned admission including those over 95 years of age and those with dementia (Abel et al., 2018b). They used systematic care planning including referral to the social prescribing scheme, and proactive community development that included community groups, peer support networks, and use of volunteer support to help as 'community connectors'. The practice has been able to demonstrate a progressive reduction, by 7.9 cases per quarter (95% confidence interval, 2.8–13.1; $p = 0.006$), in unplanned hospital admissions across the whole population during a 4-year study period. Other initiatives looking at hospital avoidance done throughout the wider region, and without the crucial aspects of community development, were unable to demonstrate such an effect. The observational nature of the study precludes any causative conclusion; however, such an association provides some empirical evidence of effect. It is also questionable the extent to which social prescribing fits within a model of compassionate communities where the focus is on developing assets from the inside rather than prescribing them 'onto' people. The outcome measure of hospital admissions and the labelling of them as 'unnecessary' is also fraught with tension and can breed a culture of avoidance and frustration when there is sometimes no alternative.

Another study by Aoun and colleagues (2018) aimed to demonstrate the use of a compassionate community model in delivering bereavement support. In a population-based cross-sectional investigation of people's bereavement experiences via postal survey, they showed that informal sources of support including family, friends and funeral providers were used most frequently. Along with being used less frequently, professional sources of support also had the highest proportion of perceived unhelpfulness. Such an association is limited in this study by the nature of a survey which prevents a deeper clarification of meaning and precludes the use of random sampling. Nonetheless, in a field where public health approaches are very much in their infancy it goes some way in making the case for a change in approach.

Examples of practice have also emerged from independent charities. Here, community development workers, compassionate community champions, and death doulas provide links between existing community efforts to support death, dying, and bereavement (Patel, 2016; Rawlings et al., 2020). These measures, and the intersection with professional services, remain theoretically underdeveloped and lack an empirical evidence base.

More recently, Kellehear (2016, 2019) has made the case for interventions at the level of local government and local councils. Describing how such bodies engage at all levels of society, he argues they therefore represent a means through which change can take place. This approach is outlined in the Compassionate Cities Charter (Kellehear, 2015) and distinguishes itself from the compassionate communities approach through its focus on civic rather than healthcare bodies or community groups. The result is a much broader remit for sustainable social and cultural change.

Evidence for such an approach can be found in De Leeuw's (2009) evaluation of the European Healthy Cities project. Although distinct from Kellehear's idea of a compassionate city, this idea is characterized as a social movement that employs a wide range of political, social, and behavioural interventions for the development of urban population health. De Leeuw argues that decisions made in the light of good evidence of effectiveness are typically based on interventions with a medical as opposed to social focus. Healthy cities and indeed compassionate cities are difficult to define while it is unclear on what general or specific outcomes they should be evaluated on. Can the clamour to display evidence dismiss the question of what is relevant and important to know in the first instance?

A greater conceptual understanding can help deliver us at this point and can be achieved by drawing lessons from case studies, stories from the experiences of member cities. This is exactly what is outlined in De Leeuw's paper and leads to intriguing questions such as, have cities been effective in forming successful partnerships with other sectors? How do healthy cities influence local structures and processes? Their evaluation reflects a range of research issues including implicit and explicit theoretical frameworks, methods, and methodologies. Crucially, healthy cities are regarded as a package that must be evaluated in context with individual elements, assessed as part of an evolutionary endeavour to compile relevant evidence of effectiveness and experiences.

More specific to compassionate cities, Pfaff and colleagues (2020) have developed the 'Health Impact Change Model' in order to try and unpack the complexities associated with implementing and evaluating similar interventions in Canada. Its widespread use is yet to be seen; however, when placed in conjunction with the work from healthy cities provides the necessary direction and approach required when looking to evaluate the effectiveness of such work.

The intersection between public, professional, and lay services and the implications for responsibility and the moral landscape

Despite the apparent success of the described compassionate communities, it remains clear that we need a greater understanding as to how the techniques they employ seek to engage and empower communities. The models described thus far pose interesting questions as to the relationship between formal and informal care networks. Evidence relating to how this relationship is negotiated and the subsequent impact of this on how care of the dying person is responsibilized is limited. Understanding this better and within the conceptual context of death as a shared social process is necessary to appreciate how communities and professional services might work together to meet the overall aims of building a community's capacity to provide end of life care.

The relationship between formal and informal care networks for people dying at home has been explored empirically by Horsfall and colleagues. In one study they sought to better understand how the two groups work together (Horsfall et al., 2013). Using qualitative methods including ten focus group discussions across urban, rural, and regional Australia, they found that formal providers of care are aware and supportive of the vital role informal networks play in caregiving at the end of life. While there was found to be goodwill towards supporting informal networks, this did not translate into meaningful actions to establish, support, or maintain them. Indeed, formal care is often provided from the 'service provider as expert' position rather than a community development position. The paper therefore provides good evidence for the need to reframe how professionals work in and engage with citizen spaces. Another study in the UK looked to understand general practitioners' perceptions of a new public health approach (Abbey et al., 2020). Using semi-structured interviews and thematic analysis, the authors identified areas of potential collaboration but also highlight discrepancy between professionally driven approaches to genuine community created and owned initiatives.

At a more theoretical level, Kellehear's description of a compassionate city is suggestive of some degree of civic responsibility for end of life care. Here responsibility may lie more in creating an accepted space for citizens to perform some of the 'work' of caring as described by Horsfall and colleagues (Horsfall, 2018). Organizations are then able to respond to local needs rather than vice versa, leading in theory to more equitable care. Compassionate communities sit within and are interdependent upon this framework and are therefore understood to share some responsibility for end of life care, yet the specifics of what they are responsible for and the nature of the motivations to assume such responsibility are unclear. There is perhaps scope for a compassionate community to collectively define death and dying in social terms, thus helping to organize supportive structures grounded in this philosophy; however, this notion has not been theoretically developed yet alone scientifically evaluated.

Where responsibility is not clearly understood, power struggles can ensue, leading to fragmented care, service gaps, and moral distress (Pesut et al., 2014). Responsibility also has a complex relationship with notions of motivation. While on the one hand it is a powerful motivational force, on the other, it can also be crippling if a person or community is responsibilized for a situation that is beyond their capacity to hold. Fostering altruistic traits from within a community as a motivational force and combining this with notions of responsibility therefore has the potential to overwhelm a community. In addition, it cannot be assumed that *all* people in *all* communities are altruistic. While compassion can be fostered via the responsibilities held at a civic or organizational level to garner further support, the reality is that while communities bring companionship, practical support, and comfort they also bring ignorance, rejection, and patronization (Rosenberg, 2011). Furthermore, altruism is difficult to implement systematically and can therefore lead to bias. For example, the collective altruism to support a dying child may not be in short supply when compared to caring for an older person dying of dementia.

If motivation is instead modelled on social exchange theory and reciprocity (Dowd, 1975), that is, that a compassionate act is exchanged for another or some other form of 'capital', there are still inherent tensions. For example, many people at the end of life are unable to reciprocate acts of care thus eliminating the purposed motivation and giving rise to the need of professional services who perform acts of care in exchange for a wage (Gott et al., 2018). In such an approach, care may be seen as 'commodified' and is subject to market rules. This is in direct contradiction to death as a '*shared social process*' and paves the way for professional involvement.

At the level of the patient and the professional, there is a more defined, although not black and white, locus of responsibility. The difficulty arises when responsibility is viewed at a population level. Very quickly it becomes clear professional services cannot carry this responsibility and for two important reasons. Firstly, and most obviously, demand far outstrips capacity. Secondly, and more importantly, professional palliative care services hold a benign, yet enduring paternalism that is a philosophical and structural barrier to a paradigmatic shift towards conceptualizing death as a shared social process (Rosenberg, 2011). Framing the problem in public health terms is a logical step to fostering the human resource 'communities' offer while building political capital, but conceptually the locus of responsibility remains rooted in the biomedical domain. This represents an enduring tension across the literature on health-promoting palliative care.

At the level of the family or an inner circle of care, the culturally embedded norms of kinship present duty as a concept that is many ways independent of responsibility and more in line with some form of obligation (Finch and Mason, 1990). Parent–child relations are in some cases founded on norms of obligation; how these norms are created and how they operate within a compassionate community is relatively unexplored yet likely to have a crucial impact. In this complex and under-researched area, there are perhaps clear principles which can be referred to when considering the 'proper' thing to do; however, there is no clear consensus regarding what is reasonable to expect, rather the responsibility is to be negotiated rather than seen as a specific rule to follow.

Issues such as responsibility, duty, and motivation are operationalized by a public health approach to palliative care, yet the theoretical and practical details are poorly defined. While it is generally accepted that the principles of prevention and harm reduction demand greater public responsibility, it could also be argued that they create professional or bureaucratized systems that demand compliance rather than empower shared responsibility; for example, an office space may demand a responsible officer for first aid, fire, or other occupational health hazards which then negates the need for collective responsibilities of such issues.

There is some evidence from the literature that under the paradigm of shared social responsibility, reciprocity is not defined in terms of simple dyadic transactions. For example, where an act of care or compassion is unreciprocated due to ill health of the recipient, then the benefactor will seek reward elsewhere in the community (Sawyer et al., 2019). Where these pathways are cultivated, this can, in theory, lead to the building of community capacity and the transference of knowledge, skill, and experience. There is therefore a fluidity to the idea of responsibility and the sharing of roles may need to be more commonplace. Traditionally described in the biomedical literature as a source of burden and distress (Stajduhar et al., 2010), the sharing of roles can also be perceived as a fulfilling and rewarding process (Horsfall et al., 2014).

Conclusion

We have traced the origins and development of palliative care and public health as distinct specialties and mapped their now closer association in terms of a new public health approach to end of life care. We have described the range of approaches and perspectives inherent within such a relationship and gone on to critically evaluate the emerging practice and evidence base, integrating rival theories from a range of disciplines along the way.

What is clear is the enormous potential this body of work holds. For palliative care services it has the potential to invigorate questions relating to access and equity in care provision while addressing the growing need for models of care that accommodate old age, frailty, and multimorbidity. Beyond palliative care services it has a role in leading the field of medicine and healthcare into an era represented by co-production and co-design through collaborative practice. This has the potential to recognize people's voices in terms of what matters to them, establish what is truly important to measure, and perhaps bring the notion of healing and 'whole person' care back into medicine.

Such a change is, however, not to be assumed. Ideas relating to a new public health approach to palliative care have been generating academic, political, and social interest for some 20 years now; however, we are yet to see a consistent and sustained change in approach from providers. This is likely in no small part due to the inherent tensions that arise when death is modelled as an exclusively social process with shared responsibility a key theoretical feature. Conceptual blurring of key terms and inconsistencies in terminology provide fertile ground for the misrepresentation of core philosophies while a more critical approach to the use of terms such as social capital is rarely employed by empirical work from within the field of palliative care. At the same time, traditional academic methods of standardization and evaluation are insufficient to address complex social systems. There is therefore a need to better engage with literature from other disciplines where core concepts have already been widely critiqued. This will allow for an evidence base to develop that pertains to the specific approaches that exist within the overarching term of new public health approaches to palliative care.

As evidence for new public health approaches continues to grow and political capital is garnered, we must heed the past lessons from a budding palliative care movement and rethink how we best demonstrate the value of this work. Do we conform to the model of evidence-based practice, showcasing compassionate communities and compassionate cities as an intervention or entity to be standardized and evaluated? Or do we see them as a lens through which people can view and evaluate their own actions helping to build trust, membership, and know-how in order to develop community capacity in real terms? The questions are multiple and profound yet their importance at this stage cannot be overstated.

REFERENCES

Abbey, E., Craig, C., and Mayland, C. 2020. General practitioners' perceptions of compassionate communities: a qualitative study. *BMC Palliative Care*, 19, 1–8.

Abel, J. 2018. Compassionate communities and end-of-life care. *Clinical Medicine (London, England)*, 18, 6–8.

Abel, J. and Kellehear, A. 2016. Palliative care reimagined: a needed shift. *BMJ Supportive & Palliative Care*, 6, 21–26.

Abel, J., Kellehear, A., and Karapliagou, A. 2018a. Palliative care—the new essentials. *Annals of Palliative Medicine*, 7, S3–S14.

Abel, J., Kingston, H., Scally, A., Hartnoll, J., Hannam, G., Thomson-Moore, A., et al. 2018b. Reducing emergency hospital admissions: a population health complex intervention of an enhanced model of primary care and compassionate communities. *British Journal of General Practice*, 68, e803–e810.

Abel, J., Sallnow, L., Murray, S., and Kerin, M. 2016. *Each Community is Prepared to Help: Community Development in End of Life Care—Guidance on Ambition Six*. London: National Council for Palliative Care.

Abel, J., Walter, T., Carey, L. B., Rosenberg, J., Noonan, K., Horsfall, D., et al. 2013. Circles of care: should community development redefine the practice of palliative care? *BMJ Supportive & Palliative Care*, 3, 383–388.

Aoun, S. M. 2019. Bereavement support: from the poor cousin of palliative care to a core asset of compassionate communities. *Progress in Palliative Care*, 28, 107–114.

Aoun, S. M., Abel, J., Rumbold, B., Cross, K., Moore, J., Skeers, P., and Deliens, L. 2020. The Compassionate Communities Connectors model for end-of-life care: a community and health service partnership in Western Australia. *Palliative Care and Social Practice*, 14, 2632352420935130.

Aoun, S. M., Breen, L. J., White, I., Rumbold, B., and Kellehear, A. 2018. What sources of bereavement support are perceived helpful by bereaved people and why? Empirical evidence for the compassionate communities approach. *Palliative Medicine*, 32, 1378–1388.

Ashton, J. and Seymour, H. 1988. *The New Public Health*. Milton Keynes: Open University Press.

Barry, V. and Patel, M. 2013. *An Overview of Compassionate Communities in England*. London: Murray Hall Community Trust and National Council for Palliative Care.

Bourdieu, P. 1986. The forms of capital. In: Richardson, J. (ed.) *Handbook of Theory and Research for the Sociology of Education*, pp. 241–258. New York: Greenwood.

Bristowe, K., Hodson, M., Wee, B., Almack, K., Daveson, B., Koffman, J., et al. 2016. 'What makes it worth the investment to say it?'—Care experiences of lesbian, gay, bisexual and/or trans people facing life-limiting illness: a qualitative interview study. *BMJ Supportive & Palliative Care*, 6, 388.

Bunce, A. 2018. Developing a compassionate community (Compassionate Inverclyde). *International Journal of Integrated Care*, 18, 1–2.

Burbeck, R., Candy, B., Low, J., and Rees, R. 2014. Understanding the role of the volunteer in specialist palliative care: a systematic review and thematic synthesis of qualitative studies. *BMC Palliative Care*, 13, 3.

Burt, J. and Raine, R. 2006. The effect of age on referral to and use of specialist palliative care services in adult cancer patients: a systematic review. *Age and Ageing*, 35, 469–476.

Christakis, N. A. and Fowler, J. H. 2007. The spread of obesity in a large social network over 32 years. *New England Journal of Medicine*, 357, 370–379.

Christakis, N. A. and Fowler, J. H. 2008. The collective dynamics of smoking in a large social network. *New England Journal of Medicine*, 358, 2249–2258.

Coleman, J. S. 1988. Social capital in the creation of human capital. *American Journal of Sociology*, 94, S95–S120.

Commission into the Future of Hospice Care. 2013. *Future Ambitions for Hospice Care: Our Mission and Our Opportunity*. London: Help the Hospices.

Conway, S. 2008. Public health and palliative care: principles into practice? *Critical Public Health*, 18, 405–415.

Cronin, P. 2016. Compassionate communities in Shropshire, West Midlands, England. In: Wegleitner, K., Heimerl, K., and Kellehear, A. (eds.) *Compassionate Communities: Case Studies from Britain and Europe*, pp. 30–45. Abingdon: Routledge.

De Leeuw, E. 2009. Evidence for Healthy Cities: reflections on practice, method and theory. *Health Promotion International*, 24, i19–i36.

Dempers, C. and Gott, M. 2017a. The status of a public health approach to palliative care at New Zealand hospices. *Progress in Palliative Care*, 25, 75–81.

Dempers, C. and Gott, M. 2017b. Which public health approach to palliative care? An integrative literature review. *Progress in Palliative Care*, 25, 1–10.

Douglas, C. 1992. For all the saints. *BMJ*, 304, 579–580.

Dowd, J. J. 1975. Aging as exchange: a preface to theory. *Journal of Gerontology*, 30, 584–594.

Etkind, S., Bone, A., Gomes, B., Lovell, N., Evans, C., Higginson, I., et al. 2017. How many people will need palliative care in 2040? Past trends, future projections and implications for services. *BMC Medicine*, 15, 1–10.

Finch, J. and Mason, J. 1990. Filial obligations and kin support for elderly people. *Ageing and Society*, 10, 151–175.

Fletcher, A., Bonell, C., and Sorhaindo, A. 2011. You are what your friends eat: systematic review of social network analyses of young people's eating behaviours and bodyweight. *Journal of Epidemiology & Community Health*, 65, 548–555.

Francis, R. 2013. *Report of the Mid Staffordshire NHS Foundation Trust Public Inquiry: Analysis of Evidence and Lessons Learned*. London: The Stationery Office.

Glaser, B. G. and Strauss, A. L. 1966. *Awareness of Dying*. New Brunswick, NJ: Transaction Publishers.

Gomez-Batiste, X., Mateu, S., Serra-Jofre, S., Molas, M., Mir-Roca, S., Amblas, J., et al. 2018. Compassionate communities: design and preliminary results of the experience of Vic (Barcelona, Spain) caring city. *Annals of Palliative Medicine*, 7, S32–S41.

Gott, M., Morgan, T., and Williams, L. 2020. Gender and palliative care: a call to arms. *Palliative Care and Social Practice*, 14, 2632352420957997.

Gott, M., Wiles, J., Moeke-Maxwell, T., Black, S., Williams, L., Kerse, N., et al. 2018. What is the role of community at the end of life for people dying in advanced age? A qualitative study with bereaved family carers. *Palliative Medicine,* 32, 268–275.

Grindrod, A. 2020. Choice depends on options: a public health framework incorporating the social determinants of dying to create options at end of life. *Progress in Palliative Care,* 28, 94–100.

Grindrod, A. and Rumbold, B. 2018. Healthy End of Life Project (HELP): a progress report on implementing community guidance on public health palliative care initiatives in Australia. *Annals of Palliative Medicine,* 7, S73–S83.

Hazelwood, M. A. and Patterson, R. M. 2018. Scotland's public health palliative care alliance. *Annals of Palliative Medicine,* 7, S99–S108.

Hinton, J. M. 1964. Problems in the care of the dying. *Journal of Chronic Diseases,* 17, 201–205.

Holt-Lunstad, J., Smith, T. B., and Layton, J. B. 2010. Social relationships and mortality risk: a meta-analytic review. *PLoS Medicine,* 7, e1000316.

Horsfall, D. 2018. Developing compassionate communities in Australia through collective caregiving: a qualitative study exploring network-centred care and the role of the end of life sector. *Annals of Palliative Medicine,* 7, S42–S51.

Horsfall, D., Leonard, R., Noonan, K., and Rosenberg, J. 2013. Working together-apart: exploring the relationships between formal and informal care networks for people dying at home. *Progress in Palliative Care,* 21, 331–336.

Horsfall, D., Noonan, K., and Leonard, R. 2014. Bringing our dying home: how caring for someone at end of life builds social capital and develops compassionate communities. *Health Sociology Review,* 21, 373–382.

Hospice UK. n.d. Compassionate Neighbours [Online]. Available: https://www.hospiceuk.org/what-we-offer/community-volunteering-hub/case-studies/compassionate-neighbours

Huang, H. Y., Kuo, K. M., Lu, I. C., Wu, H., Lin, C. W., Hsieh, M. T., et al. 2019. The impact of health literacy on knowledge, attitude and decision towards hospice care among community-dwelling seniors. *Health & Social Care in the Community,* 27, e724–e733.

Hunter, R. F., De La Haye, K., Murray, J. M., Badham, J., Valente, T. W., Clarke, M., et al. 2019. Social network interventions for health behaviours and outcomes: a systematic review and meta-analysis. *PLoS Medicine,* 16, e1002890.

Johansson, S., Leonard, R., and Noonan, K. 2012. Caring and the generation of social capital: two models for a positive relationship. *International Journal of Social Welfare,* 21, 44–52.

Kawachi, I., Kim, D., Coutts, A., and Subramanian, S. 2004. Commentary: reconciling the three accounts of social capital. *International Journal of Epidemiology,* 33, 682–690.

Kearney, M. 1992. Palliative medicine—just another specialty? *Palliative Medicine,* 6, 39–46.

Kellehear, A. 1999. Health-promoting palliative care: developing a social model for practice. *Mortality,* 4, 75–82.

Kellehear, A. 2005. *Compassionate Cities: Public Health and End-of-Life Care.* Abingdon: Routledge.

Kellehear, A. 2007. The end of death in late modernity: an emerging public health challenge. *Critical Public Health,* 17, 71–79.

Kellehear, A. 2015. The Compassionate City Charter: inviting the cultural and social sectors into end-of-life care. In: Wegleitner, K., Heimerl, K., and Kellehear, A. (eds.) *Compassionate Communities: Case Studies from Britain and Europe*, pp. 76–87. Abingdon: Routledge.

Kellehear, A. 2016. Commentary: public health approaches to palliative care—the progress so far. *Progress in Palliative Care,* 24, 36–38.

Kellehear, A. 2019. Compassionate cities: global significance and meaning for palliative care. *Progress in Palliative Care,* 28, 115–119.

Kelley, M. L., Prince, H., Nadin, S., Brazil, K., Crow, M., Hanson, G., et al. 2018. Developing palliative care programs in Indigenous communities using participatory action research: a Canadian application of the public health approach to palliative care. *Annals of Palliative Medicine,* 7, S52–S72.

Koffman, J., Burke, G., Dias, A., Raval, B., Byrne, J., Gonzales, J., et al. 2007. Demographic factors and awareness of palliative care and related services. *Palliative Medicine,* 21, 145–153.

Kübler-Ross, E., Wessler, S., and Avioli, L. V. 1972. On death and dying. *JAMA,* 221, 174–179.

Kumar, S. 2013. Models of delivering palliative and end-of-life care in India. *Current Opinion in Supportive and Palliative Care,* 7, 216–222.

Kumar, S. 2020. Community participation in palliative care: reflections from the ground. *Progress in Palliative Care,* 28, 23–28.

Kumar, S. K. 2007. Kerala, India: a regional community-based palliative care model. *Journal of Pain & Symptom Management,* 33, 623–627.

Künemund, H. and Rein, M. 1999. There is more to receiving than needing: theoretical arguments and empirical explorations of crowding in and crowding out. *Ageing and Society,* 19, 93–121.

Latkin, C. A. and Knowlton, A. R. 2015. Social network assessments and interventions for health behavior change: a critical review. *Behavioral Medicine,* 41, 90–97.

Leadbeater, C. and Garber, J. 2010. *Dying for Change.* London: Demos.

Leonard, R., Horsfall, D., and Noonan, K. 2010. Models of caring from India and Australia and their relationship to social capital. *Nepalese Journal of Public Policy and Governance,* 26, 15–25.

Leonard, R., Horsfall, D., and Noonan, K. 2015. Identifying changes in the support networks of end-of-life carers using social network analysis. *BMJ Supportive & Palliative Care,* 5, 153–159.

Lewis, J. M., Digiacomo, M., Luckett, T., Davidson, P. M., and Currow, D. C. 2013. A social capital framework for palliative care: supporting health and well-being for people with life-limiting illness and their carers through social relations and networks. *Journal of Pain and Symptom Management,* 45, 92–103.

Librada Flores, S., Herrera Molina, E., Boceta Osuna, J., Mota Vargas, R., and Nabal Vicuna, M. 2018. All with You: a new method for developing compassionate communities-experiences in Spain and Latin-America. *Annals of Palliative Medicine,* 7, S15–S31.

Librada-Flores, S., Nabal-Vicuna, M., Forero-Vega, D., Munoz-Mayorga, I., and Guerra-Martin, M. D. 2020. Implementation models of compassionate communities and compassionate cities at the end of life: a systematic review. *International Journal of Environmental Research and Public Health,* 17, 6271.

MacDonald-Wallis, K., Jago, R., and Sterne, J. A. 2012. Social network analysis of childhood and youth physical activity: a systematic review. *American Journal of Preventive Medicine,* 43, 636–642.

Marie Curie Memorial Foundation. 1952. *Joint National Cancer Survey Committee of the Marie Curie Memorial Foundation and the Queen's Institute of District Nursing. Report on a National Survey Concerning Patients with Cancer Nursed at Home.* London: Marie Curie Memorial Foundation.

McLoughlin, K., Rhatigan, J., McGilloway, S., Kellehear, A., Lucey, M., Twomey, F., et al. 2015. INSPIRE (INvestigating Social and PractIcal suppoRts at the End of life): pilot randomised trial of a community social and practical support intervention for adults with life-limiting illness. *BMC Palliative Care,* 14, 65.

Mills, J., Rosenberg, J. P., and McInerney, F. 2015. Building community capacity for end of life: an investigation of community capacity and its implications for health-promoting palliative care in the Australian Capital Territory. *Critical Public Health,* 25, 218–230.

Mitchell, S. L., Kiely, D. K., and Hamel, M. B. 2004. Dying with advanced dementia in the nursing home. *Archives of Internal Medicine,* 164, 321–326.

Morgan, L. M. 2001. Community participation in health: perpetual allure, persistent challenge. *Health Policy and Planning,* 16, 221–230.

Murray, S. A., Kendall, M., Boyd, K., and Sheikh, A. 2005. Illness trajectories and palliative care. *BMJ,* 330, 1007–1011.

Murray, S. A. and Mason, B. 2010. Palliative care looking towards 2020. *Australasian Medical Journal,* 3, 318–324.

Noonan, K. 2018. Death literacy—developing a tool to measure the social impact of public health initiatives. *Annals of Palliative Medicine,* 7, AB007.

Noonan, K., Horsfall, D., Leonard, R., and Rosenberg, J. 2016. Developing death literacy. *Progress in Palliative Care,* 24, 31–35.

Patel, M. 2016. Compassionate communities in Sandwell, West Midlands, England. In: Wegleitner, K., Heimerl, K., and Kellehear, A. (eds.) *Compassionate Communities: Case Studies from Britain and Europe,* pp. 46–59. Abingdon: Routledge.

Paul, S. and Sallnow, L. 2013. Public health approaches to end-of-life care in the UK: an online survey of palliative care services. *BMJ Supportive & Palliative Care,* 3, 196–199.

Payne, S. 2007. Public health and palliative care. *Progress in Palliative Care,* 15, 101–102.

Pesut, B., Duggleby, W., Warner, G., Fassbender, K., Antifeau, E., Hooper, B., et al. 2017. Volunteer navigation partnerships: piloting a compassionate community approach to early palliative care. *BMC Palliative Care,* 17, 2.

Pesut, B., Robinson, C. A., and Bottorff, J. L. 2014. Among neighbors: an ethnographic account of responsibilities in rural palliative care. *Palliative & Supportive Care,* 12, 127–138.

Pfaff, K. A., Dolovich, L., Howard, M., Sattler, D., Zwarenstein, M., and Marshall, D. 2020. Unpacking 'the cloud': a framework for implementing public health approaches to palliative care. *Health Promotion International,* 35, 160–170.

Portes, A. 1998. Social capital: its origins and applications in modern sociology. *Annual Review of Sociology,* 24, 1–24.

Putnam, R. 2000. *Bowling Alone: The Collapse and Revival of American Community.* New York: Simon & Schuster.

Rawlings, D., Litster, C., Miller-Lewis, L., Tieman, J., and Swetenham, K. 2020. The voices of death doulas about their role in end-of-life care. *Health & Social Care in the Community,* 28, 12–21.

Reeves, D., Blickem, C., Vassilev, I., Brooks, H., Kennedy, A., Richardson, G., et al. 2014. The contribution of social networks to the health and self-management of patients with long-term conditions: a longitudinal study. *PLoS One,* 9, e98340.

Rosenberg, J. 2011. Whose business is dying? Death, the home and palliative care. *Cultural Studies Review,* 17, 15–30.

Rosenberg, J. P., Horsfall, D., Leonard, R., and Noonan, K. 2015. Informal caring networks for people at end of life: building social capital in Australian communities. *Health Sociology Review,* 24, 29–37.

Rosenberg, J. P., Mills, J., and Rumbold, B. 2016. Putting the 'public' into public health: community engagement in palliative and end of life care. *Progress in Palliative Care,* 24, 1–3.

Rumbold, B. and Aoun, S. 2014. Bereavement and palliative care: a public health perspective. *Progress in Palliative Care,* 22, 131–135.

Sallnow, L. 2017. Collective social capital: a study of new public health and end-of-life care. Doctoral thesis, University of Edinburgh.

Sallnow, L., Kumar, S., and Numpeli, M. 2010. Home-based palliative care in Kerala, India: the Neighbourhood Network in Palliative Care. *Progress in Palliative Care,* 18, 14–17.

Sallnow, L. and Paul, S. 2015. Understanding community engagement in end-of-life care: developing conceptual clarity. *Critical Public Health,* 25, 231–238.

Sallnow, L., Richardson, H., Murray, S. A., and Kellehear, A. 2016a. The impact of a new public health approach to end-of-life care: a systematic review. *Palliative Medicine,* 30, 200–211.

Sallnow, L., Tishelman, C., Lindqvist, O., Richardson, H., and Cohen, J. 2016b. Research in public health and end-of-life care—building on the past and developing the new. *Progress in Palliative Care,* 24, 25–30.

Saunders, C. 1998. Foreword. In: Doyle, D., Hanks, G. W. C., and Macdonald, N. (eds.) *Oxford Textbook of Palliative Medicine,* 2nd ed., pp. v–viii. Oxford: Oxford University Press.

Saunders, C. 2006. *The Evolution of Palliative Care. Cicely Saunders—Selected Writings 1958–2004.* Oxford: Oxford University Press.

Sawka, K. J., McCormack, G. R., Nettel-Aguirre, A., Hawe, P., and Doyle-Baker, P. K. 2013. Friendship networks and physical activity and sedentary behavior among youth: a systematized review. *International Journal of Behavioral Nutrition and Physical Activity,* 10, 130.

Sawyer, J. M., Asgr, R., Todd Fordham, F. N., and Porter, J. D. H. 2018. A public health approach to palliative care in the response to drug resistant TB: an ethnographic study. *BMC Palliative Care,* 17, 120.

Sawyer, J. M., Sallnow, L., Kupeli, N., Stone, P., and Sampson, E. L. 2019. Social networks, social capital and end-of-life care for people with dementia: a realist review. *BMJ Open,* 9, e030703.

Sawyer, J. M. and Taylor, R. 2018. Palliative medicine: has there been mission rift? *European Journal of Palliative Care,* 25, 6–8.

Stajduhar, K., Funk, L., Jakobsson, E., and Ohlen, J. 2010. A critical analysis of health promotion and 'empowerment' in the context of palliative family care-giving. *Nursing Inquiry,* 17, 221–230.

Stjernsward, J. 2007. Palliative care: the public health strategy. *Journal of Public Health Policy,* 28, 42–55.

Szreter, S. and Woolcock, M. 2004. Health by association? Social capital, social theory, and the political economy of public health. *International Journal of Epidemiology,* 33, 650–667.

The Economist Intelligence Unit. 2015. *The 2015 Quality of Death Index: Ranking Palliative Care Across the World.* London: The Economist.

Townsend, P. 1962. *The Last Refuge: A Survey of Residential Institutions and Homes for the Aged in England and Wales.* London: Routledge.

Van Oorschot, W. and Arts, W. 2005. The social capital of European welfare states: the crowding out hypothesis revisited. *Journal of European Social Policy,* 15, 5–26.

Vanderstichelen, S., Cohen, J., Van Wesemael, Y., Deliens, L., and Chambaere, K. 2020. The liminal space palliative care volunteers occupy and their roles within it: a qualitative study. *BMJ Supportive & Palliative Care,* 10, e28.

Wakefield, S. E. and Poland, B. 2005. Family, friend or foe? Critical reflections on the relevance and role of social capital in health promotion and community development. *Social Science & Medicine,* 60, 2819–2832.

Wegleitner, K. and Schuchter, P. 2018. Caring communities as collective learning process: findings and lessons learned from a participatory research project in Austria. *Annals of Palliative Medicine,* 7, S84–S98.

Whitelaw, S. and Clark, D. 2019. Palliative care and public health: an asymmetrical relationship? *Palliative Care,* 12, 1178224218819745.

Williams, A. M., Eby, J. A., Crooks, V. A., Stajduhar, K., Giesbrecht, M., Vuksan, M., et al. 2011. Canada's Compassionate Care Benefit: is it an adequate public health response to addressing the issue of caregiver burden in end-of-life care? *BMC Public Health,* 11, 335.

Williams, L. A., Giddings, L. S., Bellamy, G., and Gott, M. 2017. 'Because it's the wife who has to look after the man': a descriptive qualitative study of older women and the intersection of gender and the provision of family caregiving at the end of life. *Palliative Medicine,* 31, 223–230.

World Health Organization. 1986. *Ottawa Charter for Health Promotion.* Ottawa: WHO/Canadian Public Health Association/ Health Canada.

World Health Organization. 2014. *WHA67, Resolution; Strengthening of Palliative Care as a Component of Comprehensive Care Throughout the Life Course. Sixty-Seventh World Health Assembly, Geneva.* Geneva: World Health Organization.

23 The evidence of the importance of informal care networks

Rosemary Leonard and Debbie Horsfall

Introduction

In this chapter, we focus on informal care networks for people at the end of life. These networks are a subset of social networks which reflect two dimensions: first, they are informal rather than formal networks meaning they are comprised of patients, carers, and other people engaging with the health system rather than the networks among professional care providers; second, they are primarily concerned with the emotional and physical work of caring for each other at times of death, dying, loss, and caregiving.

Informal social networks consist of those relationships one circulates within, be they family and friends, work colleagues, virtually, the neighbourhood, local spiritual groups, or leisure clubs. Many overlap and others are quite distinct. Networks of care come together, usually from these more general social networks, in times of need to support people how and where they want to be supported. This is not a new idea and has been around in the gerontology, disability, social work, and childcare literature for over 20 years (Prosser and Moss, 1996; Bibgy, 1997; Keating et al., 2003). It is, though, a new idea in the palliative care field.

Where there has been attention on networks for end of life care, the focus has been on networks of formal service providers. In the UK, primary care networks were established in 2019. These are networks of primary healthcare providers such as general practitioners and pharmacists. Also, the literature talks about 'integrated networks' which usually means integration across different services with the aim of providing continuity of care.

However, from a new public health perspective, informal networks of care are, we believe, a natural fit as they place relationships and connections as central to all models of care. Here, professionals' work is to identify, mobilize, initiate, and/or maintain these networks and then provide expertise and build resources as needed by the networks already surrounding individuals (Brown and Walter, 2014). In this way, caring and dying become *everyone's business* (Abel et al., 2016)—at least the business of the network.

The useful distinction between care networks and social or support networks was drawn by Keating and colleagues (2003). According to them, a person's support network usually comprises kin and friendship ties and there is a reciprocal expectation that this network provides 'emotional and tangible' support to each other over a period of time and holds within it a series of 'nested dependencies' (Kittay, 2011). Keating and colleagues argue that a care network is a 'functional subset' (2003, p. 121) of this. Care networks emerge from the support network to provide specific help and assistance because of a particular need—in this case, dying. It is Keating and colleagues' definition of care networks which is informing us in this chapter.

Why are informal networks necessary?

There will continue to be a large and growing need for informal home-based caring

Informal caring is extensive and estimated at approximately $15 billion worth of unpaid work annually in Australia (Carers Australia, 2020). It is the second most common reason for early retirement after one's own health needs (over 115,000 retired with an average age of 56 years) (Australian Bureau of Statistics, 2019). Additionally, institutionalized care at the end of life is not a universally viable solution. It is too expensive and found to be uncaring and at times unsafe (Royal Commission into Aged Care Quality and Safety, 2020). The bulk of end of life caring is conducted in the home and most people express a desire to be cared for and die at home (Palliative Care Australia, 2010). The average length of community-based palliative care is 119 days of which 117 days of care are provided by family, friends, neighbours, and community members at home during the dying process (Rumbold, 2009).

In the 'Caring at End of Life' (CAEOL)project research, approximately 90% of caring networks enabled the dying person to die in their place of choice—at home. This was achieved as the caring networks supported the primary carer to keep on caring by protecting the carer—and each other—from social isolation and physical and emotional exhaustion (Horsfall et al., 2015; Sallnow and Paul, 2015; Sallnow et al., 2016). Overwhelmingly, research participants agreed that without a strong network of support caring in the home to the point of death, this would not have been possible.

Nature of care work: complex, demanding, and emotional

Perhaps one of the distinguishing features of caring for the dying at home is that end of life care can involve complex and demanding care tasks (Visser et al., 2004) within an atmosphere of heightened emotions and lack of community-based knowledge about death and dying as a result of institutionalization (Howarth, 2007; Kellehear, 2007). As such, what is required are competent and compassionate care networks comprising both formal and informal carers to step up and share the work be it physical, emotional, spiritual, or medical. In reality, many of the tasks that need to be done are tasks of everyday living: taking children to school, shopping, paying bills, making sure there is enough food for the myriad of visitors who flow in and out of the home at such times, and having the right medications at hand when needed. And these require no special skill, just life experience and the ability and willingness to help (Abel et al., 2016).

An effective caring network can replace the burden of caring with positive experiences

Most of the literature about home-based caregivers at the end of life discusses burden, isolation, stigma, financial cost, and the overall negative effects on carers' physical and mental health (Veloso and Tripodoro, 2016). This is especially so in the biomedical research literature (Hagell et al., 2017) with informal, usually primary, carers being cast as potential hidden patients. We do not doubt that this burden can be the dominant experience of many carers. However, there is also evidence that caring at the end of life is rewarding and provides meaning and purpose to people's lives (Zapart et al., 2007) in addition to possibly increasing a person's social relationships and positive attachment to place (Woodman et al., 2016; Leonard et al., 2017; Horsfall et al., 2019). Positive experiences of caring are often due to the fact that when informal care networks are active, primary carers are no longer isolated in their role and are less likely to experience burnout, a leading cause of hospital admissions immediately prior to death (Woodman et al., 2016). Sallnow and colleagues (2016) found improved outcomes for carers such as decreased social isolation and fatigue and improved social support. Also, carers experienced less burden when a variety of tasks were shared among the network over time (Tolkacheva et al., 2011).

Clearly, though, there is a need to ensure that informal carers are comprehensively supported (Hughes, 2015). Our argument is that this may be best achieved through the mobilizing and maintaining of combined formal and informal networks of care. In her work on caring for older LGBTI people, Hughes (2009) draws on the notion of care networks as communities of practice (Lave and Wenger, 1991) which come together to engage in a particular task in our case the provision of in-home care to a dying person and their carers. This is a useful conceptualization as it draws attention to the learning potential of such endeavours as a group identity is formed and people engage in a myriad of ways in *a shared repertoire of practices* (Hughes, 2009). In this way, the social resources of the community to care at the end of life are developed.

Caring networks can have flow-on benefits to the community

Potentially, caring can increase community awareness of death and dying and increase community capacity to care. From the CAEOL research (Horsfall et al., 2015), it was clear that when a caring network functioned well and carers were comprehensively supported, everybody benefited and the effects flowed into the community. Over the period of caring, networks grew in number of participants and the relationships of the original network members could grow stronger (Leonard et al., 2015). Networks can promote a 'ripple effect' whereby those engaged in community work at the end of life took knowledge and skills they learnt into end of life care.

> It makes everyone stronger and they know what they can do as a community ... I think a lot of people realise the capabilities that they have got in personal situations and how they can help other personal situations. (Horsfall et al., 2015, Focus Group 2)

Networks were maintained after the bereavement, and people took their experiential knowledge on to other ventures: undergoing further education in ageing or death and dying, becoming a health advocate, setting up palliative care support groups, or going on to be part of another network of care. In this way, they built the death literacy of the community and increased its capacity to care in the future (Noonan et al., 2016; Leonard et al., 2021).

More broadly, home-based networked caring recognizes the multiple interdependencies we have on each other where caring about and caring for one another is underpinned by a set of ethical moral practices (Tronto, 1993) which improve the well-being of us all. These benefits go beyond caring. Experiences around death are powerful and the strong bonds that can form around it increase social capital which can be mobilized for a wide variety of goals.

Networks can facilitate better use of formal services

Larger social networks including friends were predictive of improved confidence in asking for assistance and an increased likelihood of palliative care involvement (Sallnow et al., 2016). In the CAEOL project, we found that caring networks were most effective when at least one person in the informal network had some knowledge of the health system so they were able to help access the formal support that was available (Horsfall et al., 2015).

Networks assist with grief and bereavement

Unlike most end of life services which end at the point of death, informal networks are usually maintained after the bereavement, often for several years, and people continue to support the primary carer over this period (Leonard et al., 2017). There is also evidence of the impact of peer support networks in a variety of settings on improved outcomes in bereavement, from childhood death to suicide (Metel and Barnes, 2011; Dopp and Cain, 2012).

Revealing care networks

Given the significance of informal networks, it is important to make them salient in any discussion of end of life care. Although there has been a growing recognition of the needs of home-based carers of the dying (Morris et al., 2015), most of this literature concerns the primary carer, who is usually but not always a family member. This is a limited view of in-home caring. In contrast, a network approach reveals the web of caring and supportive relationships which surround the dying person, their primary carer, and their informal caring network of friends, family, neighbours, and work colleagues (Keating et al., 2003; Leonard et al., 2015).

Visual depiction of social networks is a powerful way of communicating the importance of the network and this was the primary method we used in our research over 10 years into care networks at the end of life. Care networks have four important dimensions: the number of people involved, the strength of the relationships (density), the types of people involved, and the activities they perform.

In this section, four methods of presenting care networks are examined.

Descriptive maps drawn by researchers or clinicians

In the first example (Fig. 23.1a), we have adapted Abel and colleagues' (2016) use of the network map which looks for weaknesses in the care network which need to be addressed. Here, it is used as a tool to ask 'Who is in the network? Are they positive or negative relationships? What are they already doing? What still needs to be done? Who can do it? Who is the network coordinator?' This is an important set of questions as it makes sure that the tasks of caring are attended to holistically. It is also individualized to a particular patient and their networks of care.

In the second example (Fig. 23.1b), Young and colleagues (2016) invited students to work with people with long-term conditions to generate a map of the community of clinical practice. Although its focus is formal service provision, it does include informal carers as well. Fig. 23.1b clearly identifies the members of the community of clinical practice for the patient and their roles. The concentric circles show the importance of the services to the patient although there seems to be a mixture of dimensions: *core* and *peripheral* refer to importance whereas *occasional* refers to frequency and *active* and *transactional* describe the nature of the interaction. Another missing element is the connections among the network members. A frequent complaint from carers is that the services are uncoordinated (Rosenberg et al., 2018). Extending the map to identify connections among the community of clinical practice would identify any communication deficits which need to be addressed.

Participatory network mapping

The third method of visual depiction is participatory network mapping (illustrated in the following case studies) which requires the collective drawing of the maps by the network of carers. It involves writing the names of all the network members around the edge of a large piece of paper and then inviting the attendees to join their own name to other names with whom they are acquainted. Coloured markers can be used to indicate differences in the strength of their relationships indicating strong or weak ties between them.

There are several advantages of the group approach. The participants see the interrelationships among the group members not just with the patient or principal carer. They can describe their activities so that the researcher (or health worker) understands what a participant meant by a strong tie or a weak tie. Further, the participants can give interpretive feedback by reflecting on the maps in front of them thus providing the first level of analysis. The disadvantages may be that (1) there is group pressure to say relationships are stronger than they are or (2) to ignore serious divisions or tensions. In the first case, the participants are given clear guidance as to the meaning of tie strength in terms of behaviours, avoiding general terms such as friend or acquaintance. In the second case, it is unlikely that two factions would both attend a focus group if there were a serious division; however, the absence of one faction would limit the results.

Computer-generated maps

The fourth example is the use of a computer-generated map using a package such as NetDraw (Borgatti et al., 2002). Such programmes have a variety of ways of presenting the information. For example, the strength of relationships either through colour or the thickness of lines (called ties) between people (called nodes). The different categories of nodes can be present through shape or colour. These programmes have the strong advantage of being able to adjust the map so that people with more ties and stronger ties are placed in the middle of the map and those with fewer or weaker ties are placed on the periphery, thus giving a stronger visual representation of the importance of the various people in the network.

The data collection procedure usually employed by social network researchers is to use individual questionnaires in which participants list the names of network members and then identify the strength of their relationship to each through a Likert scale or similar method. In case studies 1 and 2, the participatory network maps were converted into NetDraw maps (Borgatti et al., 2002) which are presented as figures in later sections. For case study 4, questionnaires were used to collect data for the group analysis and later for the NetDraw representation.

Statistical analysis

Numerous statistics have been devised to summarize the key attributes of networks (Leonard et al., 2015) with various statistical packages for the analysis. As with all statistics, it is important to choose the most meaningful for the data and the research question. In the case of caring networks, size, density, transitivity, and principal carer's betweenness can be useful. They can be defined as follows:

- *Size* is the number of individuals or nodes in a network which is basic information that is always relevant.
- *Density* is the number of ties divided by the number of possible ties. An increase in density indicates people are developing more relationships within the network. If the strength of the relationships is also reported, the density can take that into account and show changes in the average strength of ties in the network.
- *Transitivity* refers to the balance and reciprocity in the relationship among three individuals. High transitivity indicates that people are connecting with each other in egalitarian and cooperative ways. If the members of the networks are only connecting with the principal carer and not each other then there will be low transitivity, indicating that the principal carer does the bulk of the communication.
- The *principal carer's betweenness* value indicates the degree to which the carer acts as the only bridge between two other individuals. A decrease in the betweenness or bridging function of the main carer indicates that she, or he, no longer needs to be the sole coordinator of the caring. People with high betweenness might be deliberately acting as gatekeepers to control the flow of information.

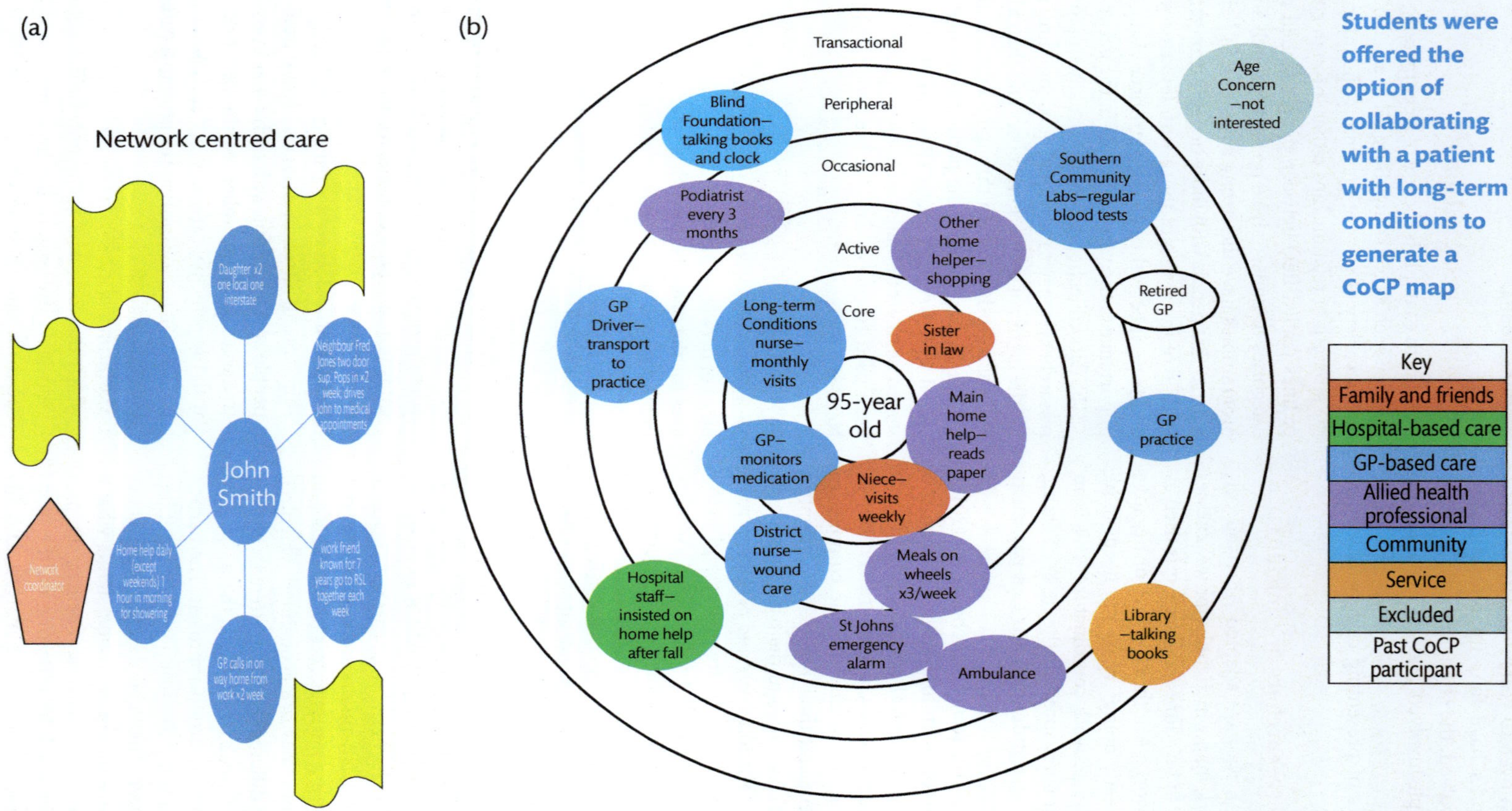

Fig. 23.1 Examples of descriptive maps drawn by researchers or clinicians.

(a) Source: data from Abel, J., Sallnow, L., Murray, S. A. & Kerin, M. 2016. *Each community is prepared to help: Community development in end of life care—guidance on ambition six.* National Council for Palliative Care UK. (b) Reproduced with permission from Young, J., et al. 2016. An exercise to map patient-centred care networks. *The Clinical Teacher*, 13, 448–450.

Case studies

The following three case studies come from the CAEOL preliminary and main projects.

Participants

For the preliminary study, participants were the caring networks of ten people who had, or were, receiving support from the not-for-profit service, Home Hospice. For the main project, there were 23 focus groups, 34 primary carer interviews, and 17 outer network interviews, people who were identified by the caring network as having an important role but were on the periphery of the network.

Procedure

The procedure had three elements; photo-elicitation, focus groups with the caring networks, and network mapping exercise conducted in the focus group of the caring network.

For the network mapping exercise, the materials were two large sheets of paper and three colours of pens. Participants were given three different coloured pens—red, blue, and yellow—representing three different strengths of relationship:

- Yellow indicated a weak tie (e.g. a person who is recognized as being seen about the area, or serving in a shop).
- Blue indicated someone who is known (e.g. the make-up of their family, their work, their interests).
- Red indicated a relationship where there is a stronger connection (e.g. regular shared work or leisure over a long period, or exchange of personal information or feelings are expressed).

Network members' initials were written in a large circle on the paper and people indicated with colour of pen their connections with other participants at time 1, when caring began. The process was repeated on the second sheet for connections for time 2, the present time. In addition, new names were added for new network members or people a participant has come to know through being part of the caring network but who were peripheral to the network. For example, a participant might have volunteered to collect children from school and thus connected with the children's teachers.

For the CAEOL main project, a variation to the procedure was introduced. Participants were asked to complete a sheet where they wrote the numbers 0, 1, 2, or 3 to indicate the strength of their connections with other members where 0 was no relationship and 1–3 were, respectively, the same as yellow, blue, red. New names could be added to the list. These lines were then drawn on to the large sheet of paper to make them visible. This procedure also reduced the effects of social desirability on the ratings.

The first level of analysis was the focus group discussion. Changes from time 1 to time 2 in the number and strength of connections between network members were immediately obvious to the participants and researchers and were discussed *in situ*.

For the next level of analysis, NetDraw in Ucinet (Borgatti et al., 2002) was used to quantify the changes in network size, density, and principal carer betweenness.

Each of the following case studies illustrates some of the diversity in the way informal care networks operate.

Case study 1: patient's husband stressed the value of privacy

Doreen[1] had died of cancer 8 months before and she had been cared for by her husband Laurie and daughter Lorraine. The other daughter, Heather, was less involved, but both had children and lived reasonably nearby. Of those who attended the focus group, Laurie and Heather's friend David were the two men while Lorraine's husband minded the children outside, but he had a few words to say at the end. The women were Doreen's daughters, sister Shirley, and a teenage granddaughter.

> Lorraine: You had neighbours who offered to help but whether the offer was taken up or not is a different thing.
>
> Laurie: We're private people. We don't believe in running over there and going in the house and then run over here and come into this one.

It was not clear that Doreen shared this concern with privacy especially as one of the photos from the photo elicitation was of the cordless phone they had bought so she could talk to her family and friends from her bed. There was quite a lot of talk about equipment to create self-sufficiency. For example, Laurie and Lorraine's husband had built a ramp for the wheelchair:

> Laurie: We were self-sufficient. If she wanted it, we got it.

There was a strong respect for the doctors and, despite having the support of Home Hospice, a not for profit that provided support for carers, when Doreen lost her mobility, she went into the palliative care unit at the hospital. This decision was reinforced by Shirley who had looked after her brother. The doctor had insisted the brother go to hospital where he died 2 days later. However, Shirley said she was glad because he had all the right care there.

The maps (Fig. 23.2) show a number of subgroups mainly around the daughters' families and friends. David, the friend of Heather, had just been part of her ten-pin bowling group when Doreen fell ill. David had been supportive and now they are close friends and David indicated a strong tie to Laurie and moderate ties to Lorraine and her husband and family.

In reflecting on the network maps, those around the table felt there had been little change because the strong family bonds were still there.

> Shirley: I think ... it has stayed much the same ... I think Laurie has been the anchor pin in this situation and it is a credit to him that my relationship and those of Doreen's brothers and sisters have stayed the same.
>
> Lorraine: People are there but it's that accepting of their help or feeling proud—'I'm fine, I'm fine'—that sort of thing. Some relationships have changed. Some may have deteriorated but I think on the whole they haven't greatly changed and perhaps Mum's death was the catalyst to bring us back together.

The general feeling was that one might expect the deterioration of relationships in a difficult period, but they had managed to avoid that. There had been tensions between the sisters about the

1 Only first names are given to protect confidentiality.

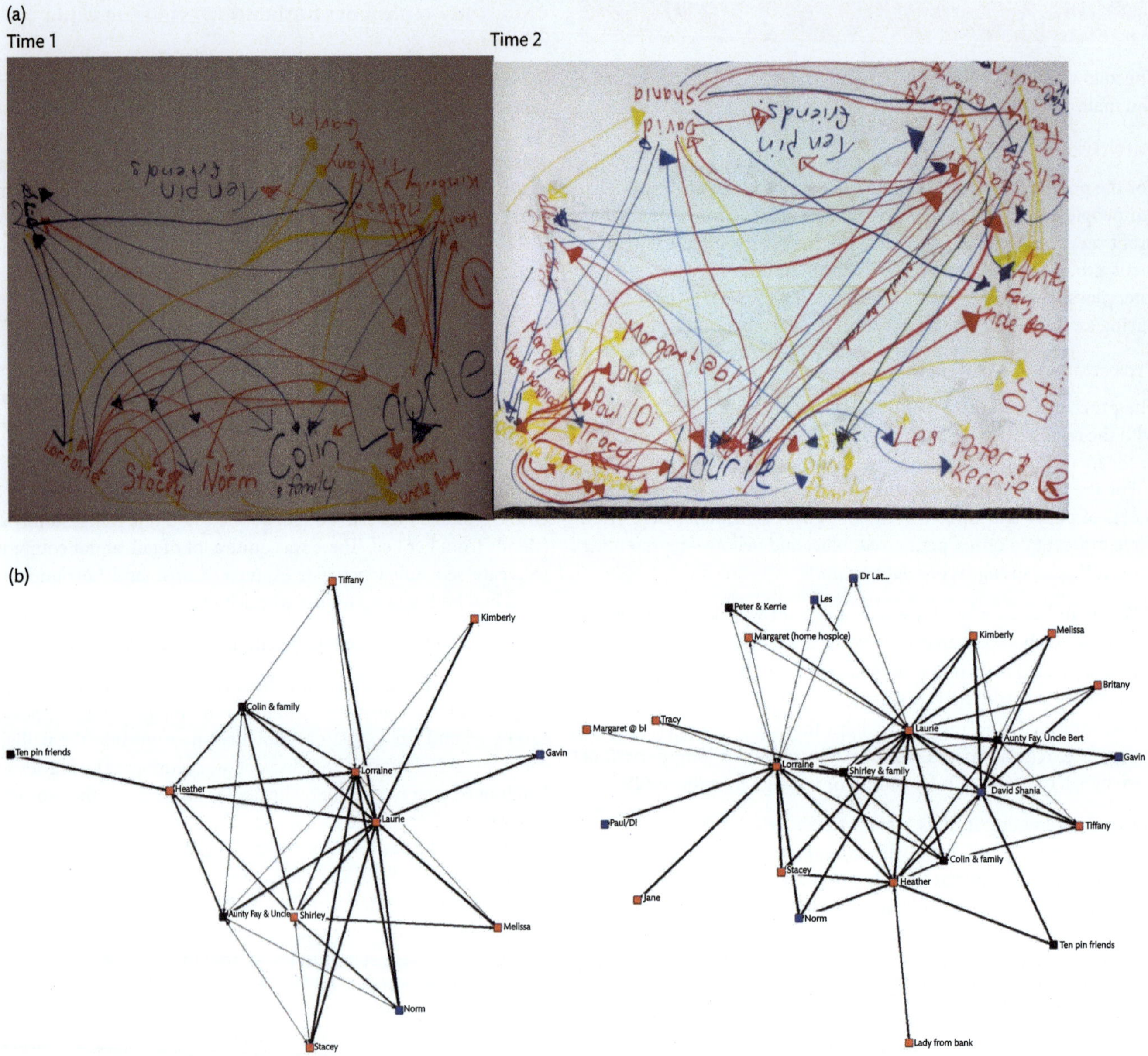

Key for participatory network mapping

Red lines—strong ties
Blue lines—medium ties
Yellow lines—weak ties

Key for NetDraw maps

Red nodes—female
Blue nodes—male
Thickest line—strongest ties
Medium thickness—medium strength ties
Thin lines—weak ties

Fig. 23.2 Case study 1 focus group network maps. (a) Time 1 when caring began and time 2 the time of the research both with participatory network maps and (b) NetDraw maps.

workload and if their mother had needed care for much longer than the 12 weeks then there could well have been signs of burnout and deep resentments. The focus group provided time for reflection and connection. At the end, the two sisters went off for a walk together.

Despite the participants' opinions, it appeared to the researchers that the map from time 2 was larger than at time 1. This was very clear in the NetDraw maps and the statistical analysis which showed that the network had grown from 13 to 24 people. With an increase in the size of the network, density decreased over time from 0.91 out of a maximum of 3 at the beginning to 0.45 out of 3 at the end. This decrease was mainly caused by most people becoming involved by connecting to Laurie alone or Lorraine and

Laurie and not to the whole family. The discussion showed that the role of these newcomers was to provide emotional support rather than practical work or hands-on care. Laurie did not accept the intrusion into the home. However, the participants were correct if the focus was solely on those who were in the original network. Considering only the original 13 members, at time 2 the density remained virtually the same as at time 1 (0.91 to 0.92 out of a maximum of 3) so there was no strengthening or weakening of the original relationships.

Other statistics also supported this pattern of a loose network with Laurie and Lorraine at the centre and little interaction among the other network members. Of all the potentially transitive triads, 52% are transitive at the beginning. When 11 people joined the network during the caring period, transitivity decreased to 36%. These new people formed more potentially transitive triads, but few new transitive triads are formed as people connect only with Laurie or Lorraine.

The results for betweenness are perhaps the most telling. Over the period of caring, Laurie's betweenness increased from 16.4 to 71.9. Lorraine's betweenness increased even more from 16.4 to 99.8 and only two other network members had even moderate betweenness at the end of caring (33.9 and 29.4), thus demonstrating how communication was not dispersed and Laurie and Lorraine were the ones doing the lion's share of communication with the network members.

As an overall reflection, we surmise that the situation for case study 1 is very likely to be commonplace. Caring was provided by immediate family with a high risk of burnout or conflict if it was prolonged. Other family and friends provided emotional support by phone or internet but very little in the way of practical support. To use Keating's (2003) terminology, they had a good social support network but an inadequate caring network. When the caring became too difficult, the patient was transferred to hospital to die. In this case the limitations on the role of the caring network were created by the head of the household's concern for privacy.

Case study 2: principal carer was encouraged to accept help

After discussions with her husband, Jo brought her mother to their home and cared for her there until she died. There were five children at home, so Jo already had a busy life. The children, neighbours, friends, and friends of Jo's mother all offered help. At first, Jo tried to be strong but an important role of the Home Hospice mentor was to encourage her to accept help.

> Mentor: She was saying how she felt really bad because the kids had had McDonalds for tea for the last five nights in a row. So we talked about that and she was telling me about ten minutes later how someone had offered to make some lasagnes for her to put in the freezer and the carer had said 'Oh no, no'. So I gently pointed out that she could of had lasagne instead of McDonalds. So through that I could talk about what's it like accepting help from people and how people offer because they really want to so it's ok to say 'Yes' to that support.

Clearly the maps (Fig. 23.3) speak for themselves and the participants had no difficulty in recognizing that the size of their network had increased; indeed it had increased from 16 to 24 members. With the increase in network size, the density decreased from 1.48 to 1.00. However, the participants reported that relationships had become stronger. When the density is calculated among the 16 individuals who had been involved from the beginning, it indeed showed an increase from 1.47 to 1.55 out of a possible 3, reflecting a slight strengthening of relationships among the initial group.

Transitivity is very high with 78% at the beginning. With more people joining the network, transitivity reduced to 62% after the caring period because the newcomers were not as well networked as the initial members.

When caring began, Jo and her close friend Nikki were highly involved in the network and acted as bridges between other people. Jo's betweenness was relatively high at time 1 at 15.8. Her friend Nikki (1) also had high betweenness at 11.9. By the end of caring, Jo's betweenness had increased to 23.5; however, the involved people had become more involved and Cassie, Donna, Madi, and Nikki all had betweenness values that were similar to Jo's.

The discussion gave insights into the various roles of the network members: washing, gardening, taking kids to dance classes, and bringing food. Even Shelley who could not bring herself to come into the home and is depicted on the edge of the network, made a valuable contribution by bringing food.

Comparing case study 2 with case study 1, we see that the networks were similar in size, but Jo had a much stronger network with higher density, and transitivity. Most significantly, in terms of carer burnout we found that whereas Lorraine and Laurie were shouldering almost all the work of connection with extremely high betweenness scores at the end of caring, Jo's inner network became more involved and there were five people with similar betweenness scores.

Case study 3: increasing strength of relationship with a service provider

In the main study, a major focus was the relationship between the informal care network, the wider community, and the formal service providers. Network maps distinguished between family, friend, community, and service providers using different-shaped nodes (circle, square, diamond, and triangle respectively). Case study 4 illustrates a network where the principal carer who was struggling with diabetes herself was looking after her mother who was dying of cancer, assisted by her family, friends, and neighbours. When caring began, the palliative care nurse was mainly connected to the daughter of the principal carer. When caring ended, he was also well connected with the principal carer and three other network members.

The carer was greatly appreciative of his commitment and he was available to come at any time she called. Even though the carer had a nursing background, she found that she needed his help with the equipment. Further, she had some very poor experiences with her mother's doctor who would not do house calls and insisted the mother be brought to the surgery for every script, even for morphine when she was in pain. The carer described a horror day when she was unwell but had taken her mother to the doctor for morphine and then left the script of the roof of the car when she drove home. Still the doctor would not write another without seeing the patient again and the carer had to warn all the pharmacies about the lost script. It was a rural area, so the choice of doctors was limited; however, this palliative care nurse found another doctor who was far more supportive.

Out of the 36 networks studied, there were only eight examples where the strength or number of ties with service providers

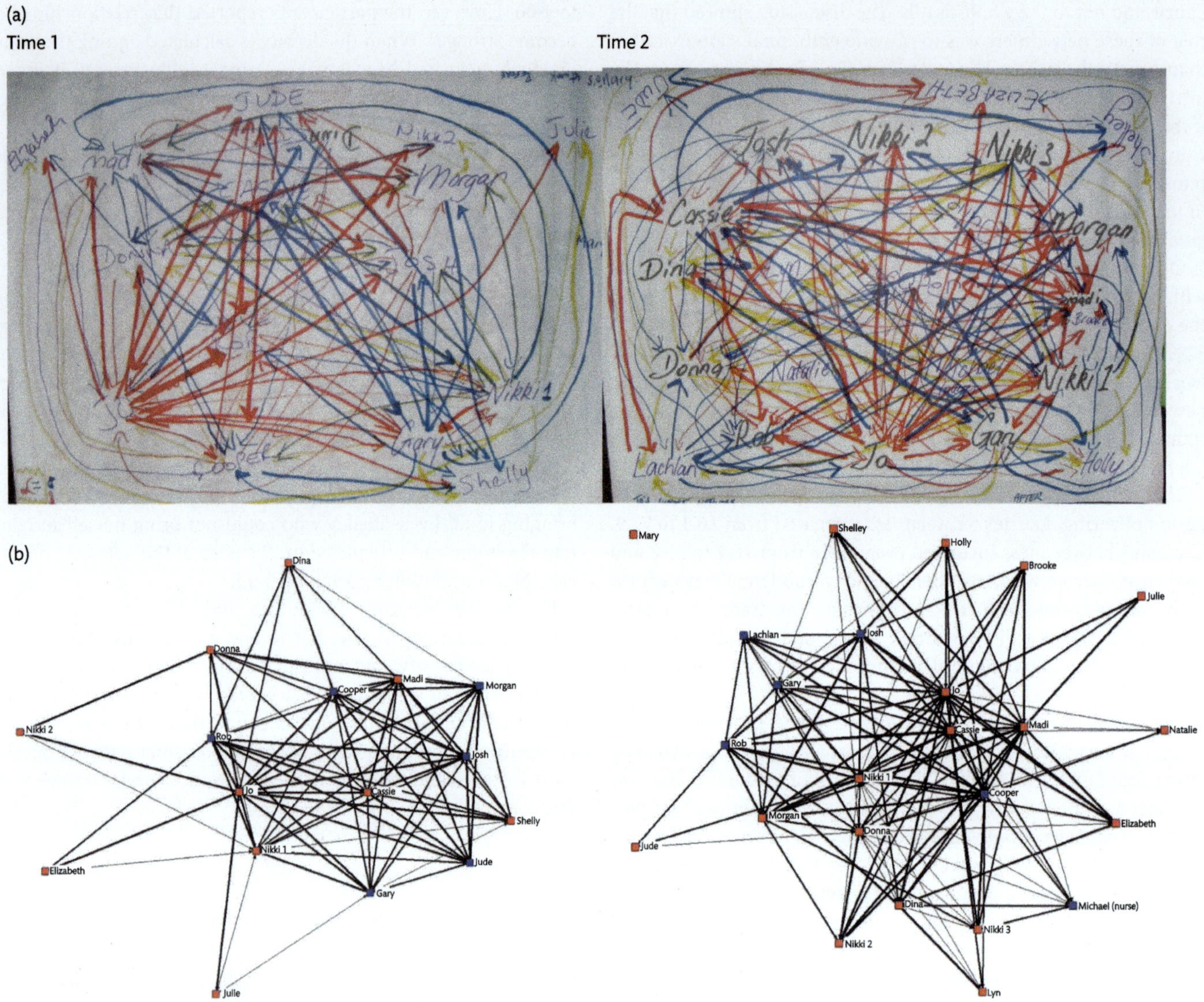

Key for participatory network mapping

Red lines—strong ties
Blue lines—medium ties
Yellow lines—weak ties

Key for NetDraw maps

Red nodes—female
Blue nodes—male
Thickest lines—strongest ties
Medium thickness lines—medium strength ties
Thin lines—weak ties

Fig. 23.3 Case study 2 focus group network maps. (a) Time 1 when caring began and time 2 the time of the research both with participatory network maps and (b) NetDraw maps.

(a) Reproduced from Horsfall, D., Noonan, K. & Leonard, R. (2011) *Bring Our Dying Home: Creating community at end of life*. Sydney: University of Western Sydney ISBN 978-0-646-55666-6, p. 43.

increased from time 1 to time 2 (Fig. 23.4). Usually the service provider was one who visited the home on a regular basis. In one case, a friend became a formal service provider which seemed to have the effect of drawing other formal service providers more closely into the network. They also felt stronger ties to those service providers who supported and empowered them and helped them work the system.

Overall insights

Size and composition of caring networks

The size of the caring network also varied but the minimum was three with seven to eight people the most frequent. Similarly, Jacobs and colleagues (2016) found that smaller networks of both formal

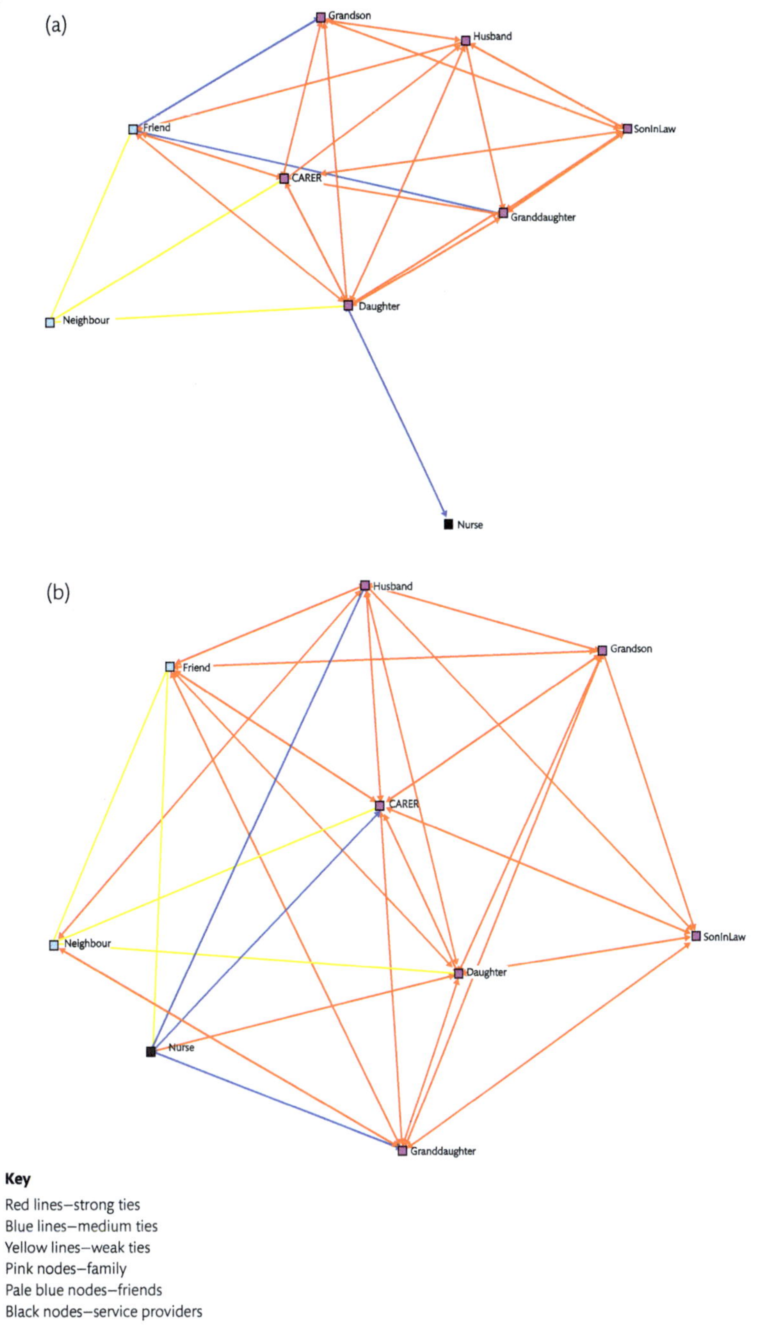

Fig. 23.4 Case study 3 focus group. NetDraw maps for (a) time 1 when caring began and (b) time 2, the time of the research.

Reproduced with permission from Leonard, R., Horsfall, D., Rosenberg, J., et al. Carer experience of end-of-life service provision: a social network analysis. *BMJ Supportive & Palliative Care*, 2020;10:e20.

and informal carers are sometimes beneficial as they are easier to organize and for communication. They comprised a variety of friends, family, neighbours, pets, work colleagues, local shops and services (e.g. pharmacist), community groups, and health services that come to the home (e.g. community nurse). Other medical service providers were usually not named as members of the caring network. Each network was unique; however, they most often contained at least one person who had a close prior experience of death—usually a hospital-based death.

Structure of caring networks

It was clear that the caring networks comprised a core or inner network and an outer network with each playing a different role and doing different sorts of tasks (Horsfall et al., 2013). The primary carer was usually, but not always, a family member. Friends were found to be as central as family. Outer networks were also essential, competent, and capable of a variety of caring roles. Service providers when mentioned were in the outer network, that is, they were seen as essential, but not central, to the caring work.

How do caring networks form?

According to Keating and colleagues: 'fundamental to understanding the caring capacity of the informal sector is to establish the ways in which social networks evolve into caregiving networks when a member has an increased care need' (2003, p. 117). We directly asked 'How did this network come together?' in our focus groups and interviews. It was clear from our data that each network was unique; they could arise spontaneously or be initiated. Family were almost always involved but equally important were friends who care (Leonard et al., 2018). Other sources were neighbours looking out for the dying person, groups that the carer or dying person already belonged to noticing their absence, and deliberately searching for help. Similarly, Jacobs and colleagues (2018) found that belief in their capacity to organize care and proximity to social networks were key to effective recruitment.

As Keating (2003) found, the care networks were indeed a subset of both the primary carers and the dying person's social support network, usually a hybrid of the two. Some networks were prompted into action by existing community groups; some just noticed or were told there was a need and then offered what they thought would be useful. In other instances, the carer directly asked their friends and family for help or the dying person would initiate a system to support their carer: 'I think John organised it so I wouldn't be alone' (Focus Group 5). Sometimes the carer approached an existing group and the group as a whole became involved coordinating their own roster of support. For family members, beliefs about family responsibilities were important motivators but for other people in the caring networks it was just the right thing to do—to show up and help out.

A key to the formation of the informal networks was communication: people needed to know that there was someone in need. Again, there was no one way this was achieved. In one instance, the local corner shop/post office owners put up a notice inviting people who were concerned to talk to the owner who could tell them that Jo and Mary could do with a hand. People used the shop/post office as an information exchange with the shop keepers being the repository of the latest news and information. In other instances, it was a matter of people being concerned enough to ask each other if they had seen Sarah lately and was she OK, thus demonstrating that everyday relationships and communication are key:

> [S]omebody else I know who suddenly had 'a death sentence' passed on him and it became known that he was not going to leave the house—he had no wife, she'd died. I said, 'Are people looking after you?' ... And he said, 'If I see another bloody casserole I'll scream'. (Focus Group 1)

Another important factor is the willingness to accept help. In the preliminary study, one group consisted only of family members and the husband/principal carer described themselves as a very private family and his daughters did the bulk of the caring. His wife, the patient, however, had a phone in her room and it seems she was in constant contact with her network. Possibly that network might have provided hands-on support had they been allowed to come to the home.

One of the hallmarks of a compassionate community is that the caring network will be much wider than the expected members such as family and close friends. So, we look forward to a time when caring networks are not simply a subset of the carer's and patient's existing social networks.

What activities do care networks do?

Part of the value of informal care networks was their flexibility. The members do not have set job descriptions and many people will do whatever they can. The activities can be grouped into six main categories: activities of daily living, emotional support, communication, life affirmation, direct care, and continuity of support after the death.

- Activities of daily living relieve the principal carers of many tasks so they can care for the patient. Activities such as shopping, cooking, cleaning, gardening, taking children to school, and walking the dog do not require any special knowledge or skill and make a huge difference to the burden of care.
- Networks can also provide emotional support for the carer and patient by simply having time to talk or sit with the patient.
- Communication activities involve updating others about the situation or sourcing services.
- Life affirmation refers to all those activities which remind everyone that the patient is still alive and still the person they have always been. Rituals, fun, shared memories, and gatherings all validate the life of the dying person.
- More specialized knowledge or skills might be needed to help with direct care for the patient such as repositioning or transferring the patient, giving medications, or obtaining specialized equipment, but the skills for most activities can be acquired without extensive training.
- Continuity of support from dying through to after the death is particularly necessary because formal services are between the domains. A home that has been busy with support workers is suddenly silent and the bereaved can feel deserted. It is the informal network that can bridge this gap and help with funeral arrangements and other gatherings and rituals, honouring the deceased's wishes and give ongoing emotional support.

Where are care networks located?

Informal caring networks can provide support for carers and patients in hospices, hospitals, aged care facilities, the patients' homes, or the carers' homes. Location makes a huge difference to the type of support that is needed and can be provided.

Care in the patients' homes keeps them connected with their familiar surroundings, memorabilia, pets, and gardens all of which not only give pleasure but help people who are dying retain their identities. It enables the patients to stay connected to their neighbours and other in their social networks. If the principal carer does not live in the same house or locally, then they can have difficulty obtaining informal help. They might not feel they can ask the patient's neighbours or friends and that it is too big an ask for their own networks to travel to the patient's house. It is also difficult for them to attend to their own homes and families.

Transferring the patient to the carer's home facilitates their access to their own networks but deprives the patient of that sense of control, ownership, familiarity, and relaxation that comes with being in one's own home. In either home, the informal network can provide the full range of support activities. Plus, there is scope for visitors to come and relax, 'have a cuppa', spend time with the carer, patient, and each other and maybe indulge in happy hour festivities or other rituals.

Facilities provide for the direct medical care of the patient, but they make it more difficult for network members to visit and give emotional support and severely restrict interaction with pets, gatherings, and rituals. So, although the person's body is cared for, their identity is difficult to maintain. Communication to others in the social networks is still needed and also practical support for principal carers to free their time to stay with the patient.

Conclusion

This chapter has demonstrated the importance of informal caring networks which are an essential ingredient for building and binding compassionate communities. People involved in informal networks learn about the challenges and joys of end of life caring. As these numbers grow, so does the community death literacy and the acceptance that end of life is everyone's business. Specific community development initiatives (Horsfall et al., 2020) have the capacity to grow the pool of people willing and capable to contribute to caring. They create a climate where people offer help and carers are given public approval for requesting help.

As a society we cannot afford to replace all home caring with institutional care, even if we wanted too so the choice is not whether there should be caring in the home, but whether carers are left to their own devices or supported to potentially make the experience one of connection and intimacy rather than burden and burnout. Death is powerful and shared caring at the end of life is an opportunity to use that power to create collective experiences which strengthen our mutual connections.

REFERENCES

Abel, J., Sallnow, L., Murray, S. A., and Kerin, M. 2016. *Each Community is Prepared to Help: Community Development in End of Life Care—Guidance on Ambition Six*. London: National Council for Palliative Care.

Australian Bureau of Statistics. 2019. *Retirement and Retirement Intentions, Australia, 2018–19*. Canberra: Australian Bureau of Statistics.

Bibgy, C. 1997. When parents relinquish care: informal support networks of older people with intellectual disability. *Journal of Applied Research in Intellectual Disabilities*, 10, 333–344.

Borgatti, S. P., Everett, M. G., and Freeman, L. C. 2002. *Ucinet 6 for Windows: Software for Social Network Analysis* (Version 6.360). Harvard, MA: Analytic Technologies.

Brown, L. and Walter, T. 2014. Towards a social model of end-of-life care. *British Journal of Social Work*, 44, 2375–2390.

Carers Australia. 2020. The value of informal care in 2020. Deloitte Access Economics. [Online] Available at: https://www2.deloitte.com/content/dam/Deloitte/au/Documents/Economics/deloitte-au-dae-value-of-informal-care-310820.pdf

Dopp, A. R. and Cain, C. C. 2012. The role of peer relationships in parental bereavement during childhood and adolescence. *Death Studies*, 36, 41–60.

Hagell, P., Alvariza, A., Westergren, A., and Årestedt, K. 2017. Assessment of burden among family caregivers of people with Parkinson's disease using the Zarit Burden Interview. *Journal of Pain and Symptom Management*, 53, 272–278.

Horsfall, D., Leonard, R., Rosenberg, J. P., and Noonan, K. 2019. People and place: co-creating an ecology of care at end of life. In: McManus, R., Cornwall, J., and Raudon, S. (eds.) *Death Down Under: Twenty-first Century Dying, Death, Disposal and Memorialisation in the Antipodes*, pp. 164–174. Newcastle-upon-Tyne: Cambridge Scholars.

Horsfall, D., Psychogios, H., Rankin-Smith, H., Read, N., and Noonan, K. 2020. *Researching Compassionate Communities in Australia: A Short-Term Longitudinal Study*. Sydney: Western Sydney University.

Horsfall, D., Yardley, A., Leonard, R., Noonan, K., and Rosenberg, J. 2015. *End of Life at Home: Co-Creating an Ecology of Care*. Sydney: Western Sydney University.

Howarth, G. 2007. Dying: institutionalization and medicalization. In: *Death and Dying: A Sociological Introduction*, pp. 115–131. Cambridge: Polity Press.

Hughes, M. 2009. The lived experience of compassionate love at end of life. Doctoral thesis, University of Tasmania.

Hughes, M. 2015. A strengths perspective on caregiving at the end-of-life. *Australian Social Work*, 68, 156–168.

Jacobs, M., Broese Van Groenou, M. I., Aartsen, M. J., and Deeg, D. J. H. 2018. Diversity in older adults' care networks: the added value of individual beliefs and social network proximity. *The Journals of Gerontology: Series B, Psychological Sciences and Social Sciences*, 73, 326–336.

Jacobs, M., Van Tilburg, T., Groenewegen, P., & Broese Van Groenou, M. 2016. Linkages between informal and formal care-givers in home-care networks of frail older adults. *Ageing and Society*, 36, 1604–1624.

Keating, N., Otfinowski, P., Wenger, C., Fast, J., and Derksen, L. 2003. Understanding the caring capacity of informal networks of frail seniors: a case for care networks. *Ageing and Society*, 23, 115–127.

Kellehear, A. 2007. *A Social History of Dying*. Cambridge: Cambridge University Press.

Kittay, E. F. 2011. The ethics of care, dependence, and disability. *Ratio Juris*, 24, 49–58.

Lave, J. and Wenger, E. 1991. *Situated Learning: Legitimate Peripheral Participation*. Cambridge: Cambridge University Press.

Leonard, R., Horsfall, D., and Noonan, K. 2015. Identifying changes in the support networks of end-of-life carers using social network analysis. *BMJ Supportive and Palliative Care*, 5, 153–1559.

Leonard, R., Horsfall, D., Noonan, K., and Rosenberg, J. 2017. Identity and end of life story: A role for psychologists. *Australian Psychologist*, 52, 346–353.

Leonard, R., Horsfall, D., Noonan, K., and Rosenberg, J. 2018. The positioning of formal service providers in support networks for caring at end-of-life at home: a social network analysis. *BMJ Supportive & Palliative Care*, 5, A6–A7.

Leonard, R., Noonan, K., Horsfall, D., Kelly, M., Rosenberg, J., Grindrod, A., et al. 2021. Developing a death literacy index. *Death Studies*, 1–13. Advance online publication. https://doi.org/10.1080/07481187.2021.1894268

Metel, M. and Barnes, J. 2011. Peer-group support for bereaved children: a qualitative interview study. *Child and Adolescent Mental Health*, 16, 201–207.

Morris, S. M., King, C., Turner, M., and Payne, S. 2015. Family carers providing support to a person dying in the home setting: a narrative literature review *Palliative Medicine*, 29, 487–495.

Noonan, K., Horsfall, D., Leonard, R., and Rosenberg, J. 2016. Developing death literacy. *Progress in Palliative Care*, 24, 31–35.

Palliative Care Australia. 2010. *Health System Reform and Care at the End of Life: A Guidance Document*. Canberra: Palliative Care Australia.

Prosser, H. and Moss, S. 1996. Informal care networks of older adults with an intellectual disability. *Journal of Applied Research in Intellectual Disabilities*, 9, 17–30.

Rosenberg, J., Horsfall, D., Leonard, R., and Noonan, K. 2018. Informal care networks' views of palliative care services: help or hindrance? *Death Studies*, 42, 362–370.

Royal Commission into Aged Care Quality and Safety 2020. *Royal Commission into Aged Care Quality and Safety Interim Report*. Canberra: Commonwealth of Australia.

Rumbold, B. 2012. Public health approaches to palliative care in Australia. In: Sallnow, L., Kumar, S., and Kellehear, A. (eds.) *1st International Conference on Palliative Care and Public Health, 2009 Institute of Palliative Medicine, Kozhikode, India*, pp. 52–68. London: Routledge.

Sallnow, L. and Paul, S. 2015. Understanding community engagement in end-of-life care: developing conceptual clarity. *Critical Public Health*, 25, 231–238.

Sallnow, L., Richardson, H., Murray, S. A., and Kellehear, A. 2016. The impact of a new public health approach to end-of-life care: a systematic review. *Palliative Medicine*, 30, 200–211.

Tolkacheva, N., Broese, M., Groenou, V., De Boer, A., and Van Tilburg, T. 2011. The impact of informal care-giving networks on adult children's care-giver burden. *Ageing & Society*, 31, 34–51.

Tronto, J. 1993. *Moral Boundaries: A Political Argument for an Ethic of Care*. New York: Routledge.

Veloso, V. I. and Tripodoro, V. A. 2016. Caregivers burden in palliative care patients: a problem to tackle. *Current Opinion in Supportive & Palliative Care*, 10, 330–335.

Woodman, C., Baillie, J., and Sivell, S. 2016. The preferences and perspectives of family caregivers towards place of care for their relatives at the end-of-life. A systematic review and thematic synthesis of the qualitative evidence. *BMJ Supportive & Palliative Care*, 6, 418–429.

Young, J., Egan, T., Williamson, M., Jaye, C., Kenrick, K., Ross, J., et al. 2016. An exercise to map patient-centred care networks. *The Clinical Teacher*, 13, 448–450.

Zapart, S., Kenny, P., Hall, J., Servis, B., and Wiley, S. 2007. Home based palliative care in Sydney, Australia: the carers' perspective on the provision of informal care. *Health and Social Care in the Community*, 15, 97–107.

24

Complexities and challenges in public health palliative care research

Steven Vanderstichelen and Luc Deliens

Introduction

The populations of industrialized and developing countries are ageing fast; people live longer and the proportions of people living beyond 65 years and beyond 80 years are increasing. Parallel to these transitions in demography, there is also transition in epidemiology of diseases and health-related problems. People are increasingly dying from chronic diseases, and especially older people who are increasingly confronted at the end of their lives with multiple organ failure. This implies that, in the next decades, more people will need some form of end of life care. At the same time, families have become smaller and the number of potential family carers is decreasing. As a consequence, healthcare systems everywhere will be put under increasing pressure to deliver effective and quality end of life care for all.

However, solutions for these major challenges will not be found only in the further development of the existing professional care systems and only a public health approach can sufficiently cope with a population-wide policy to deliver quality care for all at the end of life. Research has provided enough evidence that good end of life care for all is not being achieved; there are clear social and economic inequalities which affect, for example, place of death and access to palliative care (Cohen and Deliens, 2012). Apart from social and economic health differences, many other topics can be studied in the context of public health at the end of life or for people confronted with loss and bereavement. One could say that public health at the end of life is the collective counterpart of individual end of life patient care that is delivered by healthcare professionals such as doctors, nurses, and other paramedics. The field of public health at the end of life is wider than organized healthcare itself. There are also non-medical disciplines such as social work, educational sciences, health promotion, and spiritual caregiving involved. Furthermore, organization of healthcare, health policy, and legislation are components of public health, at the international, national, and local level.

In this chapter we describe the public health research approaches to palliative care, the appropriate research designs that will be needed to develop public health and palliative care studies, and the understanding of complexities in public health palliative care research.

What is the public health research approach to palliative care?

Palliative care is particularly concerned with the well-being and comfort of people nearing the end of their life due to serious illness or frailty. As a clinical practice, palliative care has traditionally focused on the medical and nursing interactions between individual patients with their family carers and professional caregivers (Cohen and Deliens, 2012). Palliative care research has therefore predominantly focused on clinical and health services research and has until recently predominantly painted a medicalized picture of care giving for the seriously ill or at the end of life. However, by the start of the twenty-first century, the first substantial step towards a new paradigm shift in palliative care was made by Allan Kellehear, who first conceptualized in his book *Health Promoting Palliative Care* the end of life and palliative care as a public health issue (Kellehear, 1999). In 2019, Sallnow and Paul have elsewhere provided a valuable overview of this and other key documents that have shaped the new public health movement (Sallnow and Paul, 2018). At the beginning of the twenty-first century, the World Health Organization has also recognized that palliative care should be a major public health priority (Davies and Higginson, 2004a, 2004b).

Rather than individual patient care, public health is interested in population health (Cohen and Deliens, 2012). As a field of study and practice, public health is concerned with (1) *monitoring population health* and the structural, social, and environmental factors that influence it, and (2) *promoting population health* through prevention, early intervention, and harm reduction policies and interventions. Applied to an end of life context and palliative care, public health approaches are concerned with monitoring and improving the structural, social, and environmental circumstances of individuals and communities faced with serious illness, death, dying, and loss at the population level (Cohen and Deliens, 2012). As a field of research, public health palliative care complements the traditional clinical and health services research focus on individual patient–family–caregiver interactions (Hanks et al., 2009; Ferrell and Coyle, 2010) with a particular focus on understanding the influence of social, environmental, and physical determinants of the health and well-being of populations faced with serious illness, death, dying, and loss (Sallnow et al., 2016b).

As outlined by Pivodic and Cohen (2018), public health palliative care research approaches have a focus on communities and the recognition of their involvement and empowerment as strategies to improve well-being towards the end of life; a focus on social and economic determinants of health and the inclusion of social science methods and theories; with an inclusion of non-professional actors in palliative care; and a larger focus on the impact of policy changes and the societal debate on palliative care. Importantly, the public health perspective in palliative care is focused on the full relevant population, rather than merely certain patients identified based on service use or 'biopsychosocial risk' (Sallnow et al., 2016b).

The public health perspective is increasingly being applied in the field of palliative care practice and research and today the field is commonly considered to contain two broad approaches: (1) the *traditional epidemiological research approach* to public health palliative care and (2) the *'new public health' approach* to palliative care.

Traditional public health research approaches

Traditional public health approaches to palliative care research are predominantly characterized by (post-)positivist epistemologies and encompass mainly quantitative epidemiological studies that monitor and assess the circumstances, social challenges, planning services, and policies around serious illness, death, dying, and loss (Sallnow et al., 2016b; Pivodic and Cohen, 2018). Prominent studies from this stream of research have focused on the circumstances of death and dying: quality of care for patients near the end of life (Young et al., 2009; Burt et al., 2010; De Schreye et al., 2017), quality of death and dying (Van den Block et al., 2016; Pivodic et al., 2018; Smets et al., 2018), end of life decisions (van der Heide et al., 2003; Cohen et al., 2007a; Chambaere et al., 2008, 2015a, 2015b; Dierickx et al., 2018), care setting transmissions near the end of life (Van den Block et al., 2007, 2015; Pivodic et al., 2016a), place of death (Cohen et al., 2007b, 2015; Houttekier et al., 2011; Pivodic et al., 2016b), prescription and deprescription practices (Paque et al., 2019a, 2019b), healthcare costs at the end of life (Paz-Ruiz et al., 2009; Faes et al., 2018; Maetens et al., 2019), and the need, use, and access of supportive palliative care measures and health services (Murtagh et al., 2014; Etkind et al., 2017; Morin et al., 2017; Penders et al., 2018; Maetens et al., 2019). See also Pivodic and Cohen (2018) for a comprehensive overview of epidemiological research in public health palliative care.

The 'new public health' research approach

New public health approaches are primarily characterized by their social constructivist epistemology and participatory action methodologies. These approaches developed from the community engagement movement and emerged in part in response to growing criticism of the traditional public health approach to palliative care, which holds that it reinforces the dominance of healthcare professional perspectives (Sallnow et al., 2016b), that this traditional focus on professional responses serves to disempower communities, and thereby places further demand on health services (Sallnow and Paul, 2018). This has led to what some have called a radical reframing of health as everyone's responsibility (Sallnow and Paul, 2018) and a proliferation of social change methodologies in which research and practice overlap.

New public health approaches emphasize a pursuit of equity and access (Baum, 2016). They work based on the assumption that social and environmental factors are responsible for adverse population health outcomes and they emphasize primary care as a driver for health promotion. Additionally, they emphasize the important role of all societal sectors in impacting health and that health should therefore have a place in all policies.

Finally, participation and involvement of the community are crucial in new public health approaches, including in research efforts. Prominent studies from this stream of research have focused on the impact of social relationships (Holt-Lunstad et al., 2010), social networks (Reeves et al., 2014), community engagement (Popay, 2010; O'Mara-Eves et al., 2013; Popay et al., 2015; Sallnow and Paul, 2015; Pesut et al., 2018), volunteering (Gardiner and Barnes, 2016; Dodd et al., 2018), and environmental and social determinants (Marmot, 2005) on health and well-being outcomes; the effect of community end of life care on social capital (Horsfall et al., 2012; Sallnow, 2017); support networks in end of life care situations (Leonard et al., 2015); and the role of different societal actors such as schools, hospices (Paul, 2015), and community volunteers (Seymour et al., 2013) in health-promoting palliative care and death education. See also Sallnow and colleagues (2016a) for a more detailed discussion of this important emerging evidence that connects new public health approaches in practice to positive health outcomes.

A systematic review by Sallnow and colleagues (2016a) shows a range of beneficial health and well-being outcomes associated with new public health approaches to end of life care practice. Another more recent systematic review by Collins and colleagues (2021), however, points out that research has hitherto predominantly focused on evaluating community outcomes and that evidence on health system outcomes remains scarce, with few notable exceptions (Morita et al., 2013; McLoughlin et al., 2015; Walshe et al., 2016; Abel et al., 2018a, 2018b; Librada Flores et al., 2018). This confirms previous suggestions that there has been little systematic study of objective outcomes and the efforts made to achieve systematic change at the community level (Sallnow et al., 2016b).

What research designs are appropriate for public health palliative care studies?

Research designs describe or prescribe a framework to conduct research and may prescribe a certain population, sample methods, types of data, methods for data collection and analysis, and so on. It may also reveal certain fundamental assumptions the researchers have regarding the very nature of reality (ontology) and to what extent and how we can obtain knowledge of reality (epistemology). The ways in which research designs may be classified are therefore endless as they can be categorized based on each of these elements, as well as types of data, types of study populations, data collection methods, and so on. This chapter therefore does not intend to provide an exhaustive overview of all possible research designs in the literature, nor to provide a definitive classification of research methods, but merely an overview of the most appropriate and frequently used research designs in public health palliative care research.

For the purpose of this brief overview, a particularly useful way to think about types of research design is to classify them according to interactivity with the environment. In terms of interactivity, we can discern three groups of designs: (1) observational, (2) experimental, and (3) change-oriented designs. The public health approach does not prescribe or preclude any particular research designs. As we will see in the following sections, designs from each of these big categories are applicable and appropriate for public health palliative care research.

Observational research designs

Observational research most often intends to explore or describe phenomena, either quantitatively (in width) or qualitatively (in depth), when the phenomena to be studied are beyond the control of the researchers. As this is often the case when monitoring or assessing the circumstances influencing the health and well-being at the end of life of entire populations, observational research designs are an essential tool in the arsenal of public health palliative care researchers.

Quantitative observational research designs

Quantitative observational research designs are employed frequently in epidemiological studies to monitor the prevalence and incidence of disease, but also to investigate the effects of treatment, policy, or interventions where it is impossible to randomly assign subjects to treatment or control, whether for practical or ethical reasons (Rosenbaum, 2002). These quantitative designs are primarily interested in statistical generalizability of their findings to a large or very specific population.

Classic examples of quantitative observational research designs used in public health palliative care research are cross-sectional studies, case–control studies, and cohort studies.

Cross-sectional studies often use survey questionnaires to describe a practice or attitudes of an entire populations (or a representative sample) at a specific point in time. Cross-sectional studies can be used to describe odds ratios, and absolute and relative risk from prevalence analyses. Some of the pioneering studies in public health palliative care have been cross-sectional population-based surveys, many of which use mortality follow-back designs making use of a sample of deaths and retrospectively looking back to the medical situation prior to death, such as the Dutch and Belgian studies on End-of-Life Decisions (ELDs) (van der Heide et al., 2003; Chambaere et al., 2008, 2015a; Dierickx et al., 2018), the UK VOICES (Young et al., 2009; Burt et al., 2010) study, examining quality of care at the end of life of people dying from various conditions, and the European PACE (Van den Block et al., 2016; Smets et al., 2018) nursing home study, examining quality and costs of palliative care in nursing homes across six European countries. Cross-sectional studies have further been used to estimate the need for palliative care at the population level (Etkind et al., 2017; Morin et al., 2017), cancer mortality and survival rates at the European level (De Angelis et al., 2014; Malvezzi et al., 2015), map volunteering practices across a healthcare system (Vanderstichelen et al., 2018, 2019b, 2020a, 2020c), and examine population differences in place of death (Cohen et al., 2007b, 2015; Houttekier et al., 2011; Pivodic et al., 2016b).

Case–control studies compare two or more groups that differ in outcomes based on the assumption of a causal relationship. One of the groups serves as a control group; however, group membership cannot be randomized. Case–control studies are often retrospective, meaning they look backwards and examine exposure to risk or protection factors related to a specific outcome. They are also frequently cross-sectional in nature, meaning they take a measurement at one specific point in time. Big data studies, making use of existing administrative databases often use this design, for example, comparing people having received palliative care in the last months of life to those who did not have had access to palliative care in the last months of life. Studies that take measurements at several points in time to study changes over time are called longitudinal studies.

Cohort studies are a type of longitudinal observational research design in which groups of people with a shared characteristic are examined using multiple cross-sectional measurements. Cohort studies can be both retrospective (using already collected data) or prospective, but the unique difficulties associated with identifying people near the end of life often mean that these studies in public health palliative care are retrospective in nature (Earle and Ayanian, 2006). One example of a prospective cohort study in public health palliative care research studied the correlation between patient quality of life in palliative care and the burden of their family caregivers (Krug et al., 2016). Retrospective cohort studies have examined reporting practices of dementia diagnoses on death certificates (Perera et al., 2016), the impact of palliative home care support on quality and costs of end of life care (Maetens et al., 2019), the connection between a compassionate community initiative and unplanned emergency admissions and admission costs (Abel et al., 2018a), and patient and organizational factors that influence duration of hospice-based palliative care (Allsop et al., 2018).

Qualitative observational research

Qualitative observational research designs are interested in the theoretical generalizability of their qualitative in-depth findings regarding certain phenomena, for which large samples are not required.

Useful qualitative observational research designs used in public health palliative care research are document analysis, interview studies, and ethnography. These research designs are invaluable in exploring power differentials across and within different levels of society, the impact of structures and social networks on health and well-being outcomes, process evaluations of the development and implementation of public health palliative care interventions, and their acceptability for stakeholders.

Document analysis considers paper or digital documents as their unit of analysis. Under this umbrella term, many different approaches are possible, ranging from content analysis (Mayring, 2000; Hsieh and Shannon, 2005) used to summarize, explicate, or structure the contents of various documents, to more complex analyses of narrative and discourse (De Fina and Johnstone, 2015), used to understand underlying assumptions, associations, and power structures embedded in written text. In the wider public health literature, document analysis has seen frequent use in understanding the development and implementation of public health interventions and to generate data at different levels in a system (McGill et al., 2020). In the end of life and palliative care literature, examples are less frequent, but document analysis has been used to analyse palliative care guidance and policy at the regional (Hill et al., 2019), national (Lind et al., 2013; Nakanishi et al., 2015), and international (Van Beek et al., 2013; Pivodic et al., 2021) level. It has also proven to be a useful approach to evaluate palliative care policies in the midst of a health crisis, such as the coronavirus disease 2019 (COVID-19) pandemic (Gilissen et al., 2020).

One particular type of document analysis that feels almost too obvious to mention but that is nonetheless an extremely important tool in gathering and integrating evidence is the *literature review*. Whether it be a systematic, rapid, integrative, or realist review, these are invaluable tools to create insight into the state of the art of public health palliative care research and should not be overlooked when considering a new research question.

Interview studies are well suited to explore phenomena in depth through individual and group perspectives and experiences. Such designs often operate on constructivist epistemologies that assume meaning and knowledge are constantly constructed and negotiated by individuals, their environment, or in the interaction among and between the two. It considers knowledge as essentially a political process. Interview studies often use a mix of *individual* interviews or a mix of *collective* interviews. A focus group is one type of collective interviews. Focus group discussions stimulate the exchange of views through discussion within a group of participants, allow mutual differences or similarities to drive the conversation, and enable salient themes to emerge. Frequently, a topic list is used, but depending on the nature of the study, these may be limited to a single bullet point to launch a conversation. A moderator facilitates the discussion by introducing topics and issues for the participants to discuss among themselves and occasionally probes the participants to further explore interesting emerging topics or statements. Knowledge is generated in interaction—whether agreement or conflict—between participants.

Interviews can be structured (questionnaires), semi-structured (topic guide and prompts), or unstructured (single prompt). Interviews allow the in-depth exploration of individuals' unique experiences. They are often favoured over focus groups if the subject of a study is sensitive, when participants are considered vulnerable due to (physical or mental) health concerns, the very personal nature of the subject, or when it is expected that participants may feel constrained to talk about certain topics in a group environment. Interview study designs using interviews and/or focus groups have been used to study volunteering in palliative care in both health service and community settings and their roles regarding different types of support at the end of life for patients, family caregivers, and healthcare professionals (Faulkner and Davies, 2005; Luijkx and Schols, 2009; Vanderstichelen et al., 2019a, 2020b). They have been invaluable in exploring power dynamics in engaging communities in end of life issues (Kleijberg et al., 2021) and perceptions of palliative care among people with care needs and family caregivers (Collins et al., 2017). These methods are also often used to explore how community networks can support carers for the dying (Horsfall, 2018) and to evaluate complex public health palliative care interventions (Carduff et al., 2016).

Ethnography is a type of field research originating from cultural anthropology that examines the behaviours of participants who represent a particular 'in-group' in a natural setting and is interested in understanding their interpretation of their behaviour. To this end, it often uses participant or non-participant observational methods of data collection, which intends to allow researchers to immerse themselves in a setting so as to become part of it and arrive at a position that is as close as possible to being an insider. It involves putting participants at ease over time and generating trust. This research design often applies methods from document analysis (to analyse field notes and setting-generated documents) and interviews. While not as prevalent as other research designs, ethnography can be an appropriate design to track and identify the processes and relationships through which events, practices and things become meaningful (Cohn et al., 2013), and how behaviour manifests itself in certain contexts, for example, the manifestation of existential suffering at the end of life (Renz et al., 2018).

Experimental research designs

Experimental research focuses on the manipulation of an environment to test hypotheses and to establish, if possible, causal links between predictors and outcomes in a given setting. Many types of experiments are possible, with various levels of control, randomization, and complexity. However, the most well-known type of experiment in health sciences and palliative care, often described as the gold standard for high-quality evidence, is the *randomized controlled trial.*

Randomized controlled trials are a popular research design, particularly in clinical research, but actively manipulating independent variables may become impractical and unethical when it involves human subjects and laboratory settings are traded for natural environments such as communities. This notwithstanding, the controlled trial can still be an appropriate tool for public health palliative care research, particularly when the interventions are straightforward in design and withholding it is not ethically problematic. Randomized controlled trial have been used to evaluate health system outcomes of social and practical support interventions for people with life-limiting conditions (McLoughlin et al., 2015) and *non-randomized control trials* have been used to evaluate the impact of care networks on health outcomes including quality of care, caregiver burden, place of death, and resource use (Librada Flores et al., 2018).

However, the reason that controlled trial studies are fairly rare in public health palliative care research is that controlled trials and the dominant frameworks for their development, implementation, and evaluation—such as the Medical Research Council (Craig et al., 2008), RE-AIM (n.d.), and PRECEDE-PROCEDE (Gielen and Eileen, 1996)—represent a static, linear approach that assumes the optimization of intervention prior to implementation. In practice, when interventions are implemented and come into contact with the context, often changes occur in the context and in the intervention itself which may result in feedback loops as the intervention adapts. Such changes may be mistaken as ineffectiveness of an intervention, rather than a natural process adaption and change over time (Wells et al., 2012; Walugembe et al., 2019), and interventions may be evaluated negatively merely because protocols are not or cannot be followed as outlined prior to implementation when the intervention interacts with its context in practice. Underlying this are the assumptions of 'voltage drop' and 'programme drift'. Voltage drop will occur when interventions will yield lower benefits moving from development to implementation, and programme drift occurs when deviation from protocols leads to decreased effect or benefit (Chambers et al., 2013).

Change-oriented designs

Monitoring and observing population health and well-being at the end of life and experimenting and testing health-promoting palliative care policies and programmes are essential aspects of a well-informed public health approach to palliative care. However, public health advocates mainly have an interest in achieving lasting social changes. Particularly the 'new public health' approach to palliative care, as we saw earlier, has strong roots in the community engagement movement and an affinity with social constructivist epistemologies and *participatory action research* designs.

In change-oriented research designs, the boundaries between researcher, research population, and setting, and between intervention and context are often blurry and sometimes considered non-existent. Researchers themselves often partner with the setting and become part of the intervention. Participatory action research, particularly in the 'new public health' stream of palliative care research, works on the principle of co-creation. Co-creation can be understood as collaborative knowledge generation by academics in partnership with other stakeholders and, in the community-based health services research, has been suggested to increase research impact (Greenhalgh et al., 2016).

Participatory methods are particularly useful to bring in perspectives of those affected by the intervention in which they are involved (McGill et al., 2020) and to evaluate conceptual outcomes of interventions (Collins et al., 2021). In participatory action research, those directly affected by the intervention are not only involved in evaluating it, but also in the design, development, and implementation processes. The design has been used to engage difficult-to-reach or Indigenous communities with limited access to medical services to develop palliative care programmes (Kelley et al., 2018), to examine advance care planning peer education through volunteer perspectives on training and community engagement activities (Seymour et al., 2013), or to explore power dynamics in and creating spaces for community engagement in end of life issues through intergenerational arts initiatives (Kleijberg et al., 2020, 2021). Participatory action research is a popular design particularly in the compassionate communities literature and movement, where strong and close collaborations with local communities are core principles.

Complexity in public health palliative care research

In experimental public health palliative care research, there is no equivalent of the sterile laboratory setting in which the influence of confounding factors can be controlled. Often interventions have to be adapted to different contexts, such as in multicentre studies, and tested and implemented in live settings. As a consequence, public health studies are leading to higher complexity due to many different parts and components interacting in a dynamic and unpredictable setting (Petticrew, 2011). Additionally, in change-oriented research, researchers and participants often take on dual roles and the intervention is not merely a static result of a protocol but a dynamic product of a flexible research plan, changing community needs, social power dynamics, and community stakeholder interests. Describing and evaluating such interventions is not an easy feat. Therefore, these types of interventions are aptly called 'complex interventions'.

What is complexity and what challenges does it pose?

Several definitions of complexity exist; however, most indicate that it is an emergent attribute of a system or intervention caused by interaction of multiple parts, variability in interaction, and unpredictability in outcome (Petticrew, 2011; Wells et al., 2012; Lewin et al., 2017). According to the Medical Research Council's guidance (Craig et al., 2008), complexity of an intervention arises from the:

- Number of interacting components within the experimental and control interventions.
- Number and difficulty of behaviours required by those delivering or receiving the intervention.
- Number of groups or organizational levels targeted by the intervention.
- Number and variability of outcomes.
- Degree of flexibility or tailoring of the intervention permitted.

Others argue that, more than a function of the interaction between discrete elements, complexity should be seen as 'a dynamic and constantly emerging set of processes and objects that not only interact with each other, but come to be defined by those interactions' (Cohn et al., 2013, p. 40). Complex interventions cannot be described by linear pathways between the intervention and outcome, but are marked by non-linear pathways, multiple confounding variables, and feedback loops between intervention and context (Petticrew, 2011).

Researching complex public health interventions in palliative and end of life care, presents its own unique challenges and we may find ourselves confronted by particular sources of complexity (Sallnow et al., 2016b), namely:

- Conceptual complexity.
- Scale complexity and complexity arising from environmental dynamics.

Conceptual complexity

Measuring concepts like resilience, health, well-being, and social capital is very challenging because of their conceptual complexity. Researchers aiming to evaluate complex public health palliative care interventions such as compassionate communities and cities are faced with very similar conceptual challenges as the World Health Organization's Healthy Cities evaluators were (de Leeuw, 2013), namely, how do we measure health and well-being at the end of life? When do we consider communities as 'compassionate'?

Health itself is not a straightforward concept that can be measured directly and quantitatively in a universally meaningful way. We can monitor indicators that measure only a part of the complex concept of health, such as disease prevalence in a given population, mortality statistics, healthy behaviour, nutrition, and so on. However, as there is no discrete measure of health, such indicators are inevitably reductive as they tell only part of the story of health. Alternatively, we can define health as a function of physical or mental functionality or ability, but such an approach would define anyone living and born with disabilities as unhealthy by default. Additionally, it would mean that we consider older people as incapable of being in good health. Perhaps less problematical, but equally insufficient, we can also define health as the absence of illness—which is a purely medical conceptualization of health and itself subject to ongoing change as knowledge and scientific and medical paradigms change.

These approaches consistently fall short to capture what it means to be healthy. Therefore, we must accept that health cannot be adequately or sufficiently assessed and evaluated by quantitative and discrete evaluation methods alone. Health is relative and 'highly contextual, driven by individuals, groups and communities that constantly live and create health in a complex, changing and adaptive social and physical environment' (de Leeuw, 2013). This suggests that research into health cannot be addressed sufficiently by a gold standard, but must be responsive to this relative and context-driven nature (de Leeuw, 1989, 2013).

It is clear, particularly in the field of public health palliative care, that health must be conceptualized as relative and as broader than merely the absence of physical or mental illness. Health at the end of life and in the face of serious illness can be defined 'in a positive way as energy and vitality, the ability to do things, a general feeling of well-being, being able to maintain social relationships, or as psychosocial well-being' (Cohen and Deliens, 2012, p. 4). Other complex concepts are increasingly being explored in the public health palliative care literature, such as well-being at the end of life, community resilience (Kellehear and Young, 2007) in the face of end of life care needs, and social capital (Horsfall et al., 2012; Lewis et al., 2013). Operationalizations of these concepts can vary greatly, as these cannot be directly measured, can mean different things to different communities, and a wide range of data collections can be employed. How a certain concept should be measured or understood can be the subject of heated debate. Social capital (Portes, 1998), for instance, continues to be the subject of arguments regarding definitions (Kawachi, 2004). It can therefore be challenging and sometimes impossible to compare study findings between cities or different settings, interventions that use the same concepts but define and operationalize them differently, build on similar but competing theoretical frameworks, collect different data, etc.

Scale complexity and dynamic environments

The scale of a community-driven intervention will also lead to complexities in conducting research. Problems with standardization and replication of locally driven interventions, interactions between individuals, groups, and policy, are complex due to their scale and the long time frames required for conducting the studies.

Public health palliative care intervention studies often require long time frames to develop, implement, and evaluate. It may take a long time before an effect can be observed or registered. Moreover, often a sustainable and structural change is sought after, which may take much longer than funding agencies are capable or prepared to support.

Conducting studies in a real-life context confronts the researcher with dynamic environments, for example, recognizing different perspectives, unanticipated outcomes, evaluating processes underlying transitions, and adaptation of the intervention over time. In the same way that interventions may be complex in that they have numerous components that interact in multiple, unpredictable ways, so too are the systems in which they are implemented. The introduction of even 'simple' interventions (e.g. changing a law affecting the price of products that affect health) may cause emergent, unpredictable consequences that change the system and the impact of the intervention on the system (McGill et al., 2020). Simple interventions implemented in a complex system are equally difficult to evaluate given that complex systems respond to interventions in a way that may lead to emergent consequences that may mediate the intervention's impact (McGill et al., 2020).

Public health palliative care interventions are implemented in real-world contexts, that is, communities, cities, and countries, that are arguably the most complex systems. Additionally, such interventions cannot be meaningfully isolated from their context, with which they are inseparably intertwined. Within a given community may exist a multitude of ties between individuals, organizations, government agencies, companies, civil society actors, funders, and so on. Their agendas are in turn shaped by social, economic, geographic, cultural, and political interests, of which the intervention may be part. Making sense of these is itself a daunting task. This poses a fundamental challenge to conventional (often clinical) research designs predicated on linearity and predictability (Greenhalgh and Papoutsi, 2018) and may require a more ecological notion of complexity and complex systems (Cohn et al., 2013) which may be found in *complex systems* thinking. Complex systems attributes include non-linearity, a dynamic and unpredictable nature, and the fact that they co-evolve with their environment and produce emergent outcomes (McGill et al., 2020).

Conclusion

Public health palliative care research has rapidly developed over the last decades, and promising research designs concerning observational as well as intervention studies foretell a whole new domain of research and policy in end of life care. This chapter includes an overview of public health research approaches to palliative care, existing research designs that can be applied in these studies, and discusses the many complexities in public health palliative care research.

Whatever are the best palliative care services available in any country, in order to know which patients and people have access to them, public health palliative care research can monitor not only the quality of palliative care provision but also its accessibility. A population perspective should also be implemented when the new public health palliative care approaches are evaluating the effectiveness of community-driven models of palliative care like 'compassionate communities' or 'compassionate cities'.

There is a growing recognition of the importance of this public health research in the context of the major challenges to improve community-driven care for the seriously ill dying, caregivers, and those living with loss and bereavement. Although the scientific evidence for public health approaches in palliative care has been generated only recently, the impact of this research will evolve rapidly in the next decades and different solutions will be found for the many complexities in designing and conducting public health palliative care research.

REFERENCES

Abel, J., Kellehear, A., and Karapliagou, A. 2018a. Palliative care—the new essentials. *Annals of Palliative Medicine*, 7, S3–S14.

Abel, J., Kingston, H., Scally, A., Hartnoll, J., Hannam, G., Thomson-Moore, A., et al. 2018b. Reducing emergency hospital admissions: a population health complex intervention of an enhanced model of primary care and compassionate communities. *British Journal of General Practice*, 68, e803–e810.

Allsop, M. J., Ziegler, L. E., Mulvey, M. R., Russell, S., Taylor, R., and Bennett, M. I. 2018. Duration and determinants of hospice-based specialist palliative care: a national retrospective cohort study. *Palliative Medicine*, 32, 1322–1333.

Baum, F. 2016. *The New Public Health*. Oxford: Oxford University Press.

Burt, J., Shipman, C., Richardson, A., Ream, E., and Addington-Hall, J. 2010. The experiences of older adults in the community dying from cancer and non-cancer causes: a national survey of bereaved relatives. *Age and Ageing*, 39, 86–91.

Carduff, E., Jarvis, A., Highet, G., Finucane, A., Kendall, M., Harrison, N., et al. 2016. Piloting a new approach in primary care to identify, assess and support carers of people with terminal illnesses: a feasibility study. *BMC Family Practice*, 17, 18.

Chambaere, K., Bilsen, J., Cohen, J., Pousset, G., Onwuteaka-Philipsen, B., Mortier, F., et al. 2008. A post-mortem survey on end-of-life decisions using a representative sample of death certificates in Flanders, Belgium: research protocol. *BMC Public Health*, 8, 299.

Chambaere, K., Cohen, J., Robijn, L., Bailey, S. K., and Deliens, L. 2015a. End-of-life decisions in individuals dying with dementia in Belgium. *Journal of the American Geriatrics Society*, 63, 290–296.

Chambaere, K., Vander Stichele, R., Mortier, F., Cohen, J., and Deliens, L. 2015b. Recent trends in euthanasia and other end-of-life practices in Belgium. *New England Journal of Medicine*, 372, 1179–1181.

Chambers, D. A., Glasgow, R. E., and Stange, K. C. 2013. The dynamic sustainability framework: addressing the paradox of sustainment amid ongoing change. *Implementation Science*, 8, 117.

Cohen, J., Bilsen, J., Fischer, S., Lofmark, R., Norup, M., van der Heide, A., et al. 2007a. End-of-life decision-making in Belgium, Denmark, Sweden and Switzerland: does place of death make a difference? *Journal of Epidemiology & Community Health*, 61, 1062–1068.

Cohen, J., Bilsen, J., Miccinesi, G., Löfmark, R., Addington-Hall, J., Kaasa, S., et al. 2007b. Using death certificate data to study place of death in 9 European countries: opportunities and weaknesses. *BMC Public Health*, 7, 283.

Cohen, J. and Deliens, L. (eds.) 2012. *A Public Health Perspective on End of Life Care*. Oxford: Oxford University Press.

Cohen, J., Pivodic, L., Miccinesi, G., Onwuteaka-Philipsen, B. D., Naylor, W. A., Wilson, D. M., et al. 2015. International study of the place of death of people with cancer: a population-level comparison of 14 countries across 4 continents using death certificate data. *British Journal of Cancer*, 113, 1397–1404.

Cohn, S., Clinch, M., Bunn, C., and Stronge, P. 2013. Entangled complexity: why complex interventions are just not complicated enough. *Journal of Health Services Research and Policy*, 18, 40–43.

Collins, A., Brown, J. E. H., Mills, J., and Philip, J. 2021. The impact of public health palliative care interventions on health system outcomes: a systematic review. *Palliative Medicine*, 35, 473–485.

Collins, A., McLachlan, S.-A., and Philip, J. 2017. Initial perceptions of palliative care: an exploratory qualitative study of patients with advanced cancer and their family caregivers. *Palliative Medicine*, 31, 825–832.

Craig, P., Dieppe, P., Macintyre, S., Michie, S., Nazareth, I., and Petticrew, M. 2008. Developing and evaluating complex interventions: the new Medical Research Council guidance. *BMJ*, 50, a1655.

Davies, E. and Higginson, I. 2004a. *Better Palliative Care for Older People*. Copenhagen: World Health Organization.

Davies, E. and Higginson, I. 2004b. *Palliative Care: The Solid Facts*. Copenhagen: World Health Organization.

De Angelis, R., Sant, M., Coleman, M. P., Francisci, S., Baili, P., Pierannunzio, D., et al. 2014. Cancer survival in Europe 1999–2007 by country and age: results of EUROCARE-5—a population-based study. *Lancet Oncology*, 15, 23–34.

De Fina, A. and Johnstone, B. 2015. Discourse analysis and narrative. In: Tannen, D., Hamilton, H. E., and Schiffrin, D. (eds.) *The Handbook of Discourse Analysis*, pp. 152–167. Hoboken, NJ: John Wiley & Sons, Inc.

de Leeuw, E. 1989. Concepts in health promotion: the notion of relativism. *Social Science & Medicine*, 29, 1281–1288.

de Leeuw, E. 2013. Evaluating WHO Healthy Cities in Europe: issues and perspectives. *Journal of Urban Health*, 90, 14–22.

De Schreye, R., Smets, T., Annemans, L., Deliens, L., Gielen, B., De Gendt, C., et al. 2017. Applying quality indicators for administrative databases to evaluate end-of-life care for cancer patients In Belgium. *Health Affairs*, 36, 1234–1243.

Dierickx, S., Deliens, L., Cohen, J., and Chambaere, K. 2018. Involvement of palliative care in euthanasia practice in a context of legalized euthanasia: a population-based mortality follow-back study. *Palliative Medicine*, 32, 114–122.

Dodd, S., Hill, M., Ockenden, N., Algorta, G. P., Payne, S., Preston, N., et al. 2018. 'Being with' or 'doing for'? How the role of an end-of-life volunteer befriender can impact patient wellbeing: interviews from a multiple qualitative case study (ELSA). *Supportive Care in Cancer*, 26, 3163–3172.

Earle, C. C. and Ayanian, J. Z. 2006. Looking back from death: the value of retrospective studies of end-of-life care. *Journal of Clinical Oncology*, 24, 838–840.

Etkind, S. N., Bone, A. E., Gomes, B., Lovell, N., Evans, C. J., Higginson, I. J., et al. 2017. How many people will need palliative care in 2040? Past trends, future projections and implications for services. *BMC Medicine*, 15, 1–10.

Faes, K., Cohen, J., and Annemans, L. 2018. Resource use during the last 6 months of life of individuals dying with and of Alzheimer's disease. *Journal of the American Geriatrics Society*, 66, 879–885.

Faulkner, M. and Davies, S. 2005. Social support in the healthcare setting: the role of volunteers. *Health & Social Care in the Community*, 13, 38–45.

Ferrell, B. R. and Coyle, N. (eds.) 2010. *Oxford Textbook of Palliative Nursing*, 3rd ed. New York: Oxford University Press.

Gardiner, C. and Barnes, S. 2016. The impact of volunteer befriending services for older people at the end of life: mechanisms supporting wellbeing. *Progress in Palliative Care*, 24, 159–164.

Gielen, A. and Eileen, M. 1996. The PRECEDE-PROCEED planning model. In: Glanz, K., Lewis, F., and Rimer, K. (eds.) *Health Behavior and Health Education*, pp. 359–383. San Francisco, CA: Jossey-Bass.

Gilissen, J., Pivodic, L., Unroe, K. T., and Van den Block, L. 2020. International COVID-19 palliative care guidance for nursing homes leaves key themes unaddressed. *Journal of Pain and Symptom Management*, 60, e56–e69.

Greenhalgh, T., Jackson, C., Shaw, S., and Janamian, T. 2016. Achieving research impact through co-creation in community-based health services: literature review and case study. *Milbank Quarterly*, 94, 392–429.

Greenhalgh, T. and Papoutsi, C. 2018. Studying complexity in health services research: desperately seeking an overdue paradigm shift. *BMC Medicine*, 16, 95.

Hanks, G., Cherny, N., Christiakis, N., Fallon, M., Kaasa, S., and Portenoy, R. (eds.) 2009. *Oxford Textbook of Palliative Medicine*, 4th ed. Oxford: Oxford University Press.

Hill, C., Duggleby, W., Venturato, L., Durepos, P., Kulasegaram, P., Hunter, P., et al. 2019. An analysis of documents guiding palliative care in five Canadian Provinces. *Canadian Journal on Aging/La Revue Canadienne Du Vieillissement*, 38, 281–295.

Holt-Lunstad, J., Smith, T. B., and Layton, J. B. 2010. Social relationships and mortality risk: a meta-analytic review. *PLoS Medicine*, 7, e1000316.

Horsfall, D. 2018. Developing compassionate communities in Australia through collective caregiving: a qualitative study exploring network-centred care and the role of the end of life sector. *Annals of Palliative Medicine*, 7, S42–S51.

Horsfall, D., Noonan, K., and Leonard, R. 2012. Bringing our dying home: how caring for someone at end of life builds social capital and develops compassionate communities. *Health Sociology Review*, 21, 373–382.

Houttekier, D., Cohen, J., Surkyn, J., and Deliens, L. 2011. Study of recent and future trends in place of death in Belgium using death certificate data: a shift from hospitals to care homes. *BMC Public Health*, 11, 228.

Hsieh, H. F. and Shannon, S. E. 2005. Three approaches to qualitative content analysis. *Qualitative Health Research*, 15, 1277–1288.

Kawachi, I. 2004. Commentary: reconciling the three accounts of social capital. *International Journal of Epidemiology*, 33, 682–690.

Kellehear, A. 1999. *Health Promoting Palliative Care*. Melbourne: Oxford University Press.

Kellehear, A. and Young, B. 2007. Resilient communities. In: Monroe, B. and Oliviere, D. (eds.) *Resilience in Palliative Care—Achievement in Adversity*, pp. 223–238. Oxford: Oxford University Press.

Kelley, M. Lou, Prince, H., Nadin, S., Brazil, K., Crow, M., Hanson, G., et al. 2018. Developing palliative care programs in Indigenous communities using participatory action research: a Canadian application of the public health approach to palliative care. *Annals of Palliative Medicine*, 7, S52–S72.

Kleijberg, M., Ahlberg, B. M., Hilton, R., and Tishelman, C. 2020. Death, loss and community—perspectives from children, their parents and older adults on intergenerational community-based arts initiatives in Sweden. *Health & Social Care in the Community*, 28, 2025–2036.

Kleijberg, M., Ahlberg, B. M., Macdonald, A., Lindqvist, O., and Tishelman, C. 2021. Navigating power dynamics in engaging communities in end-of-life issues—lessons learned from developing community-based intergenerational arts initiatives about death and loss. *Death Studies*, 45, 651–664.

Krug, K., Miksch, A., Peters-Klimm, F., Engeser, P., and Szecsenyi, J. 2016. Correlation between patient quality of life in palliative care and burden of their family caregivers: a prospective observational cohort study. *BMC Palliative Care*, 15, 4.

Leonard, R., Horsfall, D., and Noonan, K. 2015. Identifying changes in the support networks of end-of-life carers using social network analysis. *BMJ Supportive & Palliative Care*, 5, 153–159.

Lewin, S., Hendry, M., Chandler, J., Oxman, A. D., Michie, S., Shepperd, S., et al. 2017. Assessing the complexity of interventions within systematic reviews: development, content and use of a new tool (iCAT_SR). *BMC Medical Research Methodology*, 17, 76.

Lewis, J. M., DiGiacomo, M., Luckett, T., Davidson, P. M., and Currow, D. C. 2013. A social capital framework for palliative care: supporting health and well-being for people with life-limiting illness and their carers through social relations and networks. *Journal of Pain and Symptom Management*, 45, 92–103.

Librada Flores, S., Herrera Molina, E., Díaz Díez, F., Redondo Moralo, M. J., Castillo Rodríguez, C., McLoughlin, K., et al. 2018. Development and management of networks of care at the end of life (the REDCUIDA intervention): protocol for a nonrandomized controlled trial. *JMIR Research Protocols*, 7, e10515.

Lind, S., Adolfsson, J., Axelsson, B., and Fürst, C. J. 2013. Quality indicators for palliative and end of life care: a review of Swedish policy documents. *BMJ Supportive & Palliative Care*, 3, 174–180.

Luijkx, K. G. and Schols, J. M. 2009. Volunteers in palliative care make a difference. *Journal of Palliative Care*, 25, 30–39.

Maetens, A., Beernaert, K., de Schreye, R., Faes, K., Pardon, K., Annemans, L., et al. 2019. Impact of palliative home care support on the quality and costs of care at the end of life: a population-level matched cohort study. *BMJ Open*, 9, e025180.

Malvezzi, M., Bertuccio, P., Rosso, T., Rota, M., Levi, F., La Vecchia, C., et al. 2015. European cancer mortality predictions for the year 2015: does lung cancer have the highest death rate in EU women? *Annals of Oncology*, 26, 779–786.

Marmot, M. 2005. Social determinants of health inequalities. *Lancet*, 365, 1099–1104.

Mayring, P. 2000. Qualitative content analysis. *Forum: Qualitative Social Research*, 1, 20.

McGill, E., Marks, D., Vanessa, E., Penney, T., Petticrew, M., and Egan, M. 2020. Qualitative process evaluation from a complex systems perspective: a systematic review and framework for public health evaluators. *PLoS Medicine*, 17, 1–27.

McLoughlin, K., Rhatigan, J., McGilloway, S., Kellehear, A., Lucey, M., Twomey, F., et al. 2015. INSPIRE (INvestigating Social and PractIcal suppoRts at the End of life): pilot randomised trial of a community social and practical support intervention for adults with life-limiting illness. *BMC Palliative Care*, 14, 65.

Morin, L., Aubry, R., Frova, L., MacLeod, R., Wilson, D. M., Loucka, M., et al. 2017. Estimating the need for palliative care at the population level: a cross-national study in 12 countries. *Palliative Medicine*, 31, 526–536.

Morita, T., Miyashita, M., Yamagishi, A., Akiyama, M., Akizuki, N., Hirai, K., et al. 2013. Effects of a programme of interventions on regional comprehensive palliative care for patients with cancer: a mixed-methods study. *Lancet Oncology*, 14, 638–646.

Murtagh, F. E., Bausewein, C., Verne, J., Groeneveld, E. I., Kaloki, Y. E., and Higginson, I. J. 2014. How many people need palliative care? A study developing and comparing methods for population-based estimates. *Palliative Medicine*, 28, 49–58.

Nakanishi, M., Nakashima, T., Shindo, Y., Miyamoto, Y., Gove, D., Radbruch, L., et al. 2015. An evaluation of palliative care contents in national dementia strategies in reference to the European Association for Palliative Care white paper. *International Psychogeriatrics* 27, 1551–1561.

O'Mara-Eves, A., Brunton, G., McDaid, D., Oliver, S., Kavanagh, J., Jamal, F., et al. 2013. Community engagement to reduce inequalities in health: a systematic review, meta-analysis and economic analysis. *Public Health Research*, 1, 1–526.

Paque, K., De Schreye, R., Elseviers, M., Vander Stichele, R., Pardon, K., Dilles, T., et al. 2019a. Discontinuation of medications at the end of life: a population study in Belgium, based on linked administrative databases. *British Journal of Clinical Pharmacology*, 85, 827–837.

Paque, K., Elseviers, M., Vander Stichele, R., Dilles, T., Pardon, K., Deliens, L., et al. 2019b. Associations of potentially inappropriate medication use with four year survival of an inception cohort of nursing home residents. *Archives of Gerontology and Geriatrics*, 80, 82–87.

Paul, S. 2015. *Advancing Education and Support Around Death, Dying and Bereavement: Hospices, Schools and Health Promoting Palliative Care*. Edinburgh: University of Edinburgh.

Paz-Ruiz, S., Gomez-Batiste, X., Espinosa, J., Porta-Sales, J., and Esperalba, J. 2009. The costs and savings of a regional public palliative care program: the Catalan experience at 18 years. *Journal of Pain and Symptom Management,* 38, 87–96.

Penders, Y. W., Gilissen, J., Moreels, S., Deliens, L., and Van den Block, L. 2018. Palliative care service use by older people: time trends from a mortality follow-back study between 2005 and 2014. *Palliative Medicine,* 32, 466–475.

Perera, G., Stewart, R., Higginson, I. J., and Sleeman, K. E. 2016. Reporting of clinically diagnosed dementia on death certificates: retrospective cohort study. *Age and Ageing,* 45, 667–672.

Pesut, B., Duggleby, W., Warner, G., Fassbender, K., Antifeau, E., Hooper, B., et al. 2018. Volunteer navigation partnerships: piloting a compassionate community approach to early palliative care. *BMC Palliative Care,* 17, 2.

Petticrew, M. 2011. When are complex interventions "complex"? When are simple interventions "simple"? *European Journal of Public Health,* 21, 397–398.

Pivodic, L. and Cohen, J. 2018. Public health and epidemiological research in palliative care. In: MacLeod, R. and Van den Block, L. (eds.) *Textbook of Palliative Care,* pp. 1–18. Cham: Springer International Publishing.

Pivodic, L., Pardon, K., Miccinesi, G., Vega Alonso, T., Moreels, S., Donker, G. A., et al. 2016a. Hospitalisations at the end of life in four European countries: a population-based study via epidemiological surveillance networks. *Journal of Epidemiology and Community Health,* 70, 430–436.

Pivodic, L., Pardon, K., Morin, L., Addington-Hall, J., Miccinesi, G., Cardenas-Turanzas, M., et al. 2016b. Place of death in the population dying from diseases indicative of palliative care need: a cross-national population-level study in 14 countries. *Journal of Epidemiology and Community Health,* 70, 17–24.

Pivodic, L., Smets, T., Gott, M., Sleeman, K. E., Arrue, B., Cardenas Turanzas, M., et al. 2021. Inclusion of palliative care in health care policy for older people: a directed documentary analysis in 13 of the most rapidly ageing countries worldwide. *Palliative Medicine,* 35, 369–388.

Pivodic, L., Smets, T., Van den Noortgate, N., Onwuteaka-Philipsen, B. D., Engels, Y., Szczerbińska, K., et al. 2018. Quality of dying and quality of end-of-life care of nursing home residents in six countries: an epidemiological study. *Palliative Medicine,* 32, 1584–1595.

Popay, J. 2010. Community empowerment and health improvement: the English experience. In: Morgan, A., Davies, M., and Ziglio, E. (eds.) *Health Assets in a Global Context: Theory, Methods, Action,* pp. 183–195. New York: Springer.

Popay, J., Whitehead, M., Carr-Hill, R., Dibben, C., Dixon, P., Halliday, E., et al. 2015. The impact on health inequalities of approaches to community engagement in the New Deal for Communities regeneration initiative: a mixed-methods evaluation. *Public Health Research,* 3, 12.

Portes, A. 1998. Social capital: its origins and applications in modern sociology. *Annual Review of Sociology,* 24, 1–24.

RE-AIM. n.d.. RE-AIM—Reach Effectiveness Adoption Implementation Maintenance. [Online] Available at: http://www.re-aim.org

Reeves, D., Blickem, C., Vassilev, I., Brooks, H., Kennedy, A., Richardson, G., et al. 2014. The contribution of social networks to the health and self-management of patients with long-term conditions: a longitudinal study. *PLoS One,* 9, e98340.

Renz, M., Reichmuth, O., Bueche, D., Traichel, B., Mao, M. S., Cerny, T., and Strasser, F. 2018. Fear, pain, denial, and spiritual experiences in dying processes. *American Journal of Hospice and Palliative Medicine*®, 35, 478–491.

Rosenbaum, P. R. 2002. *Observational Studies,* 2nd ed. New York: Springer.

Sallnow, L. 2017. Collective social capital: a study of new public health and end-of-life care. Doctoral thesis, University of Edinburgh.

Sallnow, L. and Paul, S. 2015. Understanding community engagement in end-of-life care: developing conceptual clarity. *Critical Public Health,* 25, 231–238

Sallnow, L. and Paul, S. 2018. New public health approaches to end-of-life care. In: *Textbook of Palliative Care,* pp. 1–10. Cham: Springer International Publishing.

Sallnow, L., Richardson, H., Murray, S. A., and Kellehear, A. 2016a. The impact of a new public health approach to end-of-life care: a systematic review. *Palliative Medicine,* 30, 200–211.

Sallnow, L., Tishelman, C., Lindqvist, O., Richardson, H., and Cohen, J. 2016b. Research in public health and end-of-life care—building on the past and developing the new. *Progress in Palliative Care,* 24, 25–30.

Seymour, J. E., Almack, K., Kennedy, S., and Froggatt, K. 2013. Peer education for advance care planning: volunteers' perspectives on training and community engagement activities. *Health Expectations,* 16, 43–55.

Smets, T., Pivodic, L., Piers, R., Pasman, H. R. W., Engels, Y., Szczerbińska, K., et al. 2018. The palliative care knowledge of nursing home staff: the EU FP7 PACE cross-sectional survey in 322 nursing homes in six European countries. *Palliative Medicine,* 32, 1487–1497.

Van Beek, K., Woitha, K., Ahmed, N., Menten, J., Jaspers, B., Engels, Y., et al. 2013. Comparison of legislation, regulations and national health strategies for palliative care in seven European countries (results from the Europall Research Group): a descriptive study. *BMC Health Services Research,* 13, 275.

Van den Block, L., Deschepper, R., Bilsen, J., Van Casteren, V., and Deliens, L. 2007. Transitions between care settings at the end of life in Belgium. *JAMA,* 298, 1635.

Van den Block, L., Pivodic, L., Pardon, K., Donker, G., Miccinesi, G., Moreels, S., et al. 2015. Transitions between health care settings in the final three months of life in four EU countries. *European Journal of Public Health,* 25, 569–575.

Van den Block, L., Smets, T., van Dop, N., Adang, E., Andreasen, P., Collingridge Moore, D., et al. 2016. Comparing Palliative Care in Care Homes Across Europe (PACE): protocol of a cross-sectional study of deceased residents in 6 EU countries. *Journal of the American Medical Directors Association,* 17, 566.e1–566.e7.

van der Heide, A., Deliens, L., Faisst, K., Nilstun, T., Norup, M., Paci, E., et al. 2003. End-of-life decision-making in six European countries: descriptive study. *Lancet,* 362, 345–350.

Vanderstichelen, S., Cohen, J., Van Wesemael, Y., Deliens, L., and Chambaere, K. 2019a. Perspectives on volunteer-professional collaboration in palliative care: a qualitative study among volunteers, patients, family carers, and health care professionals. *Journal of Pain and Symptom Management,* 58, 198–207.

Vanderstichelen, S., Cohen, J., Van Wesemael, Y., Deliens, L., and Chambaere, K. 2020a. The involvement of volunteers in palliative care and their collaboration with healthcare professionals: a cross-sectional volunteer survey across the Flemish healthcare system (Belgium). *Health & Social Care in the Community,* 28, 747–761.

Vanderstichelen, S., Cohen, J., Van Wesemael, Y., Deliens, L., and Chambaere, K. 2020b. The liminal space palliative care volunteers occupy and their roles within it: a qualitative study. *BMJ Supportive & Palliative Care,* 10, e28.

Vanderstichelen, S., Cohen, J., Van Wesemael, Y., Deliens, L., and Chambaere, K. 2020c. Volunteers in palliative care: a healthcare system-wide cross-sectional survey. *BMJ Supportive & Palliative*

Care, bmjspcare-2020-002321. Advance online publication. https://doi.org/10.1136/bmjspcare-2020-002321

Vanderstichelen, S., Cohen, J., Van Wesemael, Y., Deliens, L., and Chambaere, K. 2019b. Volunteer involvement in the organisation of palliative care: a survey study of the healthcare system in Flanders and Dutch-speaking Brussels, Belgium. *Health & Social Care in the Community*, 27, 459–471.

Vanderstichelen, S., Houttekier, D., Cohen, J., Wesemael, Y. Van, Deliens, L., and Chambaere, K. 2018. Palliative care volunteerism across the healthcare system: a survey study. *Palliative Medicine*, 32, 1233–1245.

Walshe, C., Dodd, S., Hill, M., Ockenden, N., Payne, S., Preston, N., et al. 2016. How effective are volunteers at supporting people in their last year of life? A pragmatic randomised wait-list trial in palliative care (ELSA). *BMC Medicine*, 14, 1–12.

Walugembe, D. R., Sibbald, S., Le Ber, M. J., and Kothari, A. 2019. Sustainability of public health interventions: where are the gaps? *Health Research Policy and Systems*, 17, 8.

Wells, M., Williams, B., Treweek, S., Coyle, J., and Taylor, J. 2012. Intervention description is not enough: evidence from an in-depth multiple case study on the untold role and impact of context in randomised controlled trials of seven complex interventions. *Trials*, 13, 1–17.

Young, A. J., Rogers, A., Dent, L., and Addington-Hall, J. M. 2009. Experiences of hospital care reported by bereaved relatives of patients after a stroke: a retrospective survey using the VOICES questionnaire. *Journal of Advanced Nursing*, 65, 2161–2174.

25

Economic perspectives on public health approaches to palliative care

Charles Normand

Introduction

The perspectives that led to the emergence of palliative medicine and palliative care have much in common with the thinking behind the new public health. Palliative care has a focus on all the needs of the patient and their family and friends, seeing the patient within a social setting, and looking to improve the experience of those with life-limiting illness by providing supports of many different kinds. In some ways, palliative care developments led to further fragmentation of service delivery near the end of life, with some new services being provided outside of normal healthcare structures and systems. The (highly desirable) focus on managing pain and other symptoms, and the focus on treating the patient and not just the disease, did not always come with a good understanding of the importance of the context within which a person lives, the many sources of support, and how these can best combine to contribute to the overall experience of a person with life-limiting illness.

In the US, the way in which the hospice benefit in Medicare was structured reinforced the idea that palliative care was an alternative to other health services, with the patient being able to access the benefit only if other types of care were excluded. It therefore came to be the final episode of care rather than an approach to meeting the needs of patients. This illustrates the importance for access to appropriate care of the ways that services are funded, and the incentives that this funding generates. This is one way in which an economist's perspective can help in understanding the intended and unintended consequences of how services are organized. Similarly, since palliative care often involves the use of charitable funds and volunteer staff as well as staff paid from normal healthcare sources, it is useful to understand how this affects what is provided, by whom, and for whom—again, a topic of interest to economists.

This chapter discusses how an economic perspective can be useful in understanding issues in palliative care, and particularly issues that are prominent in public health approaches to palliative care. It is not argued that taking an economic viewpoint solves difficult problems and answers difficult dilemmas, but it is suggested that this perspective provides useful insight and understanding. It starts with a brief summary of the history of health economics and key features of an economic perspective, and then considers some cases where an economic viewpoint can assist in making better choices.

A brief history of health economics and the economics of public health

Economics is as much a way of thinking as it is a set of tools and models. Economic questions surround us at all time: in everyday life we make choices on what clothes to buy, where to live, and what to eat—all of which are economic questions. We choose from the jobs that are available to try to achieve the best available combination of income and work satisfaction. We make choices about whether and where to go on holiday, and how to travel to work. Health economics is concerned with choices around health and healthcare. What services should be provided, for whom, by whom, who should pay, and when? Should we tax tobacco and if so, by how much? Should we subsidize sports facilities to encourage more active lifestyles? Should we screen for cancers, and if so, how and how often?

While some health choices are sensibly taken by individuals and families, many require collective action. It is hard to buy and sell a healthy lifestyles programme. Since the benefits of vaccination go far beyond those to the vaccinated people—it can prevent the spread of disease to those not vaccinated—there is a need to encourage people to be vaccinated in order to protect others. For many reasons, markets do not always work well in the contexts of health and healthcare. Typically, providers of services are better informed than users, services are often complex and have uncertain outcomes, and often there are benefits and costs that are more widely spread. For these reasons, some government role is desirable to mitigate market failures. This means that many health economic choices involve local or national government, state agencies, and community organizations. Health economics therefore aims to provide a better basis for collective choices as well as choices by individuals.

Economics starts from the viewpoint of scarcity (i.e. not all services and supports that bring benefits can be provided), and it aims to understand how resources are used, why they are used in that way, and how they could be used better. The economics of health and healthcare is concerned with uses of resources in health and healthcare, and how they could be used better, to improve further health and quality of life. Health economic analysis has grown as spending on health and social care has grown, and we have reached the stage where the increasing technical capacity to improve health has come against limitations on what resources have been devoted to promoting health and providing care.

Formal health economic analysis starting in the 1960s (Arrow, 1963), with more rapid growth from the late 1970s. Some studies aim to understand patterns of needs and access to care. Typical questions include 'To what extent do financial barriers affect access to care?' For example, to what extent do user fees affect patterns of use of family doctor services? To what extent does having private health insurance affect access to hospital care? Economist are interested in how incentives affect behaviours, especially in relation to health-damaging goods or activities. How much does tax on cigarettes reduce smoking, and what are the effects of alcohol taxes on patterns of drinking? Do sugar taxes reduce the consumption of sugar-sweetened drinks and snacks, and if so, does this reduce obesity? This is not to argue that taxation (or other financial incentives) is the only or the best way to change behaviour, but it is of interest to know to what extent we can improve health by changing financial incentives (Tambor et al., 2016; Galinowska et al., 2016).

Economists understand that people do (at least to some extent) respond to financial incentives. Use of general practitioner care in the Republic of Ireland (where most people pay the full cost out of pocket) is lower than in Northern Ireland where no user fees apply (O'Reilly et al., 2007). On the supplier side, we know that private obstetric services carry out more Caesarean section deliveries than public services despite evidence that risks and outcomes are no different (Moran et al., 2020). As mentioned previously, the structure of the Medicare hospice benefit used to require a choice between receiving care with curative or palliative intent but not both, but rules have now changed (Obermeyer et al., 2014). This discouraged an appropriate blend of service use that would both affect the disease trajectory and improve the experience of patients and their families. Studies have shown that raising the price of cigarettes does reduce smoking, especially among young smokers (Cheng and Estrada, 2020), and charges for prescription drugs do reduce filling of prescriptions, so these policies should be seen not only as mechanisms to raise money but as policies that will change behaviour (Sinnott et al., 2016).

There is an important problem in how health services can best be funded. People generally need few services when they are working and earning but are more likely to need them when they are small children or are retired and have reduced incomes. A person is likely to need most when they can least afford it and need least when they can afford to pay. Together these problems mean that, even in very market-oriented countries such as the US, governments are closely involved in regulating, financing, and providing public health and health services. When some, or all, of the funds are provided by government, there is a need to make collective decisions about what should be provided, for whom should services be provided, who should provide services, and how should the providers be paid? This has led to economic studies that aim to support better choices by public regulators, funders, and providers.

Public health poses additional challenges for economic analysis. While simple interventions such as screening and immunization are easy to cost, and it is feasible to estimate outcomes and benefits, broader, population-based activities can be hard to cost and measuring effects is more difficult. It can be hard to be precise about who benefits, when, and to what extent, and many public health strategies aim to affect a range of outcomes. In some public health interventions, there is a very long gap between the intervention and the outcome so that assessing outcomes requires modelling and estimation. If someone stops smoking in their 20s there may be a gap of 40 or 50 years before the survival benefits are realized (even if there are shorter-term health benefits). This does not make it less important to ask the questions about the costs and benefits—it just makes it more difficult to estimate them. In public health, it has long been recognized that the best outcomes arise from combinations of environmental, occupational, financial, and personal circumstances as well as more direct supports and services to individuals and families. It will always be difficult to apply simple metrics that estimated costs and benefits in this context.

Health economics: key concepts and approaches

Economics is based on a few key ideas (McPake et al., 2020). The most important ones are scarcity and opportunity cost. There is also a strong focus on the margin. Each of these will be discussed briefly to provide a context for the rest of the chapter.

Scarcity simply means that resources are not unlimited. Both as individuals and as society we cannot do or have all things that we want. The consequence of scarcity is that we must make choices. There are good ways to make choices and bad ways. Making bad choices reduces the benefits of using the available resources to individuals or society.

To an economist, cost is defined by what is lost or given up. *Opportunity cost* is the best alternative use of resources. For example, the decision to provide a very expensive new drug may be the choice not to provide other drugs to other people, or not to provide respite care for families of children with special needs, or not to support families of children with life-limiting conditions. It can be the choice to have higher taxes (and fewer holidays for those taxpayers that are affected). The opportunity cost of the drug is whatever is the best of these alternatives. The argument is simple—if the new drug is better value than any of the alternatives, it should be provided, but if any other use of resources is more useful, it should not. The challenge is to find acceptable ways to measure the value of resources used in each of the possible ways. Given the complexity of this task, there is a temptation to simplify the evaluation processes and make them more manageable, but this may lead to a failure adequately to characterize the full value of costs and benefits. Simple measurement is appropriate where the activities and outcomes are relatively simple and easy to describe but are often less appropriate when dealing with complex interventions with multiple components and complex mixes of effects.

Economists aim to work *at the margin*. They ask: how much *more* benefit would be gained for how much *more* cost? They do not ask 'Is cataract surgery good value?', but 'Would more cataract surgery be good value?' There is a good example of why this is important in the case of cancer screening. Changing from

5-yearly screening to 3-yearly screening would detect some additional treatable cases. Shifting from 3-yearly screening to annual screening would still increase the cases detected, but there would be fewer additional ones. The cost of each test would be the same, but potential benefits of each test performed would be much smaller in the shift to annual screening. It may be a good use of resources to reduce the interval to 3-yearly but is not likely to be good value to reduce it to once a year. In each case, the question is 'Is it better to use additional resources to achieve additional benefits here or in some other use?'

Normally we ask if extra resources would be justified in terms of extra benefits. However, there can be circumstances in which interventions release resources for other uses. Recent research has shown that some palliative care interventions, particularly those that support patients and families in their choices about trajectories of care, lead to savings. One study in lung cancer also showed that, on average, better support for choices saved resources *and* increased life expectancy (Temmel et al., 2017). The experiences for patients and families also improved. If an intervention saves resources, in effect it costs less than nothing—indeed, it allows some existing resources to be used for a better purpose. When this is the case, it is not necessary to show that the benefits exceed the cost—in effect there is a negative cost, so there is no economic argument against the intervention. If an intervention saves money and achieves the same or more, then it is obviously good value and does not need to compete with priorities where there are positive costs—it should just happen. This is not to say that only cost-saving interventions (that improve outcomes of leave them the same) should be chosen—it is just that they should always be chosen.

The aim of public health is to protect and improve the health of communities. Better health depends on a wide range of contextual, social, and community factors as well as interventions that are more specifically targeted at improving health of individuals or communities. The best use of resources may not be visibly in the health domain, and may include interventions in education, housing, and community development. Given the fragmented nature of most public administrations, this can form a barrier to the most efficient use of resources to improve health. It can be difficult to persuade a health service budget holder to transfer funds to an education administrator in recognition that the best health gains will come from more education spending.

A linked issue is that a desired outcome may result from *the combination* of interventions. For example, educational and social development initiatives may provide the basis for better adherence to treatments and make it possible to achieve better outcomes from supports at the individual level. A stronger local community can give people to confidence to stay at home with outreach support and avoid the need for institutional care. In some cases, availability of a service is valued even when it is not actually used—the knowledge that quick and effective action will be taken if needed can allow people to live more independent lives. These complexities pose challenges for assessing costs and benefits.

Economics applied to palliative care

Few economic studies in palliative care were undertaken before the start of the twenty-first century. Palliative care developments owe much to the drive and determination of visionary and committed people, often drawing heavily on charitable funding and voluntary activity. Recently it has been recognized that it is important to understand how resources are being used, what is being achieved, and palliative care resources could be used to greater effect. Health economists working in palliative care are very aware of the analytical challenges that arise when needs are complex, the interventions are complex, and the outcomes are hard to measure.

A complication in the economics of palliative care is the widespread use of volunteer and unpaid staff, and the widespread use of charitable funding for facilities and equipment. In financial terms, these resources appear to be free—after all, someone who works for nothing must prefer that to not working for nothing. If money is given to buy staff or equipment, the donor must prefer this to other things that could be bought with the money.

The problem with this argument is that there is still an opportunity cost to any resources used for any purpose. Even within palliative care the money spent on a building might be better spent on equipment or staff, and volunteers used for one purpose might be best used in another. For the purposes of supporting good decisions, it is always best to try to account for all costs, whoever pays, and all benefits, whoever receives. This can be difficult to accept if you are a manager or clinician who is being offered something that is not exactly what you want but is 'free'. Obviously, the best position to be in is for donations to be made without the use being specified, so that the resources can be put to the highest priority use.

Volunteers in supporting palliative care services often fill gaps around the more personal and spiritual needs of service users, having the time to listen and talk, and being able to provide interesting activity and interests. Formal care providers tend to focus on tasks and supports that have obvious, measurable, and visible effects, and sometimes there are large gaps in (often more important) activities that improve morale and quality of life. There can be advantages where volunteers are not subject to some simplistic metrics in the use of resources. Voluntary effort can be a very useful catalyst for change and can help to challenge models of care that are no longer appropriate. However, the 'mixed economy' in palliative care can also make it more difficult to develop and apply national policies since there is diversity of control of use of resources by service providers.

Although charitable funding has led to many important and useful developments in palliative care, there are instances where charitable funds can be harmful. It can be difficult for donors to know the most important needs that their contributions can help to meet. It is common for such monies to be concentrated on visible, one-off, uses, such as buildings and equipment, rather than on staff wages or consumables. Care providers can feel obliged to use a building or piece of equipment that has been donated even though this may not be a high priority use of the staffing budget.

Many of the issues discussed previously also apply more widely in healthcare and provide challenges for measurement and evaluation. Reviews of the evidence suggest that interventions aimed at strengthening community participation and engagement can be effective in terms of equity and health outcomes (Cyril et al., 2015; Martins Pereira et al., 2018). What is also clear is that success in such interventions is highly sensitive to the detail of the design of the intervention, and the ways in which participation is supported (Sarrami-Foroushani et al., 2014).

Despite the challenges in carrying out economic studies in palliative care, some important insights have come from the work. Research has identified cases where it is possible to achieve more with the same or fewer resources, as well as circumstances where additional resources could be easily justified. Two topics have been chosen to illustrate how economic thinking can be helpful in the context of public health approaches to palliative care. Studies in this chapter aim to show ways in which economic evidence can be very useful, even when it is incomplete and where measurement challenges are great.

The two topics that will be used to discuss economic issues in public health approaches to palliative care are:

- Nutrition and nutritional status near the end of life.
- The relationship between formal care and informal caregivers.

The aim is to demonstrate how an economic perspective can provide some useful understanding on how resources could be used better and how the objectives could be better met. In both topics, interventions are complex and aim to meet complex needs.

Topic 1: economic issues in public health approaches to palliative care—nutrition near the end of life

Good nutrition and hydration are critical factors in improving health and quality of life for people with life-limiting illness (Bozetti et al., 2009; Stevens et al., 2021). Poor nutrition can be the cause of poor health and poor quality of life but can also be the consequence of illness. Some diseases lead to loss of appetite or difficulty in eating. It can be difficult in some circumstances to prevent weight loss (e.g. in the case of cancer cachexia), the consequences of the loss are much worse for people who progress to this stage of disease with poor nutritional status (Vettori et al., 2021).

Ensuring the best nutritional status can involve interventions and supports at many levels. These include:

- Help to build a supportive environment in which people eat well and enjoy their food.
- Individual support for healthy eating to ensure people have adequate nutrition.
- Provision of supplements to compensate for limited quantity and range of foods.
- Enteral and parenteral feeding.

These are not mutually exclusive, and it may be useful to provide supports at various levels at the same time. In many cases the appropriate balance moves from the first towards the last. We may concentrate too much on the last of these and too little on the first, but there is evidence that all can be good value and improve nutritional status.

Better nutrition leads to a better quality of life, but better nutrition can also be associated with much lower costs of treatment and care. Evidence on the cost of disease-related malnutrition demonstrates the *scale of potential savings* from improving nutrition. Rice and Normand (2012) showed that the *additional* costs of treatment of people with poor nutritional status in acute hospitals in Ireland was equivalent to 11% of the total public health service budget. Some of this was costs for people who became malnourished after admission to hospital, but much of the cost was for hospital care of people who were admitted to hospital with poor nutritional status.

A related study (Rice et al., 2016) showed that it would be possible to release around 4% of hospital beds for other uses if malnutrition in this population were better managed. These data show that at least for some patients it would be possible to provide better support for better nutrition and still save money on care.

The additional cost of treatments for people with malnutrition can be thought of as a minimum budget for successful interventions. Any successful intervention that costs less than it saves is by definition good value. If a day in hospital costs around €800, support for better hospital nutrition that reduces the stay by 1 day would pay for itself if it costs less than this amount. This is not to argue that it is only worth improving nutrition if it saves money, but it does say that there can be no case for not spending money that saves more money.

It is likely that some interventions that improve nutrition by creating a more supportive local community are cost saving, although at present there is limited evidence. There is strong evidence that some other nutrition supports are cost saving. For example, the use of oral nutritional supplements to prevent malnutrition and to supplement feeding for those who are already malnourished is good value, both in community and nursing home settings (Elia et al., 2016a) and in hospital settings (Elia et al., 2016b). The review studies showed that the costs of oral nutritional supplements were less than 5% of total costs of care for hospital patients, and that overall their use was cost saving.

The studies of oral nutrition supplements demonstrate the advantages of successful early action to prevent malnutrition, and there is other evidence that early interventions are more effective, especially in patients with cancer. Quality of life is higher for people who are well nourished, so it can be shown that improving nutritional status can reduce costs and improve outcomes (Gillespie and Raftery, 2009; Orrevall, 2015).

There is a need for more and better studies of the best ways to intervene to improve nutrition in people near the end of life. Such studies will face challenges in measuring costs and outcomes. Some interventions might be to strengthen the support at community level, some to support healthy eating for individuals, and some may be to reverse the effects of poor diet. Some would support informal caregivers to ensure that the best possible nutrition status is maintained (see 'Topic 2'). Since there is good evidence of the financial as well as health benefits of improved nutritional status, the key gap in evidence is on the effectiveness of public health interventions in improving nutrition. The scale of the potential savings from successful improvements as well as the better quality of life for patients and families show that even interventions that improve nutrition only slightly can be good value.

There is a need to create a stronger evidence base on the effectiveness and cost-effectiveness of the many potential ways in which better nutrition would be achieved for people near the end of life. However, recognizing the scale of the harm done by poor nutrition in older people and the related cost of treatment and care provides strong arguments for finding effective interventions since many of these may be cost savings, and others may have benefits that clearly justify the costs.

Topic 2: economic issues in public health approaches to palliative care—formal care and informal caregivers

Public health approaches to palliative care understand that people with life-limiting illness live their lives and receive their support in many settings, and care is provided by both paid formal service providers and a wide range of informal supports. The experiences of people with life-limiting illness and the wider community of caregivers depend crucially on how these different elements interact and support each other.

Economic studies in palliative care have provided a better understanding of the key role of informal caregivers and the costs of providing informal care. They have also provided a better understanding of how different stages of diseases can place burdens on those with the disease and those providing support. While most people have retired before they develop life-limiting illness, in some cases such as amyotrophic lateral sclerosis, people develop the disease at younger ages and are likely to be employed, and may have time off work and loss of pay (Galvin et al., 2017; Connolly et al., 2015). Those who develop life-limiting illness at younger ages display strong preferences to be involved in choices about the supports they need and the choices about trajectories of care.

Some life-limiting illnesses significantly reduce a person's ability to care for themselves, and many people remain active for long periods. Costs related to the illness can therefore fall on the person with the illness, families, and other informal caregivers as well as formal providers of services. The capacity to support a person's needs can depend on supports outside the healthcare setting. The costs related to an illness fall mainly on (adult) children and their partners as family incomes are reduced as the illness reduces the capacity to work.

Studies of costs to families and informal caregivers demonstrate the scale of such costs. Depending on the specific needs of the person receiving care, it is common for informal care to cost between one-third to one-half of total care costs (Yi et al., 2020). This can be even higher when formal care provision is poor. It is also known that poor support of informal caregivers tends to divert them from roles that only they can do well—particularly in supporting the mental health and spiritual needs of the patient. This illustrates the point made earlier that informal caregiver input appears to be free from the perspective of managers and providers of formal care, but can often be expensive in terms of the other responsibilities of caregivers and it can be difficult for informal caregivers to make the best use of their caregiving time.

A study of the cost of caring for a child with life-limiting disease suggested that the impact of expenditures and time off work added up to around one-third of post-tax family income. Relatives and other informal caregivers take time off paid work and from other important and useful work (including caring for children), and often also incur substantial costs for travel.

Taking account of the costs of informal care and the impact on informal caregivers is important in the choices of models of care. If we only measure costs to paid staff and professionals, there appears to be a saving if more costs are transferred from formal healthcare to informal caregivers. Economists call this *cost shifting*. Overall costs may be as high or even higher, but the cost to the formal healthcare sector reduces. Some cost shifting may be desirable. If stronger community support reduces the risk of a hospital admission, then it may lower formal care costs and improve experiences of care, but costs to community organizations should be understood to ensure this improves the use of resources. People with stronger social networks tend to use fewer healthcare services and remain in better health. In particular, they are likely to make less use of primary care and are less likely to be admitted to hospital. To an extent, stronger social networks can be a substitute for formal services such as counselling. Living alone has been shown to substantially increase the risk of hospital admission, but stronger social networks can offset this.

Cost shifting can also occur between different community and informal caregiving people. Economists are interested in making the best use of all resources, so a shift of burden from family to a community organization or vice versa may be desirable if it leads to better experiences or lower costs. Combinations can be particularly effective—for example, support for better nutrition may come from a combination of meals delivered to the home and weekly lunch clubs. As discussed under 'Topic 1', spending €800 on improving nutrition pays for itself if it reduces hospital stays by 1 day.

Good decision-making should be based on an understanding of all costs and benefits, regardless of who pays the costs or enjoys the benefits. The economic evidence on costs of formal and informal care does not remove the need for judgements about the best use of care resources, but does allow the whole picture to be seen when choices are made.

Economic studies provide some better understanding of the roles taken by informal caregivers, their contributions to care and related costs, and their needs and preferences. They also provide an understanding of how formal and informal caregiving are linked and how they support each other.

Informal caregivers are usually family members, particularly spouses, partners, and adult children, although some neighbours and friends play important roles. The tasks and roles of informal caregivers depend significantly on what other supports are available. Where the basic care needs are provided by formal health and social care services, informal caregivers put their effort into emotional and spiritual support. In the absence of this input by formal care workers, the informal caregivers carry out the basic care.

The time spent by informal caregivers on providing support does not seem to depend strongly on formal care provision, but the tasks carried out do. Given the evidence that many people near the end of life have psychological needs that are not met (May et al., 2020), a likely effect of better formal care is that informal caregivers can take on the important wider support roles (which are difficult for formal services to provide). A study by Brick and colleagues (2017) of three community palliative care services in Ireland showed that there were large differences in the availability of formal support for care at home, but the hours and costs of informal caregiving did not vary to the same extent. This suggest that there is normally a fairly fixed time budget for informal caregivers. How this is used depends on what other supports are available. Similar findings come from a comparison of the end of life experience in three countries (England, Ireland, and the US) which found similar patterns, with informal care costs being much less varied than formal care costs.

Many informal caregivers want to take on the role, and there is evidence that higher costs of informal care can be associated with benefits to caregivers. Grief experiences of the caregiver following the death are generally less severe when informal care costs are higher, suggesting that the satisfaction of having done a good job in caring can reduce the levels of grief. However, this is not the case when the quality of formal care services is judged to be low.

Many caregivers are engaged in full-time or part-time work and must take time off with a loss of earnings. In other cases, they are diverted from other valuable activities, so that there is still an opportunity cost to their caregiving time. There can also be financial costs such as travel, parking, and childcare. Most studies find that the cost of informal caregiving represents between one-third and one-half of the costs of care for a person near the end of life.

In addition to financial costs, caregivers can face significant stress and burden. Better provision of formal care can reduce the burden felt by informal carers—in other words, there are measurable benefits to informal caregivers of better support, especially to meet the basic care needs of people who are near the end of life. This provides direct evidence that expenditure on formal care can bring benefits not only to the person near the end of life, but also to the rest of the care team.

Using an economic lens to analyse the relationship of formal care and informal caregiving helps to understand the choices we face. Informal care is not free, even though the burden does not fall on healthcare budgets. Cutting the cost of formal care is unlikely to show up in terms of poorer physical care but may divert informal caregivers from important roles that formal care cannot carry out.

The purpose of these two examples is to show how the perspective of economics can help in identifying where costs and benefits lie and can inform better choices in how care is provided. In many cases, shifting some resource to support social and community activities may prevent more expensive care. Recognizing that unpaid services are not free can help make better choices about the balance of formal and informal caregiving and allows us to see that some additional support for informal caregiving can make it more available and more useful. In general, formal care services have visible budgets and easily measured activity, while informal care is often less visible and less easy to measure. Costs to informal caregivers are often invisible but can be high. Support for better nutrition may involve many parties, and many different types of intervention, but we know that if successful they can significantly reduce the costs of hospital care and can be very cost-effective.

Some concluding reflections

The evidence base from economic studies in palliative care is limited, and that more focused on the economic issues in public health approaches is even more limited. As can be seen from the two topics discussed in this chapter, across palliative care there is a need to build understanding from a range of studies, and to draw on a range of evidence. This is similar to the challenges in evaluating public health interventions more widely. As discussed previously, there is evidence on the effects of community engagement on health system outcomes in general, suggesting that there may be similar benefits in public health palliative care interventions. However, it is also useful to look at ways in which the evidence on public health interventions shows the importance of the specific approaches taken and the design of interventions. It is inevitable that research around complex interventions that aim to meet complex needs will require some imagination and skill to draw on a range of relevant evidence to try to provide better evidence on which to make resource allocation choices.

Drawing on an economic perspective can allow us to understand our choices better and can often shift policy towards better use of resources. The fact that evidence is limited does not make the choices any less important. The more complex the intervention the more difficult it is to measure what is being done, at what cost, and what is the measurable benefit. Across palliative care research measuring benefits has been a challenge, given the poor sensitivity of many measurement instruments in this context and the wider impact of interventions on families and informal caregivers as well as patients.

REFERENCES

Arrow, K. J. 1963. Uncertainty and the welfare economics of medical care. *American Economic Review*, 5, 941–973.

Bozzetti, F., Arends, J., Lundholm, K., Micklewright, A., Zurcher, G., and Muscaritoli, M. 2009. ESPEN guidelines on parenteral nutrition: non-surgical oncology. *Clinical Nutrition*, 28, 445–454.

Brick, A., Smith, S., Normand, C., O'Hara, S., Droog, E., Tyrrell, E., et al. 2017. Costs of formal and informal care in the last year of life for patients in receipt of specialist palliative care. *Palliative Medicine*, 31, 356–368.

Cheng, K., Estrada, M. 2020. Price Elasticity of cigarette smoking demand in the Philippines after the 2012 Sin Tax Reform Act. *Preventive Medicine*, 134, 106042.

Connolly, S., Heslin, C., Mays, I., Corr, B., Normand, C., Hardiman, O. 2015. Health and social care costs of managing amyotrophic lateral sclerosis (ALS): an Irish perspective. *Amyotrophic Lateral Sclerosis & Frontotemporal Degeneration*, 16, 58–62.

Cyril, S., Smith, B., Possamai-Inesedy, A., and Renzaho, A. 2015 Exploring the role of community engagement in improving the health of disadvantaged populations: a systematic review. *Global Health Action*, 8, 29842.

Elia, M., Normand, C., Laviano, A., and Norman, K. 2016a. A systematic review of the cost and cost effectiveness of using standard oral nutritional supplements in community and care home settings. *Clinical Nutrition*, 35, 125–137.

Elia, M., Normand, C., Norman, K., and Laviano, A. 2016b. A systematic review of the cost and cost effectiveness of using standard oral nutritional supplements in the hospital setting. *Clinical Nutrition*, 35, 370–380.

Galvin, M., Ryan, P., Maguire, S., Heverin, M., Madden, C., Vajda, A., et al. 2017. The path to specialist multidisciplinary care in amyotrophic lateral sclerosis: a population-based study of consultations, interventions and costs. *PLoS One*, 12, e0179796.

Gillespie, L. and Raftery, A. M. 2009. Nutrition in palliative care. *British Journal of Community Nursing*, 14, 427–428.

Golinowska, S., Groot, W., Baji, P., and Pavlova, M. 2016. Health promotion targeting older people. *BMC Health Services Research*, 5, 345.

Lærum-Onsager, E., Brovold, T., Bergland, A., Pripp, A. H., and Bye, A. 2020. Associations between health-related quality of life, body mass index, health status and sociodemographic variables in geriatric patients and non-hospitalized older people: a comparative cross-sectional study. *Nutrition and Health*, 26, 141–150.

Martins Pereira, S., Araújo, J., and Hernández-Marrero, P. 2018. Towards a public health approach for palliative care: an action-research study focused on engaging a local community and educating teenagers. *BMC Palliative Care*, 17, 89.

May, P., Roe, L., McGarrigle, C., Kenny, R. A., and Normand, C. 2020. End-of-life experience for older adults in Ireland: results from the Irish longitudinal study on ageing (TILDA). *BMC Health Services Research*, 20, 118.

McPake, B., Normand, C., Smith, S., and Nolan, A. 2020. *Health Economics: An International Perspective*, 4th ed. Abingdon: Routledge.

Moran, P., Daly, D., Wuytack, F., Carrol, M., Turner, M., Normand, C., et al. 2020. Predictors of choice of public and private maternity care among nulliparous women in Ireland, and implications for maternity care and birth experience. *Health Policy*, 124, 556–562.

O'Reilly, D., O'Dowd, T., Galway, K., Murphy, A., O'Neill, C., Shryane, E., et al. 2007. Consultation charges in Ireland deter a large proportion of patients from seeing the GP: results of a cross-sectional survey. *European Journal of General Practice*, 13, 231–236.

Obermeyer, Z., Makar, M., Abujaber, S., Dominici, F., Block, S., and Cutler, D. M. 2014. Association between the Medicare hospice benefit and health care utilization and costs for patients with poor-prognosis cancer. *JAMA*, 312, 1888–1896.

Orrevall, Y. 2015. Nutritional support at the end of life. *Nutrition*, 31, 615–616.

Rice, N., Normand, C. 2012. The cost associated with disease-related malnutrition in Ireland. *Public Health Nutrition*, 15, 1966–1972.

Rice, N., Nugent, A., Byrne, D., Normand, C. 2016. Potential of Earlier Detection and Treatment of Disease-Related Malnutrition with Oral Nutrition Supplements to Release Acute Care Bed Capacity. *Irish Medical Journal*, 109, 422.

Sarrami-Foroushani, P., Travaglia, J., Debono, D., and Braithwaite, J. 2014. Implementing strategies in consumer and community engagement in health care: results of a large-scale, scoping meta-review. *BMC Health Services Research*, 14, 402.

Sinnott, S. J., Normand, C., Byrne, S., Woods, N., and Whelton, H. 2016. Copayments for prescription medicines on a public health insurance scheme in Ireland. *Pharmacoepidemiology and Drug Safety*, 25, 695–704.

Stevens, T., Keller, H., Williams, N., Downar, J., and Guthrie, D. M. 2021. Cross-sectional nutrition profile of palliative home care clients in Ontario and performance of the interRAI Palliative Care Nutrition Clinical Assessment Protocol. *JPEN. Journal of Parenteral and Enteral Nutrition*, 45, 183–192.

Tambor, M., Pavlova, M., Golinowska, S., Arsenijevic, J., and Groot, W. 2016. Financial incentives for a healthy life style and disease prevention among older people: a systematic literature review. *BMC Health Services Research*, 5, 426.

Temel, J. S., Greer, J. A., El-Jawahri, A., Pirl, W. F., Park, E. R., Jackson, V. A., et al. 2017. Effects of early integrated palliative care in patients with lung and GI cancer: a randomized clinical trial. *Journal of Clinical Oncology*, 35, 834–841.

Vettori, J. C., da Silva, L. G., Pfrimer, K., Jordão Junior, A. A., Moriguti, J. C., Ferriolli, E., et al. 2021. Older adult cancer patients under palliative care with a prognosis of 30 days or more: clinical and nutritional changes. *Journal of the American College of Nutrition*, 40, 148–154.

Yi, D., Johnston, B. M., Ryan, K., Daveson, B., Meier, D. E., Smith, M., et al. 2020. Drivers of care costs and quality in the last 3 months of life among older people receiving palliative care: a multinational mortality follow-back survey across England, Ireland and the United States. *Palliative Medicine*, 34, 513–523.

SECTION 6

Education and training

26

Pedagogical approaches for professional learning

Mary Hodgson and Heather Richardson

Introduction

Learning and education form an integral part of public health palliative care (PHPC) approaches and are central to the World Health Organization's approach (Downing et al., 2015, p. 366). Education is 'at once an element of health and a cause of health' (Hahn and Truman, 2015, p. 675). Knowledge, awareness, and skills development, intrinsic parts of education and learning, are also fundamental to the application of public health approaches for all: professionals in and out of healthcare systems, and community members and citizens who will need to be aware and maintain their health, as well as to help others act on the social determinants of health. Different styles of teaching will engender different outcomes, and an educational approach which is congruent with public health is arguably one in which *process* is paid attention to as much as *content*. This chapter considers what type of education, training, and learning would help those working in PHPC achieve their aims and practise effective approaches in public health.

In what follows, we take up the charge that the situation is urgent: that there is a significant unmet need for palliative care globally and broader adoption of a public health approach must be part of the scale of the solution. Education for citizens *and* professionals is integral to this (Bollig et al., 2019, p. 2) but here we focus on professional development. We review approaches and consider their efficacy or application towards helping public health proponents achieve aims in palliative care and move towards its future goals. Lastly, we also consider the potential for change, asking how the evidence and knowledge we, as professionals, gain is produced and in which circumstances, and how professionals, many of whom bring their passion to bear in this field, might actively utilize it, and learn from new approaches and people, in order to make the requisite changes a public health philosophy suggests.

In considering the possibilities, we first deal with the rising awareness of and application of public health approaches to palliative care for palliative care and other healthcare professionals. We review curriculum development and then consider the pedagogical approach the intentions of PHPC might involve. We consider how professionals might seek to continuously learn, to become flexible and proponents of change. For the purposes of this chapter, we draw on the description of PHPC developed by Public Health Palliative Care International in which the efforts of professionals in health and social care are combined with those of local communities to promote people's health and well-being, specifically that related to their experiences of death, dying, and loss. Its focus on health promotion and related methods highlights the value of participatory relationships, community development, partnerships, and social ecology alongside education in efforts to prevent and reduce harm. A key indicator of success according to this description lies in the ongoing enactment of actions that maintain health and well-being beyond any intervention or support provided by professionals. We suggest professionals will at least need to know about, if not know how to nurture, such actions for this to work.

Curriculum development and the rise of interest in public health palliative care

Background of public health approaches in palliative care: the curriculum question

The commensurability of public health and palliative care approaches are well established today (Whitelaw and Clark, 2019). Historically, both fields place value on education. Early public health approaches advocated translating new knowledge and skills into evidence-based, cost-effective interventions and likewise, palliative care equally has demonstrably been concerned with raising awareness, generating knowledge, and expertise development. From the earliest days of the modern hospice movement, Dame Cicely Saunders and peers privileged education and training as part of its development (Saunders, 2001) and this commitment to ensuring learning and training for professionals continued as part of professional and sector development means that today many hospices have educational departments. Equally, internationally a human rights approach to palliative care made education a central tenet of a rights-based approach, as the 2002 Cape Town Declaration stated (Brennan, 2007, p. 496).

Despite potential tensions between the fields (Whitelaw and Clark, 2019), a public health approach to palliative care is considered crucial to future efforts to address global needs for palliative care and to alleviate suffering (De Lima and Pastrana, 2016). Abel and colleagues (2018) suggest quality issues in palliative care including long-standing barriers of access can be addressed with partnerships between specialist and generalist palliative care, communities, and civic institutions working together as part of a public health approach. Relevant to this chapter, it is regarded as an opportunity to protect and improve the health and quality of the life of a community by translating new knowledge and skills into evidence-based, cost-effective interventions available to everyone in the population who needs them (Stjernsward et al., 2007). Here, priority is placed on training in order to scale the advance of a public health agenda which demands the building of networks and capacity in communities to share caring responsibilities for dying people societally, not just professionals (Abel et al., 2018b). We support the notion that palliative care training would also benefit healthcare professionals more generally (Abel et al., 2018b).

However, while both palliative care and public health approaches are aligned in valuing education, the concept of combining both for professional learning and application is relatively modern and still developing. For example, concerning its application in the field of palliative care, much is left to individual hospices, learning partnerships, or networks to engage in public health as they see fit, which means inevitably that the field is varied, especially internationally. However, good policy 'lays the groundwork' for good health systems (Stjernsward et al., 2007, p. 486).

The UK context

See Box 26.1.

Basics of the curriculum: what should professionals seek to learn about?

A curriculum for PHPC must include certain key aspects: it must accept that public health contains key methods that may be out of the usual remit of mainstream healthcare training, for example, community development. Any professional must be aware of an array of multidisciplinary contributions to addressing what Dame Cicely Saunders referred early on to as 'total pain' (e.g. psychiatry, complementary and other therapies, and the application of rehabilitative approaches) (Manford-Woolley, 2011). An educational response to total pain might then also comprise a 'total curriculum' which considers how a compassionate and holistic approach to those who are experiencing such pain might be manifested, and accepts and promotes that professionals have their own well-being, pain, and loss to consider (Woodhouse, 2011) and are multidimensional members of communities.

Box 26.1 The UK context

There is evidence of a changing commitment and broader adoption nationally in the UK. In 2008 in England and Wales, a national strategy placed priority on education, training, and continuing professional development alongside other actions to improve care. Today, national policy continues to support such public health alignment. The 'Ambitions for Palliative and End of Life Care' generated for England by the National End of Life Care Partnership (2015) confirmed a dual role for communities and clinicians to address growing demands for care at the end of life, while the Gold Standards Framework terms education and training of professionals a primary mechanism in the UK for improving people's experience. Other influential public health initiatives, such as 'Compassionate Communities', advocate training for professionals and the public (Abel et al., 2018b) suggesting that through it, quality improvements, relationship building, and network generation are intrinsic to PHPC.

Curriculum development for PHPC assumes that one of the central tenets of palliative care, that it addresses 'total pain', are already manifest in any palliative care training curriculum. However, here we note that the needs addressed by palliative care have changed significantly since the inception of the hospice movement over 50 years ago. Firstly, although Dame Cicely Saunders conceptualized total pain, the question of who could benefit from this approach has broadened significantly. Originally focused on people dying of terminal cancer, there is growing awareness of the need to extend palliative care to people dying of a whole range of other conditions that span heart failure, lung disease, progressive neurological conditions, dementia, and more (Murray and Sheikh, 2008). As people have lived longer, the notion of multiple comorbidities becomes a growing reality for many people living in the latter part of their lives, often associated with increasing disability. Many older people are living with a number of different conditions, any one of which could result in their death (Murray and Sheikh, 2008). Frailty, as a condition in its own right, is of growing concern to the palliative care community, in acknowledgement of related end of life care needs as frailty worsens (Nicholson et al., 2018; British Geriatrics Society, 2020). Finally, having a long-term physical health condition increases the likelihood of mental health problems such as depression (National Institute for Health and Care Excellence, 2009) and this likelihood is increased when people have three or more long-term conditions (Department of Health, 2011).

The field of geriatrics offers valuable insight into the care and experiences of older people with palliative care interfaces (Abel and Kellehear, 2018). Nicholson and Richardson's (2019) work on age-attuned palliative care identifies key risks that people living into late old age must master to sustain quality of life, one of the most pressing being that of continually adapting to loss. They suggest a public health lens will be most effective to guarantee it. Professionals must draw on clinical expertise, service/system adjustments, and renewed interest and commitment on the part of society. The required societal shifts in valuing older people and the process of ageing, increased public death literacy to enable vital conversations about future care, and promoting participation in care on the part of community members (Nicholson and Richardson, 2019) must inevitably engender a public health approach.

Equally, the field of rehabilitation holds value for those with chronic conditions and related disability (Hastings, 1962). It focuses on how professionals fostering a culture of enablement that allows people to achieve their goals as they approach the end of their life will support them to live as independently and as fully as possible with choice and autonomy.

More recent work on the notion of rehabilitative palliative care (Tiberini and Richardson, 2015) confirms the importance for palliative care professionals of integrating a culture of enablement that allows people to achieve their goals as they approach the end of their life. This newer paradigm aims to optimize people's function and well-being and to enable them to live as independently and fully as possible with choice and autonomy. This culture is everyone's business (Tiberini and Richardson, 2015) and, as such, strongly resonates with PHPC.

Dame Cicely Saunders was early to recognize the psychological and social elements of pain and suffering in her description of total pain (Clark, 2014). There is growing evidence of the relationship between long-term illness including that which is terminal in nature and mental health problems such as depression. As importantly, practical developments in end of life care that draw on public health principles, namely community action, recognize the importance of addressing mental illness alongside palliative care needs (Philip et al., 2018).

Community development and social ecology: learning about public health approaches

Community development and social ecology are two areas which have valuable insight to offer on an end of life experience which is changing in nature, and also in public health, where there is increasing focus on community-centred ways of working to support health improvement, health protection, and healthcare public health (see Public Health Matters Blog, 2018). Public health by definition is focused on the promotion, protection, and restoration of health by organized community action; and its concentration is on the factors that affect the health of any individual as part of a broader community (Hastings, 1962). Any education and learning related to the furthering of PHPC approaches must not just address the theoretical, but also consider how to motivate and consider change. There are three key areas that public health proponents tend to consider enacting. They are health promotion, community development, and social ecology, and these are important for professionals to understand, if not know how to practise. They chime with traditional approaches for public health creating opportunities for policy development, a broader epidemiological approach to identifying priorities for action and similar. They invite integration of principles across the two approaches to achieve greater impact, in particular opportunities to draw together community development and professional/organizational development (e.g. see the World Health Organization's (2016) guide for programme managers on planning and implementing palliative care services).

Health promotion approaches are best known for positive ways of sharing messages and knowledge about health, and their efficacy and traditional application are important for professionals training in this field to bear in mind, especially considering the goal of death literacy and a growth in recognized need for advanced care planning to take place before the diagnosis of a serious illness, and in the context of epidemics such as coronavirus disease 2019 (COVID-19). Health promotion will share information and knowledge with communities, often using simple community engagement techniques to spread messages about health. While there is variance, approaches such as behaviour change theory or randomized controlled trials are testing this field. Health promotion has been criticized for failing to understand the nature of the changes that need to be made, and for having less impact than other methods on behaviour (Dawkins-Moulton et al., 2016), as well as being a 'top-down' mode of intervention (Laverack and Labonte, 2000).

Community development itself is a large disciplinary field, but there are some key principles to be aware of. A basic aim of community development is that it seeks to build capacity in people. Our definition of community capacity building focuses on activities, resources, and support that strengthen the skills, abilities, and confidence of people and community groups to take effective action and leading roles (Skinner, 2006). There is a general consensus that any community member should have the ability to act on their own health and change actions but how does this happen? Community development approaches suggest that the most effective actions anyone can take may be more efficacious and sustainable if people are leading their own health maintenance rather than it be an institutional intervention 'doing to' people.

The work of Cormac Russell, and others in this field, with its focus on assets, helps professionals understand that communities already possess capacity (sometimes unknown to professionals). Strengths-based approaches explore what works well for people in their lives, building on this as an opportunity, rather than focusing on people as having deficits or needs that need fixing (Kunnen et al., 2013). Those familiar with palliative care will appreciate that there is not much about death itself that anyone can fix, but that a good-quality experience of the death process for the person and their household might be better furthered if it better responded to people's own values, goals, strengths, and desires. Community development is seen as one way of achieving this, with professionals not fixing but co-facilitating (Boyle et al., 2010), and initiatives acting beyond institutional support (Kellehear, 2013) which will be important for community development goals and capacity building to focus on.

Social ecology approaches offer a wider application because they are more likely to take a whole system approach. They consider the interplay of individuals, organizations, and systems, and negative or restorative practices that again address social determinants of health and work systemically. Social ecology approaches make several assertions but the most important is perhaps that individual health is related to society and environmental circumstances and helps professionals understand how to take an approach that maps networks and systems. They can also help understand how 'complex' people really are as individuals (Pask et al., 2018). As we have discussed earlier, becoming aware of the methods will be useful for enacting a public health approach.

Power and social justice: understanding how curriculum development could enhance health equity

In addition to understanding the experiences any person might have, Abel and colleagues (2018) emphasize the value of taking a holistic approach to the way citizens experience and interpret the world, what power relations exist, and how we might address them. They note that palliative care tends to assume more about personal challenges than social network challenges (Abel et al., 2018) or socioeconomic circumstances such as social determinants of health. Here the curriculum for PHPC has opportunities to recognize how people's socioeconomic positionality, culture, and experiences of governance, for example, racial injustice, intersect with social and psychological distress, as well as people's experiences of the healthcare system and its institutions. Understanding of this context could be addressed through social and critical theory including that which discusses power and agency, helping offer vital insight into deploying a PHPC approach. All are crucial to understanding how public health might be successful if inequalities are to be addressed.

And while health equity is a long-established societal challenge, there is also less discussion of it within a social justice framework, despite the fact that calls have long been made for health to be seen as a social justice issue, on the grounds that good health is not simply necessary for human well-being but is also important to allow individuals to exercise a range of human rights, and necessary for well-functioning societies (Prah, 2010). Here we define social justice as the lens we must view end of life through and the actions we must take to create a fairness in society related to end of life. A social justice framework forming part of the curriculum approach would help professionals in this field understand more drivers of health, surveillance, preventive measures, environmental improvements, and so on, and recognize that death is a specific social justice issue as Reimer-Kirkham and colleagues (2016) argue. The barriers to accessing care among structurally vulnerable people at the end of life include the need to focus on day-to-day survival, difficulties identifying those who need palliative care, professional risks and safety management, and the cracks of a siloed system (Stajduhar et al., 2019). Reimer-Kirkham and colleagues (2016) highlight the dual vulnerability of many people who are dying, on the grounds that they both need palliative care services and experience deficits in the social determinants of health. They argue for a reorientation of palliative care to explicitly integrate the premises of health equity. Their conclusion is one consistent with the aims of PHPC—to adopt approaches to care that consider social determinants of health and factors that influence access to it (Reimer-Kirkham et al., 2016). Here it will also be important to recognize concepts such as structural violence which help us understand how the values, norms, and behaviour of systems and institutions themselves may not work for people or may perpetuate inequalities (Farmer et al., 2006).

There has also been little discussion within the speciality of palliative care regarding social capital, power, and agency (Lewis et al., 2013) and how these shape experiences of dying and loss, which are fundamental to issues of access to services, sustaining levels of care, quality of life, and well-being. One area that has seen some recent focus is the acknowledgement that disadvantaged groups lack the social capital that might help them act on their health (Sallnow, 2017). Social capital can be described as the networks people have and can utilize to their advantage to help them access resources (Putnam, 2000), an area there is growing evidence on as a useful health intervention if not beneficial for health promotions. For example, relating to the observation that any person can be part of a social network and that these can both be useful for health promotion and for maintaining well-being and experience of dying, as well as loss, there is increasing focus on the importance of networks (e.g. the social ecology approach). There is also increased observation that social isolation is a major affliction at end of life and has impacts on a person's experience and ability to cope (Ettema et al., 2010) that we must address collectively. The simple question of who can best address social isolation—fellow citizens or professionals—has led to many befriending or peer support schemes that work well across the dying to bereavement process (Abel and Kellehear, 2016).

As a result, attention could be paid to the importance of development of relationships and networks as improved resource acquisition and information flow for citizens. However, it is important to recognise that social capital is not neutral in value or intent. As Bourdieu (1986a) argued, at times, social resources or networks are used or withheld by some at the expense of others. This suggests that work in this area should not be merely focused on some groups acquiring more and better links, as this is often blocked to them (Green, 2016), but understanding the complexity of how power, privilege, and agency play out in relationships. If everybody has power, after Foucault (1998), then how are they able to exercise it, at whose expense, and can they do so equally? Here concepts such as hegemony or Bourdieu's (1972, 1986b) concepts of 'doxa' (very simply, the things that never get discussed) and cultural capital help us understand the very useful question of which agents in society have had most ability to influence a healthcare agenda—and what has been missing from it. What never gets discussed? These are especially important ethical questions for healthcare to explore as it relates to equitable practice at the end of life (Pelto-Piri et al., 2013). Certain types of knowledge and actions have been privileged and other types have been considered pejoratively (Foucault, 1998; Moezzi et al., 2017) and not included. For a public health aim to be effective, it must know those people it seeks to enable and must question what the impacts of professionalization of dying have been and how it has created gaps in knowledge that have impacted people's abilities to act for themselves to create good health or influence agendas. Including these considerations and debates in the curriculum may help professionals consider how the relationships between professionals and citizen could evolve to tackle the unchallenged, taken for granted assumptions, complementing what is already known or deepening perspectives.

Finally, we follow Abel and colleagues (2018) in recommending the involvement of community members (and specifically those with lived experience of death, dying, and loss) in generating the curriculum. All the considerations we raise about curriculum inclusion also inevitably raise questions of how a PHPC curriculum could be bolstered by the contribution of community members. For example, community members can provide insight into their experiences of death, dying, and loss. Stories and case studies will help people learn how it feels to be a patient or bereaved, experience helplessness, or any other condition associated with death, dying, and loss. Citizens having input to the curriculum will help professionals understand the nuances and dynamics of lived experience. Community members can also advise on how professionals might operate across different sociocultural and value settings, especially as it relates to public health and community engagement. Communities can share their death care and the actions they take. This requires some reflexivity on the part of professionals and an openness to explore new forms of knowledge and consider community knowledge as a powerful healthcare asset in its own right (Corburn, 2007). Yet such inclusive curriculum development will help professionals understand the opportunities available to them to increase personal agency to the benefit of people previously disadvantaged.

Learning from citizen stories: participatory storytelling for social change

See Box 26.2.

Pedagogical approaches: the changing public health palliative care environment?

With PHPC firmly valuing education for all, what educational processes will benefit and foster it? What is less well documented than curriculum is the *approach* to education and training for

> **Box 26.2** Learning from citizen stories: participatory storytelling for social change
>
> One way to engage with this opportunity is to appreciate the value of storytelling as evidence, for communicating knowledge and creating relationships. There is growing interest in its use as an intervention around public health perceptions and behaviours (Smith et al., 2015; McCall et al., 2019), and descriptive evidence of the place of stories in relation to community engagement, as a precursor to planning change in relation to end of life care (Richardson, 2013). Storytelling has long been a part of setting in place and authorizing ways of seeing the world and actions that can be taken (De Certeau, 1984) as well as sharing knowledge, facilitating learning between people. Stories are not just neutral entities (Moezzi et al., 2017): they have a purpose and an audience and can be understood as a social action (Cruikshank, 1988). This way they can help people understand their own situation and the viewpoints of others, and possibly reframe long-held perspectives. For example, a story can portray a situation as an opportunity rather than a problem, an important aspect of PHPC. A story of a user pathway or experience through diagnosis, for example, would be instructive as to the requirements users have when they navigate often-bewildering information and communicate with professionals.

professionals best suited to improving public health at the end of life, and the relationships and learner dispositions that would best benefit the adoption of public health, and so we attend to this question in the remainder of this chapter. Pedagogy (the approach) is important to consider because it dictates the nature of the relationship a learner has with others, knowledge generation, solutions they identify, and the change outcomes that occur (Gray et al., 2019), all of which are important for a PHPC approach.

Our starting point is that whatever the pedagogical approach taken, learning is a relationship: between a teacher and a student, co-learners, and a learner's engagement and dialogue with the information and knowledge they gain or share. The way in which that relationship evolves will be based on learner needs and preferences, and those of the institution or style of professional development. Not every learner learns in the same way, and needs vary, which to be inclusive requires pedagogical adaptation (McKinnon, 2020), for example, to a diverse learning population or to meet changing societal needs.

By considering specific pedagogical principles, public health has the potential to create future shifts for professionals in their own behaviour and outlook. The way they train and learn will help to engender this shift. We suggest professionals in palliative care provision, long-used to establishing roles in which there is replicability and a focus on what is known, consider iterative approaches to developing new skills and insights and related experimentation in order to progress the future of public health. We look at formal training approaches, continuous learning, and how learning through participatory methods will help further. We are interested here in the potential of education to create changes which may best help professionals learn and apply their learning to the real-world setting they will operate in, assuming that advancing PHPC is their goal.

Learning communities

There are a number of leading approaches to teaching in education and all have relevance and validity for professional learners. Most training opportunities will privilege a mixture of approaches, for example, a didactic approach that focuses on a lead educator sharing knowledge with learners that they can be examined on to ensure that people have basic knowledge requirements and competencies, alongside other ways of gaining knowledge that seek more emphasis on collaboration, analysis, reflection, and experience-based learning. For example, many professionals may train in higher education largely through this approach, then find that further training in their roles in placements as students or workers, as a way of 'learning by doing'. They may identify themselves as being able to progress in their careers by seeking opportunities to train, upskill by attending courses, and gaining more knowledge.

Here we are less concerned with formal qualifications gained through professional education and more with the attributes of learners and innovators who can pursue a public health approach. On one hand, to readers, the curriculum and its content may appear more relevant than the learning approach. However, as our discussion of community development articulates, any professional seeking to understand the emphasis of PHPC on training, must also consider and know about pedagogical approaches in order to enact them. Some aspects of traditional PHPC community education have been traditional in pedagogical application, for example, health promotion, which largely focuses on knowledge transmission and transfer. Questions about developing the capability of citizens through health promotion arguably best fits with the concept that education is a shared public good: knowledge becomes an asset to be gained. Here the educator deposits information into a student as if it is 'neutral', what Freire described as a banking model of education (Matthews, 2014).

Paying attention to the learning environment is important. The fora and modes through which people come together to learn are important to pay attention to and the relational elements of learning are long known to be important to facilitate retention and help people learn. Co-learning and the relationships engendered enrich the learning setting and are often consciously planned for as a part of a 'learning community' (West and Williams, 2018) or community of practice. There is some debate about learning communities, with some critique of how they can be overly valorized and normative, so not allowing for new questions or new behaviours to be introduced, or, inversely, sites of contestation.

In many palliative care working contexts generative learning is the norm, for example, multidisciplinary forums, clinical supervision, or action learning sets which emphasize group critical thinking and problem-solving between professionals (Cho and Egan, 2009). For example, action learning brings people together in a group to problem solve proactively as members of a learning communities. Reciprocal learning approaches, for example, help people in different parts and roles of systems to contribute what they know, engage critically, and learn from one another. This is a more inclusive learning (Rodriguez-Falcon et al., 2010) style relevant to when professionals and citizens come together to learn, or in the approach any institution takes to public education. It is also very relevant to adopting public health approaches for palliative care.

These approaches between them are not a rejection of the acquisition of new knowledge from credible sources. They are advantageous because as well as mastery of knowledge, they also focus on critical skills development such as reflection, problem posing, exploring what knowledge could be generated through relational approaches such as dialogue, reflexivity, and relationship building between learners. Such an approach is intentional, rather than incidental.

Likewise, there are opportunities for PHPC proponents to develop learning through experimentation. Learning skills such as listening, trial and error, and iteration, and the resilience to continue with iterative approaches, where outcomes are unclear, will be important. Experimental processes are long regarded to be a means of building confidence in learners and capacity. John Dewey's (1897) well-known approach to learning combines method and outcome in 'learning by doing', known to create significant impact in professional settings (e.g. Heales et al., 2017). In other words, individuals learn by taking actions and reflecting on them.

As Meadows (2008) argues in her approach to systems, 'the way you learn is through experiment ... in a world of complex systems, it is not appropriate to charge forward with rigid undeviating directives'. Regardless of who the learner is, the skills they will learn through innovating and experimenting will continue to enable them to act on a real situation, to reflect on it, and in so doing to advance their learning. This has short- and long-term benefits, helping people gain critical skills on which they can draw, with application to a range of situations currently and in the future.

Continuous learning

Our second suggestion for a learning approach that fosters PHPC is the simple assertion that learning organizations thrive and respond well to changing societal needs. Where learning is an ongoing process for everyone regardless of qualifications, seniority, or existing capability, organizations tend to see good results for people (Watson et al., 2018). If Kellehear's (2013) proposal that end of life care become everybody's business is successful, then tomorrow's professionals will start learning about it at school, continue to learn about it in the workplace, and be capable in it throughout their working careers. This will require ongoing learning support. In the context of facilitating PHPC, the relationships through which people learn and work will often be multiple in nature and, as a result, rich and variable in their offer, and the multidisciplinary nature of palliative care, let alone PHPC, means that professionals gaining the disposition and critical skills to learn will be very useful.

Furthermore, continuous learning happens beyond the formal setting. Lifelong learners are constantly adapting in response to what they witness in their professional practice and broader lives and are encouraged to do so. This approach is not only for individuals who want to learn, but also collective, for organizations. Such 'continuous learning' helps individuals develop within organizations, or organizations develop their practice. It is formal, informal, and non-formal learning (non-formal refers to learning that is not defined as such but provides a learning experience) (Laal and Salamati, 2012).

This method is argued to support new problem-solving and creative capacity on the part of a wide group of people and the sharing and development of skills between its members (Laal and Salamati, 2012). Alongside personal development, the expectation is of organizational change that will support these individuals, including a culture and approach that recognizes the opportunity for experimentation, and the value of personal talent, relationships, and tacit knowledge alongside that generated through formal learning.

Organizational learning approaches which facilitate continuing professional development also play a part in the delivery of quality improvement, innovation, and change, which would benefit those seeking to develop public health practices within their workforce (Qalehsari et al., 2017), to expand knowledge held by their local communities and to facilitate greater participation in relation to death, dying, and loss across the different systems involved in end of life.

To facilitate a local or national PHPC approach, organizations will need to create a knowledge base about working according to public health principles—learning from their projects, from the change they initiate (whether incremental or transformational) and their experiences. They will also want to share their learning and consolidate and review it: both within and beyond the organization, in order to gain traction, and to make public health approaches mainstream and sustainable. Ensuring that institutional learning and knowledge is shared and developed will help not only the application of a PHPC approach but also practice development and innovation styles.

Organizations that adopt a continuous learning approach for all staff will often enjoy benefits beyond improvements specific to care delivery. Professionals are also likely to be working not just in organizations but as part of a range of systems involved in health, social, and hospice care and residential/housing services including care homes. These entities are often complex in their own right and also at their intersections—with each other, the individuals for whom they care, other internal players, and the communities in which they exist. While challenging, it is these very intersections that generate the energy, creativity, and opportunity key to the success of public health approaches (Farag, 2018). Where individuals familiar with different systems learn together, they can better understand the intersections and their possibilities—generating more joined-up thinking and collaboration in practice. Cross-sectorial learning is one way to maximize these opportunities and, for this reason, valuable for any kind of professional development.

Further developing learning partnerships by involving community members as faculty could generate a more contextual and relevant understanding for professionals (Manford-Woolley, 2011). Learning from community members as instructors will help professionals gain insight and perspective that would help them throughout their careers. Learning from community members would help in service development, improvements in developing feedback and quality methods, as well as provide deeper learning for professionals on the diverse needs and wants of community members. Bringing community members and 'service users' into sessions as faculty will also have change outcomes for community members, suggesting that the shared outcomes for all will have potential for the change PHPC seeks.

An example: community members as educators

See Box 26.3.

Learning to create change

Finally, attention is paid to the potential of education for professionals to help create the kind of societal change PHPC seeks, after the work of Freire's (1968) critical pedagogy, by introducing the possibility of co-learning with community members to create change through dialogue. While for professional education focus is given largely to those inside institutions with paid roles, it is worthwhile

Box 26.3 Example: St Christopher's Hospice

At St Christopher's Hospice in London, UK, where both authors work, volunteers and community members are an active part of teaching faculty for professionals. They have taken part in teaching on topics such as 'community', 'peer support', and how to have challenging conversations. They are helped to understand how they might construct a learning outcome, but have no direction except topic: they share their own content and give examples and analysis from personal experience. The outcomes are noted by staff to be insightful, profound, and helpful, for example, sessions on supporting dementia make clear that community members and professionals both have knowledge and ability to innovate and that working together would enhance the healthcare system. Community members have started to have invites from other staff to talk and share their knowledge. Sessions from carers help professionals understand the experience of living through a situation. This is not something professionals can be told as much as learn for themselves. The outcomes are broader: immediately after each session community development projects saw a rise in referrals of patients and invitations to community members to be more involved in health care. Community members have enjoyed the experience, and have not only stayed as active participants but considered how it has helped them to speak to wider audiences and learn about themselves.

noting how professionals can be active agents in fostering change through specific pedagogical methods.

In a participatory action research approach, a variety of people come together to share experiences and identify challenges and ambitions and challenges as a basis for generating new shared plans for change. Here learning, framed as a form of participatory action in that it shares ideas, raises awareness, creates essential dialogue, and stimulates action (Morales, 2016), is an activity that leads to new forms of purpose and contribution, as well as people gaining more control.

In this approach, all those involved in learning have a key role in shaping the agenda because it is focused on listening, acknowledgement, and recognition of the views and perspectives of others and the positionality they bring to bear on the content they share (Freire, 1999). By comparison to other learning processes, information is not divorced from context or people's positions. Dialogue between members is based on recognition of power relations and the status quo (Freire, 1999). People join as their intersectional selves: doctors join as doctors, carers as carers, all members of different communities and perspectives.

Importantly, this is an opportunity to say the unsaid, to shift agendas between all. In doing so, the context each different learner provides on their life, experience, and perceptions, how they pose problems and explore them, can facilitate greater understanding of problems, and opens up the dialogue on the possibilities (Dawkins-Moulton et al., 2016). For both groups this process generates knowledge creation and empathy with one another, and any actions that derive from this co-learning have a strong chance of being more applicable to people's needs and wants.

These approaches have been deployed in public health approaches previously (Baum et al., 2006). They help explore the basics to the transformative change in power in the wider death care system. It can help community members' outcomes to be viewed as having the potential to act to redress the poor experience of end of life care experienced by many (including access issues).

The benefits of such an approach for professionals are that in meeting a range of people interested in changing end of life they have an opportunity to explore agendas and interests beyond those they have identified. They are also invited to jointly recognize opportunities for change that are upstream and that begin prior to an experience of serious illness and in generations that can expect to live well for a considerable time before starting to plan for the end of their life. For example, the dialogue about problems may situate individual complexities in the structural or organizational, in which professionals play a role. Here education becomes a mode of transformation that deals directly with inequity between systems and communities and within community death care systems. Viewing themselves as community members too could ease the stress for professionals of roles in which there is little deviation offered and an emphasis on (compassionate) neutrality (Cottam, 2018). For example, methods, such as 'forum theatre', in which scenarios are acted on but audience members intervene or suggest alternatives (Darder et al., 2017), or 'appreciative enquiry', in which problems are named and decisions are made, will not only benefit the insight and learning capability of any professional but help them consider the challenges and difficulties of their role, make the unsaid explicit, and see the possibilities for a new way of doing things.

Ensuring that they do so could also help the cross-learning of various professionals in a system; appreciating the expertise and tacit knowledge deployed by various healthcare workers too who contribute to healthcare systems but do not have power within them, as healthcare labour is itself stratified and bound by power relationships (Downing et al., 2015). We note that social justice is not just an agenda for citizens but also relates to healthcare workforces and inequity therein. It could help get better support for healthcare support workers, for example (Manford-Woolley, 2011) or help better recognize the contribution of volunteers. This approach will help organizations seeking to deal with more general issues related to engagement with, and the diversity of, its workforce, its connections with its communities, and its learning culture and priorities. The emphasis on participatory relations, community development opportunities, partnerships, and social ecology within the organization itself, or its systems, are best facilitated through a workforce that reflects those it serves, that identifies itself as part of the community and which has insight into its own construction of knowledge and meaning.

Opening up cross-learning in this way to a broader community where professionals of all kinds learn with citizens of all kinds (or indeed are taught by them) meets interest in a generative curriculum with an inclusive learning style. Yet we include a note of caution: those responsible for shaping the curriculum and enabling such learning will need to attend to the inherent and complicated issues of power and resource that affect the degree to which individuals can participate, and speak out when they do. They must ensure that the agenda is established by all rather than pre-established by some. Issues discussed should move beyond broad philosophical considerations on the part of the intellectually elite within the community and instead address what is important to all who participate. This position calls for a different frame on the part of training institutions, professional colleges, employers, and professionals about what success looks like and how it is best assessed.

Box 26.4 Case study: St Joseph's Hospice

Libby Sallnow (2018) highlights how professionals benefit from learning with citizens. In her doctoral research she evaluates and explores the change in relationship between staff and citizens taking part in a project seeking to adopt a public health approach to end of life at St Joseph's Hospice, London, UK. She describes how the project, seeking to redress power dynamics and widen participation in end of life care, created an environment and a set of interactions which allowed for greater equity and for relationships characterized by reciprocity and mutuality, giving rise to greater agency on the part of individuals traditionally disadvantaged within the system of palliative care, framing a notion of shared social capital described as 'collective'. In doing so, Sallnow evidences the learning that took place among professionals too, which many have continued to take into other professional roles. One of the authors of this piece, Heather Richardson, who was at the time clinical director and one of the driving forces behind the project, describes walking through the hospice one day after the process had begun, and hearing a community member who had taken part in the project invite another to sit down and join them with the words 'Welcome to my hospice', as a profound learning experience.

A case study: a hospice and citizens learning together?

See Box 26.4.

Reflections and final thoughts

Reviews of palliative care education programmes in the literature have clarified the need to consider more than the acquisition of new knowledge as a successful outcome to such learning, with due consideration also of changes in attitude and behaviour aligned with the needs of people who need palliative care (Mason and Ellershaw, 2008; Gryschek et al., 2020). To do this, the learning experience needs to facilitate the skills, critical skills, and relation building required. In Table 26.1, we suggest indicators for successful quality learning in relation to PHPC.

None of these indicators focus on compliance with standards of care or even competencies on the part of professionals. Here we have invited people to consider the inclusion of the lives, experiences, stories, and perceptions of community members in professional training and insight gathering. Community members, people with lived experience, and a multidisciplinary group of professionals all add richness to the learning opportunity whatever role they play in it. This approach reflects the participatory nature of PHPC that brings together a broad range of people who recognize that, regardless of professional background, training, and expertise, they are all mortal, and that investment is required on all their parts to reduce the all too present experiences of a poor death and bereavement for themselves and others around them. We suggest that this approach will help us achieve the bigger ambition we hold in relation to a community in which all participants can expect to learn—building capacity alongside skill and knowledge on the part of citizens and professionals.

We also strongly suggest that the field of PHPC invest in its learning processes to help it advance the opportunities it offers to people who are dying or who face loss. More must be done to support professionals who wish to pursue a public health approach to end of life care: when people have the opportunity to recognize the potential for the transformative qualities for working in partnership with others, it is likely they will continue to pursue this goal throughout their careers. However, this can be a challenge and supportive learning infrastructures, opportunities, and relationships must be facilitated by those who lead institutions in which people work.

Our review of current educational opportunities in PHPC has included some approaches that could be seen as radical although we suggest that in so doing we are bringing together PHPC intentions with the design to achieve better health outcomes. To engage citizens with the idea of health maintenance, social movements, and action for health, and taking care of themselves early and often, professionals must also 'allow' for these things to happen, and look for every opportunity for practice development that supports and fosters them. Every interaction will be an opportunity or a reinforcement. This can work both ways. Trust, accountability, and shared leadership are essential here and so the way that people train and learn these skills is also as important as the content they consume. How people view each other will be vital to the quality of the outcome. If there is a somewhat binary approach—in which professionals see themselves separate to community members and at liberty to choose which aspects of their experience and expertise they draw on to shape their practice—then learning on the part of all present will be limited. Instead, we urge all who participate to see each other as experts in the field of death, dying, and loss, who can support high-quality learning from a variety of perspectives. This approach allows critical learning on the part of all who attend, building capacity across the board and creating a more nuanced ecology of learning.

Those of us engaged in training or leadership of such organizations must consider this if we wish to meet the scale of need for palliative care globally. If we meet professionals where and when they start to critically engage with the world, at school, in their professional training, as they tend to their first dying patient, we will have more chance to bring more people into palliative care, and foster these positive attitudes, rather than trying to change established and embedded power relationships and hierarchies too late for it to benefit the greater good at the scale we need.

Table 26.1 Indicators for successful quality learning in relation to PHPC

Structures	Processes	Outcomes
Curriculum reflecting end of life needs and aspirations	Learning agenda negotiated by whole group	Insight into complementary approaches
Group with mix of players not just professional	Engagement from range of organizations and groups	Awareness about power and access
Dialogue created by whole group	Listening and learning from all	Sense of agency for all to initiate changes
Evidence that is broad, including stories	Experimentation with different approaches and skills	New skills for all focused on co-creation
Priority setting for problems and actions	Change plans	Real-life changes

REFERENCES

Kellehear, A. 2013. Compassionate communities: end-of-life care as everyone's responsibility. *QJM: An International Journal of Medicine*, 106, 1071–1075.

Abel, J. and Kellehear, A. 2016. Palliative care reimagined: a needed shift. *BMJ Supportive & Palliative Care*, 6, 21–26.

Abel, J. and Kellehear, A. 2018. Palliative curriculum re-imagined: a critical evaluation of the UK palliative medicine syllabus. *Palliative Care*, 11, 1178224218780375.

Abel, J., Kellehear, A., and Karapliogou, A. 2018. Palliative care—the new essentials. *Annals of Palliative Medicine*, 7, S3–S314.

Baum, F., MacDougall, C., and Smith, D. 2006. Participatory action research. *Journal of Epidemiology & Community Health*, 60, 854–857.

Bollig, G., Brandt, F., Ciurliobnis, M., and Knopf, B. 2019. Last aid course: an education for all citizens and an ingredient of compassionate communities. *Healthcare*, 7, 19.

Bourdieu, P. 1986a. *Distinction*. London: Routledge & Kegan Paul.

Bourdieu, P. 1986b. The forms of capital. In: Richardson, J. (ed.) *Handbook of Theory and Research for the Sociology of Education*, pp. 241–258. Westport, CT: Greenwood Press.

Boyle, D., Slay, J., and Stephens, L. 2010. *Public Services Inside Out: Putting Co-Production into Practice*. London: NESTA.

Brennan, F. 2007 Palliative care as an international human right. *Journal of Pain and Symptom Management*, 33, 494–499.

British Geriatrics Society. 2020. *End of Life Care in Frailty: Identification and Prognostication*. London: British Geriatrics Society.

Cho, Y. and Egan, T. 2009. Action learning research: a systematic review and conceptual framework. *Human Resource Development Review*, 8, 431–462.

Clark, D. 2014. Total pain: the work of Cicely Saunders and the maturing of a concept. [Online] Available at: http://endoflifestudies.academicblogs.co.uk/total-pain-the-work-of-cicely-saunders-and-the-maturing-of-a-concept/

Corburn, J. 2007. Community knowledge in environmental health science: co-producing policy expertise. *Environmental Science and Policy*, 10, 150–161.

Cottam, H. 2018. *Radical Help: How We Can Remake the Relationships Between Us and Revolutionise the Welfare State*. London: Virago.

Cruikshank, J. 1988. *The Social Life of Stories: Narrative and Knowledge in the Yukon Territory*. Lincoln, NE: University of Nebraska Press.

Darder, A., Baltodano, M., and Torres, R. 2017. Critical pedagogy: an introduction. In: Darder, A., Baltodano, M., and Torres, R. (eds.) *Critical Pedagogy Reader*, pp. 1–21. London: Routledge.

Dawkins-Moulton, L., McDonald, A., and McKyer, L. 2016. Integrating the principles of socioecology. and critical pedagogy for health promotion health literacy *Interventions Journal of Health Communication*, 21, 30–35.

De Certeau, M. 1984. *The Practice of Everyday Life* (Russell, S., trans.). Berkeley, CA: University of California Press.

De Lima, L. and Pastrana, T. 2016. Opportunities for palliative care in public health. *Annual Review of Public Health*, 37, 357–374.

Department of Health. 2011. No health without mental health: a cross-government outcomes strategy. [Online] Available at: https://www.gov.uk/government/publications/no-health-without-mental-health-a-cross-government-outcomes-strategy

Dewey, J. 1897. My pedagogic creed. *The School Journal*, 54, 77–80.

Downing, J., Grant, L., Leng, M., and Namukwaya, E. 2015. Understanding models of palliative care delivery in sub-Saharan Africa: learning from programs in Kenya and Malawi. *Journal of Symptom and Pain Management*, 50, 362–370.

Ettema, E., Derksen, L., and van Leeuwen, E. 2010. Existential loneliness and end-of-life care: a systematic review. *Theoretical Medicine & Bioethics*, 31, 141–169.

Farag, D. 2018. Quoted in plenary presentation by Richardson, H. and O'Leary, S. Reinvention of hospices? Of course but how do we do it. Hospice UK conference. [Online] Available at: https://www.hospiceuk.org/what-we-offer/courses-conferences-and-learning-events/conferences/hospice-uk-national-conf/video

Farmer, P., Nizeye, B., Stulac, S., and Keshavjee, S. 2006. Structural violence and clinical medicine. *PLoS Medicine*, 3, e449.

Foucault, M. 1998. *The History of Sexuality: The Will to Knowledge*. London: Penguin.

Freire, P. 1999. *Pedagogy of the Oppressed (New Revised 20th Anniversary Edition)*. New York: Continuum.

Gray, N., Ward, J., and Fogarty, J. 2019. Transformative learning through university and prison partnerships: reflections from 'Learning Together' pedagogical practice. *Journal of Prison Education & Re-Entry*, 6, 7–24.

Green, J. 2016. Community development and social development: informing concepts of place and intentional social change in a globalizing world. *Research on Social Work Practice*, 26, 605–608.

Gryschek, G., Cecilio-Fernandes, D., Mason, S., and de Carvalho-Filho, M. A. 2020. Assessing palliative care education in undergraduate medical students: translation and validation of the Self-Efficacy in Palliative Care and Thanatophobia Scales for Brazilian Portuguese. *BMJ Open*, 10, e034567.

Hahn, R. and Truman, B. 2015. Education improves public health and promotes health equity. *International Journal of Health Sciences*, 45, 657–678.

Hastings, J. 1962. Rehabilitation and the public health. *Canadian Journal of Public Health/Revue Canadienne De Sante Publique*, 53, 279–283.

Heales, C., Hodgson, M., and Rich, H. 2017. *Humanity at Work: MONDRAGON, A Social Innovation Ecosystem Case Study*. London: The Young Foundation. Available at: https://youngfoundation.org/wp-content/uploads/2017/04/Humanity-at-Work-online-copy.pdf

Kellehear, A. 2013. Compassionate communities: end-of-life care as everyone's responsibility. *QJM: An International Journal of Medicine*, 106, 1071–1075.

Kunnen, N., MacCallum, D., and Young, S. 2013. Research strategies for assets and strengths based community development. In: Moulaert, F., MacCallum, D., Mehmood, A., and Hamdouch, A. (eds.) *International Handbook on Social Innovation: Collective Action, Social Learning & Transdisciplinary Research*, pp. 285–297. Cheltenham: Edward Elgar.

Laal, M. and Salamati, P. 2012. Lifelong learning: why do we need it? *Procedia—Social and Behavioral Sciences*, 31, 309–403.

Laverack, G. and Labonte, R. 2000. A planning framework for community empowerment goals within health promotion. *Health Policy and Planning*, 15, 255–262.

Lewis, J. M., DiGiacomo, M., Luckett, T., Davidson, P. M., and Currow, D. C. 2013. A social capital framework for palliative care: supporting health and wellbeing for people with life limiting illness and their carers through social relations and networks. *Journal of Pain and Symptom Management*, 45, 92–103.

Manford-Woolley, K. 2011. Palliative care education. In: Baldwin, M. and Woodhouse, J. (eds.) *Palliative Care Education in Key Concepts in Palliative Care*, pp. 149–153. London: SAGE Publications Ltd.

Mason, S. R. and Ellershaw, J. E. 2008. Preparing for palliative medicine; evaluation of an education programme for fourth year medical undergraduates. *Palliative Medicine*, 22, 687–692.

Matthews, C. 2014. Critical pedagogy in health education. *Health Education Journal,* 73, 600–609.

McCallm, B., Shallcross, L., Wilson, M., Fuller, C., and Hayward, A. 2019. Storytelling as a research tool and intervention around public health perceptions and behaviour: a protocol for a systematic narrative review. *BMJ Open,* 9, e030597.

McKinnon, J. 2020. The pedagogy of adaptation: using specialised disciplinary knowledge to develop creative skills. *Journal of Perspectives in Applied Academic Practice,* 1 54–60.

Meadows, D. H. 2008. *Thinking in Systems: A Primer* (Wright, D., ed.). River Junction, VT: Chelsea Green Publishing.

Moezzi, M., Janda, K., and Rotmann, S. 2017. Using stories, narratives and storytelling in energy and climate change. *Research Energy Research & Social Science,* 31, 1–10.

Morales, M. P. E. 2016. Participatory action research (PAR) cum action research (AR) in teacher professional development: a literature review. *International Journal of Research in Education and Science (IJRES),* 2, 156–165.

Murray, S. A. and Sheikh, A. 2008. Palliative care beyond cancer: care for all at the end of life. *BMJ (Clinical Research Edition),* 336, 958–959.

National End of Life Care Partnership. 2015. Ambitions for palliative and end of life care: a national framework for local action 2015–2020. [Online] Available at: https://www.nationalvoices.org.uk/sites/default/files/public/publications/ambitions-for-palliative-and-end-of-life-care.pdf

National Institute for Health and Care Excellence. 2009. Depression in adults: recognition and management. Clinical guideline [CG90]. [Online] Available at: https://www.nice.org.uk/guidance/cg90

Nicholson, C., Davies, J. M., George, R., Smith, B., Pace, V., Harris, L., et al. 2018. What are the main palliative care symptoms and concerns of older people with multimorbidity? —A comparative cross-sectional study using routinely collected phase of illness, Australia-modified Karnofsky Performance Status and Integrated Palliative Care Outcome Scale data. *Annals of Palliative Medicine,* 7, S164–S175.

Nicholson, C. and Richardson, H. 2019. Age-attuned hospice care: an opportunity to better end of life care for older people. St Christopher's Hospice. [Online] Available at: https://www.stchristophers.org.uk/wp-content/uploads/2018/10/Age-attuned-Hospice-care-document.pdf

Qalehsari, M. Q., Khaghanizadeh, M., and Ebadi, A. 2017. Lifelong learning strategies in nursing: a systematic review. *Electron Physician,* 9, 5541–5550.

Pask, S., Pinto, C., Bristowe, K., van Vliet, L., Nicholson, C., Evans, C., et al. 2018. A framework for complexity in palliative care: a qualitative study with patients, family carers and professionals. *Palliative Medicine,* 32, 1078–1090.

Pelto-Piri, V., Engström, K., and Engström, I. 2013. Paternalism, autonomy and reciprocity: ethical perspectives in encounters with patients in psychiatric in-patient care. *BMC Medical Ethics,* 14, 49.

Philip, R. R., Philip, S., Tripathy, J. P., Manima, A., and Venables, E. 2018. Twenty years of home-based palliative care in Malappuram, Kerala, India: a descriptive study of patients and their care-givers. *BMC Palliative Care,* 17, 26.

Prah, R. J. 2010. *Health and Social Justice.* Oxford: Oxford University Press.

Public Health Matters Blog. 2018. Health matters: community centred approaches for health and wellbeing. [Online] Available at: https://publichealthmatters.blog.gov.uk/2018/02/28/health-matters-community-centred-approaches-for-health-and-wellbeing/

Putnam, R. 2000. *Bowling Alone: The Collapse and Revival of American Community.* New York: Simon & Schuster.

Reimer-Kirkham, S., Stajduhar, K., Pauly, B., Giesbrecht, M., Mollison, A., McNeil, R., et al. 2016. Death is a social justice issue: perspectives on equity-informed palliative care. *ANS. Advances in Nursing Science,* 39, 293–307.

Richardson, H. 2013. A public health approach to palliative care in East London: early developments, challenges and plans for the future. In: Sallnow, L., Kumar, S., and Kellehear, A. (eds.) *International Perspectives on Public Health and Palliative Care,* pp. 110–122. Abingdon: Routledge.

Richardson, H. and Cooper, M. 2020. *The Lantern Model: A Contemporary Model of Nursing at the End of Life.* London: St Christopher's Hospice.

Rodriguez-Falcon, E., Evans, M., Allam, C., Barrett, J., and Forrest, D. 2010. *The Inclusive Learning and Teaching Handbook.* Sheffield: University of Sheffield.

Russell, C. 2020. We don't have a health problem, we have a village problem. *Community Medicine,* 1, 1–12. Available at: https://www.nurturedevelopment.org/wp-content/uploads/2018/09/we-dont-have-a-health-problem-we-have-a-village-problem8259.pdf

Sallnow, L. 2017. Collective social capital: a study of new public health and end-of-life-care. Doctoral thesis, University of Edinburgh. [Online] Available at: https://era.ed.ac.uk/handle/1842/33037?show=full

Saunders, C. 2001. The evolution of palliative care. *Journal of the Royal Society of Medicine,* 94, 430–443.

Skinner, S. 2006. *Strengthening Communities: A Guide to Capacity Building for Communities and the Public Sector.* London: Community Development Foundation.

Smith, B., Tomasone, J. R., Latimer-Cheung, A. E., and Martin Ginis, K. A. 2015. Narrative as a knowledge translation tool for facilitating impact: translating physical activity knowledge to disabled people and health professionals. *Health Psychology,* 34, 303–313.

Stajduhar, K. I., Mollison, A., Giesbrecht, M., McNeil, R., Pauly, B., Reimer-Kirkham, S., et al. 2019. 'Just too busy living in the moment and surviving': barriers to accessing health care for structurally vulnerable populations at end-of-life. *BMC Palliative Care,* 18, 11.

Stjernsward, J., Foley, K. M., and Ferris, F. D. 2007. The public health strategy for palliative care. *Journal of Pain and Symptom Management,* 33, 486–493.

Tiberini, R. and Richardson, H. 2015. *Rehabilitative Palliative Care: Enabling People to Live Fully Until They Die.* London: Hospice UK. Available at: https://www.hospiceuk.org/what-we-offer/clinical-and-care-support/rehabilitative-palliative-care/resources-for-rehabilitative-palliative-care

Watson, D., Tregaskis, O., Gedikli, C., Vaughn, O., and Semkina, A. 2018. Well-being through learning: a systematic review of learning interventions in the workplace and their impact on well-being. *European Journal of Work and Organizational Psychology,* 27, 247–268.

West, R. E. and Williams, G. 2018. I don't think that word means what you think it means: a proposed framework for defining learning communities. *Educational Technology Research and Development,* 65, 1569–1582.

Whitelaw, S. and Clark, D. 2019. Palliative care and public health: an asymmetrical relationship? *Palliative Care,* 12, 1178224218819745.

Woodhouse, J. 2011. Stress and palliative care. In: Baldwin, M. and Woodhouse, J. (eds.) *Palliative Care Education in Key Concepts in Palliative Care,* pp. 223–227. London: SAGE Publications Ltd.

World Health Organization. 2016. *Planning and Implementing Palliative Care Services: A Guide for Programme Managers.* Geneva: World Health Organization. Available at: https://apps.who.int/iris/bitstream/handle/10665/250584/9789241565417-eng.pdf

27

Public health palliative care education

Children and schools

Sally Paul

Introduction

Public health palliative care recognizes that illness, caregiving, death, and loss are not just medical issues but social issues that affect every one of us, adults and children alike. Yet children are a population whose views, needs and capacity to both engage with and respond to these experiences are often unheard, unmet, and unrecognized. This absence of children's perspectives poses a significant challenge in how we holistically understand, support, and enhance children's experiences of illness, caregiving, death, and bereavement. Public health palliative care education offers an important contribution to address this challenge by placing an emphasis on children within wider social systems, specifically educational communities, that shapes how they engage with these experiences.

From this perspective, public health palliative care education with and for children is broad in its focus. It recognizes the significance of meaningful support for children, their parents/carers, and the education staff, at times of illness, caregiving, and bereavement, but looks beyond individual experiences to the role and capacity of education communities to proactively prepare its members to look after themselves and others. In this chapter, I discuss why children's experiences of caregiving, death, and loss are relevant to public health palliative care. I then go on to highlight the role of school communities in public health, specifically focusing on the concept of health-promoting schools (HPSs) and how this shapes our understanding of health-promoting palliative care schools (HPPCSs). Lastly, I discuss some examples of public health palliative care education with children, considering some of the challenges and opportunities for developing work in this area.

Please note that the term child and/or children is used throughout the chapter to denote anyone of under the age of 21 years. While I recognize that it may be preferable to also use the term young people, or people in general, this term was selected for ease of reading.

Children's experiences of illness, caregiving, death, and bereavement

Children are not immune to the experience of illness, caregiving, death, and bereavement. On the contrary, research suggests that by the age of 8 years most children have experienced a bereavement of either a parent, sibling, grandparent, or other close relative (Paul and Vaswani, 2020). Importantly, this figure is an underestimate of the true extent of childhood bereavement as it does not include deaths that occur in children's wider networks, such as the death of teachers, neighbours, distant relatives, and so on (Paul and Vaswani, 2020). Moreover, it is based on Scottish data from 2004 to 2015 and does not reflect the occurrence of bereavement for children during the coronavirus pandemic, or living in countries where there is extreme conflict, natural disasters, lack of access to healthcare, sanitation, and so on. Likewise, a considerable number of children look after someone living in their house on either a sporadic or regular basis, due to mental health, disability, substance use, long-term illness, or frailty related to ageing. As such, the term young carer is used to define children who provide substantial physical, household, medical, and/or emotional support (Smyth et al., 2011, p. 146).

Large-scale surveys suggest that between 2% and 8% of children aged under 18 years are young carers (Leu et al., 2019) and there is some evidence to suggest that this figure is as high as 22% (Joseph et al., 2019). These numbers, however, are also an underestimate due to the challenges associated with identifying children who are caring, such as children not recognizing themselves as carers (Joseph et al., 2019) or that caring is often hidden because of concerns about stigma, family loyalty, or family separation (Banks et al., 2002). Nonetheless, despite the challenges around identifying the actual number of children affected by bereavement or caregiving, it is apparent that these experiences feature in children's lives.

Research related to children's experiences of caregiving and loss frequently focus on the negative impact that they can have on a child's social, emotional, and physical health, educational outcomes, and future functioning. For example, both experiences have been found to place children at increased risk of anxiety or depression, social isolation, school absences, bullying, and academic under-achievement (Cohen et al., 2012; Jamieson and Highet, 2013; Burns et al., 2020). As such, the significance of appropriate, timely, and targeted support is recognized as important in developing improved coping and well-being (Ribbens McCarthy, 2006; Jones et al., 2015; Joseph et al., 2020). Professional services will be useful for some children; however, it is argued that this can result in a fragmented approach to support across healthcare services (e.g. in relation to somatic symptoms), school personal (e.g. in relation to academic difficulties, absenteeism, behaviour problems at school), or community support services (e.g. specialist carer or bereavement support, mental health services) (Burns et al., 2020, p. 402). Moreover, not all children require specialist intervention (Currier et al., 2007; Aldridge, 2008) and, in relation to bereavement, it has been suggested that providing professional support too soon may result in the withdrawal of other support networks (Rumbold and Aoun, 2014). This is significant given that support from family, friends, and school is a key protective factor for children (Ribbens McCarthy, 2006; Scott et al., 2019; Gough and Gulliford, 2020). Children are more likely to seek support from their social networks, but a lack of social support can negatively impact a child's coping, for example, by compounding feelings of isolation and loneliness (Rowling, 2003; Andriessen et al., 2019; Gough and Gulliford, 2020). Moreover, a child's social context has also been found to influence exposure to bereavement and caregiving, for example, low income is linked to higher rates of illness, caregiving, and bereavement (Aldridge, 2008; Paul and Vaswani, 2020). Children's personal experiences of illness, caregiving, death, and loss are thus influenced by the social, economic, and environmental context and, as such, the associated risks to individual and community health arguably situate these experiences as a public health issue (Rumbold and Aoun, 2014; Burns et al., 2020; Paul and Vaswani, 2020).

Aside from personal experience, illness, death, and loss are also part of ordinary life for children (Coombs, 2014; Davies, 2017; Paul, 2019). Children see, read, or hear about the impact of illness and dying in relation to people in their wider community (such as neighbours, friends, schoolteachers, and so on), as well as in books, films, video games, history and science lessons, and in the media (Paul, 2019). Yet, these experiences are not consistently acknowledged or recognized as a common part of a child's life by adults or in their education (Paul, 2019). It has been suggested that some adults often fear discussing death and bereavement with children believing such conversations might cause unnecessary harm or upset (Jackson and Colwell, 2001; Puolimatka and Solasaari, 2006; Smith and Hunter, 2008). This is significant given that the importance of informing, including, and promoting self-efficacy when someone is ill or dies has been found to support children's coping (Monroe and Kraus, 2010; Smith and Hunter, 2008; Gough and Gulliford, 2020). Moreover, children are not systematically taught about death and grief, despite such education being argued as essential in preparing children for loss (Rodríguez Herrero et al., 2020) and that children can, and want to, talk about these issues (Paul, 2019). Thus, children's exposure and engagement with death and loss is influenced by wider social norms, relationships, and individual needs (Paul, 2019). This reflects literature on children and childhood more broadly, which recognizes that the experiences and perceptions of children are not only shaped by their personal involvements and individual characteristics but also by 'the attitudes, ideas and expectations of both the immediate and wider social context' (Hill and Tisdall, 1997, p. 3). This is significant because other research suggests that attitudes and behaviours developed during childhood can follow into adulthood (Langford et al., 2015). Thus, if children are not systematically engaged with or taught about illness, caregiving, death, and loss, this could have future implications for how they both understand these experiences and look after themselves and others. There is then a need to move beyond understanding and responding to these experiences as individual and psychological processes or experiences to recognizing and responding to them within the context of their social environment: for most children, after the family, this social environment involves their school community (Rowling, 2010). Public health palliative care draws attention to the significance of social context in shaping children's experiences of illness, caregiving, death, and loss and, as such, offers an important contribution to how we understand and support these experiences.

Schools and public health

It is estimated that 90% of children worldwide attend primary schools and 80% of children attend secondary schools (UNICEF, 2021). Schools are therefore viewed as one of the most important settings for enhancing children's intellectual, social, emotional, and physical growth and evidence suggests that doing so not only improves children's ability to learn but also that education improves future health (Langford et al., 2015). Moreover, promoting healthy behaviours through school settings has been found not only to benefit children themselves but also their families, peers, and wider school community (Lee et al., 2019). This draws attention to schools as working environments for a variety of staff (teaching staff, administrators, caretakers, social workers, educational psychologists, nurses, librarians, and so on) and an interface between the public and private lives of families. As such, schools are recognized as anchor institutions: that is, trusted leaders in their communities due to their deep connections (economic, social, and cultural) with the communities they are both located in and serve (Taylor et al., 2014). Schools are thus well positioned to promote health and tackle health inequalities and have a long history as settings for public health interventions. This has included more traditional public health measures, such as the provision of preventative healthcare services through immunization programmes, hearing and vision assessments, and oral and dental care, as well as interventions typically associated with new public health, such as health education and promotion activities in relation to malnutrition and obesity, sexual health, substance abuse, and so on (Gard and Pluim, 2014).

Following *The Ottawa Charter for Health Promotion* (World Health Organization (WHO), 1986), the WHO gave focus to a settings-based approach to health promotion that identified the social and cultural role and impact of settings, such as cities, schools, colleges, hospitals, workplaces, and prisons, in influencing health (Whitelaw et al., 2001). In 1992, the European Network of Health Promoting Schools specifically developed the concept of HPSs as a strategic response to affect the risks associated with education, economic, political, and social conditions (Barnekow and Rivett, 2000). A HPS involves all members of the school community working together to strengthen its capacity as a healthy setting for living, learning, and working (WHO, 1996). It is a whole school approach that moves beyond traditional approaches to health education by taking a broader focus to promoting health (Langford et al., 2015). The WHO's (1996) definition for a HPS thus gives focus to the formal and informal health curricula alongside 'the creation of a safe and healthy school environment, the provision of appropriate health services and the involvement of the family and wider community in efforts to promote health' (p. 2). As such, the WHO (1996) define six elements of a HPS, these include:

1. School health policies.
2. The physical environment.
3. The school's social environment.
4. Community relationships.
5. Personal health skills.
6. Health services.

Focus is given to a holistic approach to health that involves sustained positive changes, developing and embedding health education, policy, and practice within specific cultural and community contexts.

The concept and practice of HPSs has been adopted worldwide and is recognised as providing a useful framework for addressing loss and grief from a preventative, community owned, perspective (Rowling 2003, Kennedy et al. 2021). Nonetheless, HPSs continues to attract the same critiques of public health activities more broadly due to their narrow focus on preventing and controlling illness, disease, and disability, and avoiding the experiences of death, dying, and loss and their associated social epidemiology (Kellehear and Young, 2007). This can leave individuals and communities unprepared and socially unsupported to cope with the inevitability of illness and loss (Kellehear and Young, 2007). Public health palliative care education draws attention to this omission by recognizing death as part of the life span. It refers to a broader definition of health that is not defined by the absence or avoidance of illness, disease, injury, or death, but instead situates well-being at the centre. This definition of health is what Huber and colleagues (2011) refer to as 'the ability to adapt and self-manage in the face of social, physical, and emotional challenges' (p. 1). Public health palliative care education thus identifies the relevance of HPSs but suggests a reorientation of current practice to one that acknowledges the need for and capacity of school communities to address educational and support needs in relation to meaningful care and support at end of life and into bereavement.

A model for public health palliative care education: health-promoting palliative care schools

Public health palliative care education aims to support school communities to develop education on and for experiences of illness, caregiving, death, and loss. It recognizes that these experiences are fundamentally social and, as such, places emphasis on both information giving (raising awareness about illness, caregiving, death, and loss) and action (education for life and death). Public health palliative care education with children should not therefore only occur in school settings, but instead related activities should be addressed across the multiple social domains in which children live, play, and interact. However, school communities, as discussed previously, provide a unique setting from which to support the health and well-being of children, their families, and the wider school community. As such, focus here is given to the significance of, and capacity for, school communities to normalize illness, caregiving, death, and loss and in doing so work towards creating lasting social changes which foster a shared responsibility for, and increased compassion around, end of life and bereavement (Kellehear, 2005, 2016a). Within this context, a HPPCS is a public health palliative care education approach that specifically works to promote openness and challenge stigmas related to illness, caregiving, death, and loss that promote community members to draw on their own resources and supports to adapt and cope. This requires embedding policy and practices, promoting skills, and developing learning that proactively prepares children for all life's stages. It recognizes the agency of children to both influence and be influenced by their school community and emphasizes community and collective responsibility for caring for each other at times of illness, caregiving, death, and loss. As such, HPPCSs give focus to the importance of building on the strengths and the capacity of school communities, promoting positive decision-making and meaningful care and support.

Drawing on the WHO's core features of a HPS, Table 27.1 sets out a range of indicators for HPPCSs.

The indicators identify the role that school communities play in promoting well-being at times of illness, caregiving, dying, death, and loss for children, their families, and school staff with early intervention and harm reduction as key principles. They highlight the significance of policy, education, and partnership working to co-create conditions within school communities, those in which children learn and staff work, that are conducive to children, their families, and supporting each other at times of illness and loss. Implicit across the indicators is the role of leadership within the school, and education services more broadly, to provide strong support and governance to both adopt and roll out school-agreed plans, policies, and curricula. While established policies and procedures can be critiqued for being a fundamentally top-down approach, they also offer organizational support and reinforcement to encourage changes to both individuals and organizational behaviour (Patterson et al., 2018). Focus is thus given to health equity, recognizing education as a social determinant of health, whereby developing death and grief literacy is integral to enhancing well-being.

The indicators refer to what Whitelaw and colleagues (2001) call a comprehensive model of health promotion due to the recognition that solutions lie not only within direct and tangible activities (such as the development and delivery of death and grief education or bereavement policies) but also within 'the multitude of day-to day processes and practices which constitute the whole' (p. 344). Likewise, Kennedy and colleagues (2017) argue that 'in prioritising well-being for all school community members there is a need for these issues to be community owned rather than *only* individually evaluated' (p. 121). Thus, emphasis is also placed on influencing and/or changing established cultures within school systems about how caregiving and bereavement experiences are responded to and, as such, draws focus to the significance of relationships within and between children, families, and staff.

Practice examples of public health palliative care education in schools and/or with children

This section builds on the earlier sections by discussing four practice examples of how public health palliative care education with children has been developed. The first two examples highlight activities which use a HPPCS approach, whereas examples three and four demonstrate different models of public health palliative care education.

Table 27.1 Indicators for health-promoting palliative care schools

Core features of health-promoting schools (WHO, 1996)	Health-promoting palliative care schools (HPPCS)
School health policies	• Curricula is inclusive of death and grief education that develops children's knowledge, attitudes, and skills around illness, caregiving, death, dying, and loss and the factors that enable them to make positive choices to care for themselves and others through the life course • Policies, procedures, and practices are implemented that support helpful attitudes, values, and support around illness, caregiving, death, and loss. This includes specific policies in place for pupils and staff at times of illness, caregiving, or bereavement that acknowledge diversity and difference • Training, education, and/or information is provided for children, teachers, and parents/carers around how to talk about caregiving, illness, death, dying, or loss, as well as how to support themselves and others when these experiences occur
The physical environment	• A safe environment is provided to discuss and/or seek support about caregiving, illness, death, dying, or loss • Conditions and/or spaces are created within the school that are conducive to those who are ill, caregiving, and/or experiencing loss. This might include access to a safe and quiet place for children, staff, or families; procedures which facilitate access to support; and opportunities to remember
The school's social environment	• An ethos and culture are established in the school that creates openness around experiences of illness, caregiving, death, dying, and loss • Children, staff, and parents/carers care for themselves and others at times of illness, caregiving, dying, death, and loss • Accessible mechanisms to seek support are developed
Community relationships	• Positive relationships are developed among and between children, staff, families, palliative care service, carer organizations, bereavement services, and wider community networks • Community links are strengthened, through connections and partnership working with families, the community, schools, organizations, and other stakeholders • Expert support and advice is provided when needed both within, from, and to school communities to support the well-being of children, their families and staff around illness, caregiving, dying, death, and loss
Personal health skills	• Capacity is developed among children, their families, and staff, including death and grief literacy, to prevent maladaptive coping • Children, their families, and staff know how to offer support and get support for themselves and others at times of illness, caregiving, and loss • Learning outcomes and experiences are included in formal and informal curricula to develop children's knowledge and life skills for health and well-being at times of illness, caregiving, and loss
Health services	• Establishes partnerships with local palliative care services, carer groups, and bereavement services to provide guidance, education, and support as necessary • Informal support networks within the school are co-created with children, their families, and staff • Referral pathways for informal and specialist support at times of illness, caregiving, and bereavement are clearly mapped out and accessed as necessary for children, their families, and staff

Example one: Compassionate Schools Project, Plymouth, England

In 2018, Plymouth (the largest city on England's south coast) signed up to the Compassionate Cities Charter (Kellehear, 2016b) in which organizations and groups across the city work together to create a city 'informed and compassionate towards those facing end of life or experiencing bereavement' (St Luke's Hospice Plymouth, 2021a). As part of this commitment, St Luke's Hospice Plymouth, Plymouth City Council, and the University of Plymouth created a schools' network to develop a whole school approach to ensuring that children and the wider school community feel supported at times of illness, death, and bereavement. The project was led by a community development worker, employed by St Luke's Hospice, Plymouth. Following consultation with participating local schools, the Youth Council, bereaved young people, and other relevant stakeholders, several innovations were developed and piloted at five schools and colleges that included:

- Compassionate friends training: delivered to school staff by St Luke's education team about effective communication with those affected by death, dying, and bereavement using the Listen, Empathy, Notice, and Do (LEND) model (St Luke's Hospice Plymouth, 2021a).
- Compassionate champions training: delivered by St Luke's education and social care team to equip school staff with the skills and knowledge to deliver compassionate friends training to other staff in their school communities as well as take a leadership role in this area.
- Compassionate buddies training: delivered to students by St Luke's education team in conjunction with other partner organizations, such as the University of Plymouth Conservatoire forum theatre students, to build their skills and confidence in supporting peers who may be affected by death, dying, and bereavement.
- Development of a school's bereavement policy.
- 'Time out' cards that young people can give to teachers to let them know that they need time away from the class and allocated 'safe spaces' to access support material and take time out.
- Stickers for young people to place in their homework books to alert teachers that they are struggling and would like some support.
- Development of lessons plans, aligned with school curricula, to provide teaching and learning around bereavement, death, and dying. This included developing a session on loss and grief which can be adapted for primary and secondary school-aged children and young people using forum theatre sessions to talk about the signs of grief and helpful useful responses, using the LEND model.

- Development of an award scheme for schools to sign up to that met the full criteria of a Plymouth Compassionate School and is recognized as taking a whole school approach to death, dying, and bereavement.

The initial evaluation of the project revealed that the compassionate friends and compassionate buddies developed increased confidence around talking about death, dying, and bereavement and also knowledge of how to access support services (St Luke's Hospice Plymouth, 2021b). The work is ongoing, and forms part of the council's Healthy Child Quality Mark programme helping participating schools demonstrate safeguarding of bereaved children and young people. St Luke's Hospice Plymouth hopes to recruit a full-time compassionate schools coordinator to engage with all schools in the locality. This is dependent on funding being secured and includes finalizing an online compassionate schools guidance and resource pack and broader support for young people during school holidays through allocated safeguarded 'compassionate cafes'.

Example two: The Resilience Programme, Falkirk, Scotland

The Resilience Programme was initially developed as part of a doctoral study that used action research to explore, implement, and evaluate models of best practice to promote education and support around death and bereavement from a health promotion perspective (Paul et al., 2019). The research was funded by Strathcarron Hospice due to the management team's interest in exploring how to work more effectively with school communities. Two primary schools were recruited to take part and school staff, hospice staff, parents/carers, and children, aged 9–12 years, worked in partnership to increase understanding about current practice in the schools related to death and bereavement and develop practices as appropriate. Several practice innovations were developed, and continued to be implemented, that were of relevance to the school curriculum, policy, and training:

Bereavement training

School staff participants recognized that they were not educated on childhood bereavement yet believed that it was part of their role to acknowledge and respond to children's bereavement experiences (McManus and Paul, 2019). In response, research participants designed at 2.5-hour workshop to develop the capacity of school staff to respond to bereavement issues. This training was piloted and evaluated with the two schools involved in the research. In response to the initial evaluation, the hospice management team decided to roll out the training free of charge to all schools in the hospice catchment area. A subsequent evaluation of the wider training found that prior to training, 24% of participants (n = 195) rated their confidence as high in relation to acknowledging a bereavement with a child: post training, this rose to 79% (McManus and Paul, 2019).

Curriculum design: The Resilience Project

Participants recognized that children were not systematically educated about death and grief as a normal part of the lifecycle and that children had a variety of related questions. One participating school established a working group to design an education programme on loss, death, and grief which addresses specific experiences and outcomes within the national curriculum. In 2015, this programme was delivered to all children in the school, from age 3 to 12 years. While the school deemed the pilot a success, the working group noted that it failed to address the specific questions (about death) posed by children participating in the initial research. An offshoot of the programme was thus developed (The Resilience Project: Educating and Supporting Children around Death, Dying, and Bereavement), for children 9–12 years, that consists of five lessons covering the subjects of death, loss, and grief (Quinn and Paul, 2018). It is now a core part of the school's curriculum.

Policy development

In the process of developing the innovations, it was discovered that there was no bereavement policy for schools in the locality. The policy team within the education services subsequently established a team of school staff and designed a 'service circular' on how to manage bereavement in schools. The service circular was disseminated to all schools in the locality.

The expertise of hospice staff was input into each of the practice innovations at various stages of design; however, these activities now run independently from the hospice, unless the schools need to access training for staff or specialist pre/post-bereavement support.

Example Three: Studio DöBra, Sweden

Studio DöBra was initiated as a doctoral study and is part of national research programme, DöBra (a pun which literally means 'dying well' but figuratively 'awesome'), which uses a health promotion approach to support conversations about end of life issues at individual, community, and societal levels (Lindqvist and Tishelman, 2016). It is a community-based intergenerational arts project that aims to create opportunities for children and older people to interact and exchange ideas and experiences about dying, death, and loss. Using community-based participatory action research, Studio DöBra works with community organizations to co-create knowledge and ideas about developing intergenerational arts projects through collective reflective practice. The community organizations included after-school centres connected to primary schools, a library, activity centres for elderly people, an artistic organization, and municipal organizations for culture and elder care (Kleijberg et al., 2020). In partnership, the organizations developed the content of the intergenerational workshops as well as supporting the recruitment of participants and the provision of a space to hold the project activities (Kleijberg et al., 2020).

The Studio DöBra programme involved participants taking part in a series of five workshops encompassing a variety of collaborative arts activities, such as collages, sculptures, drawings, and games, with end of life-related issues (Kleijberg et al., 2021). This includes exploring questions such as 'Where do we end up after we die?' or 'How does grief feel?' The story of the project is then shared through a final exhibition of artwork (Kleijberg et al., 2021). To date, two Studio DöBra programmes have been facilitated with a total of 32 participants (eight children and eight adults per group). Community and academic partners have worked together to create a 'toolbox' that aims to support the development of similar initiatives (Donat Magnin et al., 2019).

The programme is undergoing evaluation as part of the action research methodology (Kleijberg et al., 2020, 2021). The findings highlight that, while there were no predefined learning outcomes related to end of life issues, participants learnt from each other through sharing their own end of life experiences 'on their own terms' (Kleijberg et al., 2020, p. 2034). Moreover, the project enabled a developing sense of community through new activities and intergenerational connections which participants were keen to continue (Kleijberg et al., 2020). Challenges, however, were identified regarding both the recruitment of elderly participants and the sustainability of the programme, both of which related to the dependency of children and older adults on what Kleijberg and colleagues (2021) refer to as the 'adults-in-between', who have a key role in both introducing the topic of death to these age groups, supporting the agency of the children and older adults, and maintaining the intergenerational spaces.

Example four: public awareness campaigns

Globally there are numerous examples of public health awareness campaigns that aim to raise awareness of childhood bereavement and young carers while simultaneously induce behaviour change through supporting the public to better understand how to help children at times of caregiving and grief (Seymour, 2018). These campaigns are thus focused on improving outcomes for children at a population level and focus is frequently given to the role of school communities. They usually involve national and local collaborations to deliver a range of organized activities that recognize and address barriers to support at individual and community levels, such as unequal access to care or health literacy skills (Seymour, 2018).

Children's Grief Awareness Day is perhaps the most well-established example of a public awareness campaign, which happens annually in November. It was created in 2008 by the Highmark Caring Place in the US to help children experiencing grief feel less isolated and more supported through transforming the culture around children and grief. It has since been adopted by organizations around the world, including Ireland, the UK, Canada, and Australia, and ranges from a 1-day campaign to a whole week of activities that seek to recognize and take action around children's grief. For example, in 2021 the US campaign saw the launch of *GriefTalk*, an initiative to encourage and support honest conversations around the topics of death and grief. Likewise, in the UK, the theme *SayTheWords* was used to encourage a variety of activities related to identifying and acknowledging loss with and by children. This theme was supported by directing teachers to lesson plans on grief or encouraging schools to complete an audit tool aimed to support grieving pupils. Public awareness campaign for young carers are either part of wider annual carer campaigns, for example, in Australia, or those specifically for young carers, as in the UK. These campaigns aim to raise public awareness of carers, the associated challenges, and the need for support. In the UK, from 2021 onwards, the focus of the campaign moved from awareness to action to give greater emphasis on encouraging the public to acknowledge and support young people involved in caregiving.

Challenges and opportunities

The examples outlined in previous sections demonstrate several ways in which public health palliative care education can engage with children about illness, caregiving, death, and loss. The examples show that schools provide a useful site to connect with children about these issues but also to influence and shape behaviours, beliefs and supports, for both children and the wider school community. According to Rowling (2003), bringing death and dying into schools from a preventative, health-promotion perspective depends on several competing factors, including curriculum priorities; the skills, comfort, and motivation of teaching professionals; the learning environment; and the learning context. Curriculum priorities is a key challenge. While education on, and for, death and bereavement can be incorporated at any stage of schooling, both as a discrete or transversal topic (Rodríguez Herrero et al., 2020), to date, evidence suggests that there is insufficient curricula focus to support such teaching (Tompkins, 2018; Rodríguez Herrero et al., 2020). As such, education for and about death is not intentionally incorporated into school curricula but instead relies on the willingness and skills of individual teachers and/or schools which is, by essence, inequitable. This is against a backdrop of competing curricular priorities and a staff force who are not consistently trained in, or supported to, engage with such issues. Research regularly highlights that a key barrier for schools in engaging with illness, caregiving, death, and loss is that staff feel ill-prepared and ill-equipped to do so (Rowling, 2003; McManus and Paul, 2019). Thus, while school staff clearly have skills in working with children, there is a reticence to engage these skills around education and support relating to illness, caregiving, death, and loss. As such, death and grief education necessarily involves self-development of teachers and cooperation with parents/carers as well as effective communication with children (Rodríguez Herrero et al., 2020). Embedding training for staff at all levels, including pre and post qualification for teachers, so that death and grief education and support can be fully embedded into the culture of education should therefore be a key priority (Rodríguez Herrero et al., 2020). This, in turn, needs to be supported by distinct policy development in relation to support for staff and children. Death is a sensitive issue that can elicit powerful emotions and, as such, ensuring that staff, children, and their families can access meaningful support (social and specialist) if and when needed is essential, and a key focus within public health palliative care approaches.

While public health palliative care education invites schools to proactively prepare children, and the wider school community, for illness, caregiving, death, and loss, schools frequently attend to presenting problems. For example, it is common for school staff to engage with bereavement training or look at developing a bereavement policy once a bereavement occurs in the school, rather than proactively preparing for these experiences. This can result in a range of disjointed practice and policy provision both within and across school communities and thus there is a need to ensure that school communities can identify benefits of public health palliative care as part of their core business of education. Arguably, this should not be difficult given the prevalence and impact of illness, caregiving, death, and loss on children and within school communities; yet these issues are not common parlance and largely remain hidden. Moreover, the school setting is not an 'independent and controllable entity' (Whitelaw et al., 2001, p. 343) but subject to a variety of competing political, social, and educational demands and thus leadership is essential in promoting public health palliative care approaches. Specialist palliative care providers may have a role here. They are viewed as being in a unique position to initiate and/or provide leadership in developing public health palliative care activities due to their expertise in end of life and bereavement issues (Street,

2007; Kellehear and O'Connor, 2008; Paul et al., 2019). Moreover, in counties such as the UK and New Zealand, working with schools is a popular form of community engagement for specialist palliative care services (Paul and Sallnow, 2013; Dempers and Gott, 2017). Yet there are several barriers to developing such work due to funding, service vision and purpose, local need, and clarity around the key goals of a public health approach (Paul and Sallnow, 2013; Dempers and Gott, 2017). As such, while numerous examples exist of specialist palliative care services working with school communities, in line with the WHO's definition of a HPS (1996), a consistent challenge remains in ensuring that positive changes are sustained and are not dependent on the service or the enthusiasm and commitment of a few staff members. The current focus in schools on addressing presenting issues potentially presents an opportunity for specialist services, such as those providing palliative care, bereavement support, or support for carers to engage with schools in these issues and to support and develop informal care networks. Moreover, the examples provided identify numerous opportunities for partnership working in relation to training, curricula, and policy development, building social support networks, and providing specialist services. Nonetheless, it is essential that external agencies with an intervention role create strong, supportive, and enabling relationships, led by the needs of the school community.

Public health palliative care education in schools is a long-term process that requires attention to the development of policies, curricula, resources, staff training, and internal and external supports, alongside creating spaces and practices which acknowledge diversity and promote choice rather than prescribing certain behaviours. This relates to a change in ethos and culture as opposed to purely implementing practice strategies and, as such, Kennedy and colleagues (2020) argue that opportunities should be created for school communities to explicitly discuss their experiences and preferences for attitudinal and cultural change. It involves employing a participatory style of working rather than expert positions and includes fully recognizing the rights and agency of children. This type of approach takes time and it is important to note that three of the examples provided were initiated by someone (a staff member or researcher) with a remit and resources to develop work with children as part of a public health approach.

Finally, while schools may provide a key site for public health palliative care education, it is important to acknowledge that not all children go to school and that children exist as part of other communities. As such, public health palliative care education needs to look both within and beyond schools to the broader networks of children's lives. In relation to HPPCSs, focus thus needs to be given to considering how related activities can transcend the school building and interact with the wider family and community lives of children and staff. To date this expansion is currently underexplored.

Conclusion

This chapter has argued that illness, caregiving, and bereavement are common features in children's lives and reframing these experiences as a public health issues places emphasis on a multilayered approach to education, care, and support that firmly positions children within the families and communities in which they live. School communities provide a valuable setting for public health palliative care due to the link between health and education and the impact that schools have in mediating children's experiences. I have argued that HPPCSs offer a useful framework from which to develop meaningful engagement and holistic practices whereby children, and the wider school community, can gain information and skills to improve their health and well-being both now and into the future (Street, 2007). Reforms to school curricula, policy, and training will be integral to promoting systemic change that fosters a compassionate school community at times of illness, caregiving, death, and loss.

REFERENCES

Aldridge, J. 2008. All work and no play? understanding the needs of children with caring responsibilities. *Children & Society*, 22, 253–264.

Andriessen, K., Lobb, E., Mowll, J., Dudley, M., Draper, B., and Mitchell, P. B. 2019. Help-seeking experiences of bereaved adolescents: a qualitative study. *Death Studies*, 43, 1–8.

Banks, P., Cogan, N., Riddell, S., Deeley, S., Hill, M., and Tisdall, K. 2002. Does the covert nature of caring prohibit the development of effective services for young carers? *British Journal of Guidance & Counselling*, 30, 229–246.

Barnekow, V. and Rivett, D. 2000. The European Network of Health Promoting Schools – the alliance of education and health. *Health Education*, 100, 61–67.

Burns, M., Griese, B., King, S., and Talmi, A. 2020. Childhood bereavement: understanding prevalence and related adversity in the United States. *American Journal of Orthopsychiatry*, 90, 391–405.

Cohen, D., Greene, J. A., Toyinbo, P. A., and Siskowski, C. T. 2012. Impact of family caregiving by youth on their psychological well-being: a latent trait analysis. *Journal of Behavioral Health Services & Research*, 39, 245–256.

Coombs, S. 2014. Death wears a T-shirt – listening to young people talk about death. *Mortality*, 19, 284–302.

Currier, J. M., Holland, J. M., and Neimeyer, R. A. 2007. The effectiveness of bereavement interventions with children: a meta-analytic review of controlled outcome research. *Journal of Clinical Child and Adolescent Psychology*, 36, 253–259.

Davies, H. 2017. Embodied and sensory encounters: death, bereavement and remembering in children's family and personal lives. *Children's Geographies*, 17, 552–564.

Dempers, C. and Gott, M. 2017. The status of a public health approach to palliative care at New Zealand hospices. *Progress in Palliative Care*, 25, 75–81.

Donat Magnin, A., Libäck, C., Arvidsson Berglund, F., Hallén, H., Oad, K., Sulin, K., et al. 2019. Studio DöBra Toolbox: using arts to support conversations between children and older adults about dying, death and loss. Sweden. [Online] Available at: https://www.xn--dbra-5qa.se/en/dobra-toolbox/studio-dobra-toolbox/

Gard, M. and Pluim, C. 2014. *Schools and Public Health: Past, Present and Future*. Plymouth: Lexington Books.

Gough, G. and Gulliford, A. 2020. Resilience amongst young carers: investigating protective factors and benefit-finding as perceived by young carers. *Educational Psychology in Practice*, 36, 149–169.

Hill, M. and Tisdall, K. 1997. *Children and Society*. New York: Addison Wesley Longman Limited.

Huber, M., Knottnerus, J. A., Green, L., Horst, H. V. D., Jadad, A. R., Kromhout, D., et al. 2011. How should we define health? *BMJ*, 343, d4163.

Jackson, M. and Colwell, J. 2001. Talking to children about death. *Mortality*, 6, 321–325.

Jamieson, L. and Highet, G. 2013. Troubling loss: children's experiences of major disruptions in family life. In: Ribbens McCarthy, J., Hooper, C.-A., and Gillies, V. (eds.) *Family Troubles? Exploring Changes and Challenges in the Family Lives of Children and Young People*, pp. 135–150. Bristol: Policy Press.

Jones, A., Deane, C., and Keegan, O. 2015. The development of a framework to support bereaved children and young people: the Irish Childhood Bereavement Care Pyramid. *Bereavement Care*, 34, 43–51.

Joseph, S., Kendall, C., Toher, D., Sempik, J., Holland, J., and Becker, S. 2019. Young carers in England: findings from the 2018 BBC survey on the prevalence and nature of caring among young people. *Child: Care, Health and Development*, 45, 606–612.

Joseph, S., Sempik, J., Leu, A., and Becker, S. 2020. Young carers research, practice and policy: an overview and critical perspective on possible future directions. *Adolescent Research Review*, 5, 77–89.

Kellehear, A. 2005. *Compassionate Cities: Public Health and End-of-Life Care*. Abingdon: Routledge.

Kellehear, A. 2016a. Commentary: public health approaches to palliative care – the progress so far. *Progress in Palliative Care*, 24, 36–38.

Kellehear, A. 2016b. The Compassionate City Charter: inviting the cultural and social sectors into end-of-life care. In: Wegleitner, K., Heimerl, K., and Kellehear, A. (eds.) *Compassionate Communities: Case Studies from Britain and Europe*, pp. 76–87. Abingdon: Routledge.

Kellehear, A. and O'Connor, D. 2008. Health-promoting palliative care: a practice example. *Critical Public Health*, 18, 111–115.

Kellehear, A. and Young, B. 2007. Resilient communities. In: Monroe, B. and Oliviere, D. (eds.) *Resilience in Palliative Care*, pp. 223–238. Oxford: Oxford University Press.

Kennedy, C. J., Gardner, F., and Farrelly, C. 2020. Death, dying and bereavement: considering compassion and empowerment. *Pastoral Care in Education*, 38, 138–155.

Kennedy, C. J., Garnder, F. and Southall, A. 2021. The Intentionla Compassion Framework for school communities. *Health Education Journal*, 80(6):660–671.

Kennedy, C. J., Keeffe, M., Gardner, F., and Farrelly, C. 2017. Making death, compassion and partnership 'part of life' in school communities. *Pastoral Care in Education*, 35, 111–123.

Kleijberg, M., Ahlberg, B. M., Hilton, R., and Tishelman, C. 2020. Death, loss and community—perspectives from children, their parents and older adults on intergenerational community-based arts initiatives in Sweden. *Health & Social Care in the Community*, 28, 2025–2036.

Kleijberg, M., Ahlberg, B. M., MacDonald, A., Lindqvist, O., and Tishelman, C. 2021. Navigating power dynamics in engaging communities in end-of-life issues – lessons learned from developing community-based intergenerational arts initiatives about death and loss. *Death Studies*, 45, 651–664.

Langford, R., Bonell, C., Jones, H., Pouliou, T., Murphy, S., Waters, E., et al. 2015. The World Health Organization's Health Promoting Schools framework: a Cochrane systematic review and meta-analysis. *BMC Public Health*, 15, 130.

Lee, A., Lo, A. S. C., Keung, M. W., Kwong, C. M. A., and Wong, K. K. 2019. Effective health promoting school for better health of children and adolescents: indicators for success. *BMC Public Health*, 19, 1088.

Leu, A., Frech, M., Wepf, H., Sempik, J., Joseph, S., Helbling, L., et al. 2019. Counting young carers in Switzerland – a study of prevalence. *Children & Society*, 33, 53–67.

Lindqvist, O. and Tishelman, C. 2016. Going public: reflections on developing the DöBra research program for health-promoting palliative care in Sweden. *Progress in Palliative Care*, 24, 19–24.

McManus, E. and Paul, S. 2019. Addressing the bereavement needs of children in school: an evaluation of bereavement training for school communities. *Improving Schools*, 22, 72–85.

Monroe, B. and Kraus, F. (eds.) 2010. *Brief Interventions with Bereaved Children*, 2nd edition. Oxford: Oxford University Press.

Patterson, R., Peacock, R., and Hazelwood, M. 2018. A road less lonely: moving forward with public health approaches to death, dying and bereavement in Scotland. Edinburgh: Scottish Partnership for Palliative Care.

Paul, S. 2019. Is death taboo for children? Developing death ambivalence as a theoretical framework to understand children's relationship with death, dying and bereavement. *Children & Society*, 33, 556–571.

Paul, S., Cree, V. E., and Murray, S. A. 2019. Integrating palliative care into the community: the role of hospices and schools. *BMJ Supportive & Palliative Care*, 9, e31.

Paul, S. and Sallnow, L. 2013. Public health approaches to end of life care in the UK: an online survey of palliative care services *BMJ Supportive & Palliative Care*, 3, 196–199.

Paul, S. and Vaswani, N. 2020. The prevalence of childhood bereavement in Scotland and its relationship with disadvantage: the significance of a public health approach to death, dying and bereavement. *Palliative Care and Social Practice*, 14, 2632352420975043.

Puolimatka, T. and Solasaari, U. 2006. Education for death. *Educational Philosophy and Theory*, 38, 201–213.

Quinn, H. and Paul, S. 2018. The Resilience Project: educating and supporting children around death, dying and bereavement, Falkirk: St Francis Xavier's Primary School. [Online] Available at: https://www.goodlifedeathgrief.org.uk/content/resources/The_Resilience_Project.pdf

Ribbens McCarthy, J. 2006. *Young People's Experiences of Loss and Bereavement: Towards an Interdisciplinary Approach*. Maidenhead: Open University Press.

Rodríguez Herrero, P., De La Herrán Gascón, A., and De Miguel Yubero, V. 2020. The inclusion of death in the curriculum of the Spanish Regions. *Compare: A Journal of Comparative and International Education*, 1–19. Published online 11 September, DOI: 10.1080/03057925.2020.1732192.

Rowling, L. 2003. *Grief in School Communities: Effective Support Strategies*. Buckingham: Open University Press.

Rowling, L. 2010. Schools and grief: attending to people and place. In: Monroe, B. and Kraus, F. (eds.) *Brief Interventions with Bereaved Children*, 2nd edition, pp. 147–160. New York: Oxford University Press.

Rumbold, B. and Aoun, S. M. 2014. Bereavement and palliative care: a public health perspective. *Progress in Palliative Care*, 22, 131–135.

Scott, R., Wallace, R., Audsley, A., and Chary, S. 2019. Young people and their understanding of loss and bereavement. *Bereavement Care*, 38, 6–12.

Seymour, J. 2018. The impact of public health awareness campaigns on the awareness and quality of palliative care. *Journal of Palliative Medicine*, 21, S30–S36.

Smith, D. E. and Hunter, S. B. 2008. Predictors of children's understandings of death: age, cognitive ability, death experience and maternal communicative competence. *OMEGA*, 57, 143–162.

Smyth, C., Blaxland, M., and Cass, B. 2011. 'So that's how I found out I was a young carer and that I actually had been a carer most of my life'. Identifying and supporting hidden young carers. *Journal of Youth Studies,* 14, 145–160.

St Luke's Hospice Plymouth. 2021a. A compassionate city. [Online]. Available at: https://www.stlukes-hospice.org.uk/plymouth-a-compassionate-city/

St Luke's Hospice Plymouth. 2021b. Compassionate schools pilot. [Online]. Available at: https://www.stlukes-hospice.org.uk/wp-content/uploads/2021/02/Schools-Pilot-Overall-Evaluation_V2.pdf

Street, A. 2007. Leading the way: innovative health-promoting palliative care. *Contemporary Nurse,* 27, 104–106.

Taylor, H., McGlynn, L., and Luter, G. 2014. Public schools as neighbourhood anchor institutions: the Choice Neighbourhood Initiative in Buffalo, New York. In: Patterson, K. and Silverman, M. (eds.) *Schools and Urban Revitalization: Rethinking Institutions and Community Development*, pp. 109–135. New York: Routledge.

Tompkins, B. 2018. Compassionate communities in Canada: it is everyone's responsibility. *Annals of Palliative Medicine,* 7, S118–S129.

UNICEF. 2021. Primary education. [Online]. Available at: https://data.unicef.org/topic/education/primary-education/

Whitelaw, S., Baxendale, A., Bryce, C., Machardy, L., Young, I., and Witney, E. 2001. 'Settings' based health promotion: a review. *Health Promotion International,* 16, 339–353.

World Health Organization. 1986. *Ottawa Charter for Health Promotion: First International Conference on Health Promotion, Ottawa, 21 November 1986.* Geneva: World Health Organization.

World Health Organization. 1996. *Regional Guidelines: Development of Health-Promoting Schools – A Framework for Action.* Manila: World Health Organization, Regional Office for the Western Pacific.

28

Specialist training

The UK palliative medicine curriculum

Polly Edmonds

The specialty of Palliative Medicine

In the UK, Palliative Medicine became a recognized medicine specialty in 1987, under the auspices of the Royal College of Physicians, a professional body dedicated to improving the practice of medicine, chiefly through the accreditation of physicians. As outlined by David Clark (2014) in a blog considering the development of palliative medicine as a specialty, three factors came together to create a platform for the wider development of the field of palliative medicine in the 1980s: the formation of a medical association to support its practitioners (the Association of Palliative Medicine of Great Britain and Ireland); a scientific journal, *Palliative Medicine*, was established; and formal recognition was given to palliative medicine as an medical specialty. Specialty recognition was important, providing not just a standing within the medical profession and enhanced opportunities for research and research funding, but also enabling the development of education and training in palliative medicine, not just for doctors aspiring to be consultants in the specialty, but also for a range of junior doctors and medical students, with the aim of improving the quality of treatment and care for people who were dying. The UK was the first country in the world to give palliative medicine specialty status. In 2014, Clark estimated that 26 countries recognized some form of accreditation for the specialty or subspecialty of palliative medicine.

In 2004, the UK National Institute for Health and Care Excellence guidance, 'Improving Supportive and Palliative Care for Adults with Cancer', recommended that specialist multidisciplinary palliative care teams as a minimum comprise a palliative care consultant, nurse specialist, and administrative support. These recommendations were reinforced in NHS England commissioning guidance in 2016. The appointment of consultants in palliative medicine to specialist services provides a benchmark, as in order to be appointed as a consultant, doctors need to have completed an established specialty training programme or demonstrated equivalence to the level required of a doctor completing specialist training.

As a medical specialty, responsibility for postgraduate curricula and the quality of postgraduate training sits with the Joint Royal College Physicians Training Board (JRCPTB). The JRCPTB is responsible for internal medicine training and 30 medical specialties and three subspecialties, all of which have Specialty Advisory Committees (SACs), responsible for the curriculum and quality of training in their specialty. The General Medical Council (GMC) sets the UK national standards that medical training organizations are expected to meet in the delivery of training and the outcomes that doctors in training should achieve by the end of their training. The GMC approves curricula and assessment systems for training.

In the UK, doctors in training complete 2 years of Foundation training in a range of specialties following completion of medical school. After Foundation training, doctors apply competitively to broad-based specialty training: for physicianly specialties, this changed in August 2019 from core medical training to stage 1 internal medicine training. The current Palliative Medicine postgraduate training programme is an indicative 4 years in length, with the majority of trainees entering specialist training on completion of core medical (now internal medicine) training. Completion of training results in award of the certificate of completion of training in the specialty of Palliative Medicine and entry to the GMC specialist register. Until 2022, trainees are working to a curriculum that was implemented in 2010, with minor amendments approved by the GMC in 2014. This curriculum is competence based, with detailed descriptions of the knowledge, skills, and attributes required for each area of competence and covers 13 domains: introduction to palliative care; physical care; communication; psychosocial care; attitudes and responses of doctors and other professionals; culture, language, religion, and spirituality; ethics; legal frameworks; teamwork; learning and teaching; research; management; and clinical governance.

Shape of Training Review

The 2013 Shape of Training Review report, 'Securing the future of excellent patient care', has led to significant changes to training nationally and the updating of all specialty curricula. The report recommended that patients and the public need more doctors who are capable of providing general care in broad specialties across a range of different settings, driven by population changes (e.g. an increasing number of people with multiple morbidities and an ageing population), rising health inequalities, and increasing patient expectations (Shape of Training Review, 2013). In response to its recommendations, the JRCPTB grouped its specialties into group 1 specialties (dual training with internal medicine, leading to award of a dual completion of training in internal medicine and specialty) and group 2 specialties (single specialty completion of training). Palliative Medicine was confirmed as a group 1 specialty by the UK Shape of Training Steering Group in 2017.

Following the Shape of Training Review, all postgraduate medical curricula are being reviewed and updated; for this, the GMC stipulates that curricula conform to agreed standards and requirements (GMC, 2017). These standards work in conjunction with 'Promoting excellence: standards for medical education and training' (GMC, 2015). Together, they provide an integrated standards framework for the development, approval, and provision of postgraduate medical education and training in the UK. The GMC standards require curricula to describe fewer, high-level generic, shared, and specialty-specific outcomes, which will support all doctors better in understanding what is expected of them in their training programme.

Public health and the 2010 (2014 amendments) Palliative Medicine curriculum

In 2018, Abel and Kellehear published a critique of the 2010 curriculum, specifically focusing on its relationship and relevance to contemporary palliative care policy and strategy. They concluded that from the perspective of academic public health and contemporary UK public health policy, this curriculum 'fails to deliver important current content and insight for trainees'. The authors noted that the curriculum is based on a biomedical model of palliative care, with the public health and psychosocial sections of the curriculum narrowly defined and with gaps identified in relation to both public health and sociological concepts of illness, caregiving, grief, and bereavement (Abel and Kellehear, 2018) (see Table 28.1 for further details).

Development of the new (2022) palliative medicine curriculum

A new Palliative Medicine curriculum has been developed and approved by the GMC. As a new group 1 specialty, Palliative Medicine trainees will undergo 'dual training' in both the specialty and internal medicine, in line with the recommendations of the Shape of Training Review (2013). The training programme will remain an indicative 4-year programme.

In developing the new curriculum, a subgroup of the Palliative Medicine SAC worked virtually over 18 months in 2017–2019 to develop and refine the specialty-specific capabilities in practice (CiPs), supported by the Palliative Medicine SAC and the curriculum team at JRCPTB. Once the CiPs had been agreed and developed, the main body of the curriculum was developed, including the syllabus (i.e. topics, presentations, and conditions to be covered), minimum training requirements, and methods of assessment. Several iterations of the evolving curriculum were sent out for informal consultation, including to a virtual group of trainees and to a task and finish group between the SAC and national professional body, the Association of Palliative Medicine of Great Britain and Ireland. A formal stakeholder consultation process was undertaken in autumn 2019. The curriculum is now approved will be implemented in August 2022.

Development of a new palliative medicine curriculum: considering public health

Abel and Kellehear's 2018 review of the public health component of the 2010 (2014 amendments) curriculum was very timely, published at a time when the CiP descriptors and syllabus were being developed. As the curriculum lead for the SAC, I was very aware that my own knowledge of public health and consideration of the societal component of palliative care is limited, having spent all of my consultant career working in an acute hospital. Prior to this, my medical and palliative care training conformed to a traditional biomedical model, which in retrospect was overly focused on concepts of disease, diagnosis, and treatments, albeit with a holistic perspective from working in palliative care. Thinking back to my

Table 28.1 Specific observations on the 2010 UK palliative medicine curriculum

Observation	Comment
Concept of community	• Concept of community: its meaning as a social influence on health and well-being appears trivial and isolated and focused on work site • No mention of the role of palliative medical leadership in relation to school or workplace policies or advice; no mention of the potential influence of palliative medicine on church or temple activities for support in palliative, bereavement, or aged care; no mention of any outreach role for prisons or the homeless
Balance of curriculum	• Curriculum unbalanced, with focus on negative concepts, such as conflict • Relatively little or no discussion of either fear of death; or of protective factors for health and well-being at the end of life, such as love, intimacy, friendship, finding meaning, happiness, and hope
Curriculum section: public health	No requirement to understand important facets of public health, including: • Social impact and clinical epidemiology of living with advanced ageing, dying, long-term caregiving, grief, and bereavement • Key concepts of public health (prevention, harm reduction, early intervention) or their methods and their relevance to palliative care (community development, social ecology, death literacy, social marketing, health promotion) • Understanding of the effects of social supports on personal health and well-being • Awareness of importance of mapping civic and neighbourhood social supports • Application of understanding of culture and beliefs on health perceptions to death, dying, caregiving, or grief and loss • Opportunities to improve wider social support where patients and their families live and work is absent, including awareness of involvement with community leaders
Curriculum section: psychosocial care	• Concepts of grief and bereavement overly focused on negative views of 'normal' life events, affecting all • No exploration of the potential personal or societal resources to support the bereaved and promote healing

own medical and palliative medicine training, I received no formal training on psychological, environmental, public health, and social influences on health and their relevance to palliative care. As a consultant, my own clinical practice was profoundly influenced by the appointment of a dynamic palliative care social worker to our hospital team, who brought a different focus and approach to patient care; this enabled team members, myself included, to become more skilled in identifying and supporting a broad range of psychosocial issues. This was critical, working in a hospital serving a very diverse (ethnically and culturally) and deprived local community. Our team frequently utilizes a range of community services to support our patients and those close to them, including faith groups, befriending services, and third-sector organizations such as the Red Cross, alongside hospital services such as our homelessness team. However, both individually and as a service and despite having skilled and experienced palliative care social workers within the team, our close links to local hospice and palliative care services has not extended to a cogent understanding of the wider societal work undertaken by some hospices and community services and the opportunities offered through community engagement. Interestingly, the clinical service I work in is based within a large academic palliative care department, with specific public health expertise; however, the public health focus is more on epidemiology and analysis of large data sets to inform policy rather than health promotion in palliative care.

Prior to considering the limitations of the 2010 curriculum, I had not previously considered the concept of health promotion in relation to palliative care. At first glance, this appeared to be to be something of an oxymoron, working in a specialty continually working with people facing a range of losses. However, in considering further, I realize that health promotion informally underpins much of what we do in our hospital palliative care practice: supporting people to move forward from negative communication, such as 'There's nothing more we can do'; focusing on helping people realize realistic goals; supporting the concept of hope alongside preparing for the worst-case scenario; and a relentless focus on the things we *can* do. Recognizing that my own knowledge was lacking, I read around the subject and organized a video call with an expert in the field, which was fascinating. This allowed me to start reflecting on how we could weave more contemporary themes of public health and health promotion into the new curriculum to address some of the issues identified within the current curriculum. At the time of this discussion, I was very aware that the initial drafts of the 2022 curriculum were as unbalanced and biomedical in approach as previous curricula and that revisions were required.

Developing the palliative medicine specialty capabilities in practice: public health

As outlined earlier, all new medical curricula need to conform to current GMC standards. The GMC requires curricula to describe generic, shared, and specialty-specific outcomes, to support doctors in understanding what is expected of them.

These high-level learning outcomes are known as CiPs and describe professional tasks or work that are generic or within the scope of the specialty and are based on the concept of 'entrustable professional activities' (Ten Cate, 2015). These use the professional judgement of appropriately trained, expert assessors or supervisors as a defensible way of forming global judgements of professional performance. Each CiP has a set of descriptors associated with that activity or task; these are intended to help trainees and supervisors recognize the knowledge, skills, and attitudes that should be demonstrated. Doctors in training may use these capabilities to provide evidence of how their performance meets or exceeds the minimum expected level of performance for their year of training.

Box 28.1 Palliative medicine specialty capabilities in practice

Specialty CiPs:

1. Managing patients with life-limiting conditions across all care settings.
2. Ability to manage complex pain in people with life-limiting conditions across all care settings.
3. Demonstrates the ability to manage complex symptoms secondary to life-limiting conditions across all care settings.
4. Ability to demonstrate effective advanced communication skills with patients with life-limiting conditions, those close to them, and colleagues across all care settings.
5. Ability to manage, lead, and provide optimal care of the complex dying patient and those close to them across all care settings.
6. Manages delivery of holistic psychosocial care in patients with life-limiting conditions and those close to them, including religious, cultural, and spiritual care across all care settings.
7. Demonstrates the ability to lead a palliative care service in any setting, including those in the third sector.

Box 28.1 outlines the palliative medicine specialty CiPs in the new curriculum.

Each CiP has a list of descriptors attributed it; these are not meant to be exhaustive, but rather to guide trainees and supervisors to support learning. One challenge in writing the new curriculum was how to integrate the public health component of the curriculum into the descriptors, while not allowing the descriptors to become too detailed and thereby moving away from the concept of high-level learning outcomes.

As part of the development of the new curriculum and aware that none of the SAC curriculum subgroup had any specific expertise in this area, I invited experts in the field to help us develop a language that better reflected current understanding of health promotion in palliative care and the societal impact of progressive illness and dying. We hope that this has led to the integration of a more balanced and positive language when describing the public health components of the new curriculum.

Table 28.2 outlines the proposed descriptors for CiP6 (holistic psychosocial care), with those most relevant to public health and health promotion in italics. While not exhaustive, the agreed descriptors try to achieve a better balance, in this case recognizing both the negative and potential psychosocial consequences for patients and those close to them of life-limiting illness.

In other specialty CiPs, additional descriptors include:

- Recognition of the range of social problems potentially leading to poor outcomes, including increased morbidity and mortality, for example, poor public and personal support networks; poor or absent school or workplace policies; or poor or absent partnerships between health services, social care providers, and communities.
- Acknowledgement of the parallel health and well-being aspects of dying, caregiving, and bereavement, for example, growth of love,

Table 28.2 CiP6—holistic psychosocial care

6. Manages delivery of holistic psychosocial care of patients and those close to them, including loss and grief; and religious, cultural, and spiritual care across all care settings	
Descriptors	• Ability to identify, assess, and manage complex psychosocial issues affecting patients and those close to them and healthcare professionals in the context of life-limiting disease • Ability to utilize the multiprofessional team, across care settings and between services, to provide customized patient-centred care for patients with complex psychosocial issues • *User of appropriate knowledge and skill to support patients and those close to them in dealing with distress, loss, and grief, including support for those at risk of prolonged or abnormal bereavement and the needs of children (including siblings) at different developmental stages, teenagers, and young adults* • *Awareness of the range of psychological interventions that can be used to support patients and those close to them* • *Awareness of the positive and negative impacts of caring on those close to patients with life-limiting illness, including ability to work, lifestyle changes, and managing concurrent physical and mental illness* • *Awareness of need for people and those close to them to maintain social participation and support networks; to support informal carers in both the positive and enriching and challenging aspects of care giving; and of the potential for empowered, supportive informal networks to improve outcomes* • Knowledge of the responses and needs of children or adults with learning difficulties • Knowledge of and skills in recognizing and managing mental illness in patients with life-limiting conditions, including the ability to differentiate between appropriate sadness and depression • Ability to recognize and manage agitated, violent, and/or suicidal patients and/or those close to them, including liaison with psychological/psychiatric services and use of appropriate legal frameworks • Awareness of rehabilitation approaches to maximize physical and social functioning in the context of advanced life-limiting illness • Knowledge of financial and welfare benefits available • *Awareness of and ability to work alongside the community and social resources available to support vulnerable people, e.g. those that are homeless, in custody, without recourse to public funds, or those with learning or physical disability* • Knowledge and skills to elicit spiritual concerns and to recognize and respond to spiritual distress; and respects differing spiritual beliefs and practices • *Understanding of the impact of culture, ethnicity, and sexuality in response to life-limiting conditions and at the end of life, including an awareness that this may affect equity of access to services*

intimacy, and friendship; the importance of sense of meaning and well-being found in relationships during dying, caregiving, or grief; or the powerful support role of community during this time.

- The benefits of participation in reducing harm and promoting well-being and their impact on lifelong problems.
- Awareness of the potential role for palliative care services in supporting health promotion interventions, including helping to develop compassionate communities and supporting civic programmes.

To support the learning outcomes, or CiPs, the syllabus section of the curriculum contextualizes the patient population and breadth of experiences required for trainees. We added a commentary to the introduction to the syllabus component of the curriculum, highlighting why more up-to-date understanding of public health in palliative care was important for trainees. This section specifically comments that 'Palliative care as a speciality focuses on making the most of the time left for living for those undergoing the experiences of death, dying, loss and care giving, at the same time as managing the negative impacts of life-limiting illnesses'. It then goes on to explain the concepts of public health and health promotion and their relevance to palliative medicine training:

> As clinical leaders of the future, trainees also need to develop an awareness of the potential for broader community engagement, development and health promotion in end of life care, in which palliative care services have an important facilitatory role. There is evidence that community engagement initiatives improve a range of health and social care outcomes at the end of life. These include improving the relevance of services; development of knowledge, skills and capacity in communities; support for self-management and resilience in the face of death, dying and loss; reduced social isolation and its negative health consequences; reduced admissions to secondary care; improved outcomes for informal carers; and support for developing healthier attitudes to death, dying and loss (Sallnow and Paul, 2015; Sallnow et al., 2016; Abel et al., 2018). Community initiatives such as compassionate communities and primary care networks will be important in delivering sustainable services in the future and in addressing current inequalities in access to specialist palliative care services, which will become more marked as the potential need for palliative, supportive and end of life care increases in line with the predicted population changes.

Feedback on the new palliative medicine curriculum

I was not unique in having a relatively narrow, biomedical approach to palliative medicine and the new curriculum. When discussing the reworking of the public health components of the new curriculum, SAC colleagues were open in recognizing their own limitations in this area and lack of confidence in helping trainees gain expertise.

Few respondents to the October 2019 stakeholder consultation commented on the changes to the public health and health promotion components of the curriculum, but informal feedback suggests that many consultants, supervising training, feel that they have limited experience or expertise in this area. While many existing consultants may lack confidence, palliative care services are increasingly involved in a variety of community engagement strategies, but consultants have, to an extent, not recognized these as public health initiatives.

In implementing the new curriculum, we recognize that there will be a need for formal training, led by national experts for both trainees and supervisors; signposting to resources (literature, podcasts, websites, projects); and regional and local mapping of opportunities for involvement in health promotion and community engagement projects, to support trainee learning and development. The existing gap in knowledge and confidence in this field highlights the need for further training of the palliative care workforce, but also the opportunities provided through inclusion in the specialty training curriculum.

Finalizing the new UK palliative medicine curriculum

Following the stakeholder consultation process, the new curriculum for 2022 has been finalised and was approved by the GMC in 2001. In retrospect, we were lucky that Abel and Kellehear's paper critiquing the current curriculum was published in 2018, at a time when work was underway to develop the new curriculum. This gave us an opportunity to reflect on the feedback; as a curriculum working group, we were at risk of repeating the omissions and imbalances in relation to the public health component of the 2010 (2014 amendments) curriculum, primarily as a result of our own lack of knowledge in this field and cognitive biases. We were very grateful to experts in public health in palliative care, who gave their time and provided constructive feedback on curriculum drafts, including developing some of the CiP descriptors and the paragraph providing context in the syllabus.

Prior to sending the curriculum out for stakeholder consultation, all CiP descriptors were heavily edited to ensure that the learning outcomes remained 'high level' and did not become overly detailed, in line with GMC recommendations. While this included editing some of the public health descriptors, the curriculum subgroup was careful to maintain a focus on the opportunities provided by health promotion and community empowerment at the end of life. Several iterations of the curriculum were reviewed in detail by the SAC curriculum group prior to and after the formal stakeholder consultation and the final curriculum, including the public health components, has now been agreed by the SAC, prior to submission to the GMC. The GMC approval process is more focused on the process of curriculum development and its implementation rather than the content, so no significant changes were required prior to approval.

The consensus from stakeholders is that the new curriculum better reflects current palliative medicine practice and is sufficiently 'future-proofed' for the next 5–10 years, to take account of evolving practice, including in the field of health promotion and public health.

Final thoughts

The aim of the Palliative Medicine curriculum is to deliver broad-based specialty training, encompassing clinical expertise, alongside training in generic skills, including teaching, quality improvement, research, leadership, and management. The award of the certificate of completion of training (CCT) allows doctors to be appointed as consultant in the specialty. Consultants in palliative medicine often work in relatively small teams or may be single-handed and therefore often take on leadership responsibilities relatively early in their consultant careers. To be effective clinicians and leaders, palliative medicine training needs to work to a curriculum that reflects current practice and is, as much as possible, future-proofed to allow for population and service changes. The change to high-level learning outcomes, exemplified by the generic and specialty CiPs, allows more flexibility in postgraduate training and we hope will facilitate training to evolve as the specialty continues to develop over the next 10 years or so.

A review of the current curriculum has highlighted the narrow interpretation of public health concepts. In developing the new curriculum, the authors and the SAC have increased their knowledge and awareness of community engagement and health promotion at the end of life. The concept of enabling everyone to live well within their communities to the very end of their lives is in line with Dame Cicely Saunders' vision for palliative care, exemplified in her famous comment, 'You matter because you are you, and you matter to the end of your life. We will do all we can not only to help you die peacefully, but also to live until you die.' While most senior doctors working in palliative medicine in the UK will have completed the specialty training curriculum and would profess to practise holistic, patient-centred palliative care, training in the public health components of palliative care is likely to have been limited.

In some areas, palliative care services act as hubs for community empowerment and an awareness of the opportunities to support the development of informal carer and community networks can be critical to support patients reaching the end of life. The importance of community empowerment was highlighted in the 2010 Marmot Review on health inequalities (Marmot et al., 2010). The Institute of Health Equity (Marmot et al., 2020) more recently reported a slowdown in improvements in life expectancy; deteriorations in physical and mental health; and widening health inequalities, which have been brought into sharp focus by the coronavirus disease 2019 (COVID-19) pandemic. The pandemic has also highlighted the importance of community engagement and support, particularly in enabling social connection for those experiencing death, dying, loss, and bereavement, which are likely to have societal implications for some time. The significant economic impact of the COVID-19 pandemic internationally will have implications for health and social care planning and funding, potentially for generations.

The implementation of the new specialty curriculum is therefore an opportunity to increase understanding of and involvement in community empowerment initiatives to support the delivery of comprehensive models of palliative care, as part of integrated health and social care systems. As Abel and colleagues (2018) elegantly describe, community empowerment interventions have the potential to reduce unplanned hospital admissions and reduce costs across healthcare systems.

REFERENCES

Abel, J. and Kellehear, A. 2018. Palliative curriculum re-imagined: a critical evaluation of the UK palliative medicine syllabus. *Palliative Care*, 11, 1178224218780375.

Abel, J., Kingston, H., Scally, A., Hartnoll, J., Hannam, G., Thomson-Moore, A., et al. 2018. Reducing emergency hospital admissions: a population health complex intervention of an enhanced model of primary care and compassionate communities. *British Journal of General Practice*, 68, e803–e810.

Clark, D. 2014. Palliative medicine as a specialty. [Online] Available at: http://endoflifestudies.academicblogs.co.uk/palliative-medicine-as-a-specialty

General Medical Council. 2015. Promoting excellence: standards for medical education and training. [Online] Available at: https://www.gmc-uk.org/education/standards-guidance-and-curricula/standards-and-outcomes/promoting-excellence

General Medical Council. 2017. Excellence by design: standards for postgraduate curricula [Online] Available at: https://www.gmc-uk.org/education/standards-guidance-and-curricula/standards-and-outcomes/excellence-by-design

Joint Royal College Physicians Training Board. 2010, amendments 2014. Specialty training curriculum for palliative medicine. [Online] Available at: https://www.jrcptb.org.uk/specialties/palliative-medicine

Marmot, M., Allen, J., Boyce, T., Goldblatt, P., and Morrison, J. 2020. *Health Equity in England: The Marmot Review 10 Years On*. London: Institute of Health Equity. Available at: http://www.instituteofhealthequity.org/resources-reports/marmot-review-10-years-on

Marmot, M., Allen, J., Goldblatt, P., Boyce, T., McNeish, D., Grady, M., et al. *Fair Society, Healthy Lives: The Marmot Review*. London: Institute of Health Equity. Available at: http://www.instituteofhealthequity.org/resources-reports/fair-society-healthy-lives-the-marmot-review

National Institute for Health and Care Excellence. 2004. Improving supportive and palliative care for adults with cancer. Cancer service guideline [CSG4]. [Online] Available at: https://www.nice.org.uk/guidance/csg4

NHS England. 2016. NHS England specialist level palliative care: information for commissioners. [Online] Available at: https://www.england.nhs.uk/wp-content/uploads/2016/04/speclst-palliatv-care-comms-guid.pdf

Sallnow, L. and Paul, S. 2015. Understanding community engagement in end of life care: developing conceptual clarity. *Critical Public Health*, 25, 231–238.

Sallnow, L., Richardson, H., Murray, S., and Kellehear, A. 2016. The impact of a new public health approach to end of life care: a systematic review. *Palliative Medicine,* 30, 200–211.

Shape of Training Review. 2013. Securing the future of excellent patient care. Final report of the independent review led by Professor David Greenaway. [Online] Available at: https://www.gmc-uk.org/education/standards-guidance-and-curricula/guidance/shape-of-training-review

Ten Cate, O. 2015. Nuts and bolts of entrustable professional activities. *Journal of Graduate Medical Education,* 5, 157–158.

29

Using and building toolkits to support community action

Bonnie Tompkins and Dan Malleck

Declaration of Interest and Acknowledgements: Bonnie Tompkins is a co-author of Pallium's Compassionate Community Startup Toolkit. In this chapter we give some general examples of experiences we have had when assembling community resources. Some of this insight is drawn from Tompkins's work with toolkit development as part of a team at Pallium Canada. Just as collaboration can be at the heart of important work done in a community, these toolkits are also the product of collaboration.

Introduction

The last two decades have seen remarkable progress in increasing the reach of palliative care beyond the purview of medical and nursing professionals. A major factor in this change is the concept of Public Health Palliative Care (PHPC), which adapts the principles of health promotion articulated in the Ottawa Charter for Health Promotion to the area of palliative care. This work is best done not in a top-down manner where professionals work 'on' or provide information 'to' patients or community members, but rather in a collaborative process that engages the community in the various issues around death, dying, loss, and grieving. This concept of health-promoting palliative care (HPPC) as represented in Kellehear's book of the same name (1999) lays out the key areas to be addressed by using PHPC principles. The vision is for an active, engaged, and informed citizenry who are able to do the work to promote awareness, competence, and compassion in the area of death, dying, loss, and grieving (Kellehear, 1999; Rosenberg and Yates, 2010; Abel and Kellehear, 2016). These initiatives should include community engagement when designing interventions. Such community action is best effected by adopting the principles of Asset-Based Community Development (ABCD), which empowers community members to harness the strengths of their community to address issues of concern. In the ABCD process, experts, scholars, professionals, and other stewards of knowledge act as resources, but do not lead community development (McKnight and Russell, 2018). The community-centred principles of ABCD are perfectly suited to addressing the experiences of death, dying, loss, and grieving and, when merged with health promotion principles, can lead to powerful change. Abel and Kellehear (2016) argue that PHPC is a collaborative activity whereby the community works 'to fill the support spaces outside episodes of professional care'. As Kumar (2020) notes, strengthening the ability of communities to take control of palliative care helps to deal with limited availability of palliative care services, but 'it is a complex task, and is definitely not easy' (Kumar, 2020). This chapter discusses the value of toolkits in helping achieve that goal.

The trickiness of knowledge translation

Knowledge translation can be a challenge for those who are deeply embedded in their research and much of the literature explaining knowledge translation has been designed for scholars hoping to give their expertise to the general public (Graham et al., 2006; Grimshaw et al., 2012). This top-down process is not conducive to the ABCD model. One valuable resource that can help translate knowledge to action that can engage communities more actively is Health Canada's *Knowledge Translation Planner* (2017) which itself converts the 'Knowledge to Action' model developed by Graham and colleagues (2006) into a collaborative process of change. The Knowledge to Action model describes the steps for empowering non-academics to be actively involved in applying knowledge to realize change in their communities. The *Planner* converts that model into clear steps to help knowledge creators make the results of their research usable in the community.

Nevertheless, we advise care when deploying the Knowledge to Action model (and the *Planner*). First, and most important for individuals hoping to apply principles of ABCD and PHPC, these resources continue to view recipients of knowledge as addressing a 'need' (in the *Planner*) or a 'problem' (in Graham et al., 2006). Second, the equal partnership idealized in ABCD is not articulated in the model. Several steps are focused on the researchers' actions (identifying the problem, undertaking evaluation) and do not identify that the community needs to be an equal partner in this process. It is what practitioners of ABCD describe as emphasizing work 'by' a community rather than experts providing their expertise 'to' a community (McKnight and Russell, 2018). Indeed, with ABCD, community members (the 'audience') should be the main drivers of all aspects of the process. It is the community's questions and the

Box 29.1 Knowledge to Action model–dissemination and implementation plan

A. Identify need. Identify, review, and select knowledge:
   1. Identify and consult with your stakeholders and target audience(s).
   2. Define the need and the expected outcomes for your initiative.
   3. Identify the knowledge you want to disseminate and implement.
B. Adapt knowledge to local context:
   4. Identify any adaptations needed to the knowledge.
C. Identify barriers and facilitators to knowledge use. Select appropriate knowledge translation strategies:
   5. Identify the barriers and the facilitators.
   6. Choose the appropriate dissemination and implementation strategies.
D. Tailor and implement knowledge translation strategies:
   7. Define the dissemination and implementation strategies.
   8. Assess the context for your strategies.
   9. Tailor the strategies.
   10. Prepare to implement the strategies.
   11. Validate your outputs, outcomes, and indicators.
E. Monitor knowledge use:
   12. Plan to monitor knowledge use.
F. Evaluate outcomes:
   13. Plan to evaluate outcomes.
G. Sustain knowledge use:
   14. Plan for sustainability.

Reproduced with permission from Health Canada. *Knowledge to Action Planner* (2017).

issues they define that are central to change, not questions or issues (let alone 'problems' or 'needs') defined by researchers. To be sure, researchers may approach the community to see if there are issues on which they may work together, but it must be a partnership of equals. Researchers are content experts, who have valuable knowledge in a specific area of research; community members are context experts, who understand their community, its capacities, and uniqueness. Ensuring the content suits the context is fundamental to realizing positive change.

Box 29.1 lists the steps to ensure that the community is actively involved in the process, and ideally leads the initiative. Note that the *Planner* separates section 'A' into several key components of community engagement, a necessary, indeed essential, step. The simple term 'community engagement' represents a complex undertaking that requires a conscious effort to place the priorities and voices of the community at the forefront of every step.

Toolkits as essential knowledge translation resources

The Knowledge to Action model provides a blueprint for knowledge translation; toolkits provide the tools. From both the literature on toolkits as knowledge translation strategies (Barac et al., 2014; Yamada et al., 2015) and our experience, we have identified several key features of toolkits that can enhance their effectiveness in translating complex and diverse research into practical, implementable change:

- Toolkits should provide a variety of resources and 'tools' that enable users with a variety of interests and backgrounds to engage in effecting change.
- When a toolkit's intended users are community members, these tools should include templates to guide users in unfamiliar processes. Templates lighten the load on users, as well as prompt them to develop new ideas and strategies. Consider, for example, meeting agendas. If your toolkit highlights the importance of holding meetings, it is helpful to provide both a sample agenda and an agenda template that users can simply adjust to suit their context. Toolkits should be easy to access. This means recipients and users of the toolkits should have limited barriers when accessing the material.
- Toolkits should be written in language that is appropriate for the group for which they have been developed. This does not always mean they should be in simple language; toolkits written for executives or professionals would need to use different language and different writing styles than those aimed at community members.
- Toolkits should be based in research and provide lists of the resources used. This research does not need to be placed prominently, since something that places scholarship in the foreground may leave users feeling excluded or frustrated with the toolkit.
- Toolkits should be modifiable, allowing users to adapt them to their individual context.
- Finally, toolkits should include evaluation components, allowing users to evaluate the toolkit itself and also giving users advice and information on how to assess the progress of their work. Evaluation permits both community members and toolkit authors to improve on their work.

One essential criterion that we do not include in this list, because it is implicit in the process of developing toolkits, is the way that knowledge is provided and used. As noted by Barac and colleagues (2014), knowledge may be provided through education (which we define as organized courses or sessions), through sharing (community members exchanging experiences), or through other techniques and tools that are intended to result in behaviour change. It is worth remembering that toolkits and web resources are dynamic and may be changed as toolkit developers receive feedback from users, and as knowledge around toolkits broadens and deepens. The details and evaluation we provide here are based upon our assessment of the toolkits up to the autumn of 2021.

Public Health Palliative Care toolkits

The growing interest of groups engaged in building compassionate communities has resulted in the development of several important toolkits to support communities in leading this work. The following section examines the seven most comprehensive toolkits developed to aid communities in realizing the goals of PHPC.

We examined each toolkit using three sets of criteria. First, we look at the resources as effective toolkits, using the six components described in the previous section. We then consider the toolkits in relation to five areas of focus adapted from the Ottawa Charter (Kellehear, 1999) to embrace the principle of HPPC (Box 29.2). Third, we assess which health promotion methods each toolkit encourages (Box 29.3). The results of these analyses are provided in the summary statement for each toolkit.

Box 29.2 Key health-promoting palliative care areas of toolkit focus

- *Build public policies that support health*: toolkit encourages developing public policies related to palliative care and supporting the dying, along with the uptake of policies by organizations.
- *Create supportive environments*: toolkit encourages creating a supportive environment for people who are dealing with palliative care experiences.
- *Strengthen community action*: toolkit empowers the community to engage and take action to support community members who are dealing with palliative care experiences.
- *Develop personal skills*: toolkit encourages increasing personal knowledge through information and education about health but also dying and death so that they may make informed decisions.
- *Reorient palliative care services*: toolkit empowers palliative care services to reorient towards a health-promoting approach.

Source: Kellehear, A. 1999. *Health Promoting Palliative Care*. Melbourne. Oxford University Press; Rosenberg, J. P. and Yates, P. 2010. Health promotion in palliative care: the case for conceptual congruence. *Critical Public Health*, 20, 201; and Abel, J. and Kellehear, A. 2016. Palliative care reimagined: a needed shift. *BMJ Supportive & Palliative Care*, 6, 21.

Compassionate Community Startup Toolkit, by Pallium Canada (Canada)

Purpose

To support community champions when having conversations in the community about becoming a more compassionate community and to initiate the process of asset mapping.

Effectiveness as a toolkit

- *Multiple resources*: this toolkit has a variety of resources to support the user such as templates, a PowerPoint slide deck, and other communication materials.
- *Ease of access*: this is a free resource for anyone to download.
- *Accessible language*: the language appears to be accessible for the end user and there is opportunity for the local user to adjust for local context.
- *Provides research used*: the toolkit does showcase its research and also encourages the user to connect with other known experts in the field.
- *Evaluation plan*: a pilot evaluation has been completed.

Box 29.3 Health promotion methods encouraged within the toolkits

- *Participatory relations*: this toolkit encourages community members to take the lead.
- *Community development*: this toolkit encourages the community to define their own concerns and priorities.
- *Partnerships*: this toolkit encourages partnerships across the community.
- *Education*: this toolkit increases communities' understanding about key end of life topics.
- *Population health approach*: this toolkit encourages engagement in community-wide activities that promote death education and community support.
- *Ecological/settings emphasis*: this toolkit encourages integration and adaptation to suit local context.

Source: Public Health Palliative Care International. 2021. The Public Health Approach to Palliative Care. https://www.phpci.org/public-health-approach

Summary

This toolkit is focused on starting more compassionate community initiatives in Canada and has many of the key criteria for a strong toolkit used within communities. While the toolkit includes content to increase the user's understanding, it also includes templates and resources to help the user engage with the community and host meetings. It thus meets the HPPC areas of building supportive environments and community action. Considering health promotion methods, the toolkit encourages community development and partnerships with a population health approach that has an ecological/settings emphasis. The need for an internet connection may be a barrier, as would be the zip file format which some people may find difficult to use. Also, there is no evaluation other than what was done during the pilot phase.

Developing Palliative Care Programs in First Nations Communities: A Workbook, by the Improving End-of-Life Care in First Nations Communities Research Team, Lakehead University (Canada)

Purpose

To support First Nation (Indigenous) communities who wish to create a local palliative care program.

Effectiveness as a toolkit

- *Multiple resources*: this workbook meets the criteria of a toolkit because it includes a variety of resources such as guides for both the community and health care professionals, examples of job descriptions and other key outputs, a large number of templates to support interviews, surveys, project timelines, community readiness, and reports.
- *Ease of access*: this resource is free for download.
- *Accessible language*: the language appears to be accessible for the end user and there are many opportunities for users to adjust for local context.
- *Provides research used*: this resource was developed from a research project and includes references.
- *Evaluation plan*: this resource includes assessment for community readiness and evaluation throughout the development process.

Summary

This resource is focused on the creation of local palliative care programs within First Nation Communities and takes a multi-pronged approach with a variety of tools for the community (as the leaders of this work) and for health care professionals. The workbook meets the criteria for a strong toolkit as it includes many resources, examples, tools, and templates to support the initiative at the local level. It meets all the areas of HPPC which include public policy, creating supportive environments, strengthening community action, developing personals skills, and reorienting palliative care services. Considering health promotion methods, this resource uses participatory relations, community development, partnerships, population health and ecological/setting emphasis. Potential barriers include access to internet and the possibility that some users may be overwhelmed by the diverse material in this robust resource.

Compassionate Communities Toolkit, by British Columbia Centre for Palliative Care (Canada)

Purpose

To support organizations and groups interested in building compassionate communities.

Effectiveness as a toolkit

- *Multiple resources*: this toolkit includes resources and tools to talk about compassionate communities, host a meeting to assess readiness, and reflect on these meetings; it also includes case studies.
- *Ease of access*: this is a free resource for anyone to download and permits users to download a section at a time which adds accessibility for repeat users.
- *Accessible language*: the language appears to be accessible for the end user and there is ample opportunity to adjust for local context as well.
- *Provides research used*: the toolkit does not clearly indicate the research involved in the development but it does link to Public Health Palliative Care International and highlights that it was developed with the input of those leading compassionate communities.
- *Evaluation plan*: this toolkit encourages the community to evaluate and includes approaches to evaluation.

Summary

This toolkit is focused on guiding anyone interested in the compassionate communities movement and provides ideas and supports to explore based on 3 levels of difficulty, making this a robust and user-friendly toolkit. It meets many of the criteria for a strong toolkit and has included what has been learned from the movement within the province of British Columbia. It thus meets the HPPC areas of building supportive environments, community action, and developing personal skills. Considering health promotion methods, the toolkit encourages participatory relations, partnerships, education, and has an ecological/settings emphasis. However, the exclusively online format may be a barrier. The addition of templates to accompany the included sample meeting agenda would support the recommendation that community members host meetings.

Building Compassionate Communities in Australia: Tools for a Community-led Approach to End-of-Life Care, by The Groundswell Project (Australia)

Purpose

To provide information about the process communities have undertaken to build compassionate communities in the hope that users will work towards expanding the Compassionate Communities movement.

Effectiveness as a toolkit

- *Multiple resources*: this toolkit includes a tool for reflection, sends users to other sites to broaden their knowledge, and includes case studies. However, it has a limited variety of tools and templates.
- *Ease of access*: this is a free resource for anyone to download.
- *Accessible language*: the language appears to be accessible for the end user and the user is encouraged to take the language and adjust it for their local context.
- *Provides research used*: the toolkit does include the research used in its development.
- *Evaluation plan*: this toolkit encourages the community to evaluate and includes two approaches to evaluation.

Summary

This toolkit, designed to encourage others to join the compassionate communities movement, meets many of the criteria for a strong toolkit and has also included learning from those leading compassionate communities initiatives. As with the British Columbia Centre for Palliative Care toolkit, the Groundswell toolkit addresses HPPC areas of building supportive environments, community action, and developing personal skills. Considering health promotion methods, the toolkit encourages participatory relations, partnerships, education and has an ecological/settings emphasis. The need for an internet connection to access may be a barrier. The toolkit could benefit from adding templates for community members to use when starting an initiative and hosting meetings.

Scottish Compassionate Communities Toolkit, by Good Life, Good Death, Good Grief (Scotland)

Purpose

To provide information and resources for people who want to make their community supportive of neighbours who are experiencing death, dying, loss, and grieving.

Effectiveness as a toolkit

- *Multiple resources*: the website has many resources and tools for many different interests and ability levels.
- *Ease of access*: easily accessible for people with a computer and internet access.
- *Accessible language*: clearly written and well-laid-out web pages. Some material may be more detailed and complicated, but the variety of material means it can appeal to a variety of learning styles and interests.
- *Provides research used*: this website and its tools are based on a variety of experiences and a range of research. Some webpages have links to organizations upon whose work the project is built; some include direct references to research or other material.
- *Evaluation plan*: does not include an evaluation plan.

Summary

This toolkit focuses on supporting those with the desire to create a more supportive community and is an example of a quality toolkit. It has varied resources appealing to users from different backgrounds. It addresses several HPPC goals, including creating supportive environments, nurturing community action, and developing personal skills. Considering health promotion methods, the toolkit encourages community development, nurturing partnerships, and providing opportunities for education. It also has a strong ecological/settings emphasis. It is an online resource, which may be a barrier to people who do not have access to the internet or who are not comfortable using online materials. Nevertheless, in community partnerships, gaining access to online tools seems increasingly not to be a barrier.

Scottish Bereavement Friendly Workplaces Toolkit, by Good Life, Good Death, Good Grief (Scotland)

Purpose

To provide resources to help both employers and employees build a bereavement-friendly workplace.

Effectiveness as a toolkit

- *Multiple resources*: this toolkit provides a variety of links to best practices, case studies, legal information about employee rights, and information about training. It does not have many tools or templates.
- *Ease of access*: easily accessible for people with a computer and internet access.
- *Accessible language*: it is written in clear language and includes well laid-out web pages.
- *Provides research used*: there are links to various supporting reports but does not include a reference list.
- *Evaluation plan*: does not mention evaluation.

Summary

This toolkit is a useful roadmap for workplaces to become more bereavement friendly. The inclusion of legal information may be especially useful for employers. The limited number of tools means that the information provided will need to be supplemented with other resources. It represents the HPPC goals of creating supportive environments, nurturing community action, building healthy workplace policy, and developing personal skills. Considering health promotion methods, the toolkit encourages community development (here the workplace is the community) and provides opportunities for education. It also has a strong ecological/settings emphasis. The lack of an evaluation component may limit its long-term usefulness for workplaces.

Public Health Approaches to End of Life Care, by the National Council for Palliative Care (UK)

Purpose

This toolkit provides information to people who are interested in moving end-of-life care from clinical settings to communities.

Effectiveness as a toolkit

- *Multiple resources*: this toolkit provides several resources including models of community development, and activities and questions that could help facilitate discussions in a community meeting.
- *Ease of access*: the toolkit is a pdf with click-through type links directing the user through the information, and at the end of each brief overview of a concept or section it gives the user the choice of reading more detail or moving to the next section.
- *Accessible language*: although this toolkit is designed for everyone, the language is sophisticated and may not be accessible to all users. It does include a glossary that defines many important terms.
- *Provides research used*: there is a comprehensive reference list at the end of this resource.
- *Evaluation plan*: there is no section on evaluating the toolkit itself, but there is a section explaining how to evaluate compassionate city projects.

Summary

Designed to initiate discussions about PHPC, this toolkit presents an exhaustive and detailed body of information and is especially helpful for introducing professionals to the idea of compassionate communities and the Compassionate City Charter. As a toolkit co-authored by Kellehear, this resource addresses all HPPC goals but is strongest in addressing the need to build healthy public policies, nurture community action, and reorient health services. Also, this resource encourages all six health promotion methods. It is, however, text heavy, which may be a barrier for some users but since it was intended to help professionals reconsider their ideas about palliative care, it was not designed to be accessible to all users.

See Box 29.4 for some additional resources.

Box 29.4 Other resources to note

Public Health Palliative Care and the Compassionate Communities movement are constantly evolving as interest and awareness spreads. Below are some additional toolkits that support the progression of this work. To stay up to date on future toolkits and resources, visit Public Health Palliative Care International's resource page at https://www.phpci.org

- *Compassionate Community Toolkit*: the Health Promotion Department of Taiwan has been actively supporting the compassionate communities movement along with other key partners in the country. It is currently available only in Mandarin. Visit https://health99.hpa.gov.tw/material/6495 to access their 'The Compassionate Community Action Guide' and more.
- *Horizons of Hope: A Toolkit for Catholic Parishes on Palliative Care*: this partner-developed toolkit is focused on increasing the parishioners' understanding of key medical information, what this means regarding their Roman Catholic faith, and empowers them to take action at home, in their parish, and out in the community—by starting a compassionate community. Visit https://www.cccb.ca to learn more.
- Atlas *CareMap Community Workshop Toolkit*: this toolkit is one of three resources focused on helping caregivers share their caregiving experience with family, friends, and health care professionals and to increase their support network by using the Atlas CareMap tool. The workshop toolkit equips the user with everything they need to host a workshop in the community to increase the awareness of the Atlas CareMap tool and support caregivers. Visit https://www.pallium.ca/care-connections to learn more.
- *Pan-Canada Compassionate Community Evaluation Toolkit (in development)*: this toolkit will focus on empowering those leading compassionate community initiatives to increase their understanding of how to measure their results and impact and to share what they have learned. The toolkit will support the creation of evaluation plans and dissemination strategies.

Building a toolkit to empower community members to engage with Public Health Palliative Care

Having described the key components of an effective toolkit, shown the strong potential for toolkits to transfer knowledge and support communities to take action, and provided examples of some of the most well-developed toolkits, we now turn to the process of toolkit creation itself. We are framing this section around the steps from the *Knowledge Translation Planner* (Health Canada, 2017). We include examples from our own experience creating toolkits and similar resources to encourage community action.

Who should be involved in the toolkit creation?

Anyone can create a toolkit to support PHPC at the community level. Earlier in this chapter we saw how organizations at both the regional and national levels, as well as a national government, support and fund toolkits. Partnership with such organizations can be essential, since they may have the contacts, the influence, and the resources to support the toolkit development and sustainability.

How to create a toolkit

Are you ready to create your own toolkit to inspire action within the PHPC field? In this section we will walk you through how to create one, outline the tools that we use, and share examples from our toolkit development work in the hope you will feel more confident to create your own.

When we began developing community resources, we found the *Knowledge Translation Planner* to be essential for many reasons we discussed earlier. Another useful toolkit resource is 'How to Build an Implementation Toolkit from Start to Finish' by the California Social Work Education Center (CalSWEC). Links to both resources are provided at the end of the chapter.

A. Identify the issue you are hoping to impact: identify, review, and select knowledge

See Box 29.5 for a language tip.

Before putting in the time to create a toolkit, you should ensure you understand the desired change you want the toolkit to support.

Collecting the knowledge that will be the foundation for your toolkit should happen in several ways, ensuring different types of knowledge are included in the final product.

Remember that these approaches to collecting knowledge are not listed in a priority order. What you learn through one approach may affect the way you gather knowledge in another approach.

Box 29.5 Language tip

Note: the *Planner* uses the term 'need' which highlights an absence of something in people and can imply that they are powerless. Following the principles of ABCD, we prefer using language that emphasizes the assets of people and communities. We therefore look at this as an 'issue' or 'desired change' and we emphasize language that focuses on people and the community's strengths.

Literature review

Review the literature that focuses on the issue you want to address. If you have not undertaken a literature review before, we would encourage you to learn how to do this to ensure an appropriate, high-quality review. It might be helpful to include partners who have experience in this approach and access to resources, such as public health professionals or researchers who may be engaged as subject matter experts (discussed later).

Focus groups

These groups are potential toolkit users who will help you learn from the experience and perspectives of the audience for which your toolkit is being designed. This type of knowledge is key: it will help fine tune your literature research as you become more aware of the issue the community hopes to address. It will increase the uptake of the toolkit because not only will it help you understand the audience's unique context and adapt your strategies accordingly, it shows potential users that their experiences and knowledge have been valued in creating the toolkit.

Subject matter experts

Engaging people who are experts in the subject matter is another important way to ensure you have a strong foundation of knowledge upon which you will build the tools for the toolkit. Such people can be experts in content (specializing in specific areas of knowledge being used in the toolkit) or context (people who know the unique nature of the situation in which the toolkit will be used). These experts can be researchers, professionals, and members from the group that the toolkit is intended to support. Subject matter experts can be part of an advisory team or you can engage them to help with the knowledge creation process.

These three ways of gathering knowledge will fine tune and strengthen the content upon which you base the toolkit. Choosing to skip parts of the knowledge collection process can set up the toolkit for unachievable outcomes.

For example, when we began developing resources for compassionate communities, we first needed to understand how leaders of the Compassionate Communities movement inspired their community. We gathered knowledge on the movement, we spoke to those who were already leading compassionate communities to learn what they used and what they felt would have really helped them. We also engaged with people who expressed interest in starting their own compassionate community but didn't know how to begin. By performing the literature review, conducting interviews, and speaking to those who were leading compassionate communities work, we developed a greater understanding of what kind of tools and information about the movement needed to be in resources to support their work.

B. Adapt knowledge to local context

In this phase, you consider any adjustments in how the knowledge is presented and how it 'fits' the context in which you are working. You need to be sure the knowledge you will be sharing in the toolkit will be read and understood—this can make or break the effectiveness of the toolkit. You need to consider, for example, whether the information is directly related to the context in which you are working, or if you need to make specific adjustments to keep it relevant to the intended audience. Such adjustments can take many forms.

When we began building toolkits aimed at the general population, we paid careful attention to the readability level of the resources we were providing. We found that writing the content at the reading level of grade 6 (Canada) or average 11- or 12-year-old would ensure that most of the general public could read and understand it. Now we run all the content for toolkits aimed at the general public through the 'Check Accessibility' feature in Microsoft Word to make sure it is at the appropriate reading level.

C. Identify barriers and facilitators to knowledge use and select appropriate knowledge translation dissemination and implementation strategies

See Box 29.6. Identifying potential barriers must be done in consultation with the focus group, but you may also find them during your literature review and by talking with subject matter experts. The better you understand these barriers, the better you can address them in the toolkit and during its dissemination.

Barriers can come in many forms, from the language level (discussed previously) to the way the toolkit is accessed, and potential hesitations by the target audience when talking about caregiving, serious illness, death, and grieving. They also might include the absence of certain community resources that might exist in other places, such as suitable meeting locations or even people's willingness or availability to attend meetings.

Also think about the things that can aid in the uptake of the toolkit and address many of those barriers. These aids (Box 29.7) are as unique as the barriers themselves. For example, when considering holding a community meeting, will providing snacks encourage people to show up? Will meetings be held at a time when the people most affected by the issue can attend? Is your location suitable and accessible? If this toolkit is going to be used by an organization, there may be aids such as finding a champion within the organization who can encourage people to get involved. Be sure to highlight these aids in the toolkit to increase the likelihood of achieving the desired outcomes.

This is also the time to start thinking about dissemination: how can you design your toolkit for the greatest use? How will you get the toolkit 'in front' of the intended audience? When thinking about how you will build awareness of this toolkit, think about where and how the audience might learn about and access this resource.

The success of dissemination is only as good as the toolkit itself, so think about how to design the toolkit to ensure the knowledge is trusted and accessible and the tools are understandable and user friendly.

This is also the time to pilot the toolkit. Remember, the resources within the toolkit do not need to be finalized because piloting the toolkit will help you find areas that you need to improve. Try to find pilot sites that will represent as broadly as possible your intended users. Pilot sites' feedback is invaluable. If you create something people cannot easily understand (especially within a community of volunteers), they will look for another resource or, worse, become discouraged.

When we build tools that will be used in a variety of locations, we consider potential barriers that could affect the usefulness of the resource. For example, when building resources to be used throughout the country, we assemble an advisory team of people from across the country who could point out barriers and aids from the perspective of their region. One aid is to design the resources to allow for some modification by the end user. We also include instructions on how and where to adjust terminology for the best impact within the user's community. This is a best practice because it will increase both the comprehension of the material and the trust of the community, leading to greater interest and use. Other aids can include encouraging users to partner with local organizations (such as public health) which can give credibility to the initiative, and to hold meetings in neutral spaces (such as public libraries) to avoid barriers to access.

Box 29.6 Tip

Remember, we have already selected our main knowledge translation strategy—it is a toolkit. However, the toolkit is made up of different strategies which are the tools you develop that will be in the toolkit.

Box 29.7 Aids

Health Canada's guide calls these aids 'facilitators'. We find that confusing because a facilitator is a term often given to someone who leads or 'facilitates' a meeting.

D. Tailor and implement knowledge translation strategies

This section is about pulling it all together. It emphasizes making adjustments based on information from the pilot sites. These are essential components for an effective community-based toolkit, since the pilot sites will show you things you may not have anticipated and let you refine the toolkit to make it as accessible as possible. Also, this phase highlights the additional human resources needed to launch the toolkit.

There are many things you should be doing or thinking about at this point:

1. *Collect pilot site feedback and adjust as necessary.* This will help you determine if you are going to achieve the desired outcome of the toolkit, and what you need to do to fix any deficiencies in your toolkit. If several pilot sites made the same suggestion, and if it's an easy fix, do it.
2. *Finalize the knowledge to be shared.* The pilot site may request additional knowledge and you need to determine how to include it in the toolkit. In our experience, it is important to balance the need to prepare potential users against overwhelming them. One strategy we have found is to include only essential information and provide users with a list of other resources if they want to know more.
3. *Address any new barriers and potential aids.* Your pilot sites will likely point out other barriers or aids. This is a good thing because it helps you to make the toolkit more accessible and usable. One valuable approach we have used is to encourage community members to develop an asset map at one of their first community meetings. We have also seen community groups effectively employ an asset map exercise by appointing a "point person" to facilitate the activity and providing them with concise resources

to lead the group. This kind of resource is a useful aid to address a barrier (in this case the lack of familiarity with asset maps). We have also found that sometimes such tools come as a result of the piloting project and can then be included in the toolkit itself (giving appropriate credit to the pilot site).

4. *Finalize all the tools (strategies).* Now that you have completed pilot site testing, you need to determine which tools will be going into the toolkit. Pay attention to the feedback from the pilot sites. It will increase the chances of success. Make sure that all members of the review team have agreed to the changes to avoid potential costly revisions later on.
5. *Use a graphic designer (if there are funds).* Try to hand over all content at once so the designer can see the whole toolkit and be able to achieve the look and feel you are hoping for. It might cost more if you hand over pieces at different times. Make sure the designer knows who the target audience is, so they can create material that is accessible, readable, and understandable.
6. *Translate any additional content.* Often there is new content created after a pilot phase, so this needs to be translated into all languages and will also need to be edited for reading level. Don't just translate the content and launch it; you should make sure you pilot the translated toolkit in a community to ensure that the translation is accurate and appropriate.
7. *Finalize the plan to create awareness.* Here you should be thinking about the toolkit dissemination plan. This should begin about 2–3 months before your launch date and should use as many strategies as possible. Increasing awareness can take many forms. Reach out to your pilot sites, subject matter experts, partners, focus group participants and anybody who was involved in the creation of your toolkit. Use social media and other communication tools. Always ensure to use consistent messaging that could be shared through this network.
8. *Engage with other staff to support the launch.* Think about how the toolkit is going to be accessed, what staff may be contacted for support if things are not going as planned, or what staff might be fielding questions from the end users.

E and F. Planning to evaluate for knowledge use and toolkit outcomes

Evaluation can help increase the sustainability of your toolkit but if your organization does not have the resources to administer, process, and incorporate the findings, you may not be able to focus on evaluation at this time. You can go back after and evaluate when you have the resources. If you think this is the approach you might take, make sure to put a system in place to track who accessed your toolkit so you can go back and contact users later to help you to evaluate the toolkit's usefulness.

If you can support an evaluation, think about the indicators you want to assess and whether you will be able to measure them. Ideally your evaluation plan should measure the effectiveness of your dissemination plan (how well you got the toolkit into the hands of the target audience) and how effective the toolkit was at achieving the desired outcome. The information gathered from an evaluation will help you understand the toolkit's impact, learn how the knowledge is being used, and allow you to adjust the toolkit. This can be a great time to partner with an organization that can support this component of the work, such as a university or public health unit, where there is expertise in evaluation.

If you can undertake this type of evaluation, planning for it is key because there are things that you should know ahead of time. They include:

- The costs associated with running the evaluation, assessing the results, and communicating the findings.
- How the data is collected, where is it stored, and who owns the data (creating an agreement is helpful if you are partnering on this piece).
- What you are going to do with the results (data).

The information gathered by evaluations can take several forms, and each project may have different priorities. Funding agencies will expect certain types of information such as 'quantitative' data, which is represented by things that are counted: number of meetings held, number of attendants, number of communities who used the toolkit, and so on. Another useful type of data is 'qualitative' which gives greater insight and emotion to the impact witnessed. Collecting stories is an example of qualitative data and will describe connections made and changes in the community that might not be easily represented in numbers. Including this type of data will deepen the understanding of the toolkit's impact. The evaluation plan you include for users to assess their progress should then provide indicators and tools to measure both qualitative and quantitative data to gather the relevant information.

G. Sustaining knowledge use

Toolkit sustainability involves keeping the content up to date and the resources applicable. You should think about sustainability from the outset. Are you going to be able to update and adjust the toolkit in the future to make sure that the desired outcomes can be met as new information comes to light and as communities change and grow in response to the work? Be prepared to incorporate the things that you and the communities have learned into future versions of your toolkit.

A best practice for the sustainability of the toolkit is to make it as adjustable as possible at the local level. As discussed earlier, resources in the toolkit should be designed to be relatively easy for community members to fit to their local context, which also means the toolkit can be modified as the local situation changes. This adaptability is noted to increase the sustainability of the toolkit and desired outcome (Shelton et al., 2018).

Conclusion

Toolkits can be an effective way of translating complicated knowledge into accessible, informative, and, most importantly, usable material that can result in an active community that is empowered to support those dealing with death, dying, loss, and grief. The current toolkits addressing HPPC are valuable resources for realizing that change. They have all contributed to progress in community engagement and have increased the skills and ability of the community members. Nevertheless, more effort needs to be put into the area of evaluating the toolkits' effectiveness and the results of the community activities.

People who wish to build their own toolkits to drive change in communities need to keep several key guidelines in mind. Developing an effective toolkit for community action requires partnerships in which community members, those ultimate users of the toolkit, are actively engaged in the process at every step. It is important to recognize that partnerships with organizations that have valuable resources, be they a broad network that you can access to reach communities, expertise in evaluation, other types of knowledge usage, or financial support, is also a valuable part of community-based toolkit building. We cannot state strongly enough that when a toolkit is built for the use of community volunteers, providing tools they can adjust to suit their local context is invaluable. Such resources lighten their workload, which is most often provided for free. Finally, to ensure longevity, a toolkit's resources should be adaptable, and the knowledge and strategies included in a toolkit should enable the community members to take the lead and see the changes they desire grow through their own actions.

Links to resources and toolkits for building an effective toolkit

California Social Work Education Center (CalSWEC). How to Build an Implementation Toolkit from Start to Finish: https://calswec.berkeley.edu/toolkits/implementation-toolkits/how-build-implementation-toolkit-start-finish

Health Canada. Knowledge Translation Planner: https://www.canada.ca/en/health-canada/corporate/about-health-canada/reports-publications/grants-contributions/knowledge-transfer-planner.html

Toolkits

British Columbia Centre for Palliative Care. Compassionate Communities Toolkit: https://bc-cpc.ca/cpc/all-resources/community-organizations/compassionate-communities-toolkit/

Good Life Good Death Good Grief. Scottish Compassionate Communities Toolkit: https://www.goodlifedeathgrief.org.uk/content/toolkit_homepage/

Good Life Good Death Good Grief. Bereavement Friendly Workplaces Toolkit: https://www.goodlifedeathgrief.org.uk/content/workplace_home/

Improving End-of-Life Care in First Nations Communities Research Team, Lakehead University-- Developing Palliative Care Programs in First Nations Communities: A Workbook:

https://eolfn.lakeheadu.ca/develop-palliative-care-programs-workbook

National Council for Palliative Care. Public Health Approaches to End of Life Care Toolkit: https://pdf4pro.com/view/public-health-approaches-to-end-of-life-care-ncpc-521897.html

Pallium Canada. Compassionate Community Startup Toolkit: https://www.pallium.ca/toolkits/startup-toolkit/

The Groundswell Project. Compassionate Communities Toolkit: https://www.thegroundswellproject.com/compassionate-communities-toolkit-2020

REFERENCES

Abel, J. and Kellehear, A. 2016. Palliative care reimagined: a needed shift. *BMJ Supportive & Palliative Care*, 6, 21–26.

Abel, J., Kellehear, A., and Karapliagou, A. 2018 Palliative care—the new essentials. *Annals of Palliative Medicine*, 7, S3–S14.

Barac, R., Stein, S., Bruce, B., and Barwick, M. 2014. Scoping review of toolkits as a knowledge translation strategy in health. *BMC Medical Informatics and Decision Making*, 14, 121.

Graham, I. D., Logan, J., Harrison, M. B., Straus, S. E., Tetroe, J., Caswell, W., et al. 2006. Lost in knowledge translation: time for a map? *Journal of Continuing Education in the Health Professions*, 26, 13–24.

Grimshaw, J. M., Eccles, M. P., Lavis, J. N., Hill, S. J., and Squires, J. E. 2012. Knowledge translation of research findings. *Implementation Science*, 7, 50.

Health Canada. 2017. *Knowledge Translation Planner*. Ottawa: Health Canada. Available at: https://www.canada.ca/en/health-canada/corporate/about-health-canada/reports-publications/grants-contributions/knowledge-transfer-planner.html

Kellehear, A. 1999. *Health Promoting Palliative Care*. Melbourne: Oxford University Press.

Kumar, S. 2020. Community participation in palliative care: reflections from the ground. *Progress in Palliative Care*, 28, 83–88.

McKnight, J. and Russell, C. 2018. *The Four Essential Elements of an Asset-Based Community Development Process*. Chicago, IL: ABCD Institute, DePaul University.

O'Mara-Eves, A., Brunton, G., McDaid, D., Oliver, S., Kavanagh, J., Jamal, F., et al. 2013. Community engagement to reduce inequalities in health: a systematic review, meta analysis and economic analysis. *Public Health Research*, 1, 4.

Public Health Palliative Care International. 2021. The public health approach to palliative care. [Online] Available at: https://www.phpci.org/public-health-approach

Rosenberg, J. P. and Yates, P. 2010. Health promotion in palliative care: the case for conceptual congruence. *Critical Public Health*, 20, 201–210.

Shelton, R. C., Cooper, B. R., and Stirman, S. W. 2018. The sustainability of evidence-based interventions and practices in public health and health care. *Annual Review of Public Health*, 39, 55–76.

Yamada, J., Shorkey, A., Barwick, M., Widger, K., and Stevens, B. J. 2015. The effectiveness of toolkits as knowledge translation strategies for integrating evidence into clinical care: a systematic review. *BMJ Open*, 5, e006808.

SECTION 7
Conclusion

30 Conclusion

Julian Abel and Allan Kellehear

Cicely Saunders encapsulated her vision of palliative care with her quote 'You matter because you are you'. It anticipated the direction palliative care has taken over the last 70 years. Palliative care has focused on providing excellent care for the *individual with the illness* through the relief of physical, social, psychological, and spiritual suffering.

Much has been achieved through this approach. The hospice movement and the speciality of palliative medicine has had a worldwide impact. In particular, palliative care specialists have set the standard for assessing symptoms in the different domains, providing symptom relief, and giving hands-on care to those most in need, whether this be at home or in institutional care. In addition, the systematic application of palliative care methods across these multiple settings has brought huge relief for many and has highlighted those areas where there is insufficient attention paid to much suffering. The influence of palliative care has extended beyond the boundaries of the speciality. Palliative care standards inform the practice of health and social care professionals who look after people with terminal illnesses. Palliative care services provide education and training on how to care for people who are dying. Communication skills training is now a routine part of medical studies, informed by the development of breaking bad news training and extending the principles broadly into the practice of medicine.

And yet much remains to be done. Only 14% of the people in the world estimated to need palliative care receive it (World Health Organization, 2020). Six developed countries accounted for 79% of global morphine consumption, while developing countries only accounted for 6% of global opioid consumption, despite improved access to pain treatment over the past two decades (Manjiani et al., 2014). But the limitations of the current model do not rest simply with the lack of availability of medication, or palliative care specialist or generalist. Even in countries with established palliative care services, the majority of people who die do not receive adequate palliative care. Availability of services are largely restricted to those with a diagnosis of cancer. Nearly 80% of deaths are predictable and the palliative needs of those with non-cancer diagnoses do not significantly differ from those who have cancer. The different experiences of grief have a commonality irrespective of cause of death, whether this be sudden death from murder, suicide, or accidents or prolonged periods of ill health which lead to death. For many palliative care services, the focus is on the needs of patients with the solution to these needs being professional care. Families, friends, and neighbours are not routinely seen as the critical part of providing meaning, value, and care for those undergoing the experiences of death, dying, loss, and caregiving. Palliative care has become a medical speciality sometimes at the cost of cultural and social practices that have been part of human existence up until the present day.

Trying to provide equity of access to palliative care cannot be solved by increasing the professional workforce. Nor is it the best form of care. Throughout the textbook, references are made to the positive value of looking after our loved ones with a terminal illness as well as the role of the broad caring network, looking after both the person who is unwell and each other. These principles are embedded deeply in compassionate communities and the civic response outlined in the Compassionate City Charter (see Appendix A). Put simply, there is insufficient funding and trained professionals who can provide current levels of demand, never mind increasing the workforce by as much as two-thirds.

The public health approach to palliative and end of life care provides a way forward. There are two guiding principles. The first is about how we look after each other in the last phases of life. This is not just the care we give to the person with the illness who we know and love, it is also about the caring networks of family, friends, neighbours, and community members who care for them and each other, recognizing and celebrating the positive meaning and value of doing so. It is a truly social as well as a medical event, steeped in culture, history, and practice. It is not confined to the harm reduction of symptom control, but fully recognizes the positive aspects of love and friendship, the meaning that this gives to life, and how we can all do this together.

The second principle is that of equity. If palliative care is going to move forward from a specialty that is confined to the lucky minority who can benefit from its help and support, then it has to take a population-based, social approach. This cannot be dominated by and reliant upon professional care. Dying is so much more than something that is confined by professionalization.

The *Oxford Textbook of Public Health Palliative Care* provides a thorough discourse on how the next phase of palliative care development can be achieved. The principles of public health, particularly new public health, are applied to palliative and end of life care irrespective of age or diagnosis. Lack of familiarity with public health methodology can make it seem that public health palliative care is something new and not founded in a firm historical and practice traditions. As the textbook shows, this is not the case. The argument for the need of a population-based, social model of palliative and end of life care is made in the first section of the book. This is followed by Section 2 on basic concepts and theories, including new public health, community development, the fundamental role of supportive networks, and a thorough discussion of participatory relations. A repeated theme throughout the book is how professional domination has led to a schism in relationships between professional services and citizens. The needed shift to a public health model requires seeing communities as equal partners in a social *and* medical model.

From theory the textbook moves on to practice, with Section 3 on basic practice methods. Examples of public health palliative care are given in a wide variety of circumstances all over the globe, with one of the earliest and most advanced programmes being in Kerala in India. The Compassionate City Charter was developed from the principles of public health practice methodology of the Healthy Cities project. The 13-point charter focuses on how all of us in civic society can participate in palliative and end of life care as a truly social phenomenon, creating the opportunities for geographical areas of any size to organize systematic programmes to fully participate in all settings as a public health priority. Examples of what can be achieved can be found in Europe, South America, Canada, Australasia, and south east Asia, among others.

The evidence base for public health palliative care is growing but has considerable challenges and is the focus of Section 5. Applying health service research methods to the social experience of end of life care is fraught with problems, unsuitable in demonstrating the broad complexity of human relationships. New methodologies of research are needed. Simple outcome measures are not a proxy for quality, meaning, or social value. And death, dying, loss, and caregiving is an intensely personal experience as well as a community one. We all have experiences in this area multiple times in our lives, until our own personal, final one in which we die. We all want not just to minimize the suffering of ourselves and those we love, we want these experiences to be as full of meaning, full of love, and full of positive qualities as possible, mixed in with the emotions of loss and sadness. Traditional health service research is unable to capture this.

Section 6 of the textbook discusses the education and training that is needed to bring about the vision of public health palliative care into clinical practice, communities, and the civic institutions mentioned in the compassionate city charter. Death, dying, loss, and caregiving is everyone's responsibility (Kellehear, 2013). Significantly, public health palliative care has become part of the training curriculum for palliative medicine specialists in the UK. The chapter on the development of the curriculum explains about how this was achieved and the dilemma of trainers not fully understanding the subject. The textbook provides a comprehensive explanation from theory, practice, policy, research, and education perspectives. It is a complete foundation text and will need updating as the field develops further.

This will hopefully be as prophetic to the future development of palliative care as the original quote of Cicely Saunders' vision of individualized care. To 'You matter because you are you' we might add 'and we matter to each other, because we are all in this together'.

REFERENCES

Kellehear, A. 2013. Compassionate communities: end-of-life care as everyone's responsibility. *QJM: An International Journal of Medicine*, 106, 1071–1075.

Manjiani, D., Paul, D. B., Kunnumpurath, S., Kaye, A. D., and Vadivelu, N. 2014. Availability and utilization of opioids for pain management: global issues. *Ochsner Journal*, 14, 208–215.

World Health Organization. 2020. Palliative care—key facts. [Online] Available at: https://www.who.int/news-room/fact-sheets/detail/palliative-care

APPENDIX A

The compassionate city charter

A charter of actions

Compassionate cities are communities that recognize that all natural cycles of sickness and health, birth and death, and love and loss occur every day within the orbits of its institutions and regular activities. A compassionate city is a community that recognizes that care for one another at times of crisis and loss is not simply a task solely for health and social services but is everyone's responsibility.

Compassionate cities are communities that publicly encourage, facilitate, support, and celebrate care for one another during life's most testing moments and experiences, especially those pertaining to life-threatening and life-limiting illness, chronic disability, frail ageing and dementia, grief and bereavement, and the trials and burdens of long-term care. Though local government strives to maintain and strengthen quality services for the most fragile and vulnerable in our midst, those persons are not the limits of our experience of fragility and vulnerability. Serious personal crises of illness, dying, death, and loss may visit any of us, at any time during the normal course our lives. A compassionate city is a community that squarely recognizes and addresses this social fact.

Through the auspices of the mayor's office a compassionate city will—by public marketing and advertising, by use of the cities network and influences, by dint of collaboration and cooperation, in partnership with social media and its own offices—develop and support the following 13 social changes to the city's key institutions and activities:

1. Our schools will have annually reviewed policies or guidance documents for dying, death, loss, and care.
2. Our workplaces will have annually reviewed policies or guidance documents for dying, death, loss, and care.
3. Our trade unions will have annually reviewed policies or guidance documents for dying, death, loss, and care.
4. Our churches and temples will have at least one dedicated group for end of life care support.
5. Our city's hospices and nursing homes will have a community development programme involving local area citizens in end of life care activities and programmes.
6. Our city's major museums and art galleries will hold annual exhibitions on the experiences of ageing, dying, death, loss, or care.
7. Our city will host an annual peacetime memorial parade representing the major sectors of human loss outside military campaigns—cancer, motor neuron disease, AIDS, child loss, suicide survivors, animal companion loss, widowhood, industrial and vehicle accidents, the loss of emergency workers and all end of life care personnel, etc.
8. Our city will promote compassionate communities programmes to engage neighbourhoods and local streets in direct care activities for their local residents living with health crisis, ageing, caregiving, and grief.
9. Our city will create an incentives scheme to celebrate and highlight the most creative compassionate organization, event, and individual/s. The scheme will take the form of an annual award administered by a committee drawn from the end of life care sector. A 'Mayor's Prize' will recognize individual/s for that year, those who most exemplify the city's values of compassionate care.
10. Our city will publicly showcase, in print and in social media, our local government policies, services, funding opportunities, partnerships, and public events that address 'our compassionate concerns' with living with ageing, life-threatening and life-limiting illness, loss and bereavement, and long-term caring. All end of life care-related services within the city limits will be encouraged to distribute this material or these web links including veterinarians and funeral organizations.
11. Our city will work with local social or print media to encourage an annual city-wide short story or art competition that helps raise awareness of ageing, dying, death, loss, or caring.
12. All our compassionate policies and services, and the policies and practices of our official compassionate partners and alliances, will demonstrate an understanding of how diversity shapes the experience of ageing, dying, death, loss, and care—through ethnic, religious, gendered, and sexual identity and through the social experiences of poverty, inequality, and disenfranchisement.
13. We will seek to encourage and to invite evidence that institutions for the homeless and the imprisoned have support plans in place for end of life care and loss and bereavement.

Our city will establish and review these targets and goals in the first 2 years and thereafter will add one more sector annually to our action plans for a compassionate city—for example, hospitals, further and higher education, charities, community and voluntary organizations, police and emergency services, and so on.

This charter represents a commitment by the city to embrace a view of health and well-being that embraces community empathy, directly supporting its inhabitants to address the negative health impacts of social inequality and marginalization attributable to dying, death, and loss.

A city is not merely a place to work and access services but equally a place to enjoy support in the safety and protection of each other's company, in schools, workplaces, places of worship and recreation, cultural forums, and social networks anywhere within the city's influence, even to the end of our days.

APPENDIX B

Useful organizational links

Compassionate Communities UK

https://www.compassionate-communitiesuk.co.uk/what-we-do

Compassionate Communities UK is a registered charity that has been developed to work with communities to build compassion as a major value in public institutions, manifesting in the way we treat each other and the world around us.

Relationships with people and place play a central role in life. Good social relationships play a major part in helping us to live long, healthy, happy lives. In addition to building communities where compassion and kindness is part of everyday life, compassionate communities (and cities) recognize the central role that chronic ill health and mortality plays in the minds, behaviours, and social meanings that people develop when confronted with experiences of all serious illness, ageing, caregiving, and loss. They complement the efforts of all health promotion activities in national communities. The practice approach is essentially the same—that is, civic engagement and community development, public education, and changes to the social and policy environment. Compassionate communities are communities that squarely acknowledge the major but under-recognized, the least spoken about, and the often-overlooked human experiences in all communities of serious illness, ageing, dying, caregiving, and loss. The people undergoing these experiences have a right to health and well-being. Compassionate Communities UK implements strategies to address the morbidities (illnesses) and mortalities (deaths) that are consequences of the experiences of ageing, serious illness, caregiving, or loss.

Compassionate Communities UK provides a variety of different services relating to the public health approach to the spectrum of chronic disease management, disengaged members of the community, and into end of life care including bereavement:

- Provide guidance and expertise through a consultancy service.
- Provide education programmes on the public health approach to general health care and end of life care, including how to work with naturally occurring networks, build compassionate communities, and run a civic programme such as implementation of the Compassionate City Charter.
- Act as a source of guidance on policy formation at local, regional, national, and international levels.
- Formulate project plans for small-, medium-, or large-scale projects.
- Oversee or run projects on the ground.
- Formulate and provide expertise on programmes of evaluation, including reports.
- Act as research partners.

Death Literacy Institute

https://www.deathliteracy.institute

The Death Literacy Institute is a non-governmental organization business with a social mission.

The Institute vision is to help create a world where death is understood to be a normal part of life. Their mission is to create a more death literate society, one that actively supports the needs of all citizens who are dying, grieving, and caregiving. To do this, they aim to work across sectors and institutions, with people, places, and organizations to embed skills, experience, actions, and knowledge that create death literacy and achieve better outcomes. Through training and education, the Death Literacy Institute aims to support the capacity of community change-makers to take action towards new and innovative ways of practising death and loss.

As a start-up, the Institute's goal is to embed the United Nations Sustainable Development Goals (2015) into their organizational planning and development.

Their values embrace:

- Actions with integrity.
- Openness, always learning and developing.
- Acknowledging that change work takes courage and time.
- Acknowledge the Traditional Owners and Elders of the Australian lands that the Institute live and work on, and the wisdom of these community leaders.
- Sustainable business practices that are purposefully mindful of people, planet, and profit.

European Association for Palliative Care Public Health Reference Group

https://www.eapcnet.eu/eapc-groups/reference/public-health/

The reference group on public health and palliative care brings together all the major public health initiatives in palliative care in

Europe. It is a working group under the auspices of the European Association for Palliative Care and brings together researchers and clinicians with common interests in public health approaches to palliative care.

The main aim is to promote and improve palliative care via public health approaches and promote public health and health promotion as essential elements of national and international palliative care policies and strategies. It will also develop a network of public health researchers within the European Association for Palliative Care Research Network.

Institute of Palliative Medicine, Kerala

https://www.instituteofpalliativemedicine.org/index.php

The Institute of Palliative Medicine is the pioneer of the public health palliative care movement in South and South East Asia. As the first World Health Organization Collaborating Centre for Community Participation in Palliative Care and Long Term Care in developing countries, it is trying to establish community-based palliative care in different parts of India and abroad. The Institute of Palliative Medicine is instrumental in developing the 'Kerala Model' of palliative care which is popular among the palliative care fraternity worldwide. The Institute of Palliative Medicine is the training, research, and outreach arm of the Pain and Palliative Care Society. It is located in the Medical College Campus, Kozhikode, Kerala, India.

New Health Foundation

http://www.newhealthfoundation.org

The New Health Foundation is a non-profit institution for the observation and optimization of health, social care, and family and environmental support systems to improve the quality of life in advanced disease processes, high dependency, and the later stages of life. It is the key non-governmental organization in Spain for the advocacy and development of public health palliative care in civic institutions.

Public Health Palliative Care International

https://phpci.info

Public Health Palliative Care International is the main membership-based professional body that promotes practice learning and professional support for public health approaches to palliative care. This organization facilitates local and international communication between members around the world by and for those wishing to embed a public health approach to the practice of palliative care.

Aims:

- To promote the philosophy, values, concepts, and methods of health promotion into palliative care services everywhere.
- To support members in their educational and practice needs to meet their goal of health-promoting palliative care.
- To provide a regular forum in their conferences (every 2 years) for the exchange of practice wisdom in public health approaches to palliative care.
- To encourage and foster research and evaluation of health-promoting palliative care.
- To encourage palliative care to foster professional links and knowledge exchange between colleagues in public health, community health and development, health policy, health education, health promotion, and end of life care.
- To provide a global forum for communication to members involved in this common endeavour.
- To support, network, and mentor students in their efforts to further develop and evaluate this approach to end of life care.
- To collaborate effectively with all organizations that represent people affected by death, dying, loss, and care.

Public Health Palliative Care Unit, La Trobe University

https://www.latrobe.edu.au/public-health/research/centres/palliative-care-unit

The Public Health Palliative Care Unit is the world's first and oldest public health palliative care policy and practice centre based inside a university (since 1998). This Unit emphasizes the importance of developing whole of life responses to the universal issue of human mortality. Their mission is to re-engage local communities as active partners in providing end of life care and supporting end of life decision-making.

The public health orientation means that, in addressing this strategic direction, they aim to:

- Develop capacity around assets rather than perceived problems.
- Ensure these community and organizational capacities are sustainable.
- Advocate for vulnerable populations, recognizing that disability, social exclusion, and discrimination are all social determinants of health.
- Promote the participation of those who use services as well as those who provide them.
- Enable community members to take a key role in caring for their dying.
- Develop the evidence needed to support policy change.

Index